Kees J. Dik / Ilona Gunsser

Atlas of Diagnostic Radiology of the Horse

Diseases of the front and hind limbs

Kees J. Dik / Ilona Gunsser

Atlas of Diagnostic Radiology of the Horse

Diseases of the front and hind limbs

Second edition

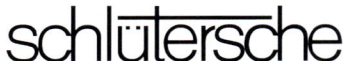

© 2002 Schlütersche GmbH & Co. KG, Verlag und Druckerei,
Hans-Böckler-Allee 7, 30173 Hannover, Germany
E-mail: info@schluetersche.de

Printed in Germany

ISBN 3-87706-651-8

A CIP catalogue record for this book is available from Deutsche Bibliothek, Frankfurt – Germany.

Preface

Front and / or hind limb lameness represents a major reason for poor performance of horses.

Despite, the introduction of new imaging modalities such as ultrasonography, computed tomography and magnetic resonance imaging, radiography will remain a crucial tool in the diagnosis and management of equine lameness.

The first edition of this radiographic atlas demonstrates common and uncommon features of the various bone and joint diseases of the equine front limb (Part 1) and hind limb (Part 2), thus providing references for equine practitioners and students as an aid for radiological diagnosis.

Such a collection will never be complete. However, the greater the variety of demonstrated appearances, the better the reference function will be effectuated.

Therefore, the second edition of this Atlas not only combines Parts 1 and 2, but also includes about 50 percent new material.

The new illustrations cover all parts of the equine front and hind limb, with emphasis on the various lesions of the foot, such as the different pedal bone fracture types, pedal osteitis, laminitis appearances and the various navicular bone lesions including the postnatal development and role of the navicular bone shape in the pathogenesis of navicular disease; fetlock abnormalities, like the variable origin of fetlock "fragments" and avulsion injuries of the proximal sesamoids; carpal disorders, such as the divers fracture types and angular deformities; as well as common and uncommon hock and stifle lesions, including the various manifestations, postnatal development and differential diagnosis of osteochondrosis.

Utrecht and Munich, September 2001

Kees J. Dik, Ilona Gunsser

Acknowledgements

Our special thanks go to Mr. A. van der Woude for preparing the photographs and schematic drawings, to miss H. L. A. Lammers for typing the manuscript and to the colleagues of the Large Animal Surgery Department for providing essential clinical background information.

We would like to thank Dr. Darryl N. Biery of the Department of Clinical Studies, School of Veterinary Medicine, University of Pennsylvania, Dr. Kathelijne Peremans, Veterinary Clinic Aan de Watergang, St-Gillis-Waas, Belgium and Prof. Dr. C. Kiesling for their kind advice and critical reading of the manuscript.

Finally we sincerely acknowledge the close cooperation with the publisher Schlütersche GmbH & Co. KG, Verlag und Druckerei and appreciate the excellent layout of the book.

Kees J. Dik, Ilona Gunsser

Contents

Contents

The Foot

Fracture

Navicular bone shape

Navicular disease

Infectious arthritis

Osteoarthrosis

Bone cyst

Laminitis

Rupture of the deep flexor tendon

Contracted foot

Buttress foot

Side bones

Puncture wound

Keratoma

Ossification of the deep flexor tendon

Calcified neurectomy scar

Schematic drawings

Fracture

Pedal bone

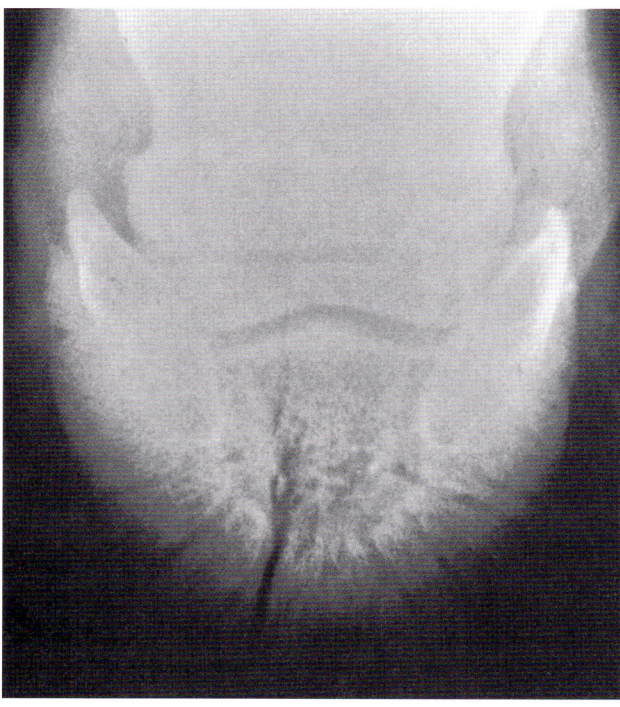

1 Pedal bone, right front, dorsopalmar view.
Warmblood, 3 years.

A sharply bordered, narrow, vertical, radiolucent zone through the midportion of the pedal bone, resulting from a recent, simple, complete, nearly sagittal, intra-articular fracture.

2 Pedal bone, right front, dorsopalmar view.
Warmblood, 7 years.

A narrow, slightly irregular, radiolucent zone through the lateral wing of the pedal bone, resulting from a recent, simple, complete, extra-articular fracture.

Additional finding: minimal ossification of both accessory cartilages.

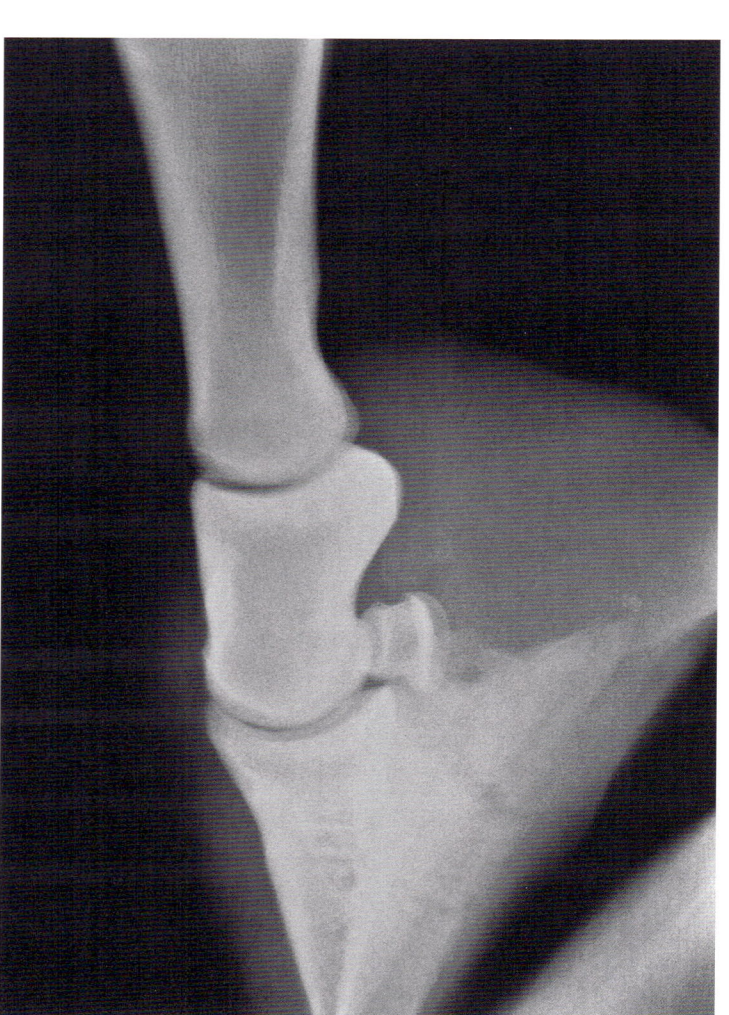

3

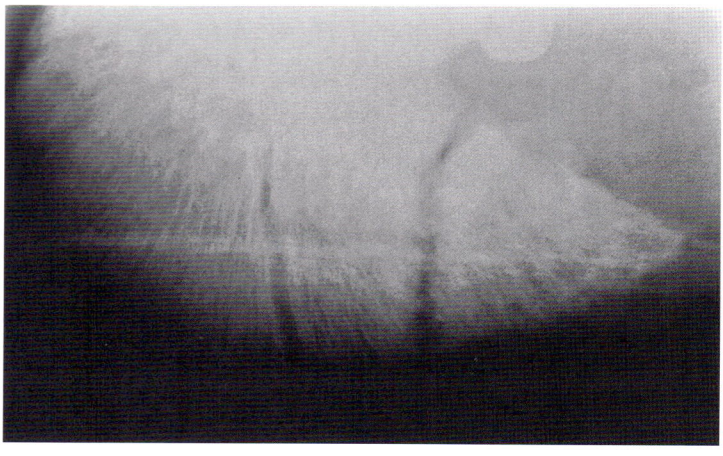

4

3/4 Pedal bone, left front, lateromedial view and dorsoproximolateral – palmarodistomedial oblique view: close-up of the lateral wing of the pedal bone.

Warmblood, 5 years.

A vertical, slightly irregular, radiolucent zone through the lateral wing of the pedal bone, indicating a recent, simple, complete, extra-articular fracture.

The fracture is most obvious on the dorsoproximolateral-palmarodistomedial oblique view (Fig. 4), but also visible on the routine lateromedial view (Fig. 3).

Pedal bone

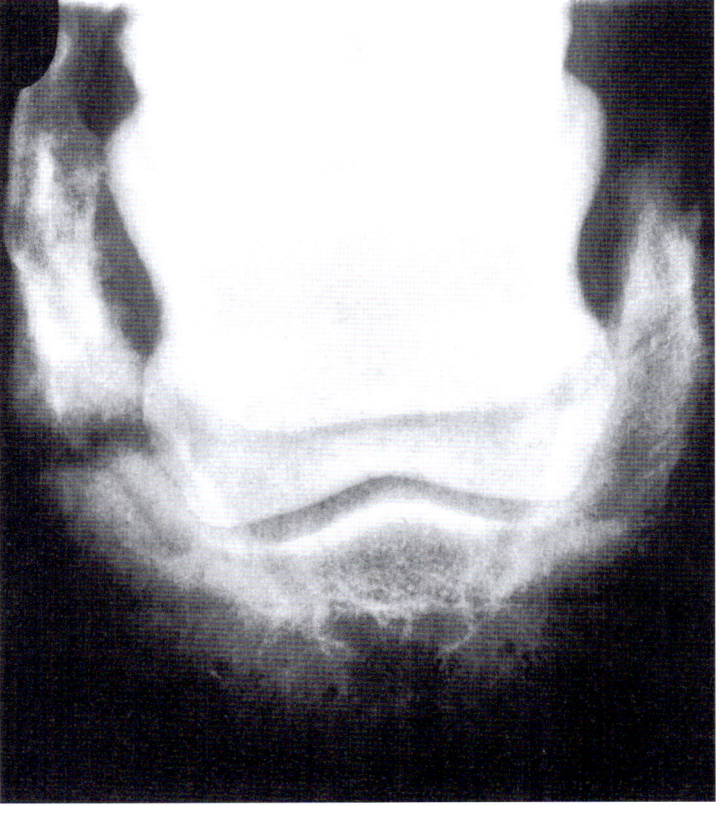

5

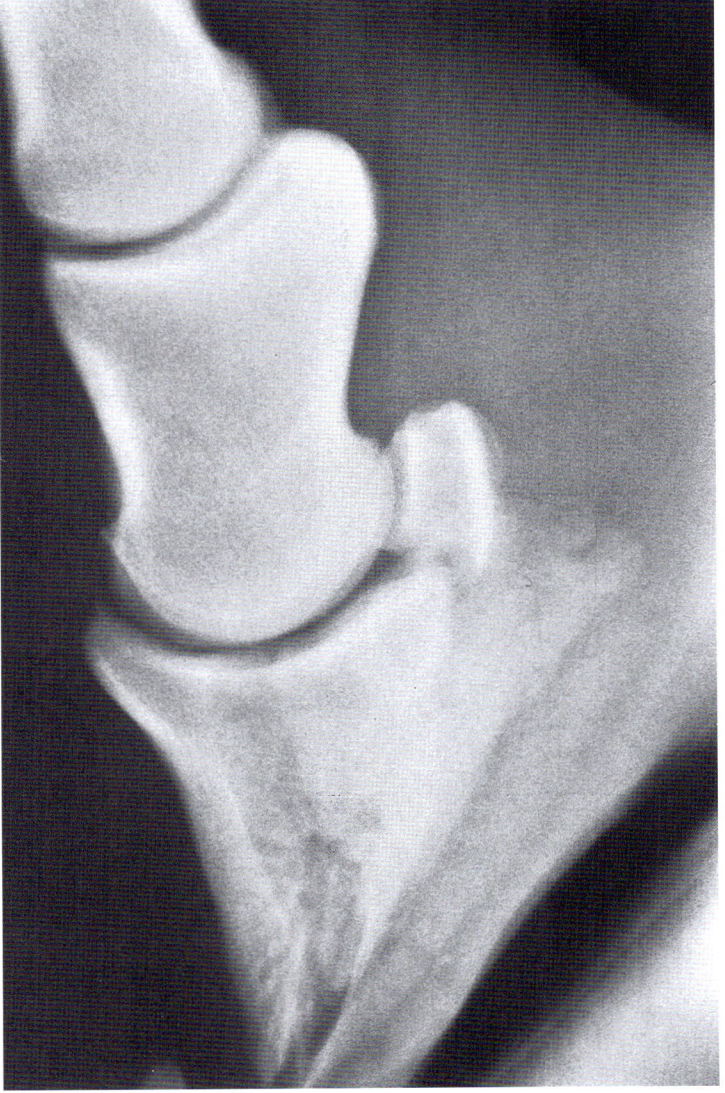

6

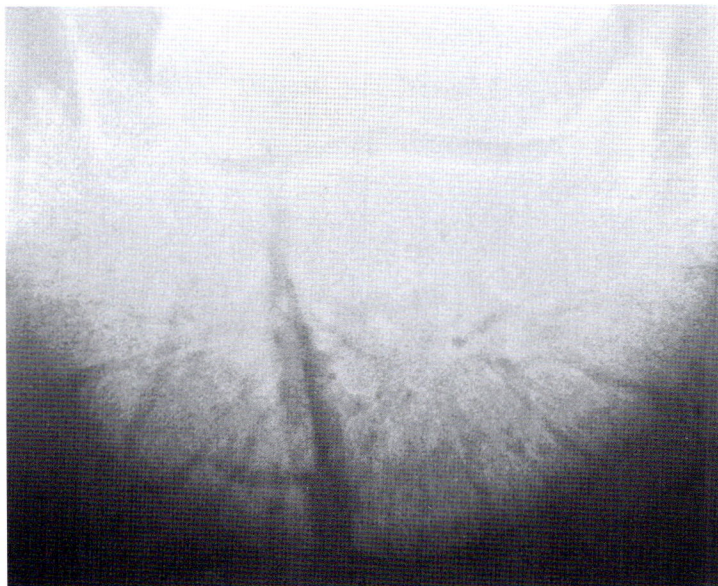

7

5 Pedal bone, right front, dorsopalmar view.

Warmblood, 8 years.

A radiolucent zone through the lateral wing of the pedal bone, due to a simple, complete, intra-articular fracture. The widened, ill bordered fracture zone indicates that the fracture is not recent.

Additional finding: extensive ossification of the lateral accessory cartilage, less extensive ossification in the medial cartilage.

6/7 Pedal bone, right front, lateromedial and dorsopalmar view.

Warmblood, 2 years.

The lateromedial view (Fig. 6) shows an obscure, wide, radiolucent zone through the dorsal portion of the pedal bone, interrupting the articular surface as well as the distal border.

The dorsopalmar view (Fig. 7) reveals a clear, wide, vertical radiolucent zone through the centrolateral portion of the pedal bone. Additional, less obvious, narrow, horizontal and oblique radiolucent lines are visible in the lateral region of the pedal bone. These changes are consistent with a recent comminuted fracture.

Fracture

Pedal bone

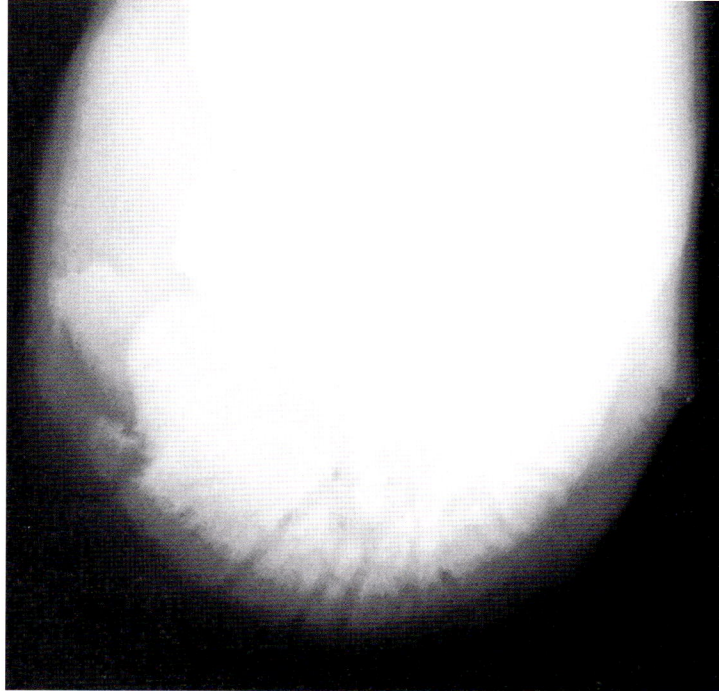

8

8 Pedal bone, left front, dorsoproximomedial-palmarodistolateral oblique view.

Foal, 5 months.

A sharply bordered, isolated bone fragment on the distomedial margin of the pedal bone, due to a recent chip fracture sustained when the animal trod on a stone.

Additional finding: the radiolucent zone palmar to the isolated bone fragment is caused by disruption of the sole.

N. B. In this foal, 5 months of age, the wings of the pedal bone are not yet ossified, explaining their absence on the radiograph.

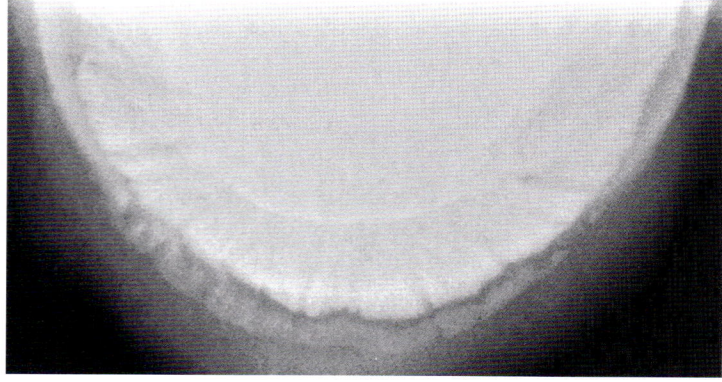

10

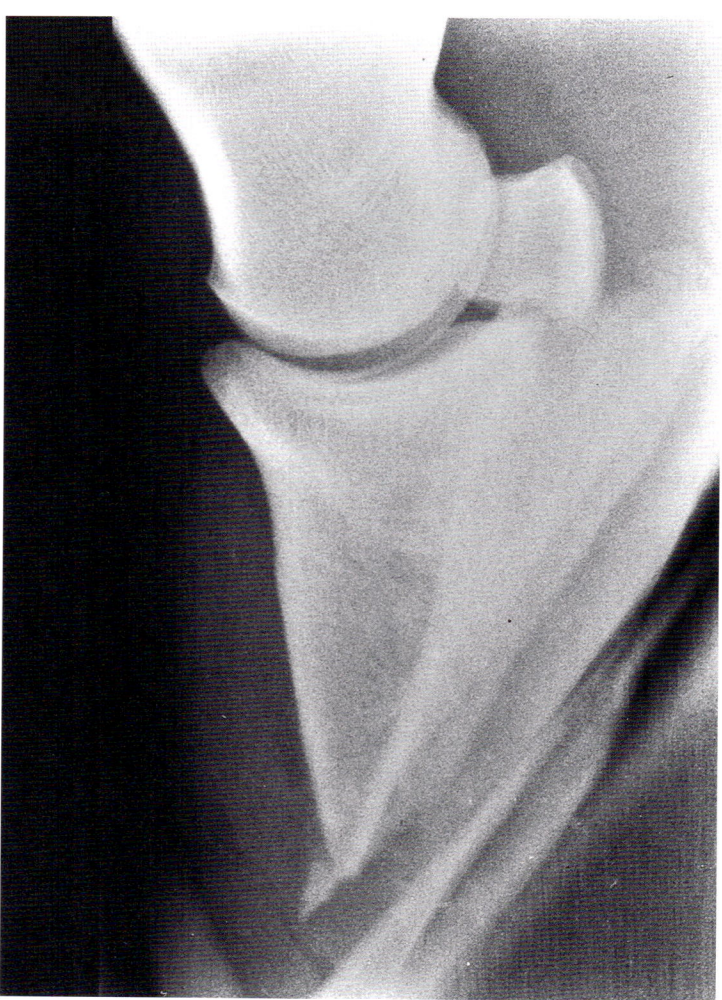

9

9/10 Pedal bone, left front, lateromedial and dorsopalmar view: close-ups.

Thoroughbred, 11 years.

The lateromedial view (Fig. 9) shows a dorsoproximally displaced bone fragment separated from the tip of the pedal bone. The pedal bone is also rotated away from the hoofwall.

On the dorsopalmar view (Fig. 10) the fragmentation is not limited to the tip of the pedal bone, but involves a large portion of the solar margin. This extensive solar margin fragmentation probably is associated with the concurrent pedal bone rotation, i.e. laminitis.

Pedal bone

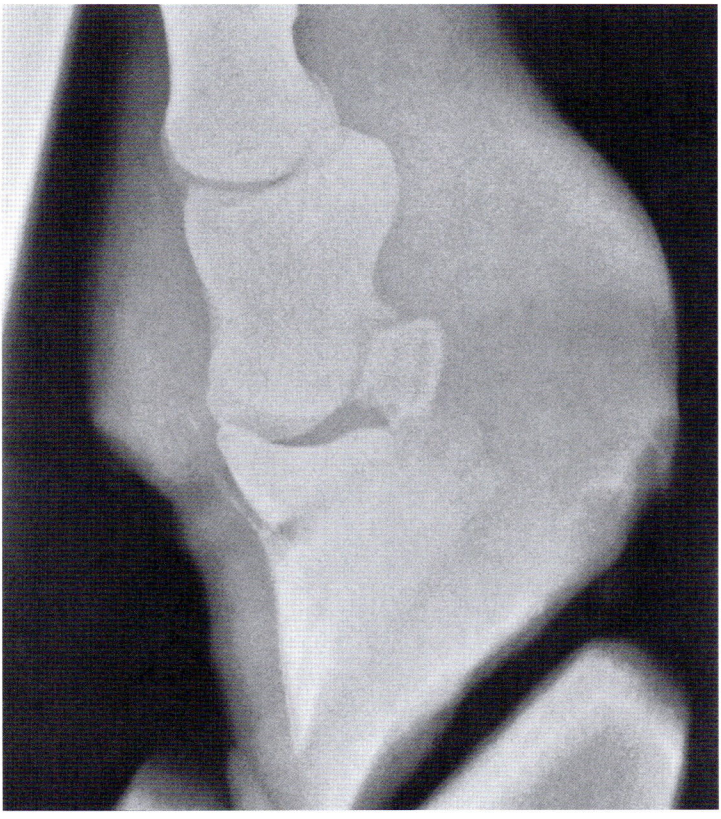

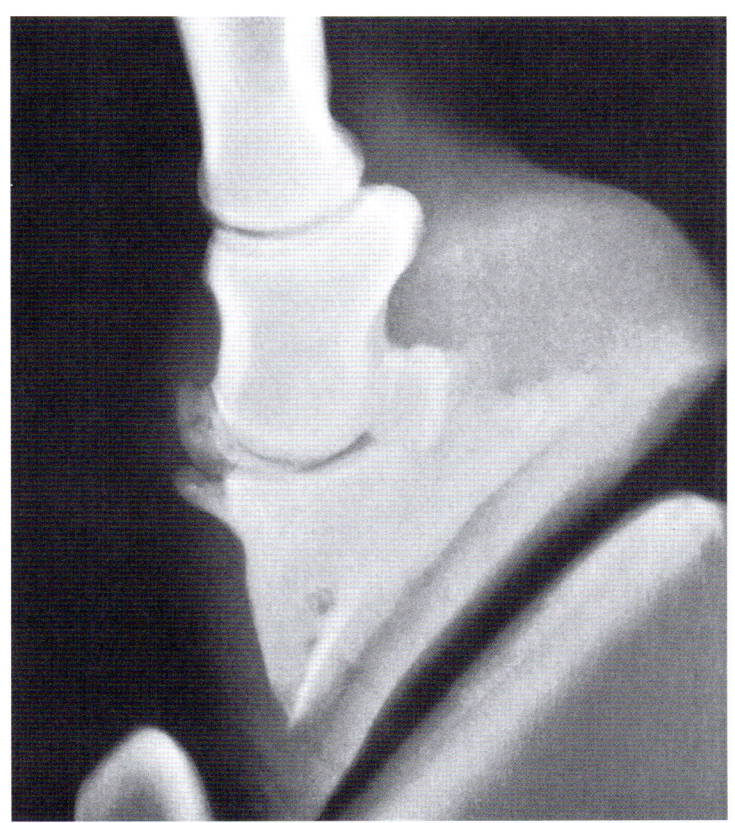

11 Pedal bone, left front, lateromedial view.

Warmblood, 1 year.

A wide, ill bordered, radiolucent zone distal to the extensor process and disruption of the dorsal surface of the pedal bone, due to a fracture associated with a puncture wound 3 weeks prior to the examination.

Additional finding: widening of the coffin joint space resulting from infectious arthritis.

12 Pedal bone, right front, lateromedial view.

Warmblood, 7 years.

A large, isolated bone fragment dorsal to the coffin joint resulting from an avulsion fracture of the extensor process. The extensive, smooth, sharply bordered new bone formation along the dorsal surface of the pedal bone distal to the isolated bone fragment indicates that the fracture is not recent.

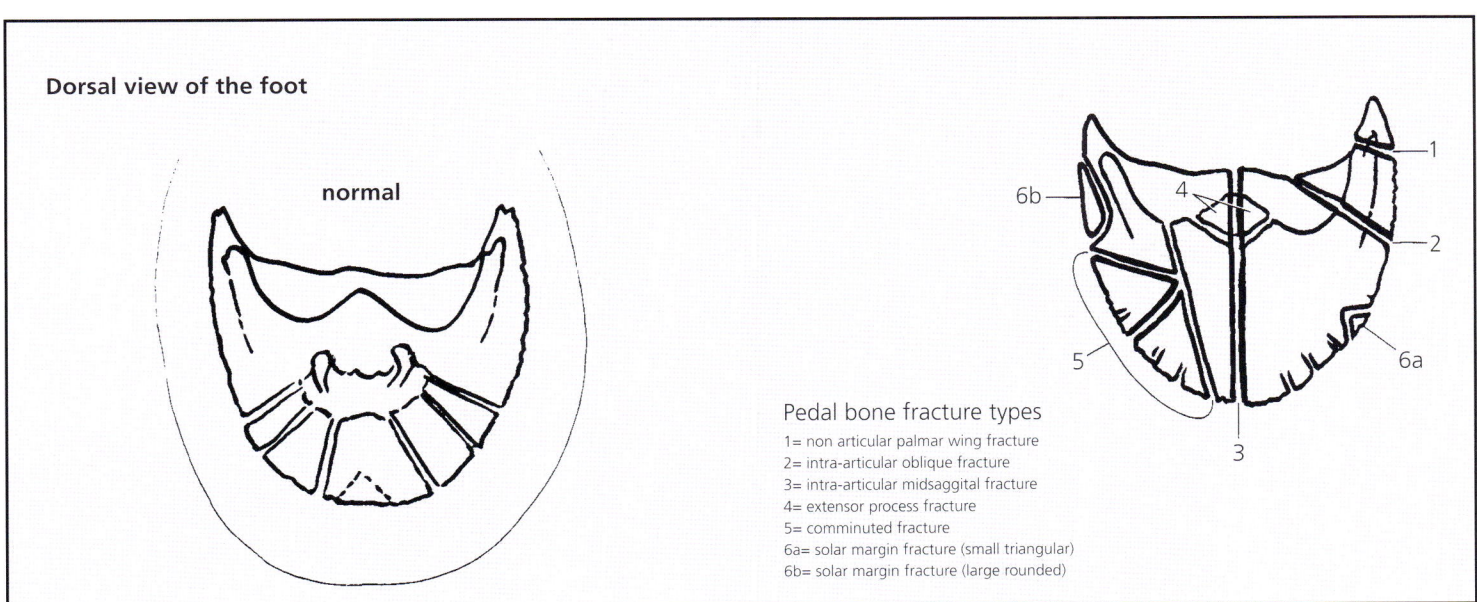

Dorsal view of the foot

normal

Pedal bone fracture types

1= non articular palmar wing fracture
2= intra-articular oblique fracture
3= intra-articular midsaggital fracture
4= extensor process fracture
5= comminuted fracture
6a= solar margin fracture (small triangular)
6b= solar margin fracture (large rounded)

13 Schematic drawings of the pedal bone.

The normal dorsal appearance of the foot versus the different pedal bone fracture types.

Fracture

Pedal bone

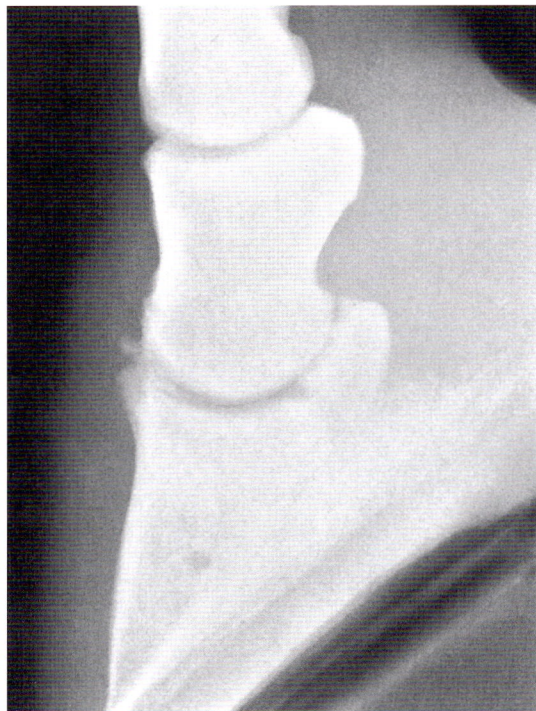

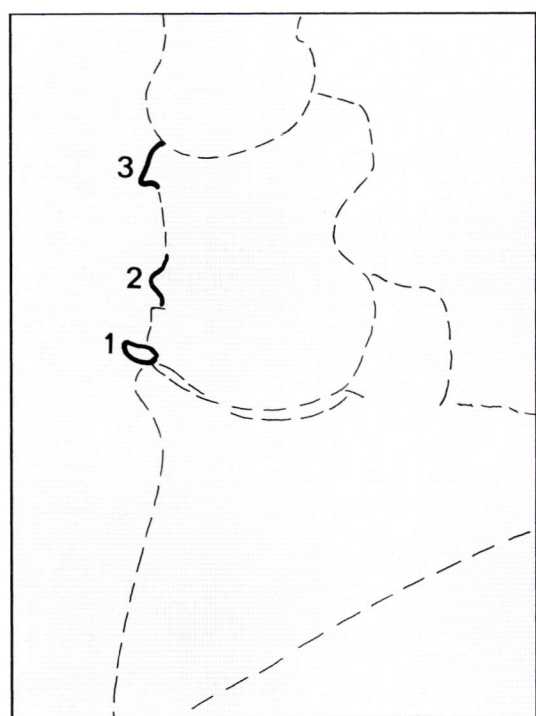

14 Pedal bone, left front, lateromedial view.

Warmblood, 6 years.

A small piece of bone **(1)** proximal to the extensor process of the pedal bone. There is neither a corresponding defect, nor new bone formation on the dorsal aspect of the second or third phalanx, suggesting that the fragment may not be the result of a fracture. A bone fragment of unknown origin is often found bilaterally; most of these fragments are not clinically significant.

14 a Schematic drawing

Additional finding: a small spur **(3)** is present on the dorsal aspect of the proximal end of the second phalanx, usually this is of no clinical significance.

N. B. The ligament insertion **(2)** overlying the dorsal aspect of the distal end of the second phalanx should not be confused with new bone formation.

Navicular bone

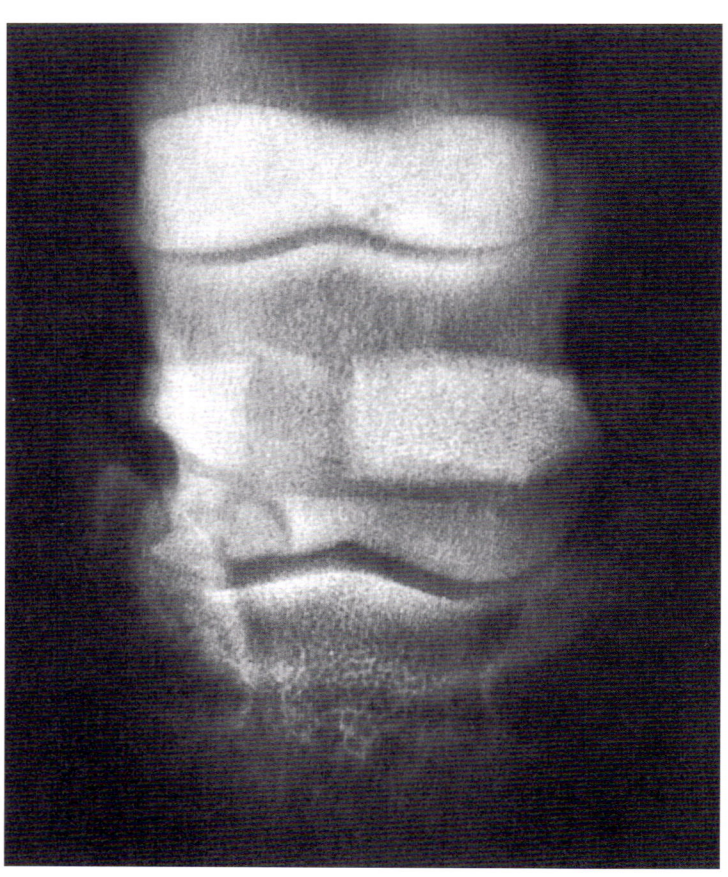

15

15 Navicular bone, left front, upright pedal view (dorsopalmar).

Warmblood, 6 years.

A wide, sagittal, sharply bordered radiolucent zone through the mediocentral portion of the navicular bone, resulting from a recent fracture.

Two indistinct, thin, bone fragments superimposing the fracture zone are visible.

Additional finding: multiple fracture fragments in the corresponding portion of the distal end of the second phalanx.

Navicular bone

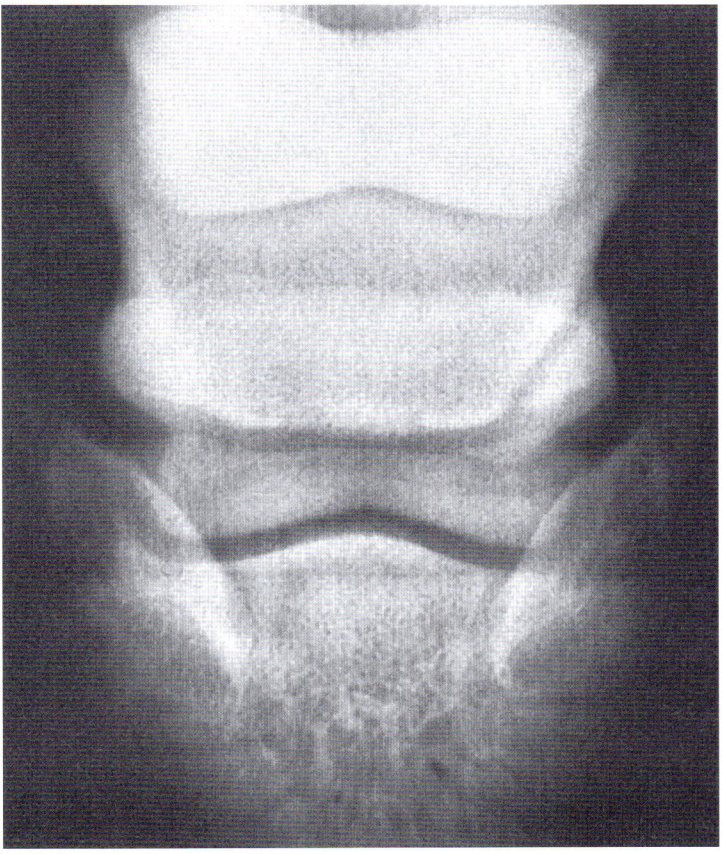

16

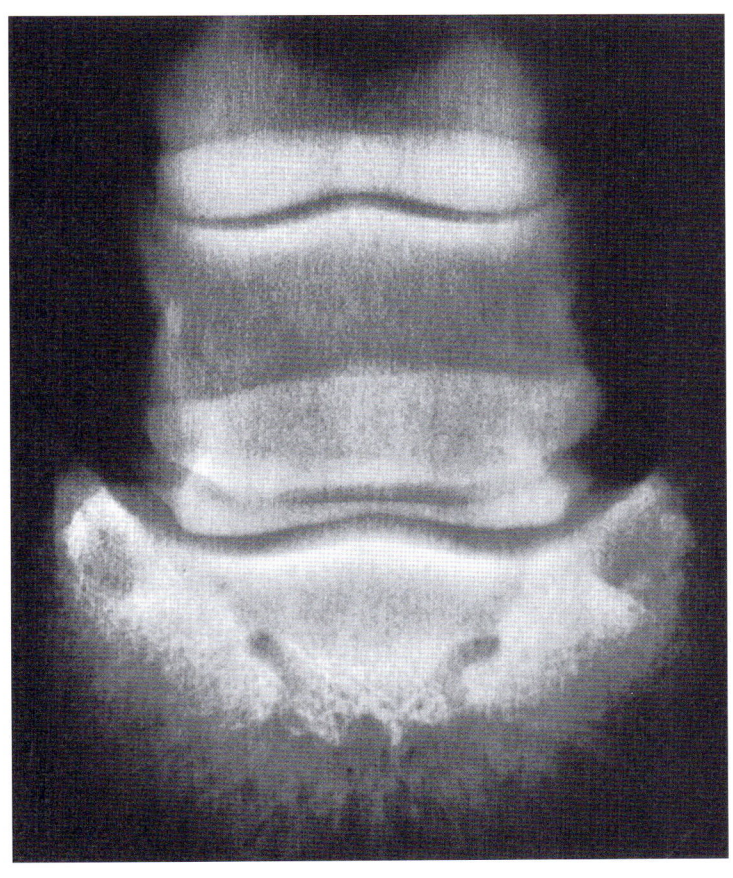

17

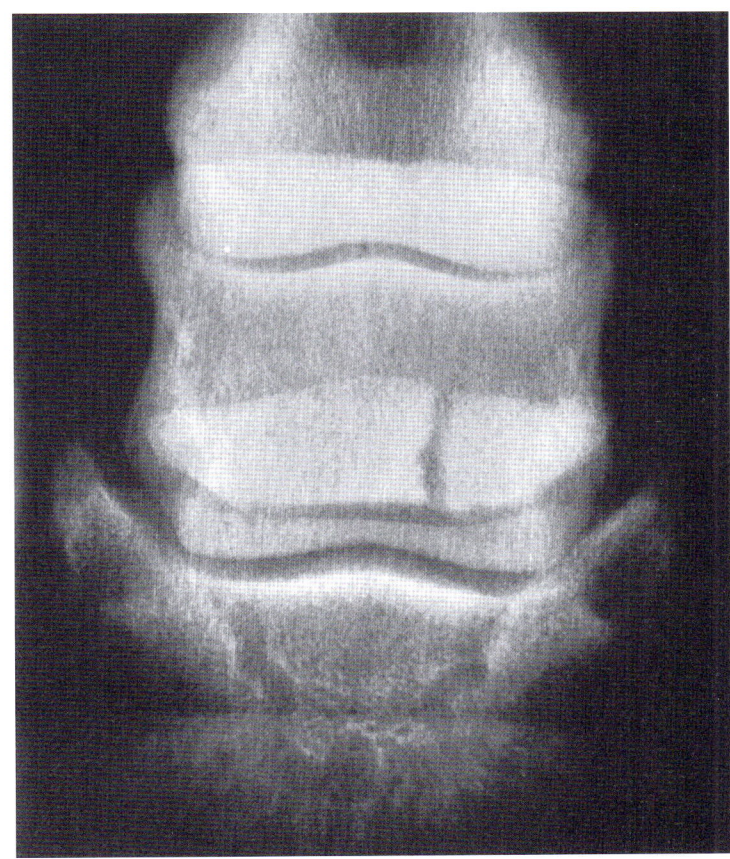

18

16 Navicular bone, right hind, upright pedal view (dorsoplantar).

Warmblood, 3 years.

An oblique, sharply bordered, radiolucent zone through the medial portion of the navicular bone, the result of a recent fracture.

17/18 Navicular bone, left front, serial upright pedal views (dorsopalmar).

Pony, 7 years.

The initial examination (Fig. 17) presents a poorly detectable, vertical radiolucent line through the laterocentral portion of the navicular bone, resulting from a recent fracture.

The second examination 10 days later (Fig. 18), demonstrates widening of the fracture line, due to bone resorption.

Fracture

Navicular bone

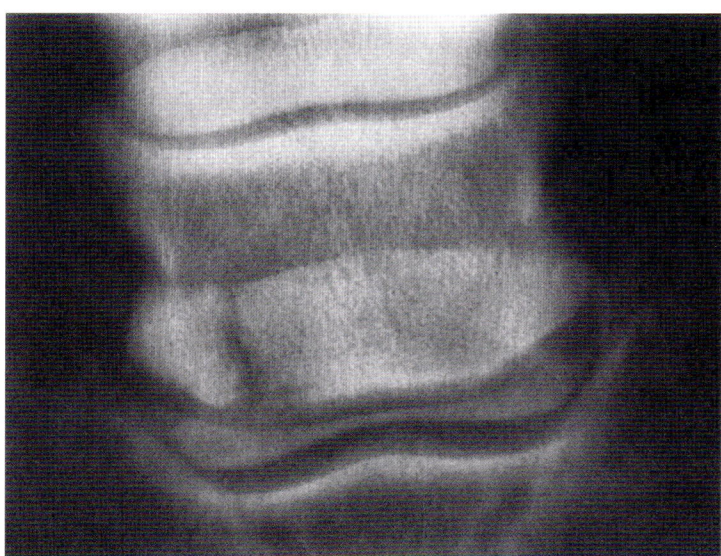

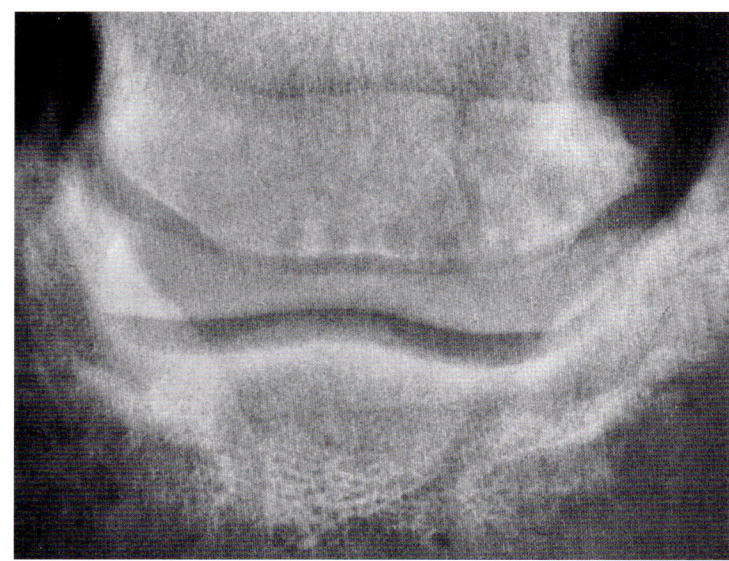

19 Navicular bone, right front, upright pedal view (dorsopalmar).

Pony, 9 years.

A wide, sagittal, ill bordered, radiolucent zone through the lateral portion of the navicular bone.

The irregularity of the fracture zone and the loss of bone density in the navicular bone adjacent to the fracture zone indicate a long-standing (non-union) fracture.

20 Navicular bone, left front, upright pedal view (dorsopalmar).

Warmblood, 6 years.

A sagittal radiolucent zone through the laterocentral portion of the navicular bone, resulting from a fracture. The irregularity of the fracture zone and the loss of bone density in the navicular bone adjacent to the fracture zone indicate that the fracture is not recent. The multiple cystic radiolucent lesions along the distal border of the navicular bone and the new bone formation along the proximal border indicate the presence of navicular disease and suggest that the fracture is pathological i.e. occurring through a weakened area of the diseased bone.

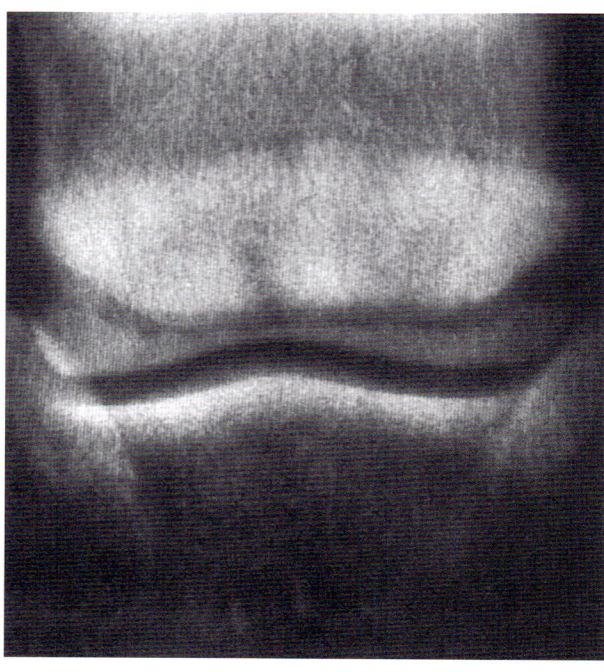

21

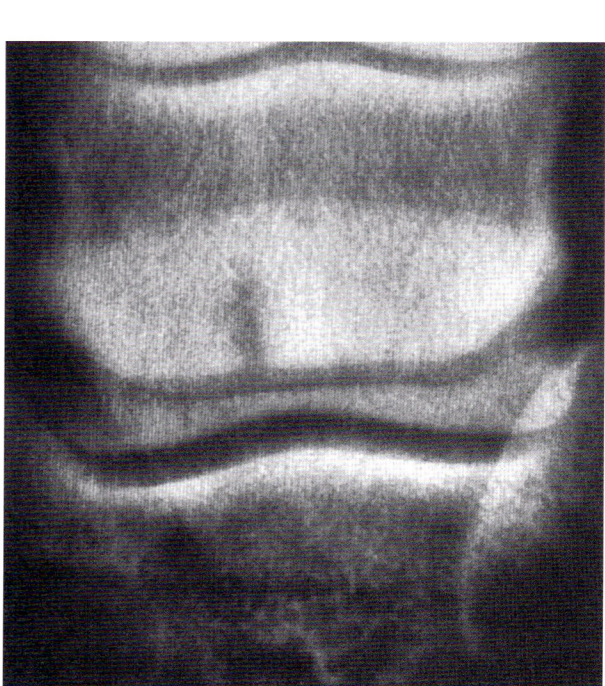

22

21/22 Navicular bone, right front, serial upright pedal views (dorsopalmar).

Pony, 7 years.

The initial examination (Fig. 21), 4 weeks after the onset of lameness, reveals an ill bordered, vertical, radiolucent zone at the distal border of the laterocentral portion of the navicular bone; increase in length of the zone is demonstrated one week later in the second examination (Fig. 22).

Such a radiolucent zone progressively invading the navicular bone represents an incomplete fracture possibly arising from local ischaemia in the navicular bone.

Navicular bone

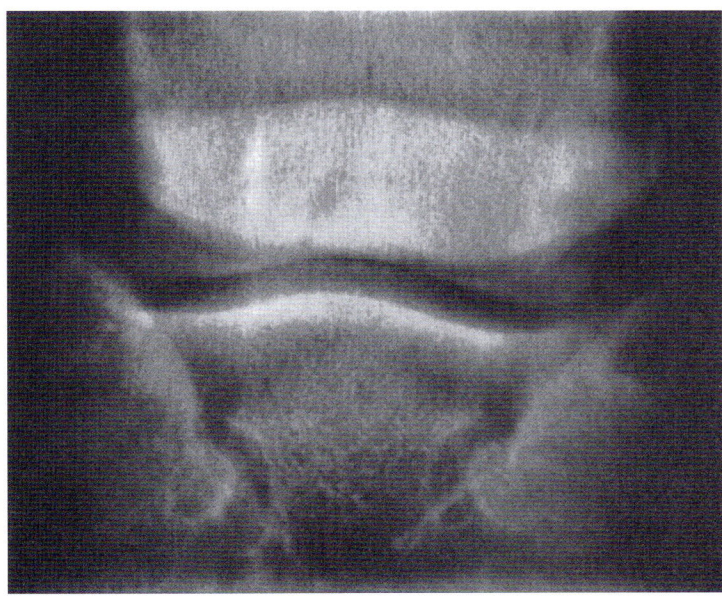

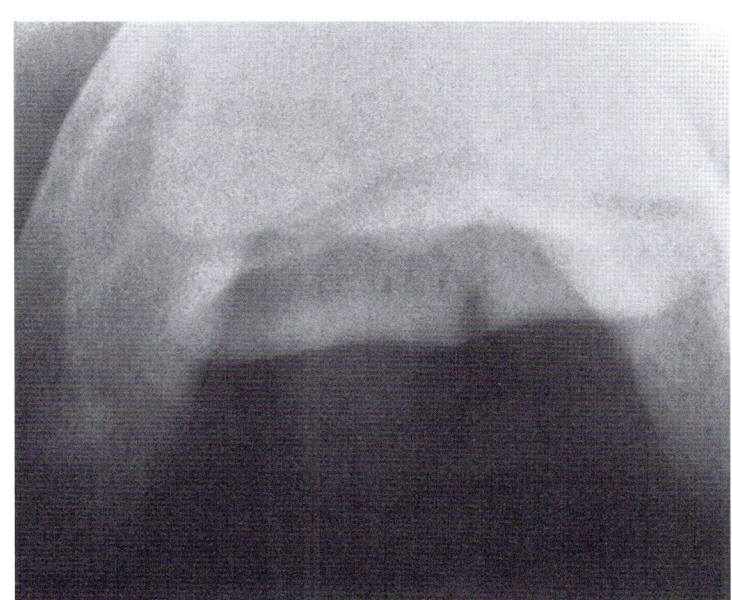

23

24

23/24 Navicular bone, left front, upright pedal view (dorsopalmar) and palmaroproximal-dorsodistal oblique "skyline" view.

Warmblood, 6 years.

The indistinct radiolucent zone in the mediocentral portion of the navicular bone visualized on the dorsopalmar view (Fig. 23) represents a slightly oblique, vertical fracture, which is more clearly demonstrated on the palmaroproximal-dorsodistal oblique "skyline" view (Fig. 24) illustrating the value of this additional projection.

Additional finding: in the dorsopalmar view the radiopaque line medial to the radiolucent zone is an artefact, resulting from dirt in the medial sulcus of the frog.

Fracture

Navicular bone

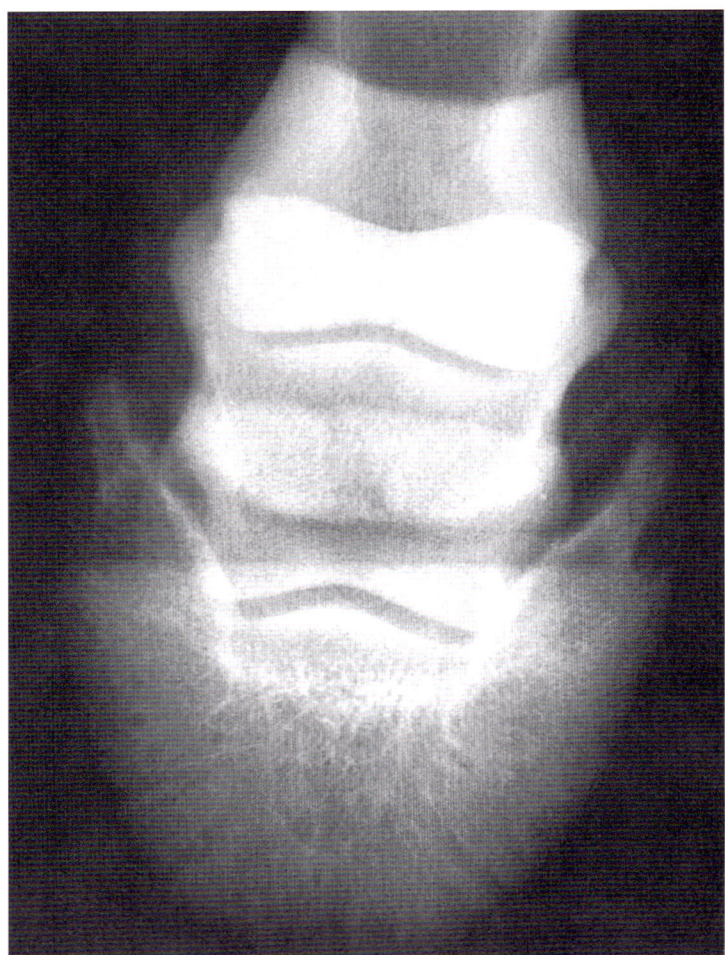

25

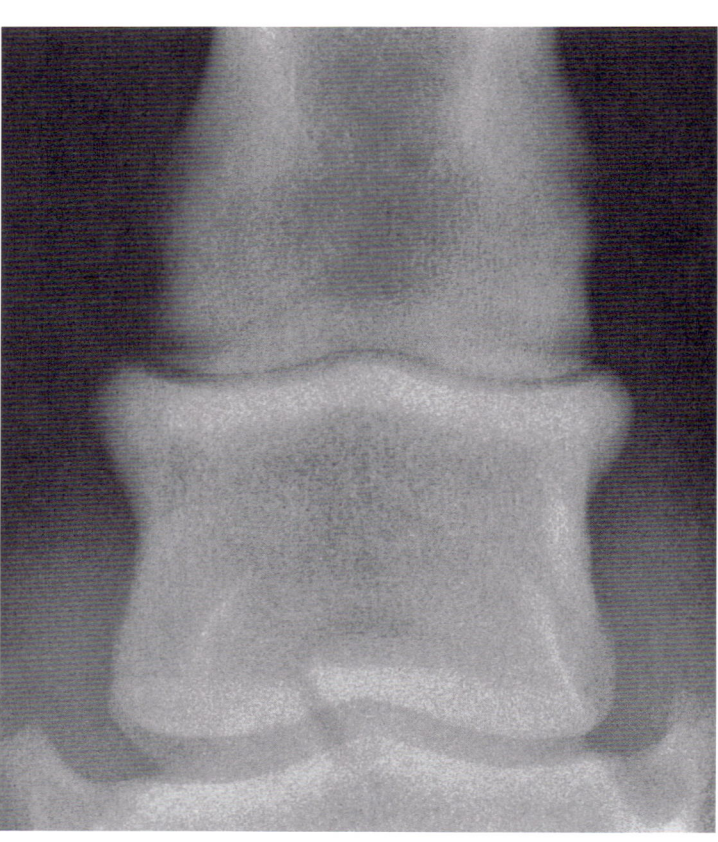

26

25/26 Navicular bone, right front, upright pedal view (dorsopalmar) and dorsopalmar weight bearing view: close-ups.

Pony, 7 years.

The upright pedal view (Fig. 25) shows an ill bordered radiolucent zone in the central portion of the navicular bone. Due to the small size of the horse it was impossible to obtain a palmaroproximal-dorsodistal oblique "skyline" view.

The weight-bearing dorsopalmar view (Fig. 26) shows disruption **(1)** of the proximal border and a radiolucent zone **(2)** through the corresponding portion of the navicular bone, indicating that the radiolucent zone on the upright pedal route projection represents a vertical-oblique navicular fracture.

26 a Schematic drawing

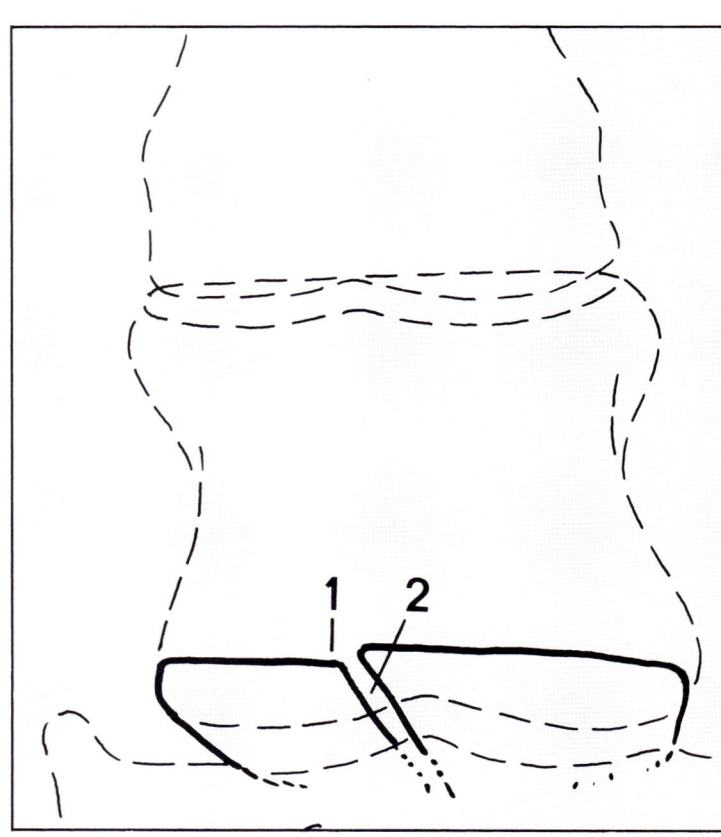

26 a

Navicular bone

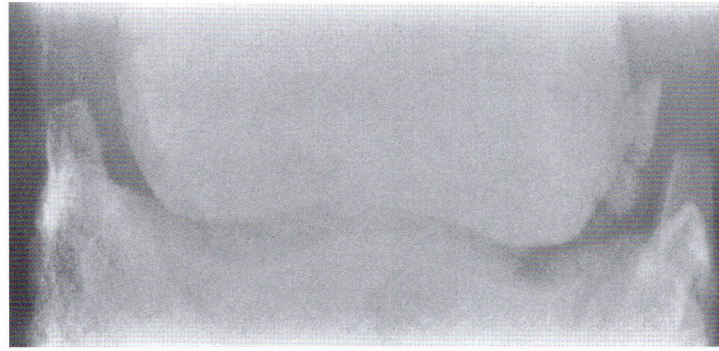

27 Navicular bone, right front, dorsopalmar upright pedal view: close-up.
Warmblood, 4 years.

Fragmentation of the medial extremity of the navicular bone resulting from a recent fracture. (The radiograph is underexposed deliberately to highlight the fragments).

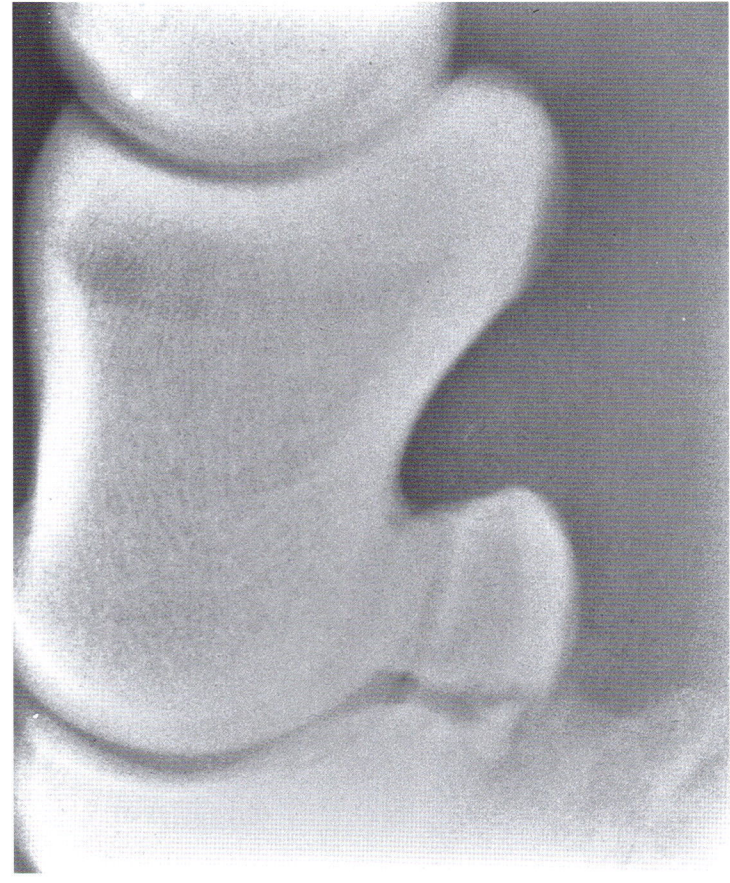

28 Navicular bone, right hind, lateromedial view: close-up.
Warmblood, 7 years.

Fragmentation of the plantarodistal border of the navicular bone indicating an avulsion fracture caused by overstretching of the impar ligament.

(Pseudo)Fracture

Navicular bone

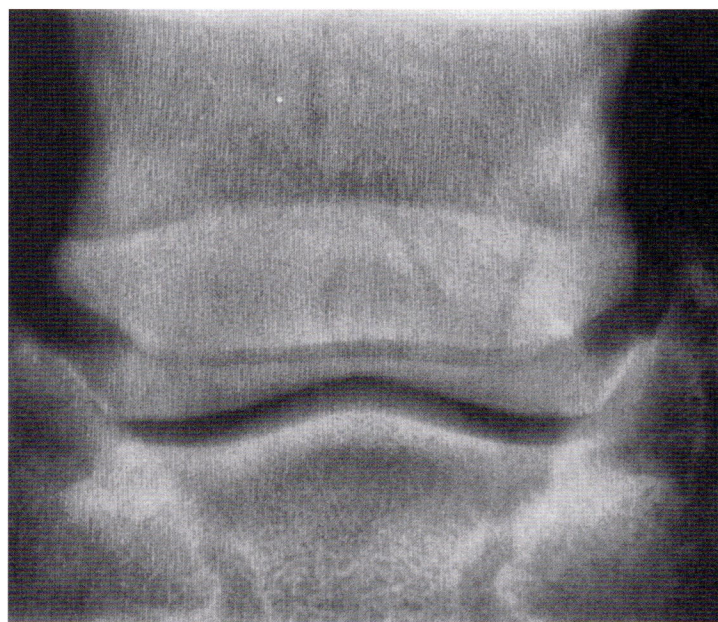

29

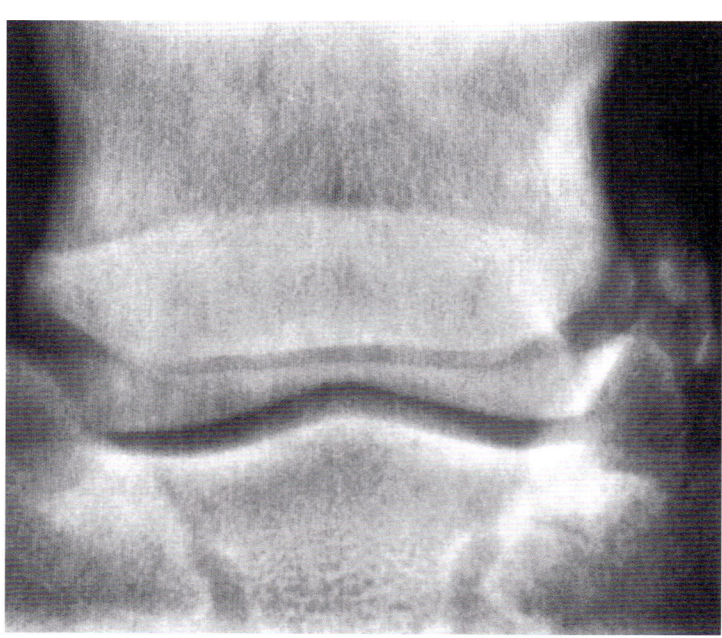

30

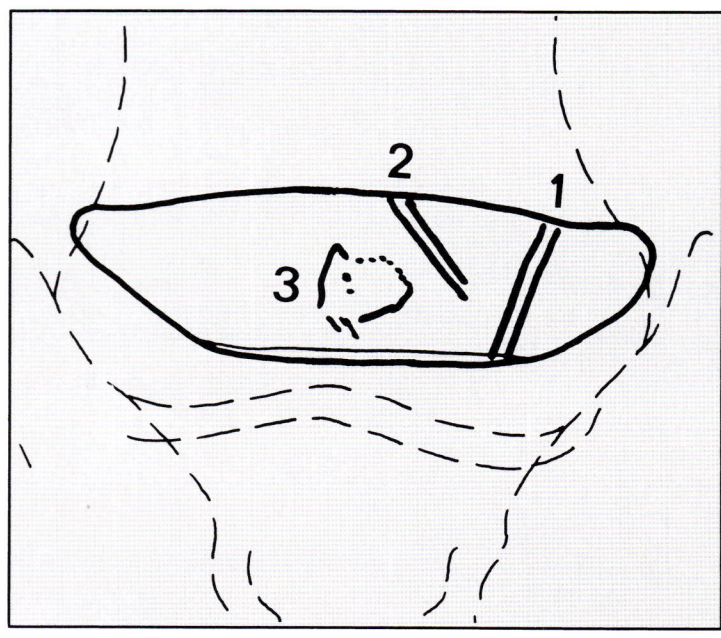

29 a

29/30 Navicular bone, right front, upright pedal views (dorsopalmar): close-ups.

Warmblood, 5 years.

The initial film (Fig. 29) shows a vertical, slightly oblique radiolucent zone **(1)** between the proximal and distal borders of the medial portion of the navicular bone.

Also present are an oblique radiolucent zone **(2)** through the mediocentral portion beginning at the proximal border and a small radiolucent area **(3)** in the central portion of the navicular bone.

Radiographic changes are no longer visible on a repeat view (Fig. 30) after cleaning and repacking the sole, indicating that the radiolucent zones present in the initial film were artefactual fracture lines caused by inadequate packing of the sole.

29 a Schematic drawing

Navicular bone

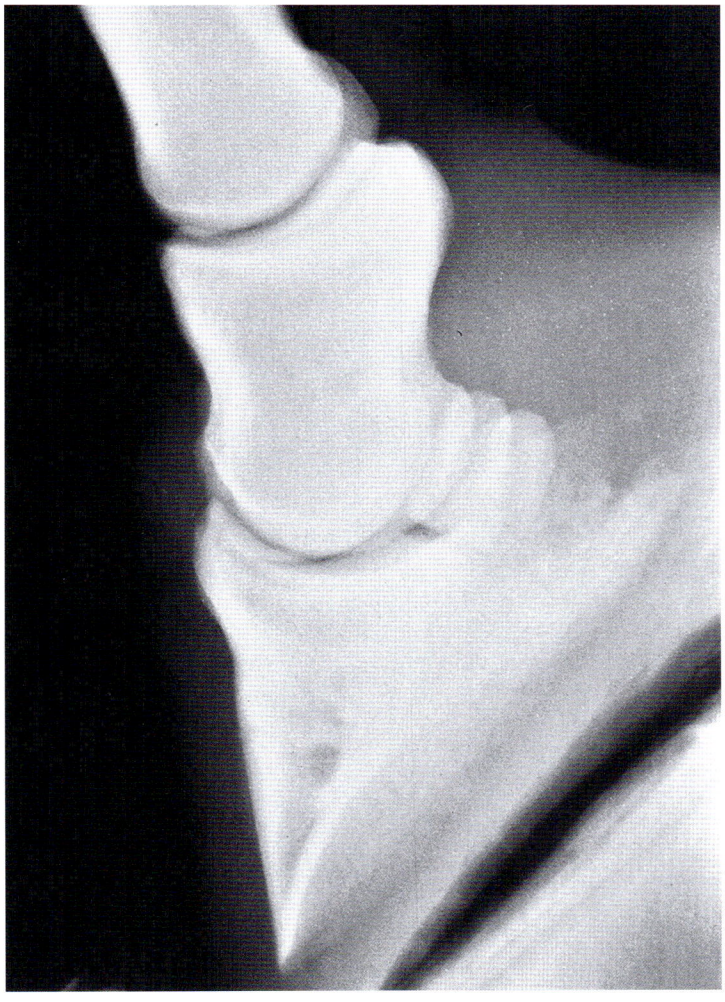

31

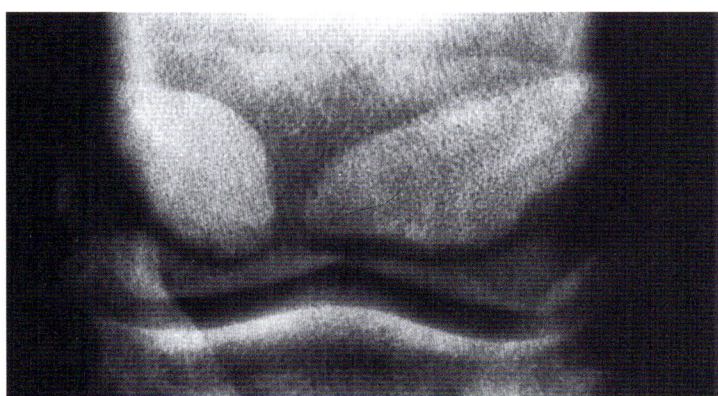

32

31/32 Navicular bone, right front, lateromedial view and dorsopalmar upright pedal view: close-up.

Warmblood, 3 years.

On the dorsopalmar upright pedal view (Fig. 32) the navicular bone consists of two, large, rounded, clearly separated fragments thus explaining the confusing double navicular bone appearance on the lateromedial view (Fig. 31).

The rounded shape of these fragments and the absence of textural radiolucencies along the "fracture zone" are in favour of a congenital malformation, i.e. a bipartite navicular bone.

Navicular bone shape: Predisposition to navicular disease

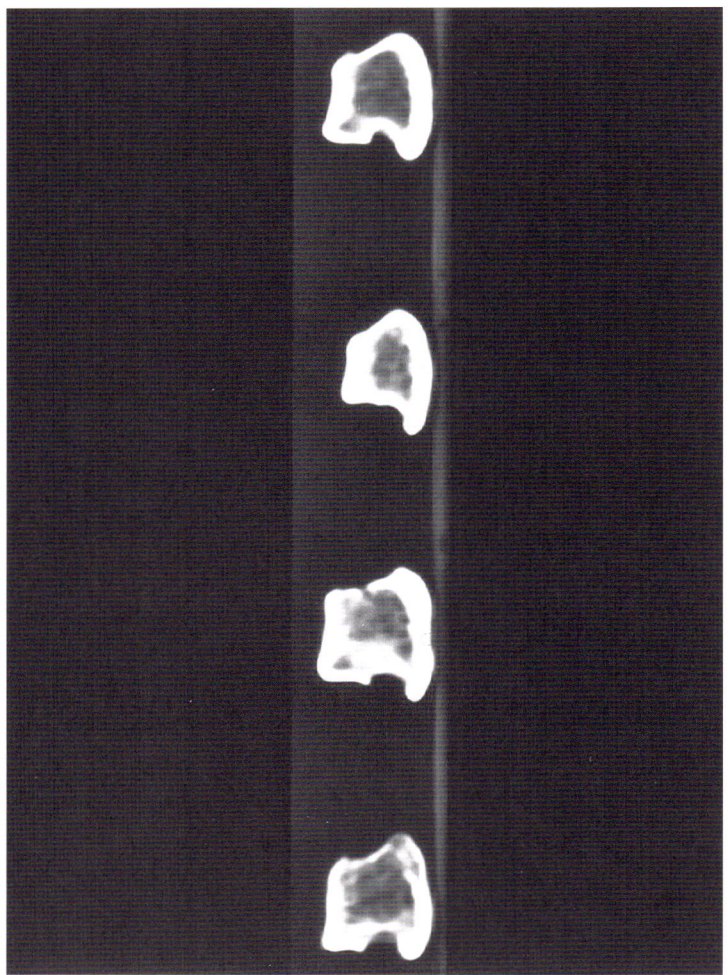

33

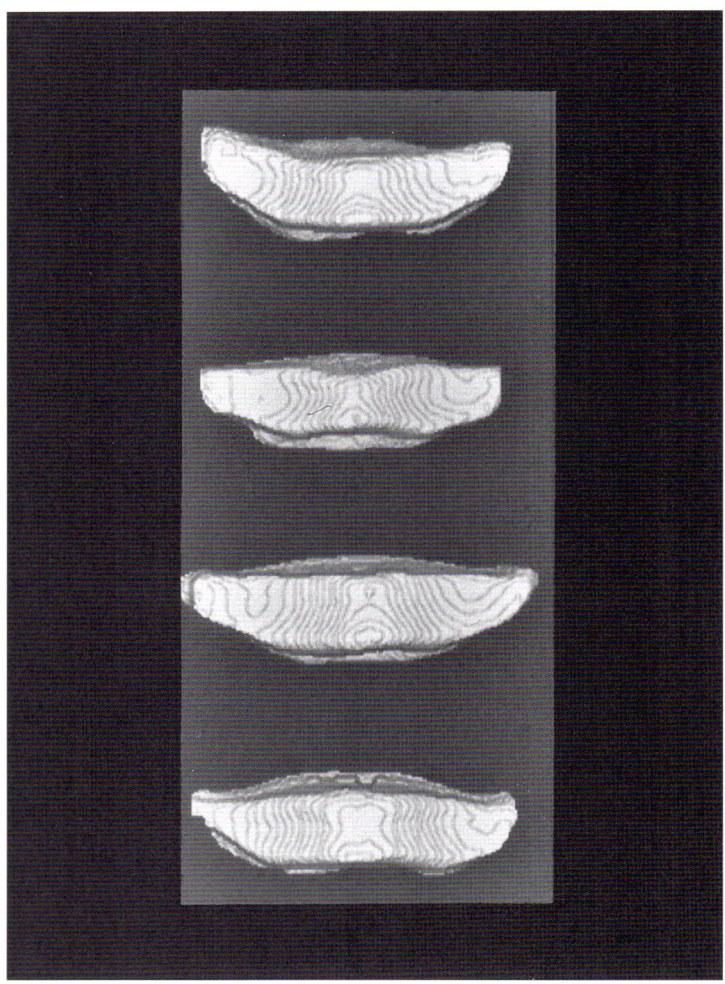

34

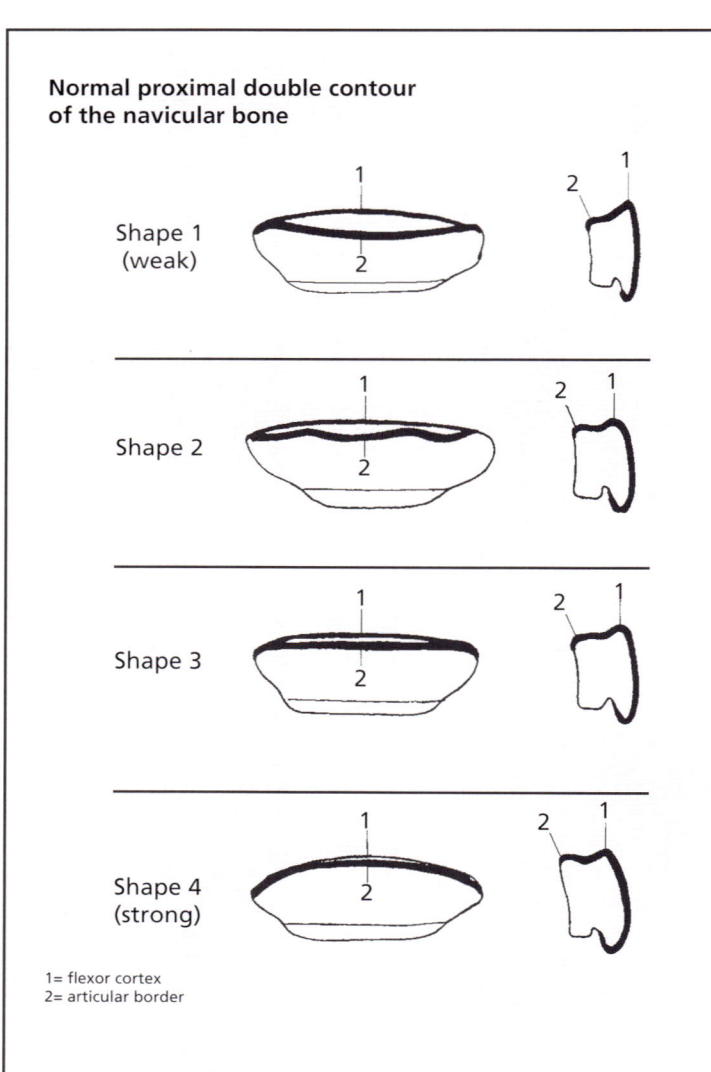

Normal proximal double contour of the navicular bone

Shape 1 (weak)

Shape 2

Shape 3

Shape 4 (strong)

1= flexor cortex
2= articular border

35

33/34/35 Navicular bone specimen, lateromedial and dorsopalmar appearances and corresponding schematic drawing:

On dorsopalmar upright pedal views (Fig. 34, 35) the proximal and distal contour of the navicular bone is commonly visualized as two lines.

The most distal line of the distal contour represents the fairly straight ridge from which the impar ligament originates; the more proximal line is the articular border which is also usually fairly straight.

The most proximal line of the proximal contour represents the flexor border, which usually has a convex shape; the more distal line corresponds with the proximal articular border. The shape of this articular border may be concave = shape 1; undulating = shape 2; straight = shape 3, or convex = shape 4.

These shapes are genetically determined and carrry different risk for the development of navicular disease, a concave articular border (shape 1) being the poorest conformation and a convex articular border (shape 4) reflecting the least susceptible shape. These shapes are not recognisable on lateromedial views (Fig. 33, 35).

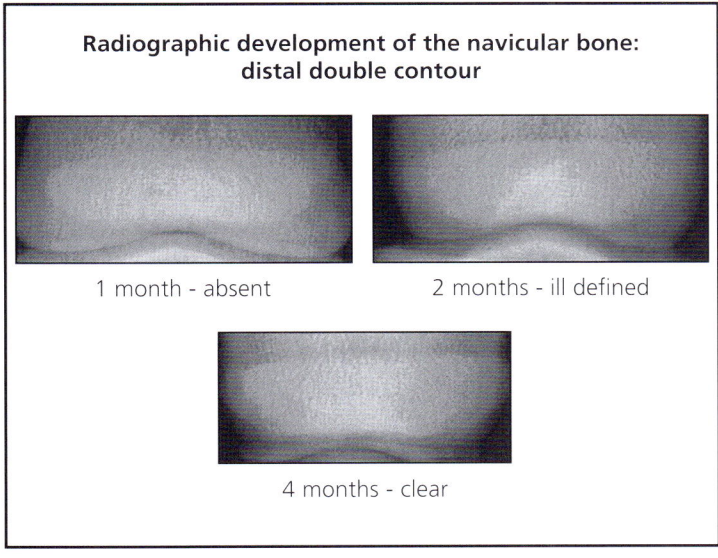

Radiographic development of the navicular bone: distal double contour

1 month - absent

2 months - ill defined

4 months - clear

36

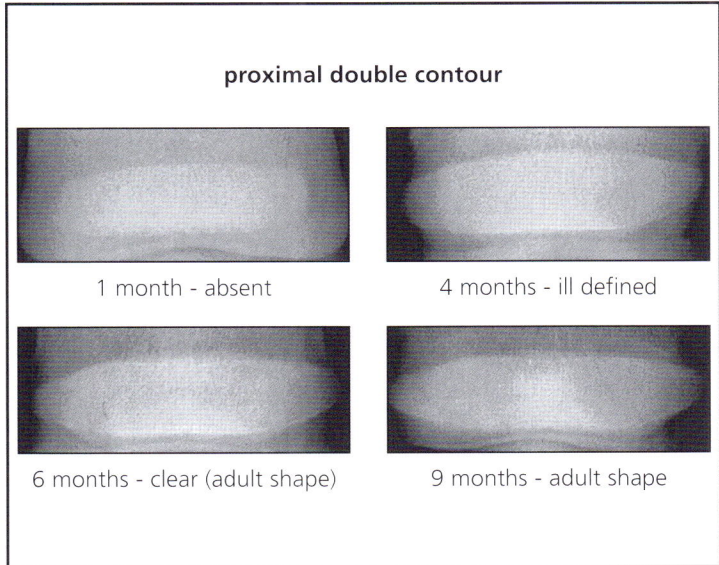

proximal double contour

1 month - absent

4 months - ill defined

6 months - clear (adult shape)

9 months - adult shape

37

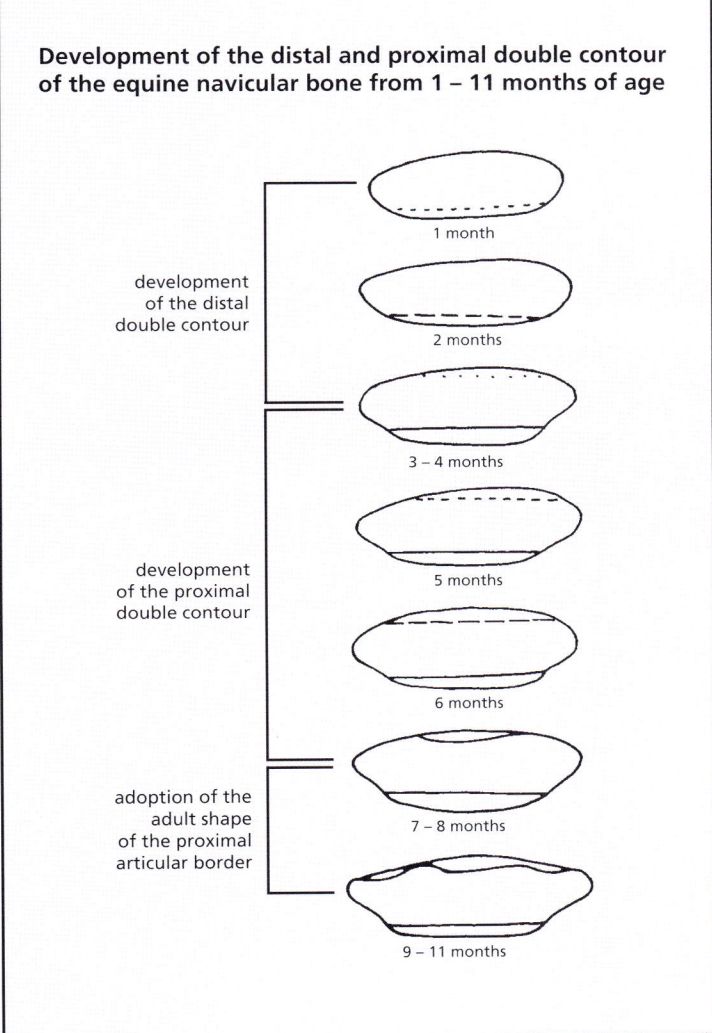

Development of the distal and proximal double contour of the equine navicular bone from 1 – 11 months of age

development of the distal double contour

1 month

2 months

3 – 4 months

development of the proximal double contour

5 months

6 months

adoption of the adult shape of the proximal articular border

7 – 8 months

9 – 11 months

38

36/37/38 Navicular bone, postnatal serial dorsopalmar upright pedal views and corresponding schematic drawing.

At birth the navicular bone has an oval radiographic appearance with a single proximal and distal outline, which represent the flexor cortex.

The subsequent development is characterized by gradual manifestation of the articular borders, thus resulting in a double distal and proximal contour.

The distal double contour develops soon after birth, the radiographic visibility of the articular border improving from ill-defined at 1 – 2 months to clearly seen at 3 months (Fig. 36, 38). After this, the proximal double contour becomes gradually manifest. Ill-defined visibility of the proximal articular border usually begins at 3 – 4 months. Clear manifestation of this line usually follows 1 – 3 months later. Adoption of the 4 adult shapes of the proximal articular border is associated with gradual extension and modelling of the extremities and becomes obvious between 9 and 11 months (Fig. 37, 38).

Nutrient foramina

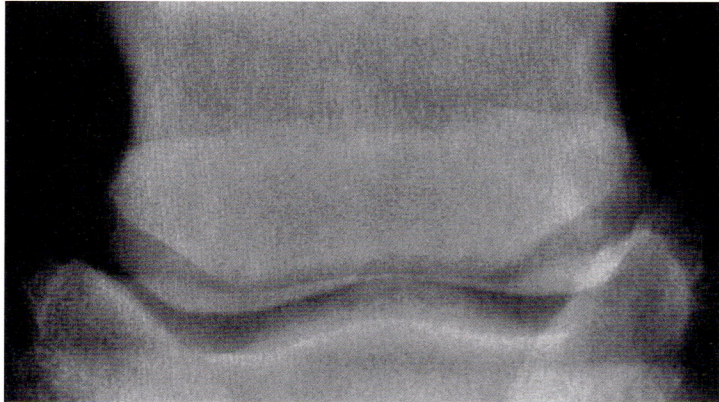

39

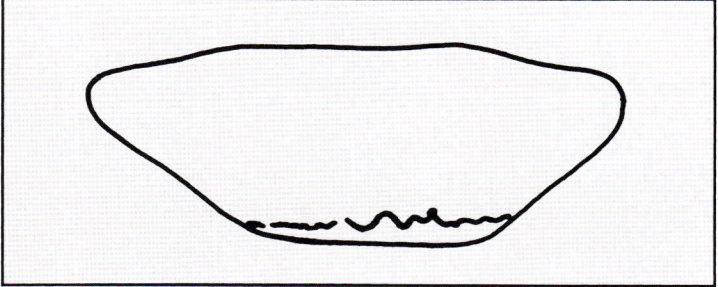

39 a

39 Navicular bone, right front.

Standardbred, 6 years.

Minimal roughening of the distal border of the navicular bone; such changes may be present in sound horses.

39 a Schematic drawing

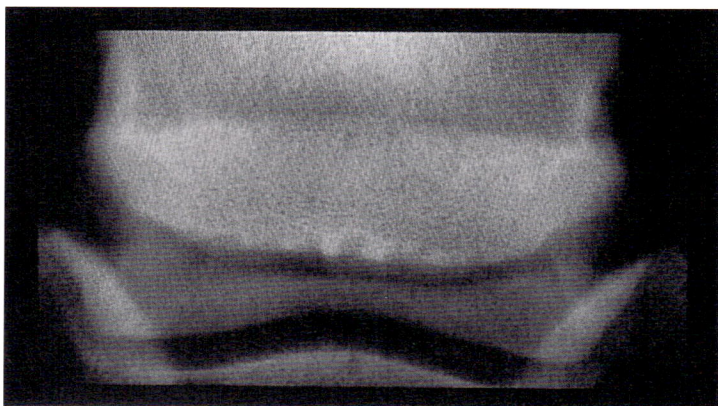

40

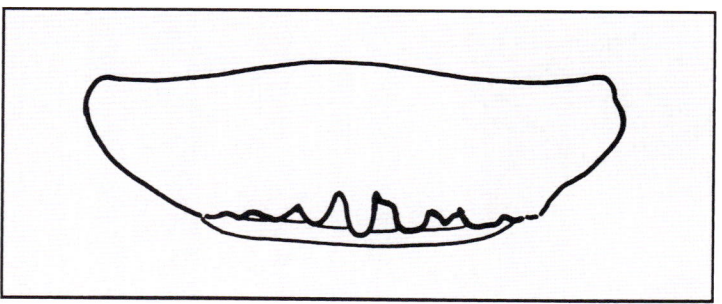

40 a

40 Navicular bone, left front.

Warmblood, 4 ½ years.

Marked "saw-toothed" appearance along the distal border of the navicular bone, due to the presence of several, short, wide, pointed and conical nutrient foramina, some which are surrounded by sclerosis.

Such an appearance is suggestive but not definitive for navicular disease, but may be present in sound horses.

40 a Schematic drawing

Nutrient foramina

41 Navicular bone, left front.

Warmblood, 5 years.

Several narrow, pointed or conical foramina, some short, one of moderate length, and one deeply penetrating the navicular bone.

The greater the number and length of the foramina the more likely are clinical signs to be present.

41 a Schematic drawing

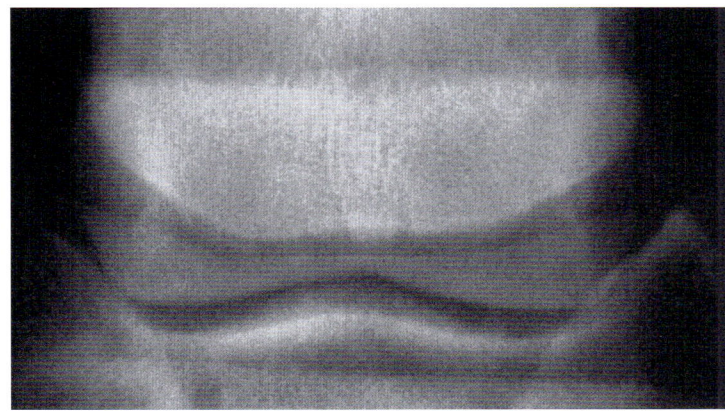

41

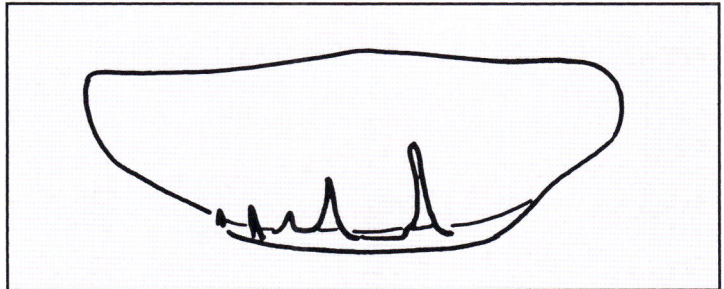

41 a

42 Navicular bone, right front.

Warmblood, 11 years.

Many rounded, inverted flask shaped nutrient foramina. Definitive changes confirming navicular disease.

42 a Schematic drawing

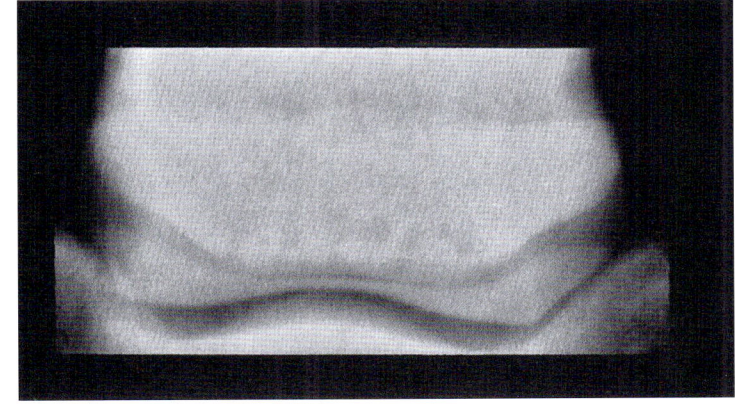

42

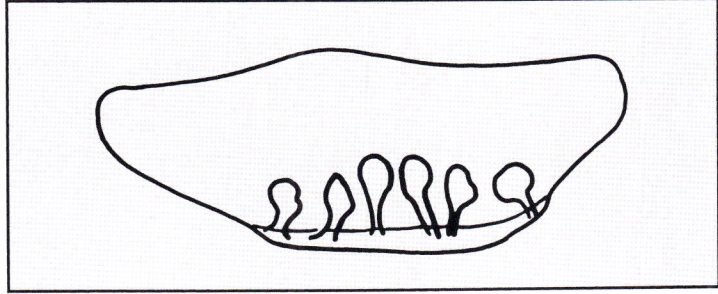

42 a

Navicular disease
Upright pedal views (dorsopalmar): close-ups.

Cyst

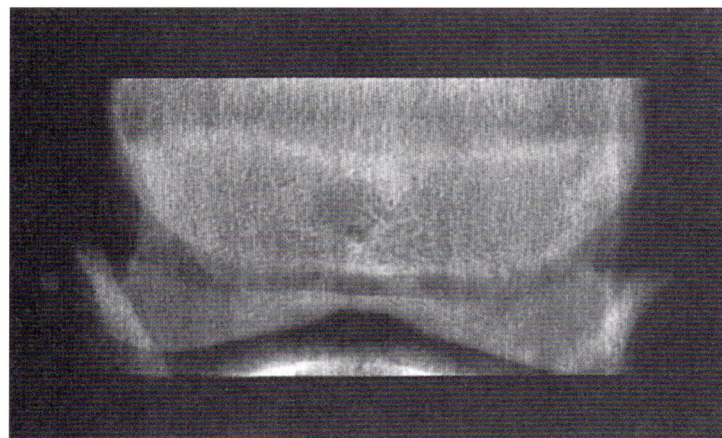

43

43 Navicular bone, right front.

Warmblood, 7 years.

A solitary, clearly defined, cystic, radiolucent area in the central portion of the navicular bone, generalized osteoporosis and many ill defined, inverted flask shaped nutrient foramina along the distal border of the navicular bone.

Cysts are definitive changes confirming navicular disease and present in lame horses.

43 a Schematic drawing

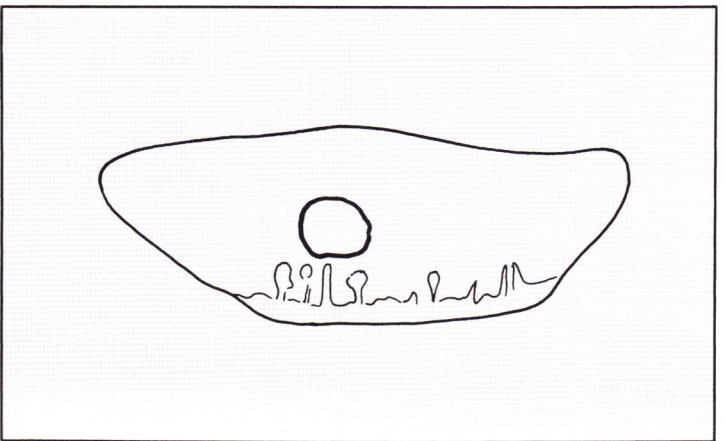

43 a

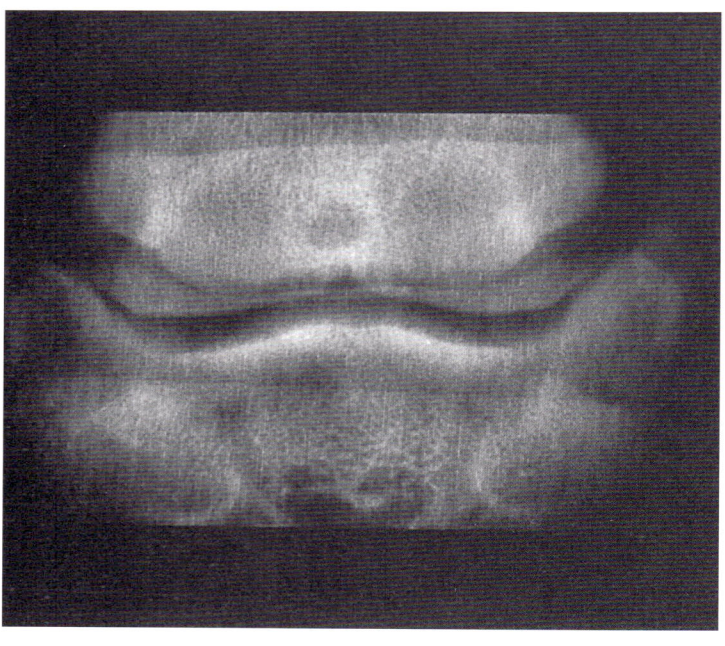

44

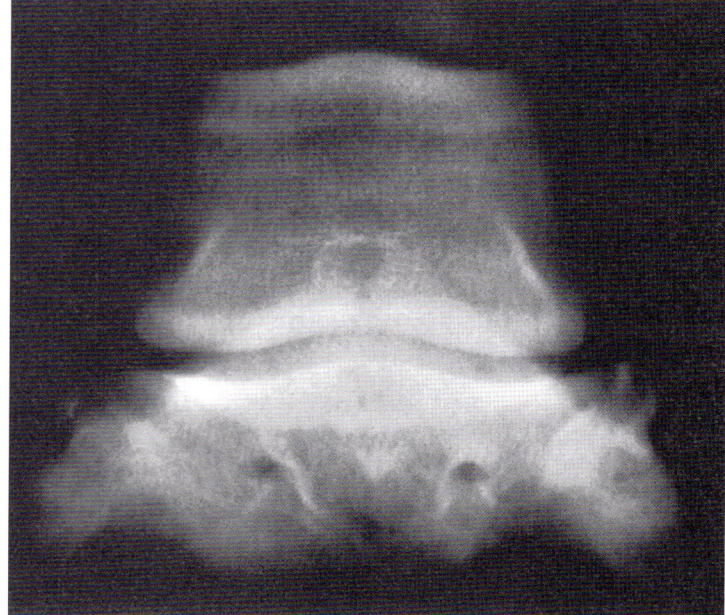

45

44/45 Navicular bone, right front, upright pedal view (dorsopalmar) and dorsopalmar weight-bearing view.

Warmblood, 8 years.

The upright pedal view (Fig. 44) shows a well defined, cystic, radiolucent lesion in the central portion of the navicular bone and roughening of the distal border.

On an additional weight-bearing dorsopalmar view (Fig. 45) the projection of the navicular bone has shifted distally and the cyst is visible proximal to the navicular bone, indicating that the cyst is located within the second phalanx.

A bone cyst in the second phalanx may be present in sound horses.

Sclerosis

46 Navicular bone, left front.

Warmblood, 6 years.

Generalized sclerosis of the navicular bone and roughening of the distal border.

Generalized sclerosis is a rare change of variable clinical significance, suggestive of navicular disease but inconclusive.

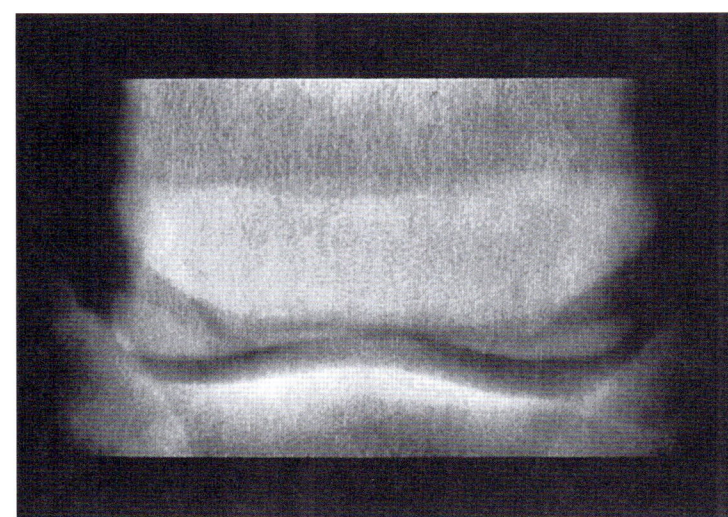

46

Enthesophytosis

47 Navicular bone, left front.

Warmblood, 7 years.

A large spur on the lateral extremity of the navicular bone and several ill defined nutrient foramina along the distal border. (The radiograph is underexposed deliberately to highlight the spur.)

Large spurs are significant changes present mainly in lame horses.

47 a Schematic drawing

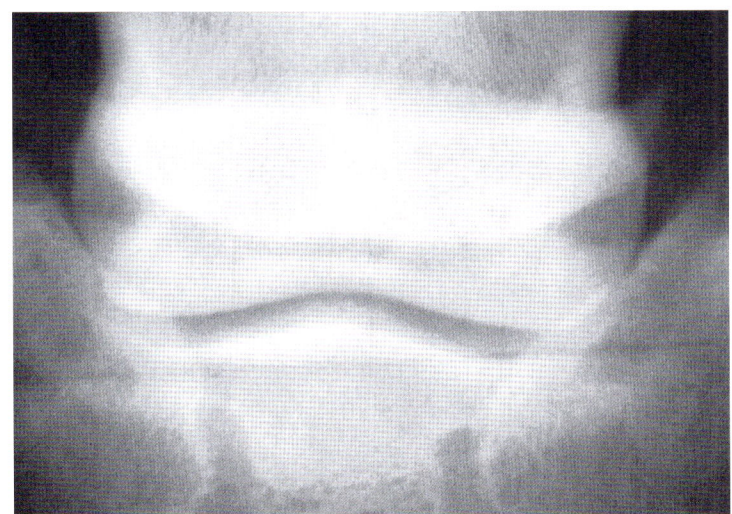

47

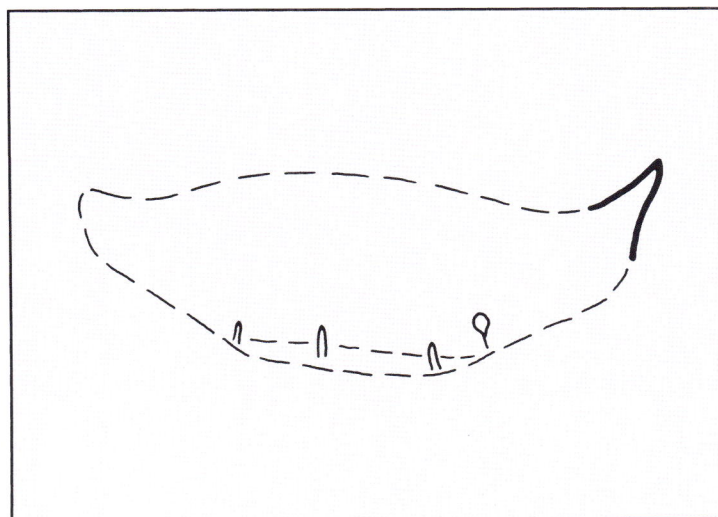

47 a

Navicular disease
Upright pedal views (dorsopalmar): close-ups.

Enthesophytosis

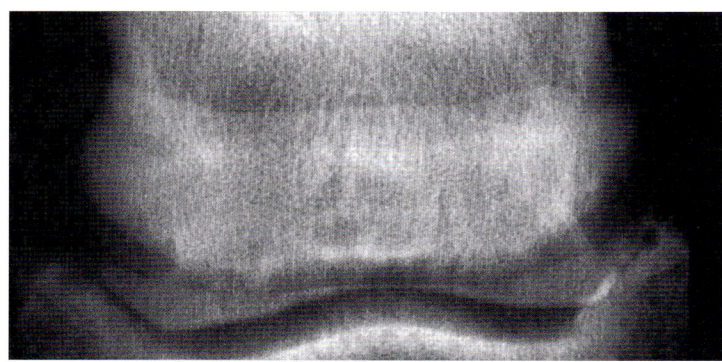

48 Navicular bone, right front.

Warmblood, 10 years.

Extensive new bone formation along the entire proximal margin, a large, indistinct, cystic, radiolucent area in the central portion and roughening of the distal border of the navicular bone.

Extensive new bone formation along the proximal border is a significant change present mainly in lame horses.

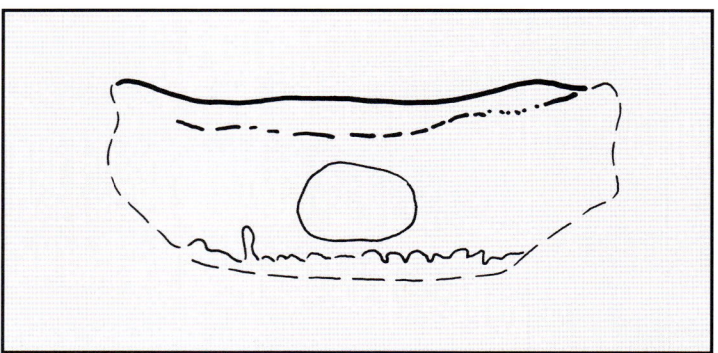

48 a Schematic drawing

Pseudoenthesophytosis

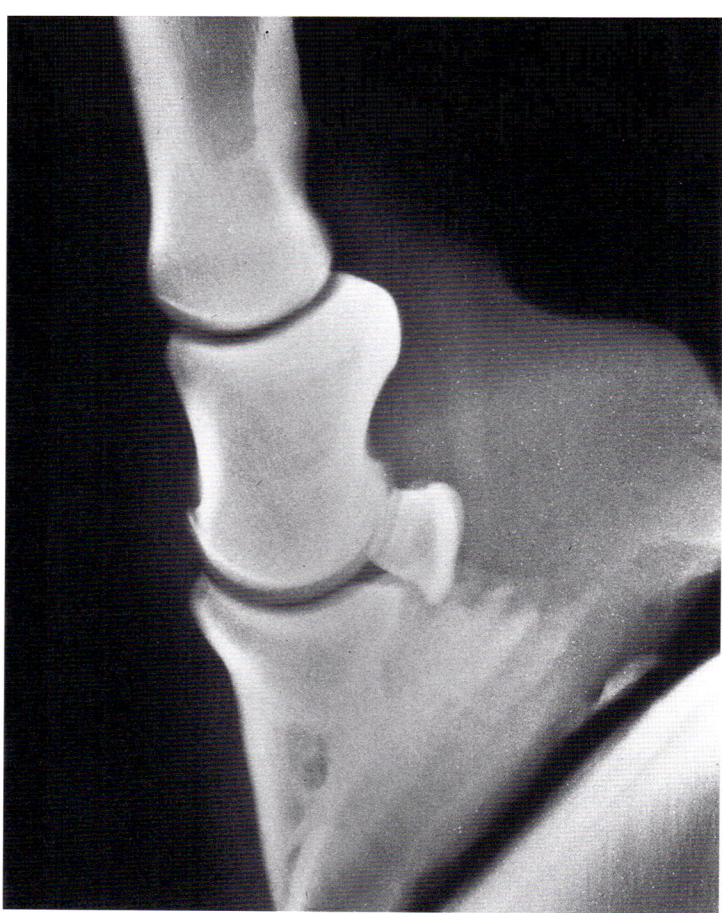

49

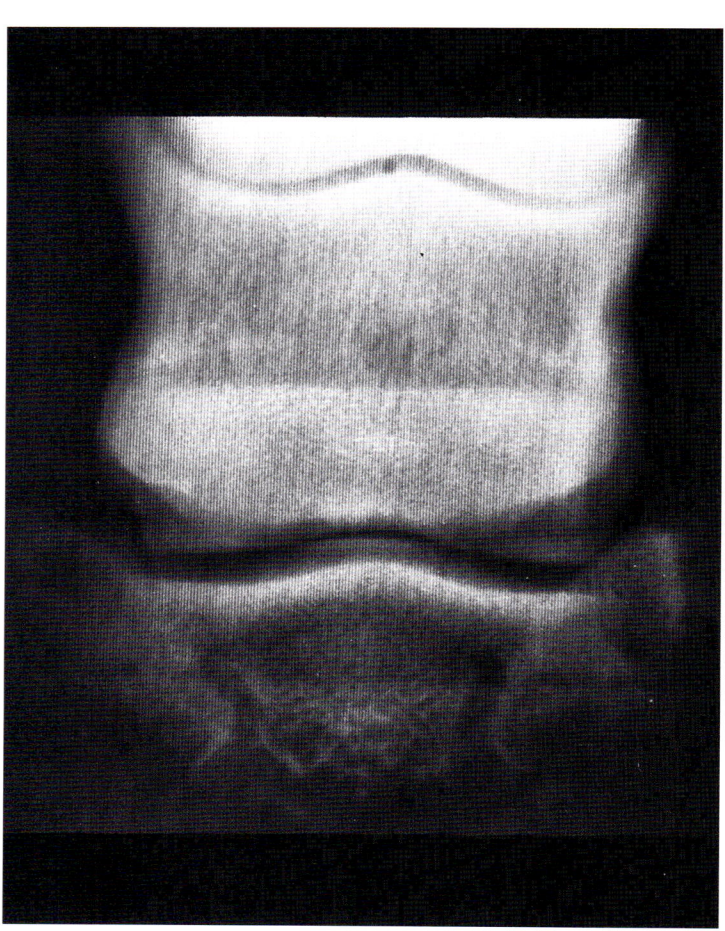

50

49/50 Navicular bone, right front, lateromedial and dorsopalmar upright pedal views.

Warmblood, 3 years.

The dorsopalmar upright pedal view (Fig. 50) shows discrete, sclerotic horizontal lines in the lateral and medial region of the second phalanx, adjacent and roughly parallel to the proximal contour of the navicular bone.

These lines may mimic new bone formation along the proximal navicular border, but actually represent prominent, abrupt palmaroproximal condylar margins of the distal articular surface of the second phalanx.

The prominent, pointed appearance of these margins and the normal appearance of the proximal contour of the navicular bone are clearly visible on the lateromedial view (Fig. 49), thus confirming the absence of navicular enthesophytosis.

Pseudoenthesophytosis

51 Schematic drawings of the navicular bone.

The normal dorsopalmar and lateromedial appearance of the navicular bone versus elongation of the proximal flexor cortex, proximal border – and extremity enthesophytosis.

Contrary to extensive new bone formation along the entire proximal margin of the navicular bone or limited to the lateral and/or medial extremity, elongation of the proximal flexor cortex usually is not associated with lameness.

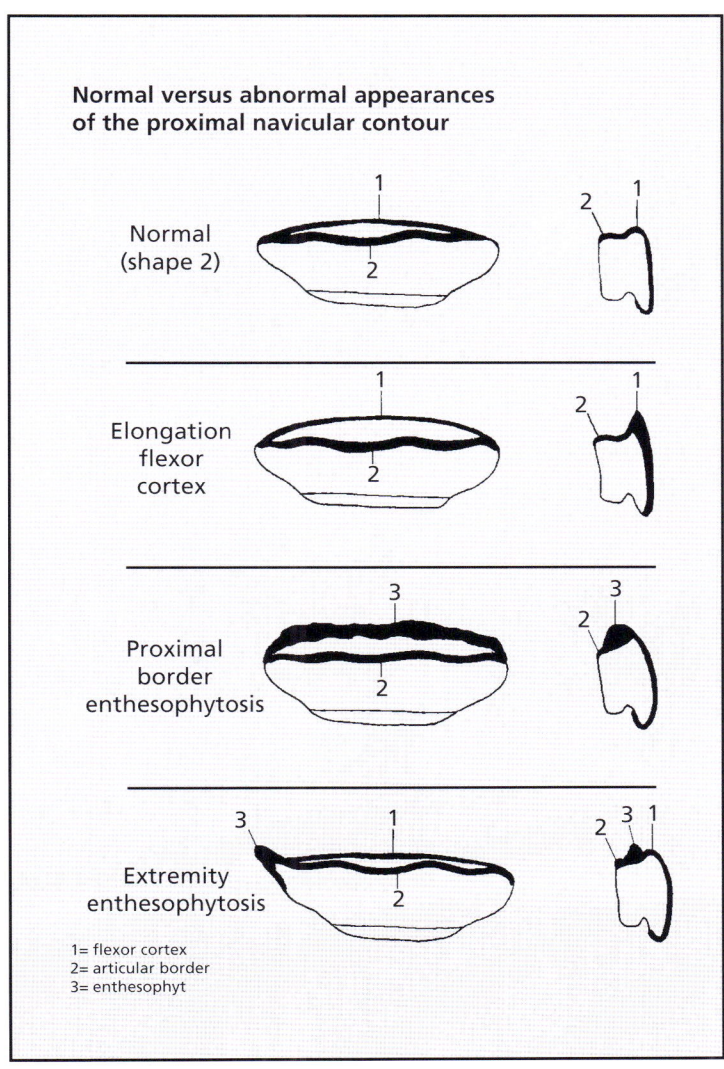

Normal versus abnormal appearances of the proximal navicular contour

Normal (shape 2)

Elongation flexor cortex

Proximal border enthesophytosis

Extremity enthesophytosis

1= flexor cortex
2= articular border
3= enthesophyt

51

Chip fracture

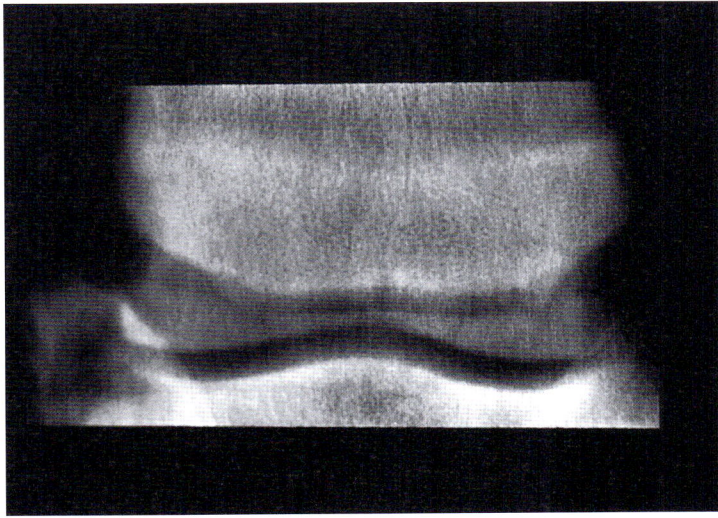

52 Navicular bone, left front.

Warmblood, 7 years.

An isolated ellipsoidal bone fragment on the distal border of the lateral part of the navicular bone, indicating a chip fracture originating from the prominent edge of the distal border. The fragment is slightly separated from the navicular bone.

The fracture "bed" is visible. Several ill defined, conical nutrient foramina of moderate length are present in the corresponding area of the navicular bone, the remaining portion of the distal border is roughened.

Chip fractures are changes of variable significance and may be present in both lame as well as sound horses.

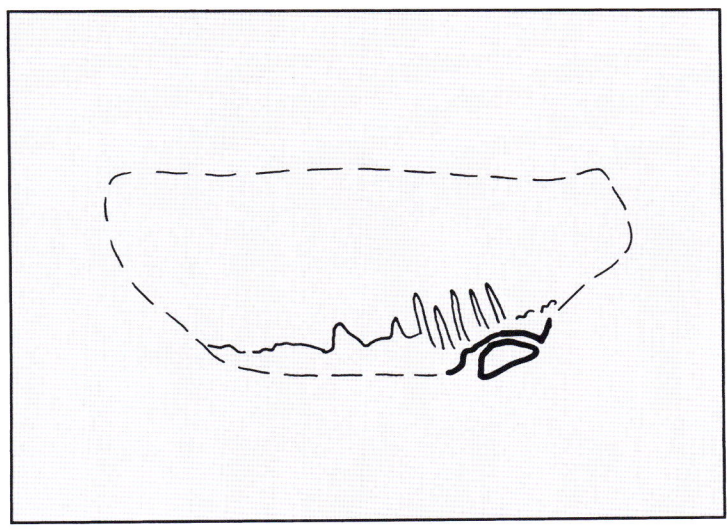

52 a Schematic drawing

Erosion of the flexor surface

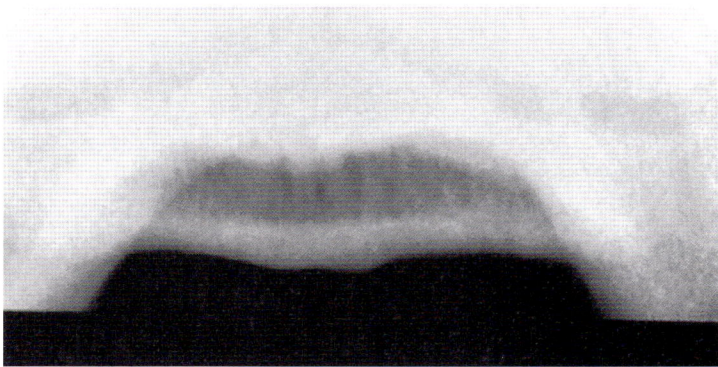

53

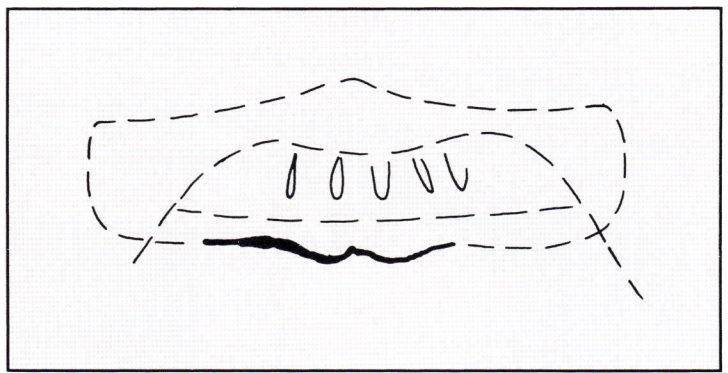

53 a

53 Navicular bone, right front.

Warmblood, 12 years.

Flattening and depression of the flexor surface of the sagittal ridge of the navicular bone.

Significant changes present mainly in lame horses.

53 a Schematic drawing

Roughening of the flexor surface

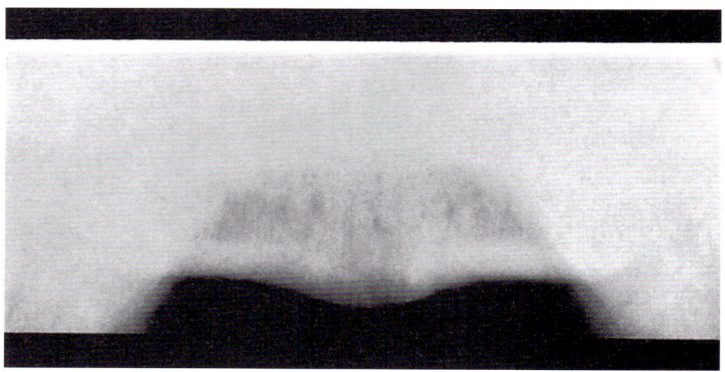

54

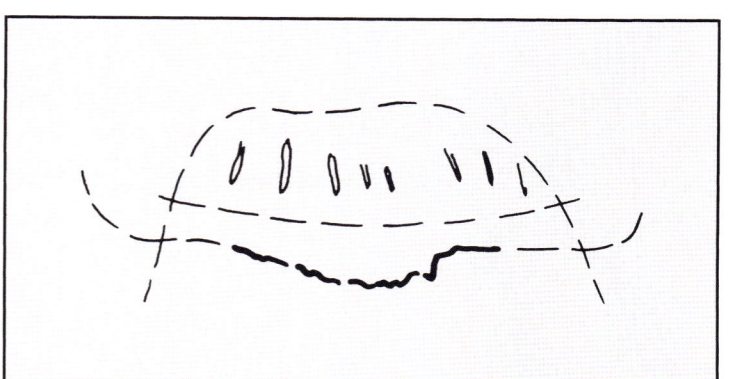

54 a

54 Navicular bone, left front.

Warmblood, 9 years.

Roughening of the flexor surface around the sagittal ridge of the navicular bone and radiolucent defects in the corresponding cortical bone of the flexor surface.

Significant changes present mainly in lame horses. (The radiograph is under-exposed deliberately to highlight the roughening of the flexor surface.)

54 a Schematic drawing

Cyst

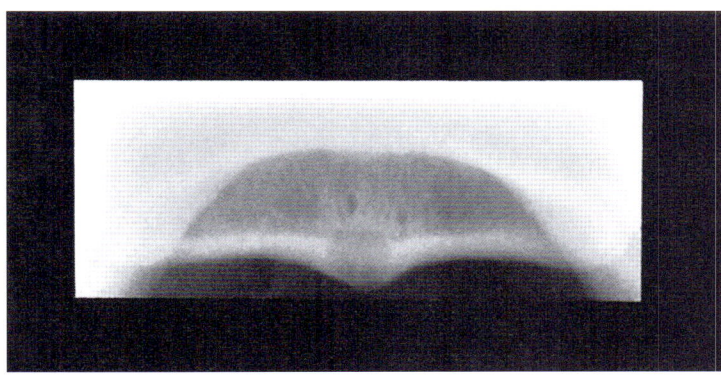

55 Navicular bone, left front.

Warmblood, 10 years.

A clearly defined, cystic, radiolucent lesion in the cortical bone of the sagittal ridge of the navicular bone and sclerosis in the corresponding area of the spongiosa.

Cysts are definitive changes confirming navicular disease and present in lame horses.

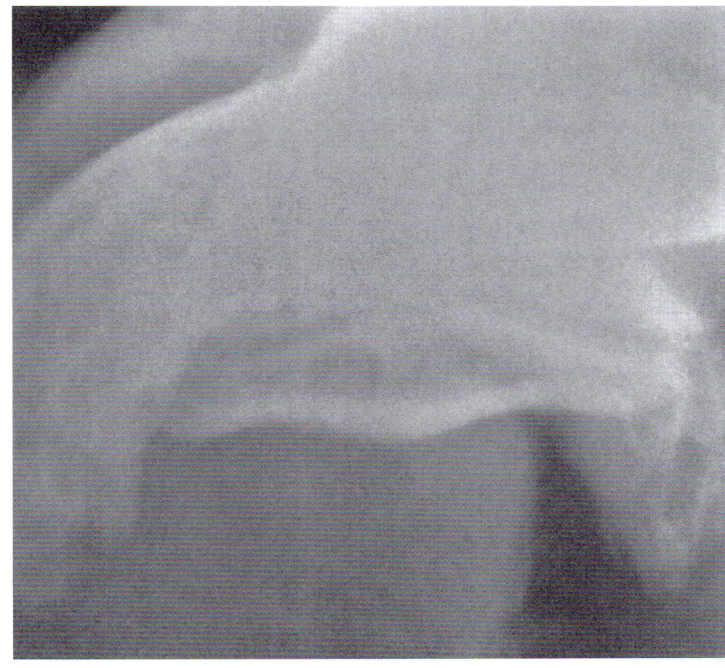

56 Navicular bone, left front.

Pony, 7 years.

A clearly defined, cystic, radiolucent lesion within the spongiosa of the navicular bone; the overlying cortical bone is intact. A cystic lesion limited to the medullary spongiosa is an unusual finding. Cystic radiolucent lesions are usually seen in the compact bone of the flexor surface near the sagittal ridge and occasionally within the compacta and spongiosa.

Sclerosis

57 Navicular bone, left front.

Warmblood, 6 years.

Generalized sclerosis of the spongiosa. The trabecular pattern of the spongiosa is lost and the sharp interface between the spongiosa and the compact bone of the flexor surface is no longer visible. Sclerosis is a change of variable significance, suggestive but not confirming navicular disease.

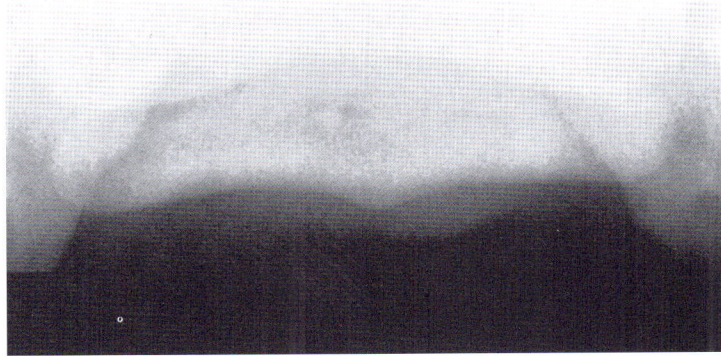

57

Infectious arthritis

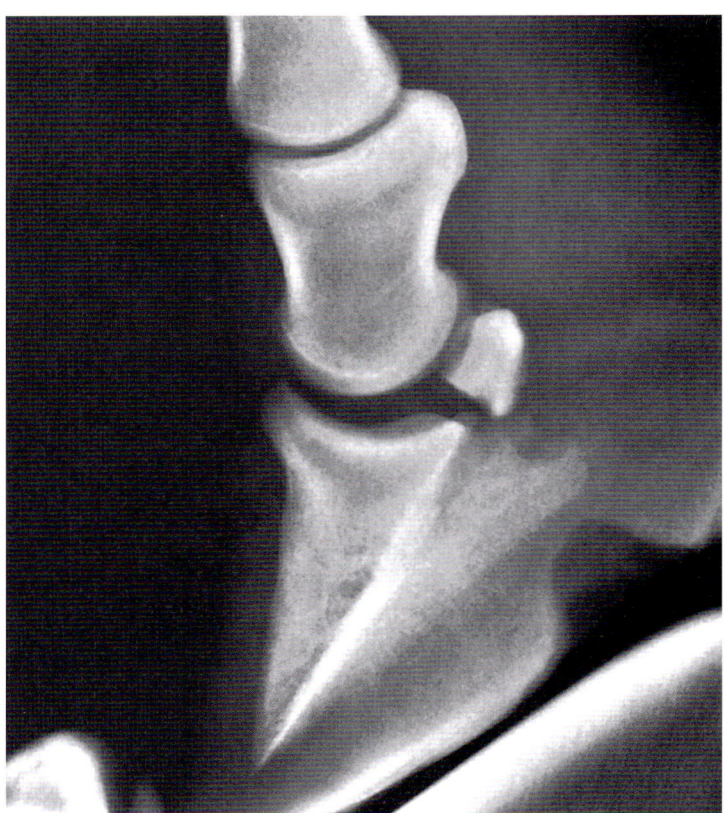

58

58 Coffin joint, left front, lateromedial view: close-up.

Standardbred, 3 years.

Extreme widening of the coffin joint space caused by infectious arthritis which resulted from nail puncture in the middle of the frog, 4 weeks prior to examination.

Osteoarthrosis
(Low ringbone)

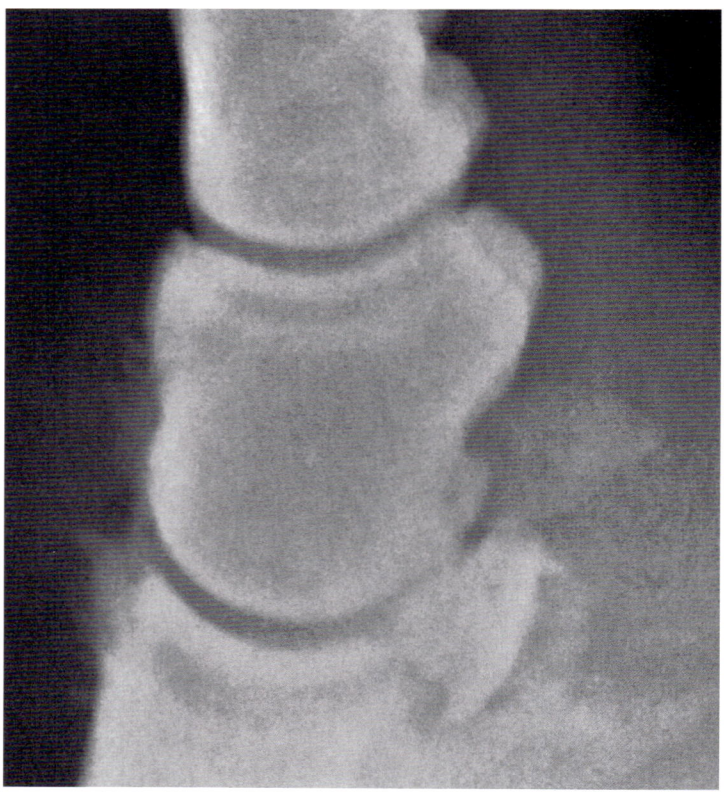

59 Coffin joint, right front, lateromedial view: close-up.

Draughthorse, 7 years.

Indistinct, irregular, ill bordered new bone formation **(1)** along the extensor process of the pedal bone and the dorsal aspect of the second phalanx, indicating active low ringbone of recent origin.

Additional finding: ossification of the accessory cartilages **(2)**.

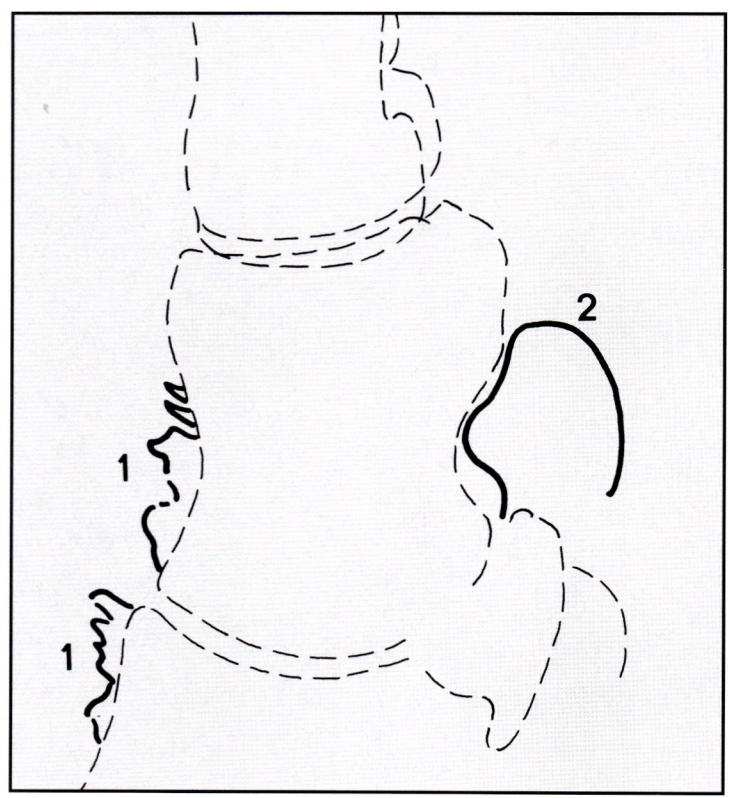

59 a Schematic drawing

Pedal bone

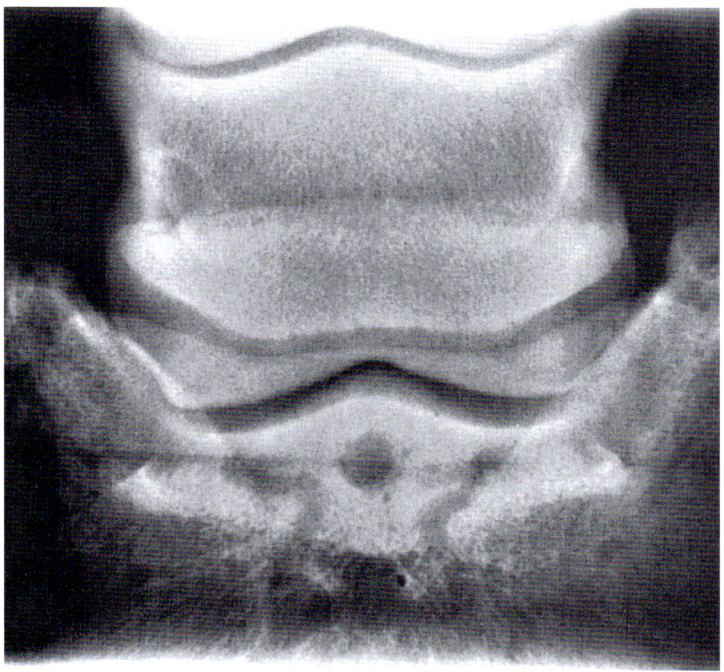

60

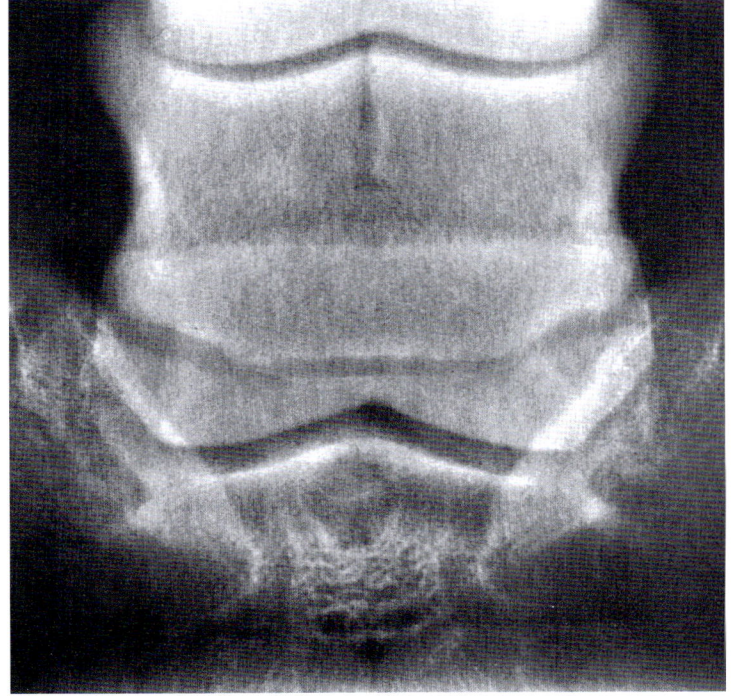

61 Pedal bone, left front, upright pedal view (dorsopalmar): close-up.
Warmblood, 14 years.

A sharply delineated, oval area of diffuse radiolucency **(1)** in the extensor process of the pedal bone, close to the coffin joint. This represents a bone cyst. The cyst is not surrounded by a sclerotic zone and there is no visible communication between the cyst lumen and the coffin joint.

N. B. The vertical radiolucent zone **(2)** in the middle of the second phalanx proximal to the navicular bone is artefactual, due to inadequate packing of the central sulcus of the frog.

60 Pedal bone, right front, upright pedal view (dorsopalmar): close-up.
Warmblood, 4 years.

A solitary, clearly defined, circular area of diffuse radiolucency, surrounded by a sclerotic zone, in the extensor process of the pedal bone. These changes indicate the presence of a long-standing bone cyst. There is no visible communication between the cyst lumen and the coffin joint.

N. B. The radiolucent area proximal to the lateral extremity of the navicular bone is artefactual, the result of inadequate packing of the lateral sulcus of the frog prior to the radiographic exposure.

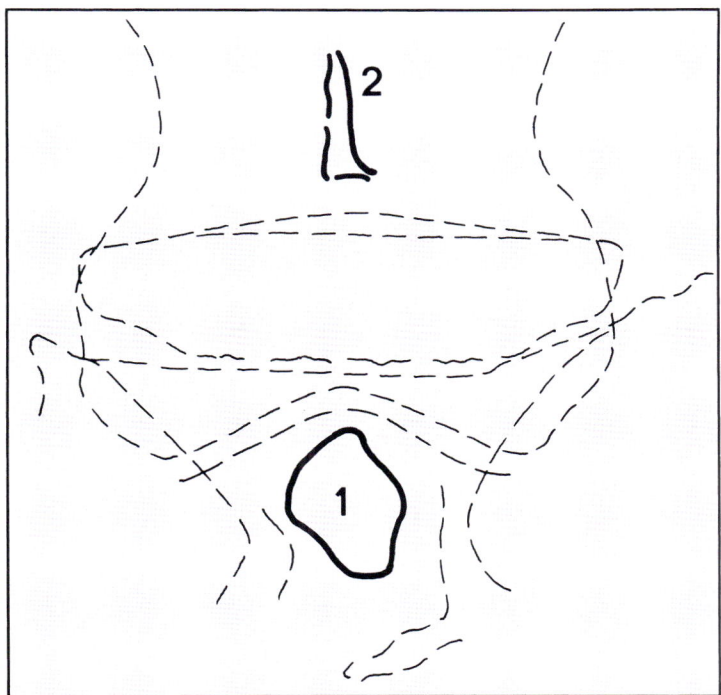

61 a Schematic drawing

Laminitis

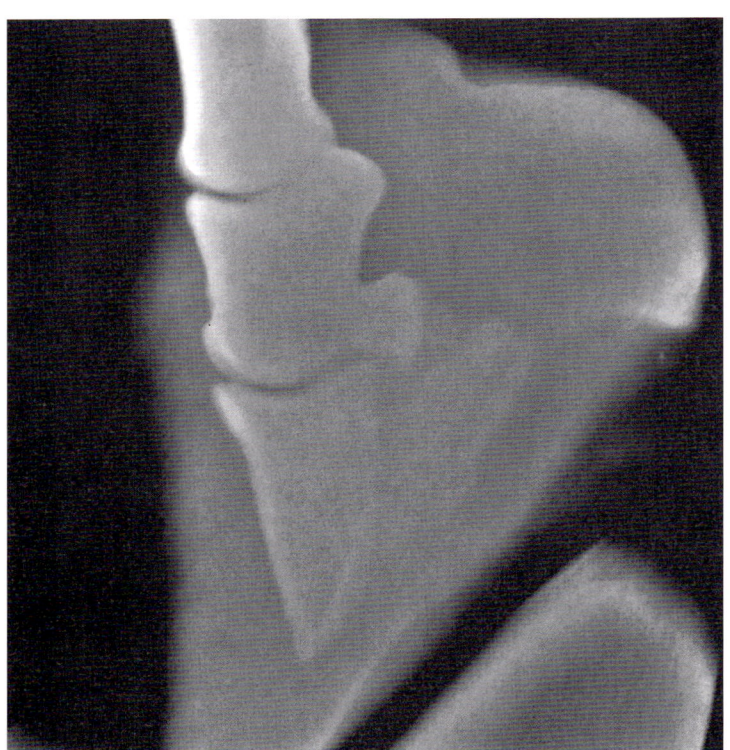

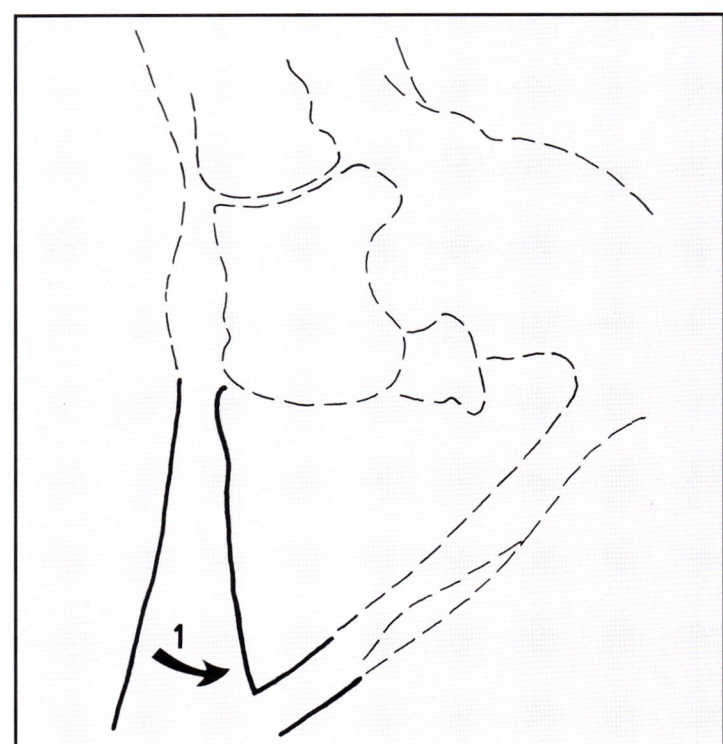

62 Pedal bone, right front, lateromedial view.

Warmblood, 5 years.

The dorsal wall of the hoof is no longer parallel with the dorsal surface of the pedal bone; the pedal bone is rotated away from the hoofwall **(1)**.

The tip of the pedal bone has not perforated the sole, due to the lesser degree of rotation and a relatively thick sole.

62 a Schematic drawing

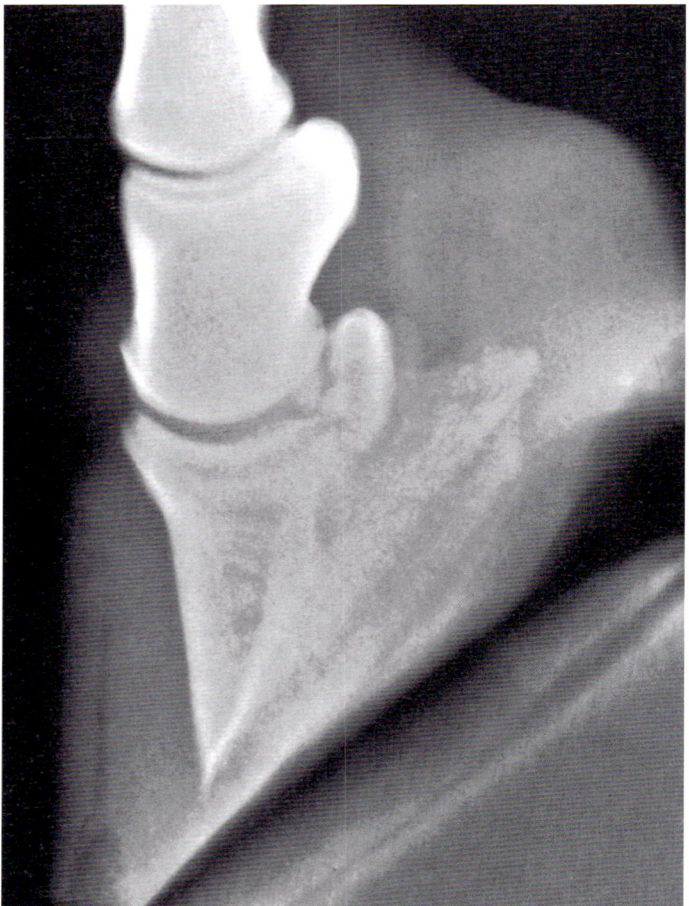

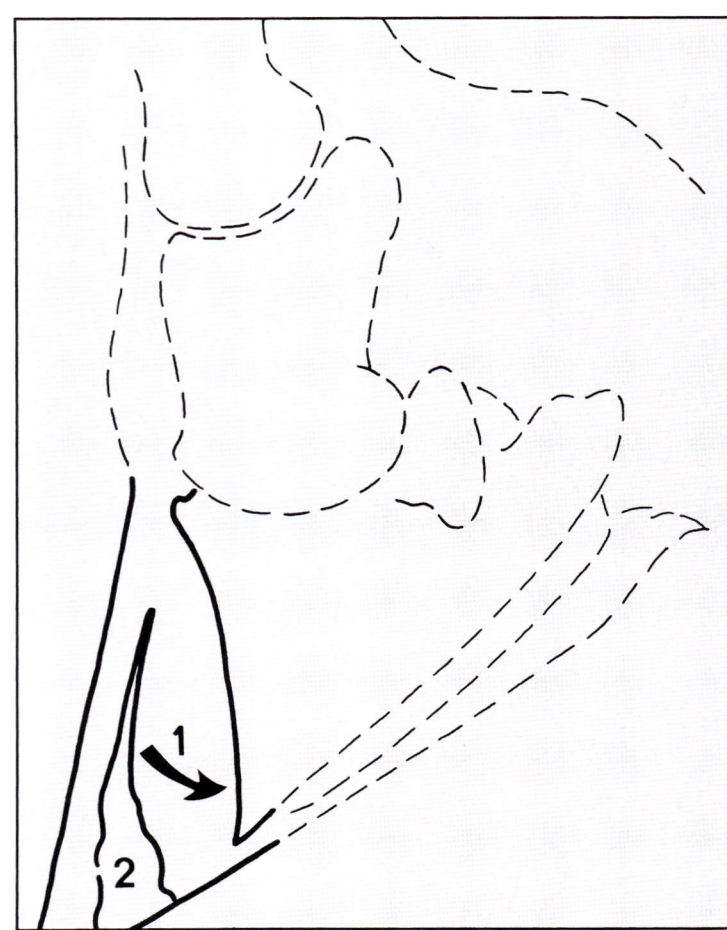

63 Pedal bone, left front, lateromedial view.

Warmblood, 4 years.

Rotation of the pedal bone **(1)** and a radiolucent zone **(2)** within the hoofwall arising from haemorrhage within the sensitive laminae, or the penetration of air, or infection along the separated white line.

63 a Schematic drawing

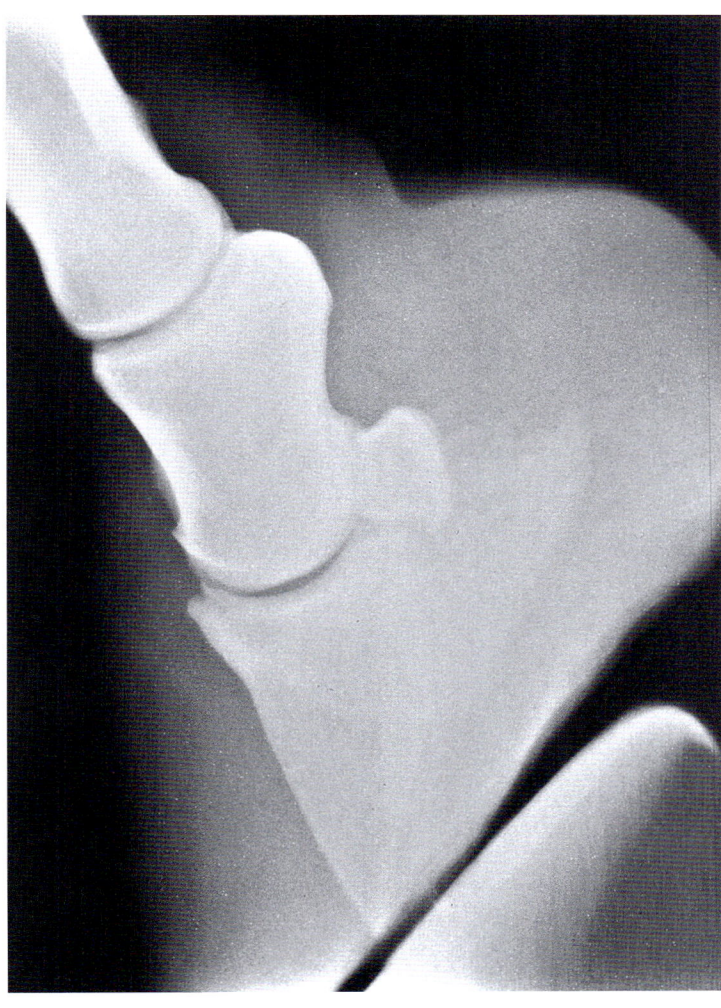

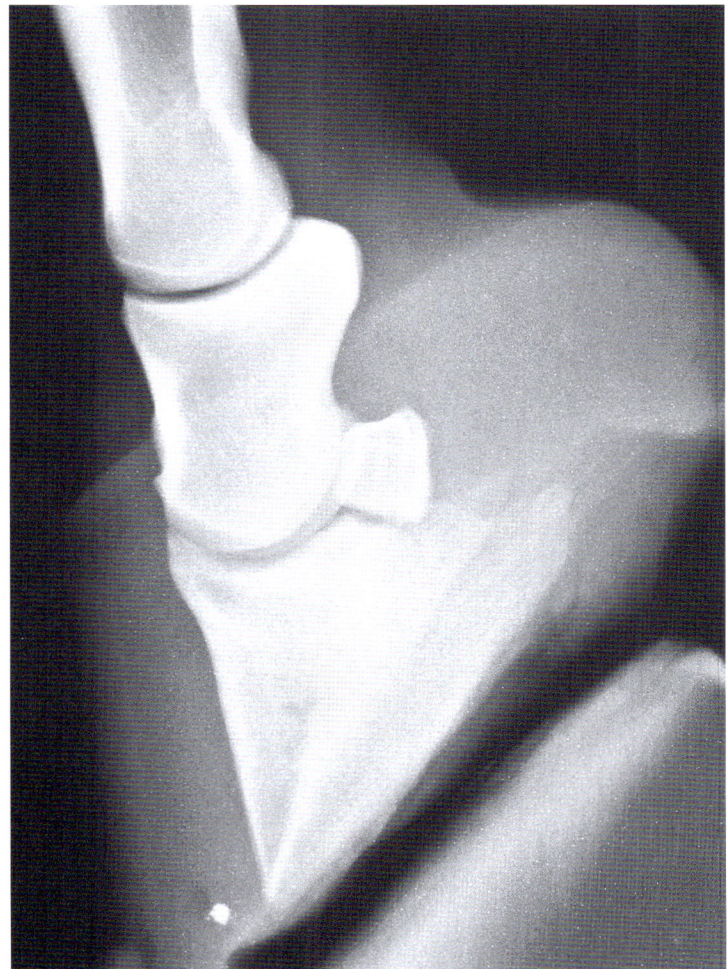

64 Pedal bone, left front, lateromedial view.

Warmblood, 7 years.

Severe downward rotation of the pedal bone, the tip of the pedal bone protruding through the slightly dropped sole.

65 Pedal bone, right front, lateromedial view

Warmblood, 5 years.

The dorsal hoofwall is not strictly parallel with the dorsal surface of the pedal bone and is also thicker than normal. This indicates rotational displacement, as well as vertical displacement, i.e. "sinking" of the pedal bone.

The increased visibility of the coronary band and the soft tissue depression immediately above the dorsal aspect of the coronary band results from swelling and sinking of the coronary band, which is associated with the distal drop of the pedal bone within the horny capsule.

A faint radiolucent line is present in the dorsal hoofwall. The sole is very thin and convex, but the tip of the pedal bone is not protruding through the dropped sole.

N. B. In Warmbloods the normal radiographic thickness of the dorsal wall is 19 ± 1.5 mm.

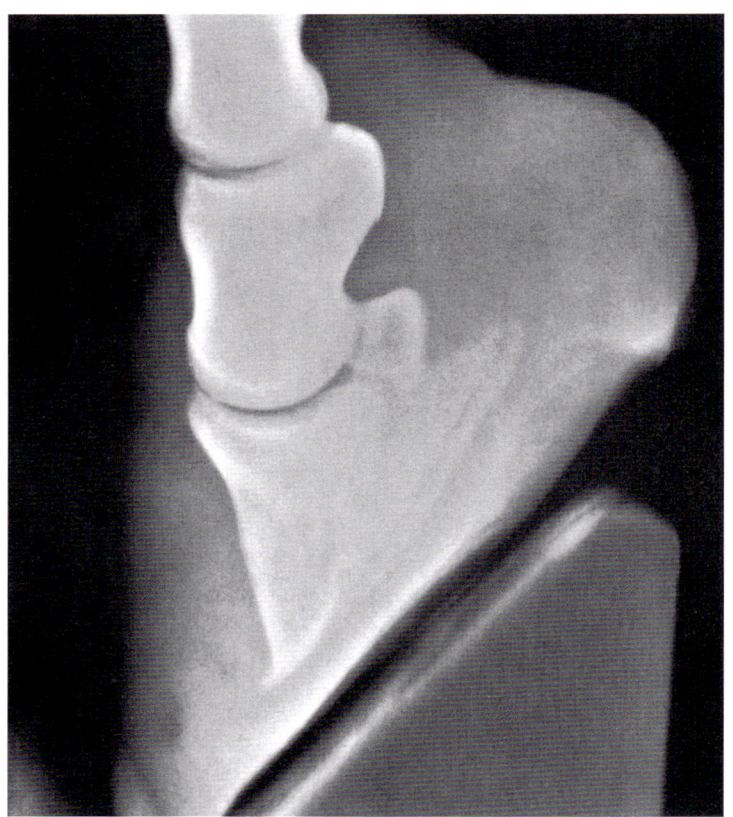

66

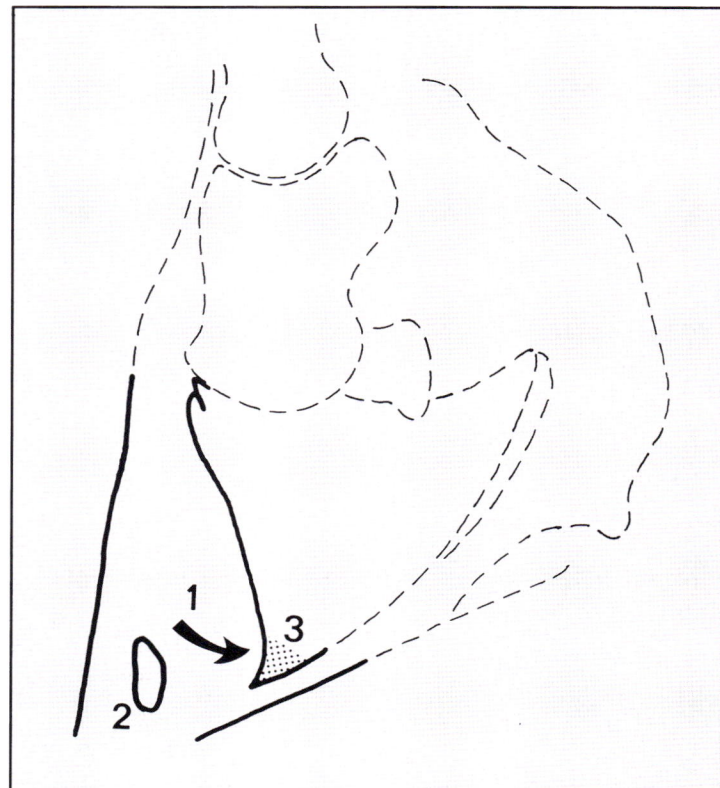

66 a

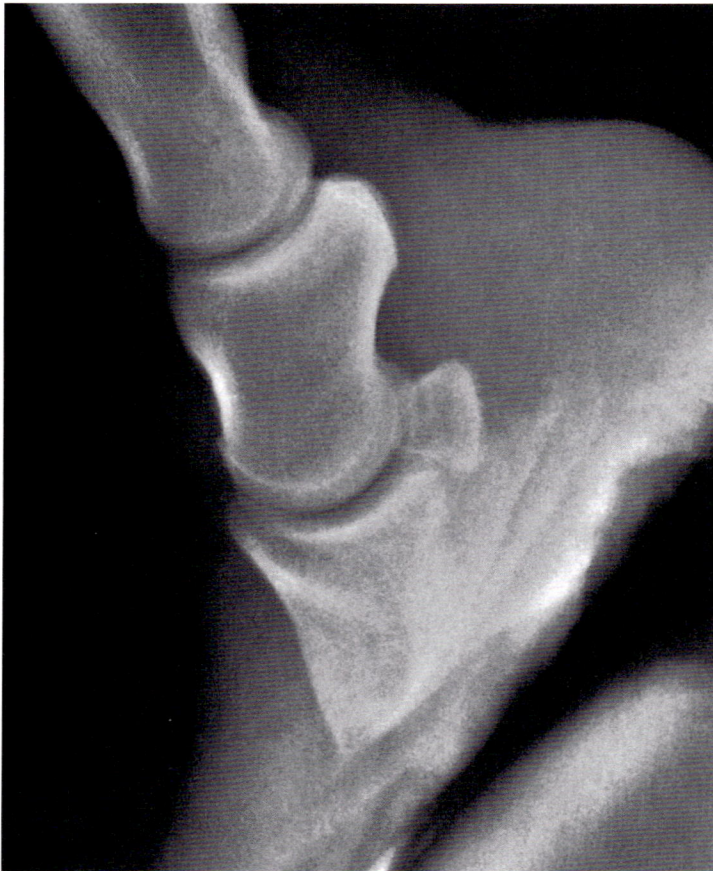

67

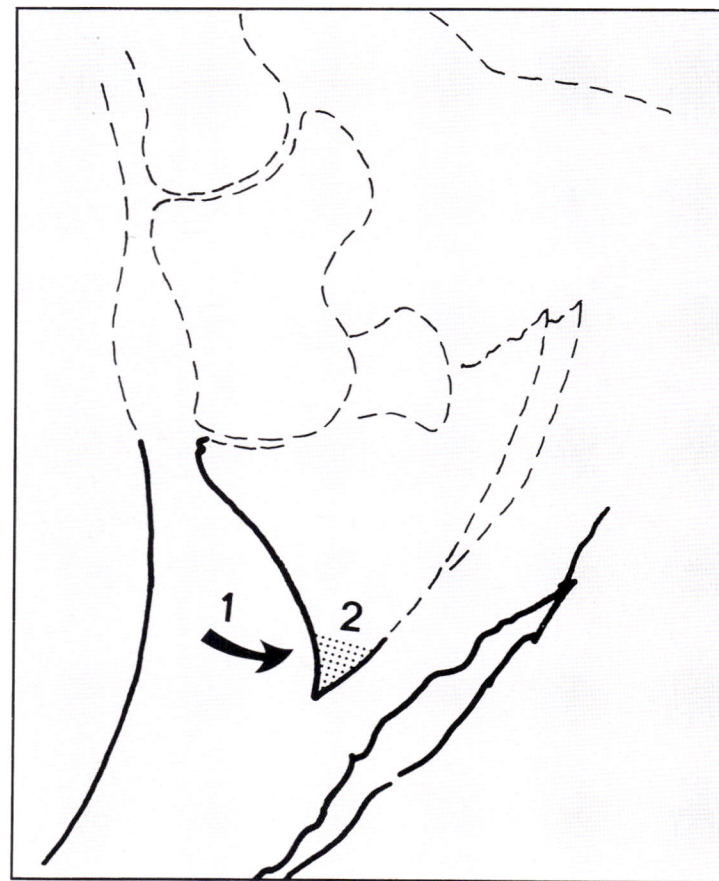

67 a

66/67 Pedal bone, right front, serial lateromedial views.

Warmblood, 10 years.

Fig. 66: Rotation of the pedal bone **(1)**, a radiolucent defect **(2)** within the hoofwall and lipping **(3)** of the dorsal aspect of the distal border of the pedal bone. This kind of deformation of the pedal bone caused by excessive pressure, is present from 4 until 6 weeks after the onset of the disease.

Fig. 67: The same horse after 21 months. The pedal bone is not only rotated **(1)** and deformed **(2)** but also shortened.

The hoof has a dropped sole and a long curved toe.

66 a/67 a Schematic drawings

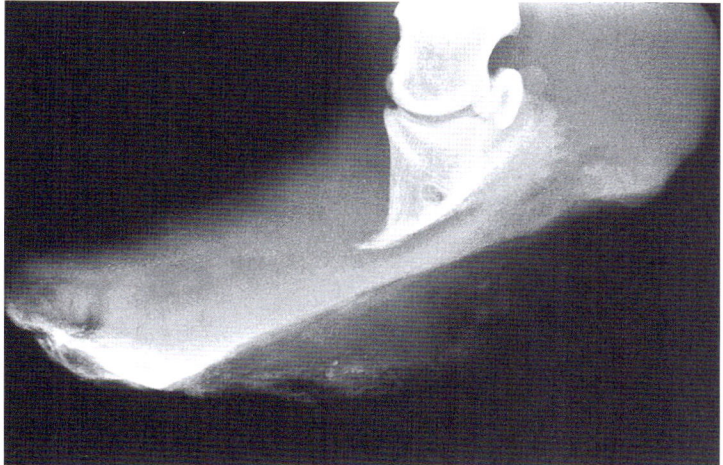

68

68 Pedal bone, right front, lateromedial view.
Pony, 17 years.
Obvious rotation and lipping of the dorsal aspect of the distal border of the pedal bone 5 years after the onset of the disease, the extreme length and deformation of the toe resulting from neglected foot care.

Rupture of the deep flexor tendon

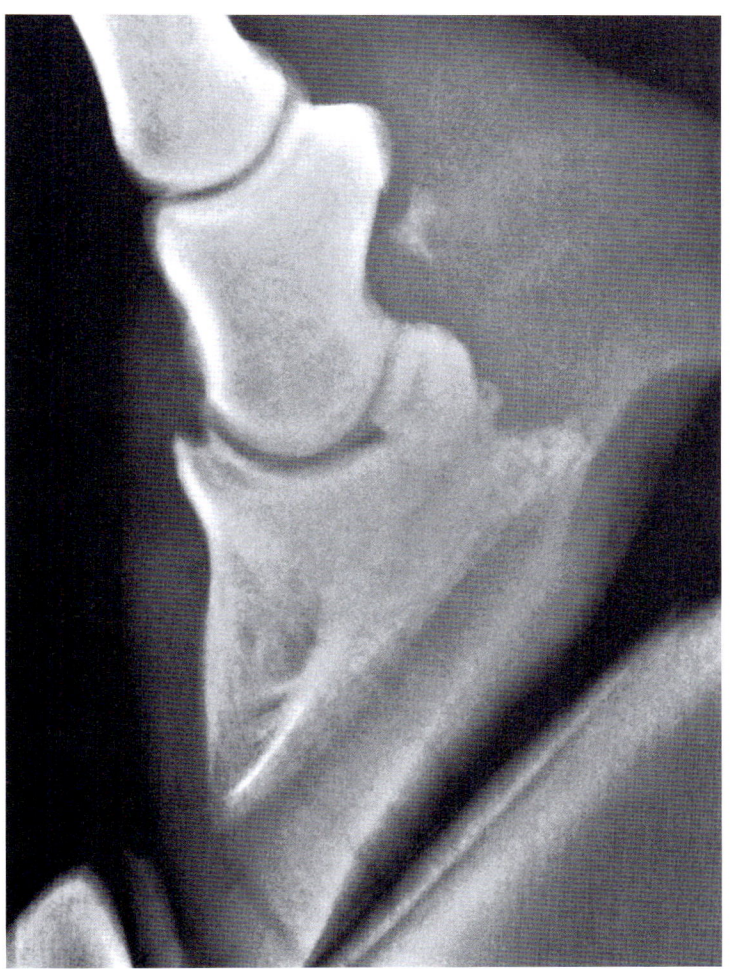

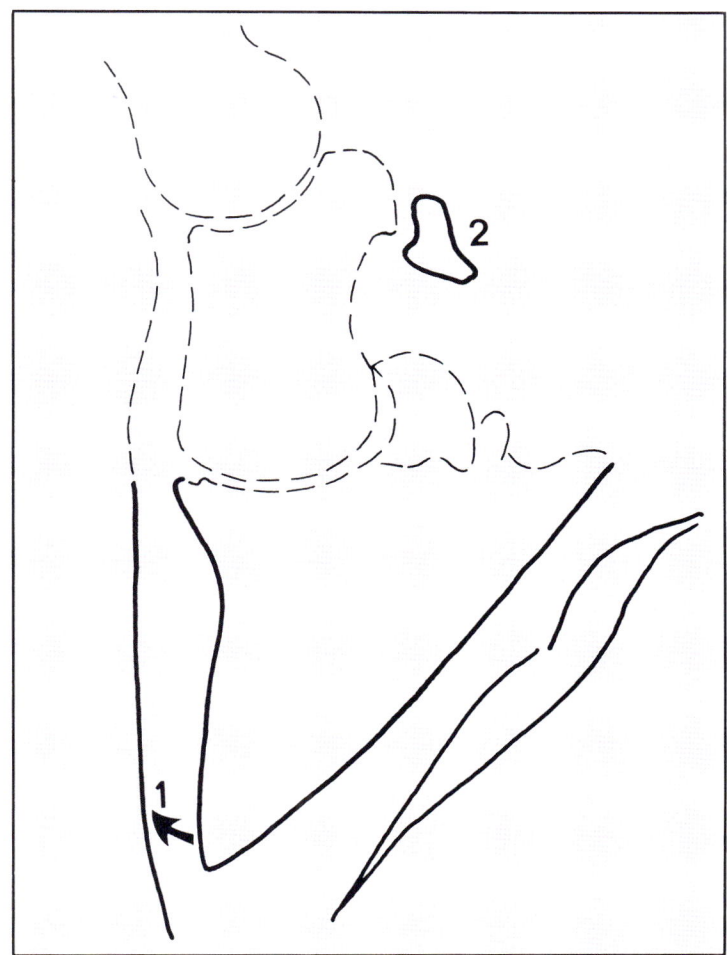

69 Pedal bone, left front, lateromedial view.
Warmblood, 8 years.
Upward rotation **(1)** of the pedal bone. The dorsal wall of the pedal bone is no longer parallel with the dorsal hoofwall, the distal border of the pedal bone is no longer at an angle between 5° and 10° to the bearing surface of the hoof but tilted in the wrong direction due to a rupture of the deep flexor tendon.

Additional finding: the sharply outlined radiopacity **(2)** palmar to the second phalanx is caused by focal calcification of the deep flexor tendon.

69 a Schematic drawing

Contracted foot

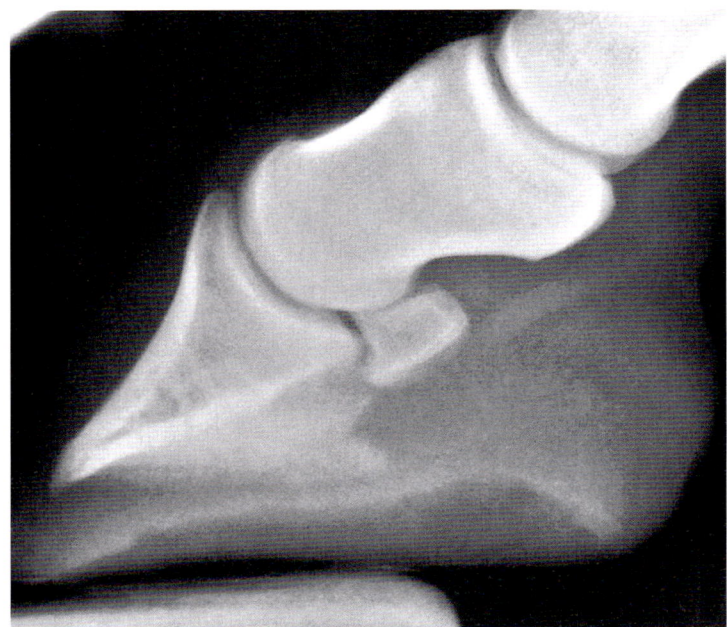

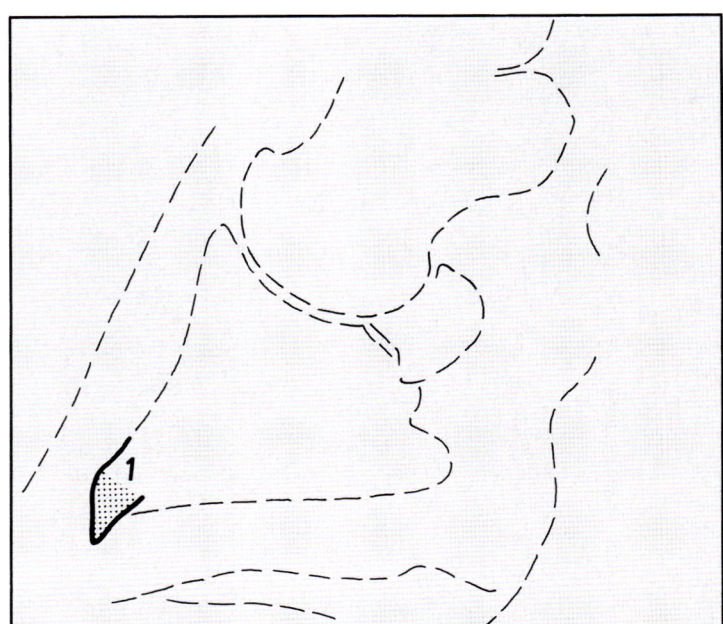

70 Pedal bone, right front, lateromedial view: close-up.

Foal, 8 months.

"Tiptoe" deformation **(1)** of the dorsal aspect of the distal border of the pedal bone, resulting from excessive pressure on the tip of the pedal bone in a long-standing case of contracted foot caused by congenital contraction of the deep flexor tendon.

70 a Schematic drawing

Buttres foot

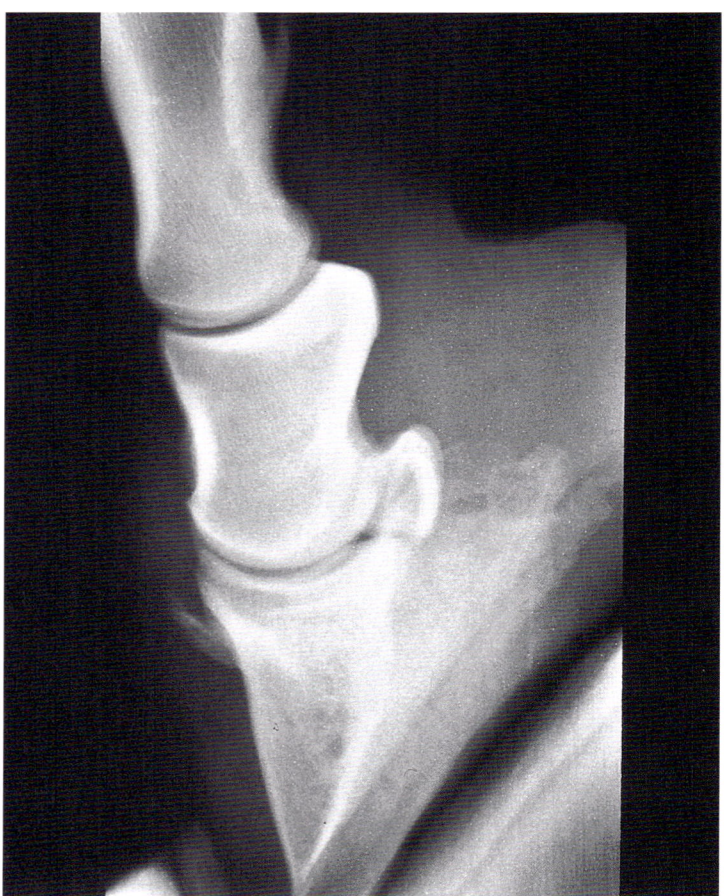

71 Pedal bone, right front, lateromedial view.

Warmblood, 6 years.

The large, pointed exostosis distal to the extensor process of the pedal bone represents enthesophyte formation at the region of insertion of the common digital extensor tendon.

Additional finding: the pointed exostosis at the palmar aspect of the first phalanx results from enthesophyte formation at the region of insertion of the oblique distal sesamoidean ligaments.

These changes are occasionally encountered in horses with very upright pasterns.

71

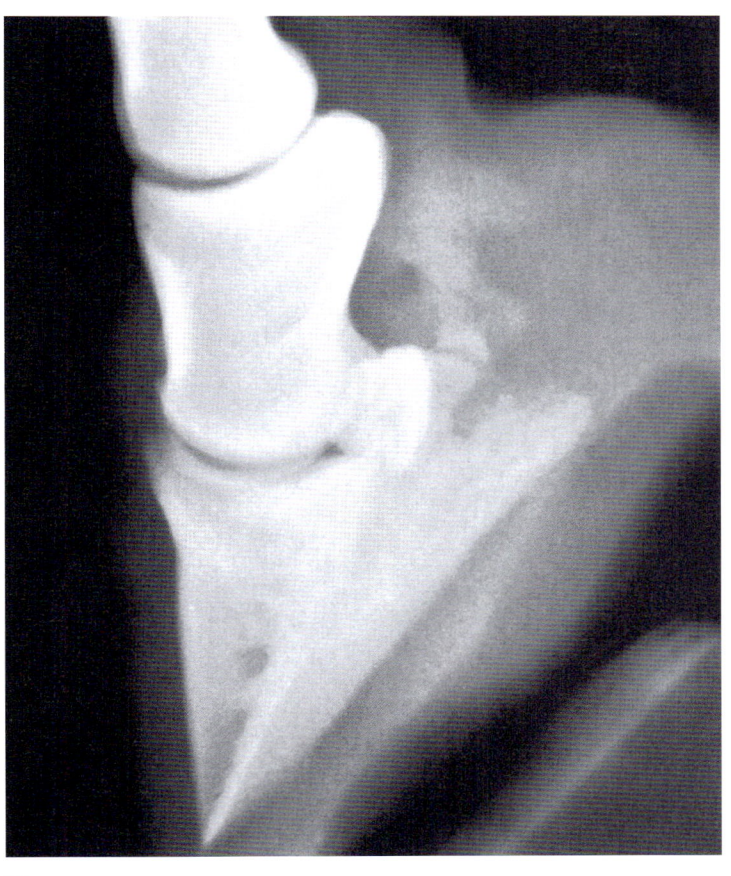

72

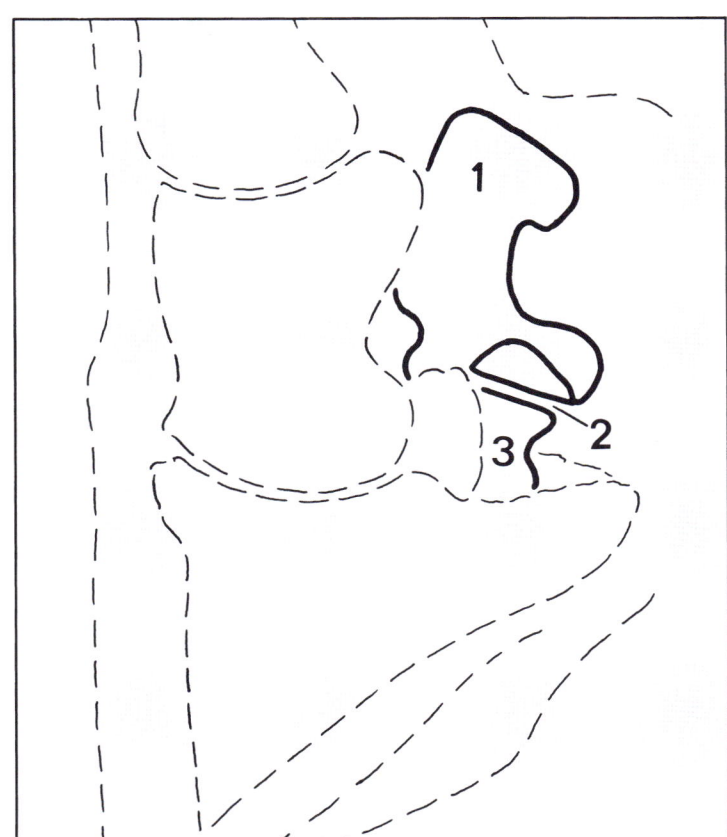

72 a

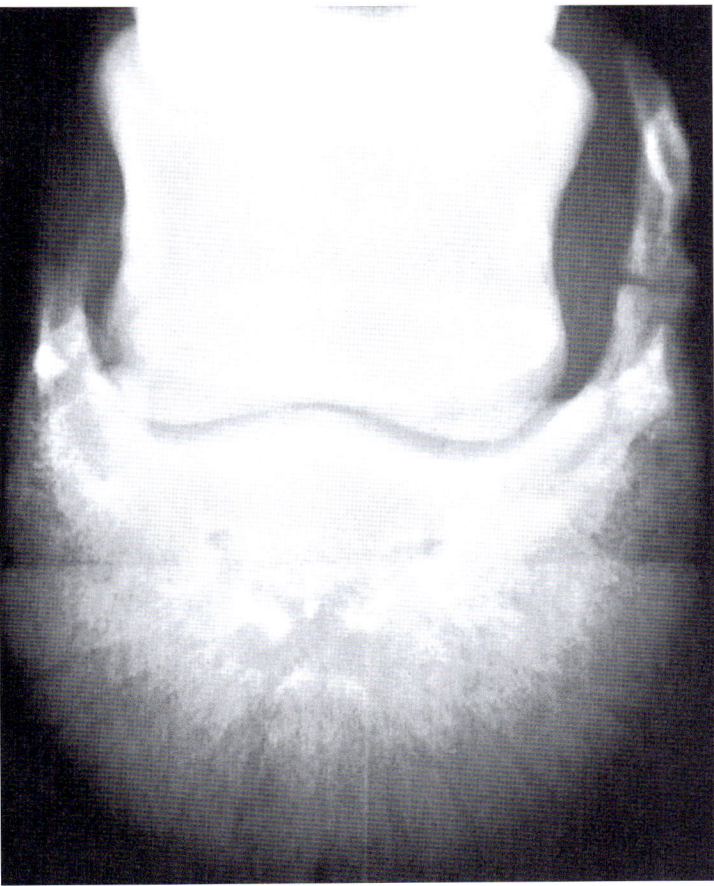

73

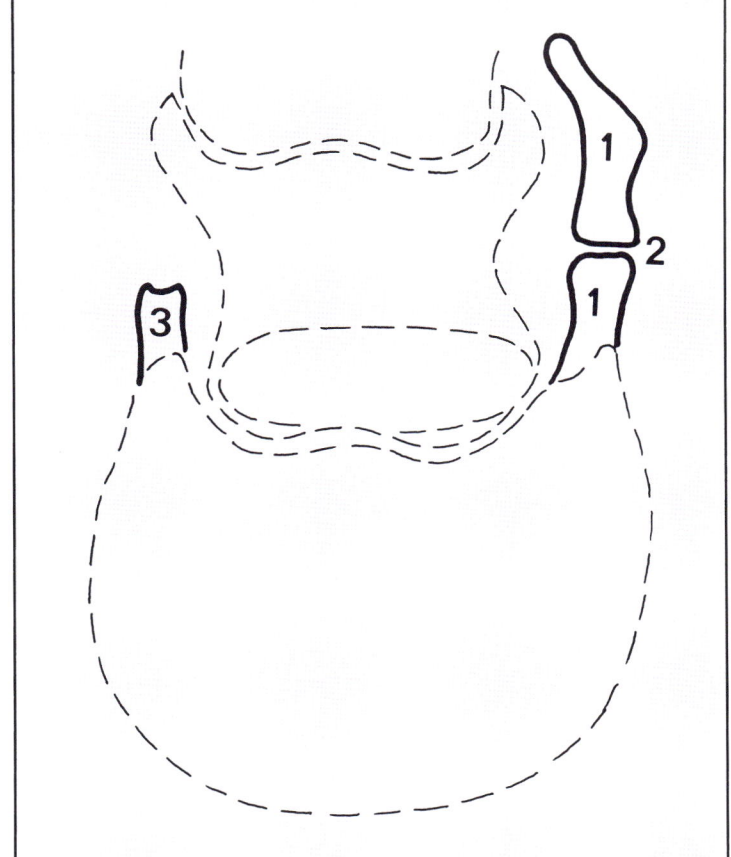

73 a

72/73 Foot, left front, lateromedial and dorsopalmar upright pedal view. Warmblood, 5 years.

Extensive ossification **(1)** of the lateral accessory cartilage. The ossification started in both the tip and the base of the cartilage. The two ossifying areas approach each other but are not completely united. The radiolucent zone **(2)** between the two ossification centres must not be interpreted as a fracture. Minimal ossification **(3)** extending just above the proximal border of the navicular bone in the medial cartilage.

72 a/73 a Schematic drawings

Side bones

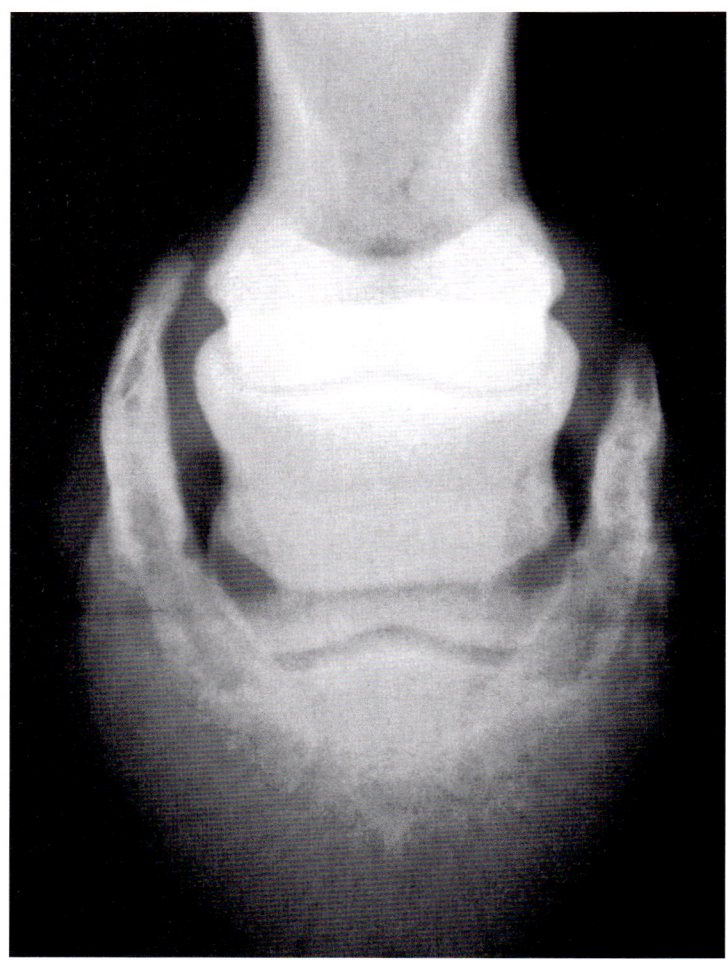

74

74 Foot, right front, upright pedal view (dorsopalmar).
Warmblood, 7 years.
Extensive ossification of both accessory cartilages.

Foreign body

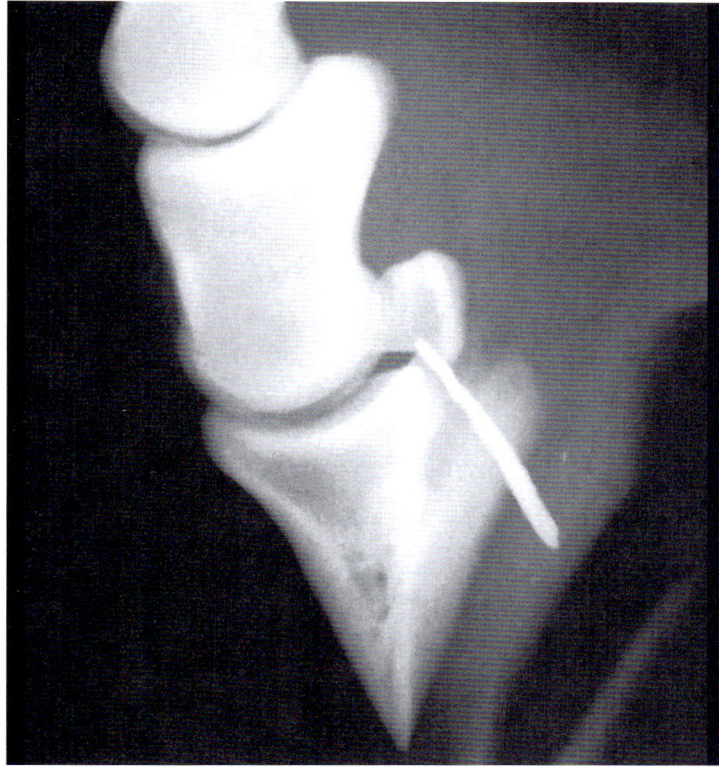

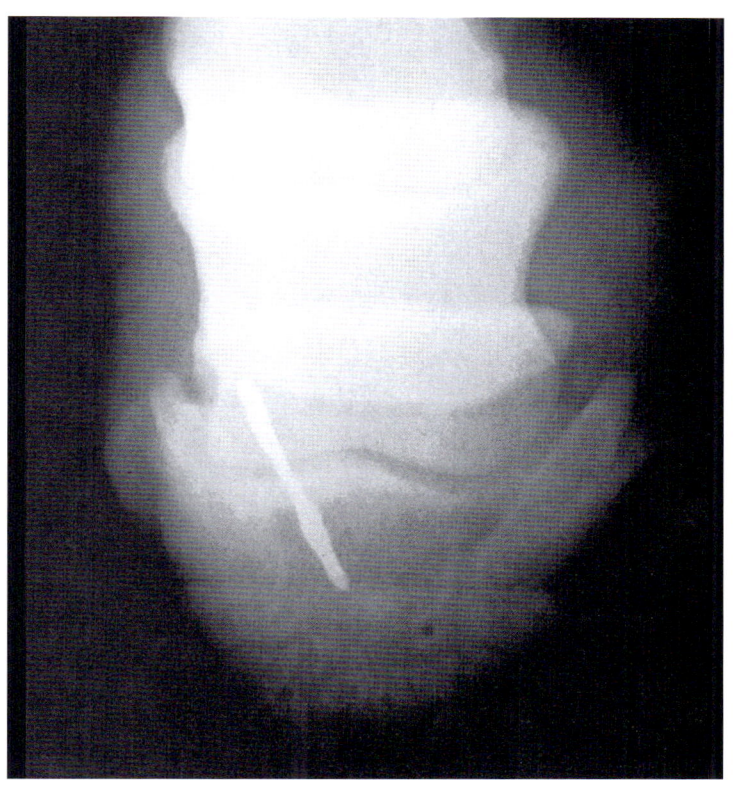

75

76

75/76 Foot, right front, lateromedial and dorsopalmar upright pedal view.
Pony, 1 ½ years.
An iron foreign body perforated the middle of the frog, punctured the distal ligament of the navicular bone and entered the coffin joint.

Sinography

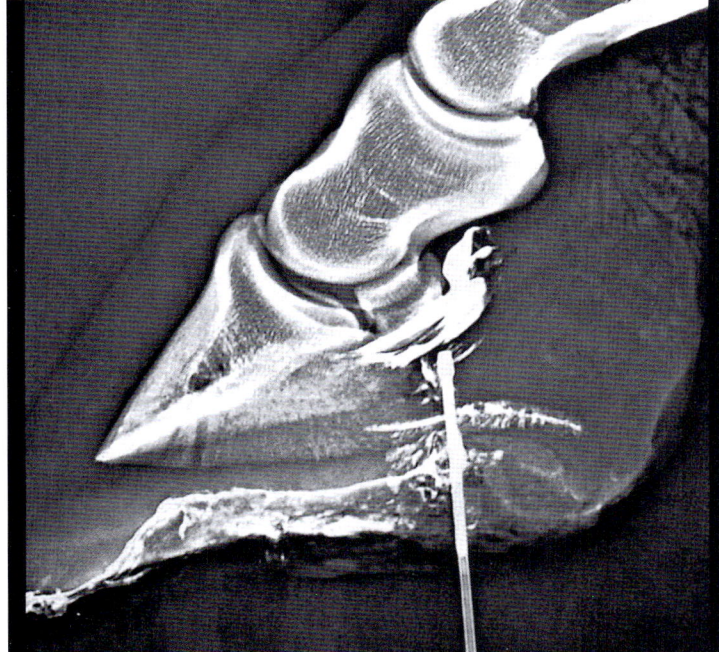

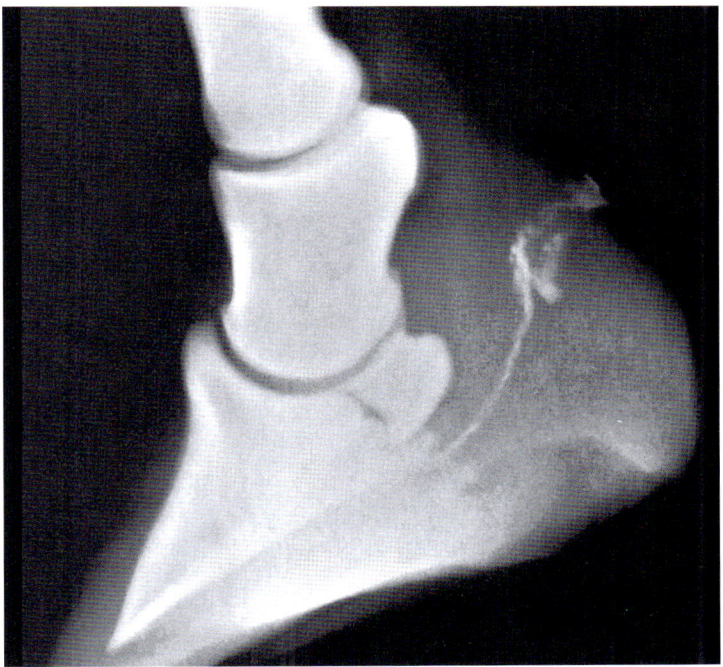

77 Foot, right hind, lateromedial view.
Warmblood, 3 years.
A recent puncture wound in the middle of the frog. The foreign body is no longer present. The puncture tract, visualized by 2 ml positive contrast material injected with a blunt needle, communicates with the navicular bursa.

78 Foot, left front, lateromedial view.
Warmblood, 5 years.
A recent puncture wound between the bulbs of the heel. The foreign body is no longer present. The puncture tract, outlined by injection of 2 ml positive contrast material, communicates with neither the navicular bursa nor the coffin joint.

Puncture wound

Infection of the navicular bone

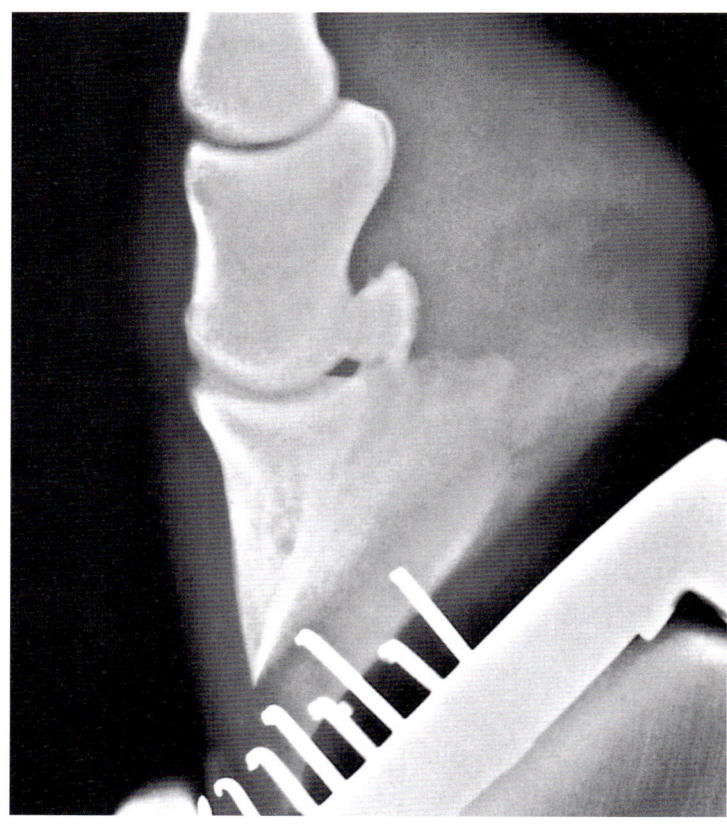

79

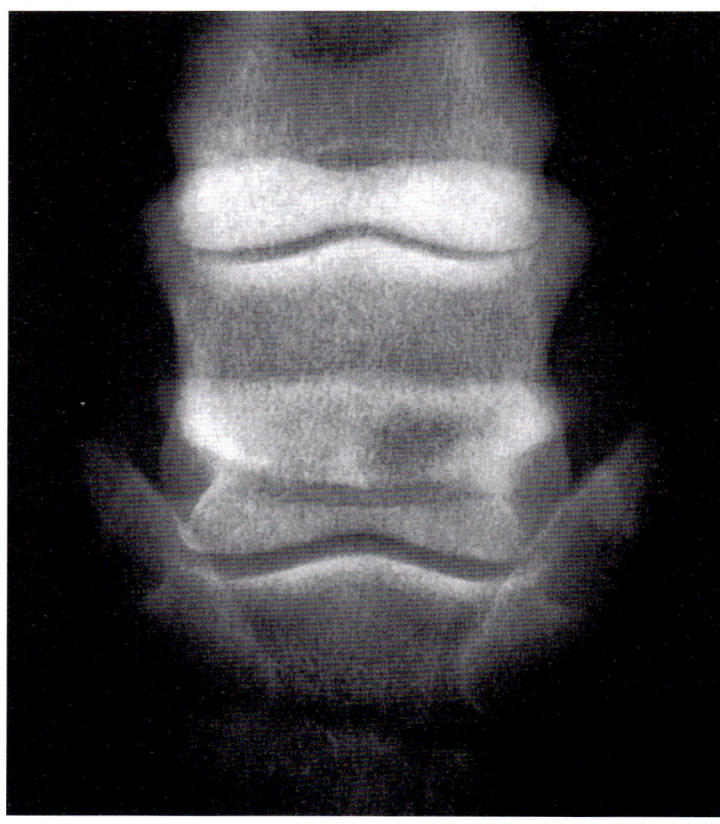

80

79/80/81 Foot, left front, lateromedial and dorsopalmar upright pedal view and palmaroproximal-dorsodistal oblique "skyline" view.

Warmblood, 2 years.

The lateromedial view (Fig. 79) shows new bone formation **(1)** along the proximal border of the navicular bone and an obscure erosion **(2)** of the flexor surface.

The dorsopalmar view (Fig. 80) has a faint radiolucency **(3)** in the laterocentral area of the navicular bone.

The skyline view (Fig. 81) reveals bone destruction (4) in the corresponding area of the flexor surface and spongiosa of the navicular bone. Minimal new bone formation results in roughening of the affected portion of the flexor surface. The destructive and productive lesions of the navicular bone are the result of a 6 weeks old puncture wound between the bulbs of the heel perforating the navicular bursa. The most detailed and valuable information is obtained by the skyline view.

Additional finding: disuse osteoporosis evident especially on the dorsopalmar view.

Infection of the navicular bone

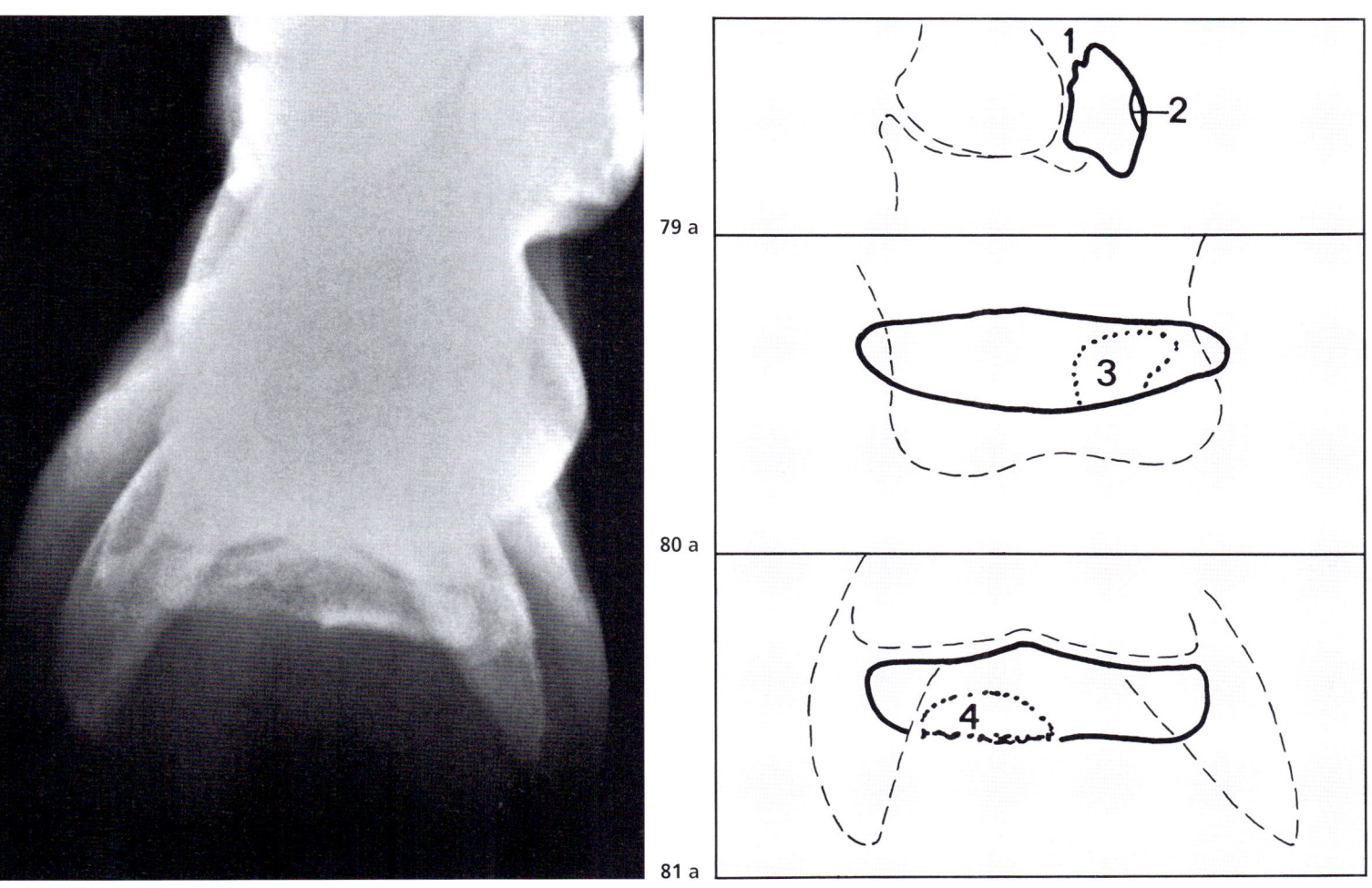

79 a

80 a

81 a

81

79 a/80 a/81 a Schematic drawings

Infection of the pedal bone

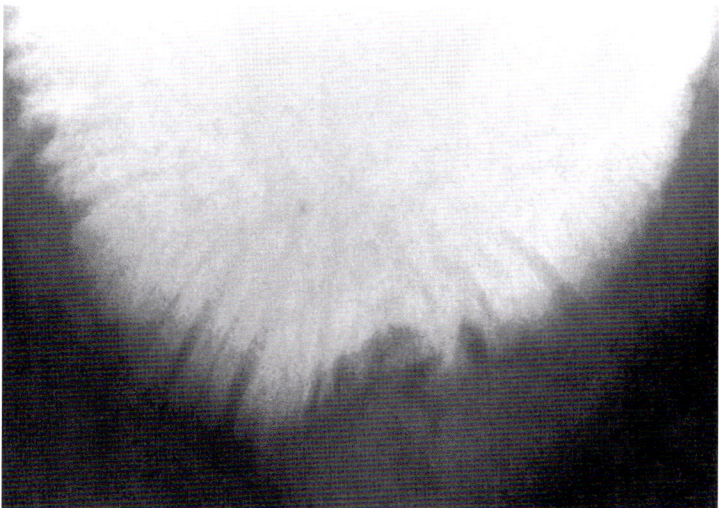

82

82 Pedal bone, right front, upright pedal view (dorsopalmar): close-up of the dorsal aspect of the pedal bone.

Warmblood, 2 years.

The frayed appearance of the distal border of the pedal bone and the radiolucent defects in the corresponding area of the hoofwall are caused by infection, due to a nail puncture of the toe, sustained 3 weeks previously.

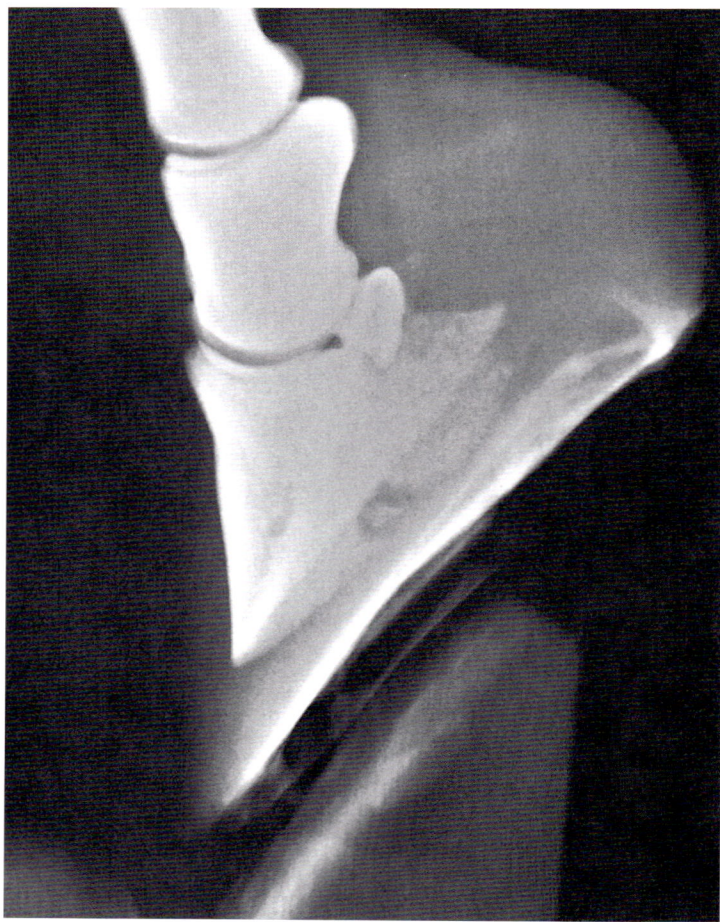

83

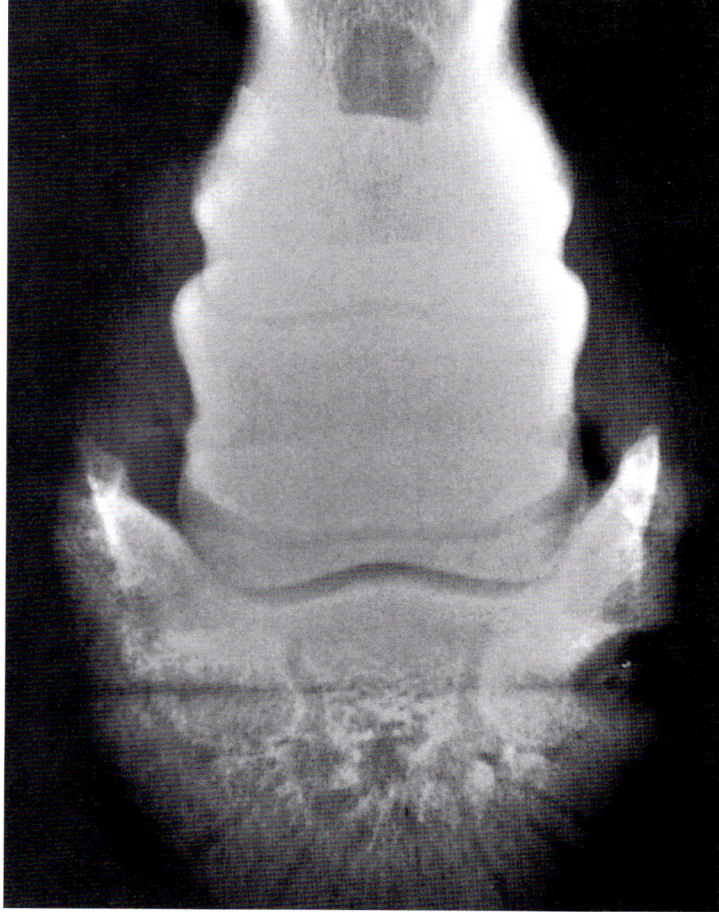

84

83/84 Foot, left front, lateromedial and dorsopalmar upright pedal view.

Warmblood, 3 years.

A well demarcated sequestrum in the centre of a semicircular osteolytic defect in the distal border of the pedal bone. The lesion is a sequel of a puncture wound of the sole which occurred 3 weeks prior to examination.

Infection of the pedal bone

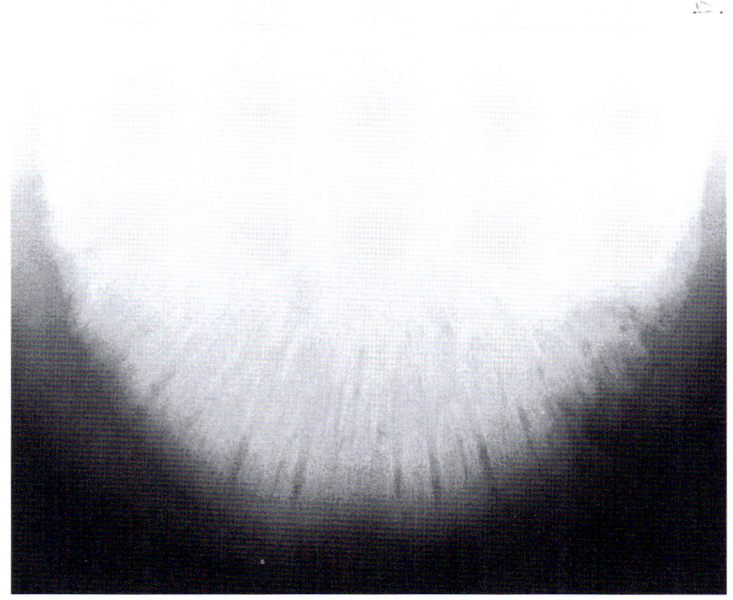

85

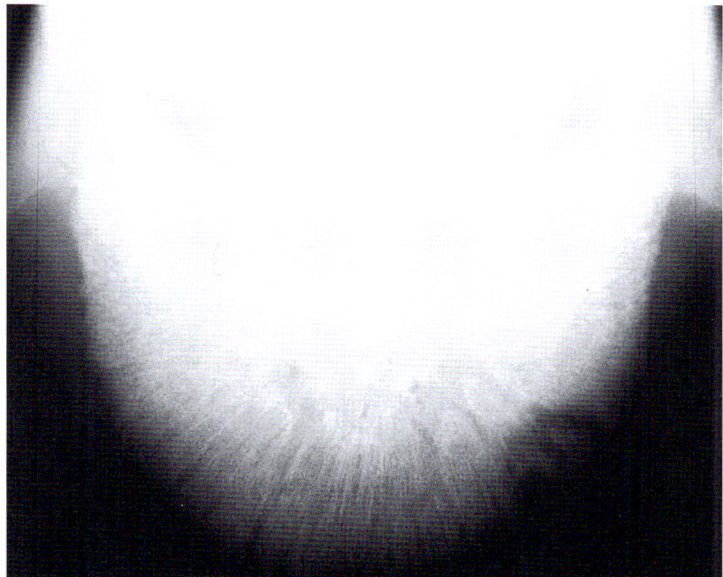

86

85/86/87 Pedal bone, left front, serial upright pedal views (dorsopalmar): close-ups of the pedal bone.

Warmblood, 8 years.

The initial examination (Fig. 85), 2 weeks after the onset of acute lameness associated with subsolar abscessation, reveals irregular radiolucency and an ill defined small solar margin fragment in the dorsolateral region of the pedal bone. These changes indicate infectious pedal osteitis with early sequestration. One week later (Fig. 86) the sequestrum formation is more obvious.

Three weeks later (Fig. 87), i.e. 6 weeks after the onset of lameness, the sequestrum has disappeared, the spontaneous resorbtion or shedding resulting in an irregular defect of the solar margin of the pedal bone. Such defects may persist through many years.

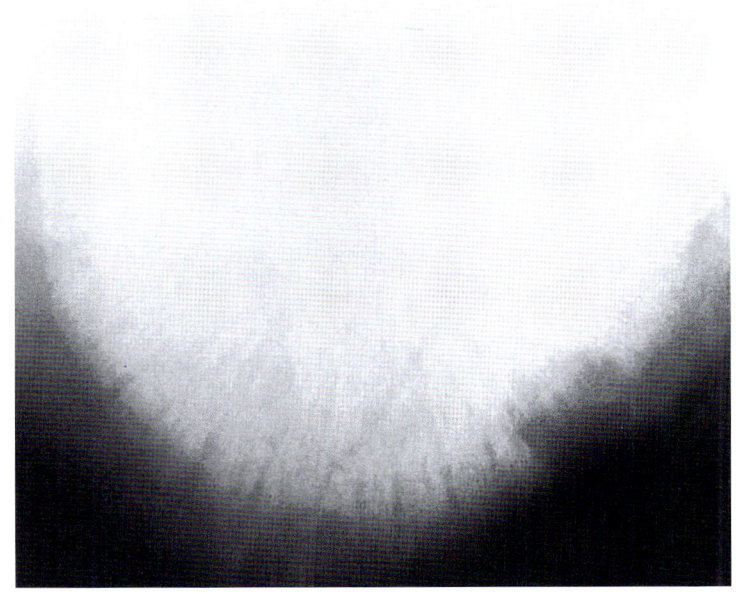

88/89 Pedal bone, right front, dorsopalmar and dorsoproximolateral – palmarodisto-medial oblique view.

Warmblood, 6 years.

A rounded radiolucent area in the lateral wing of the pedal bone adjacent to the solar margin, resulting from surgical removal of a pedal bone sequestrum 1 year prior to this examination.

87

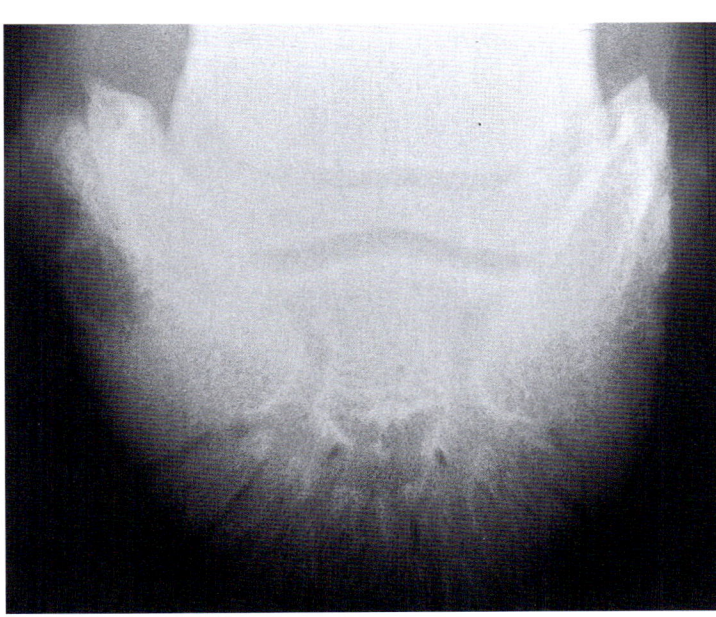

88

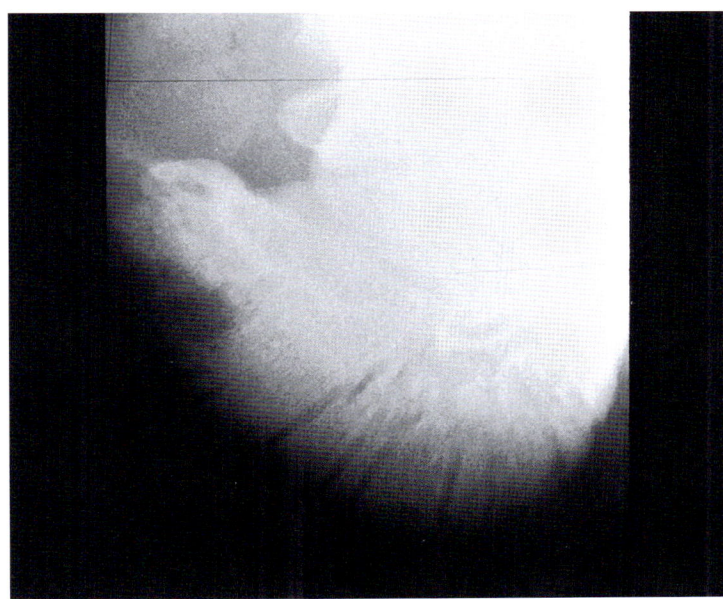

89

Puncture wound

Abscess formation

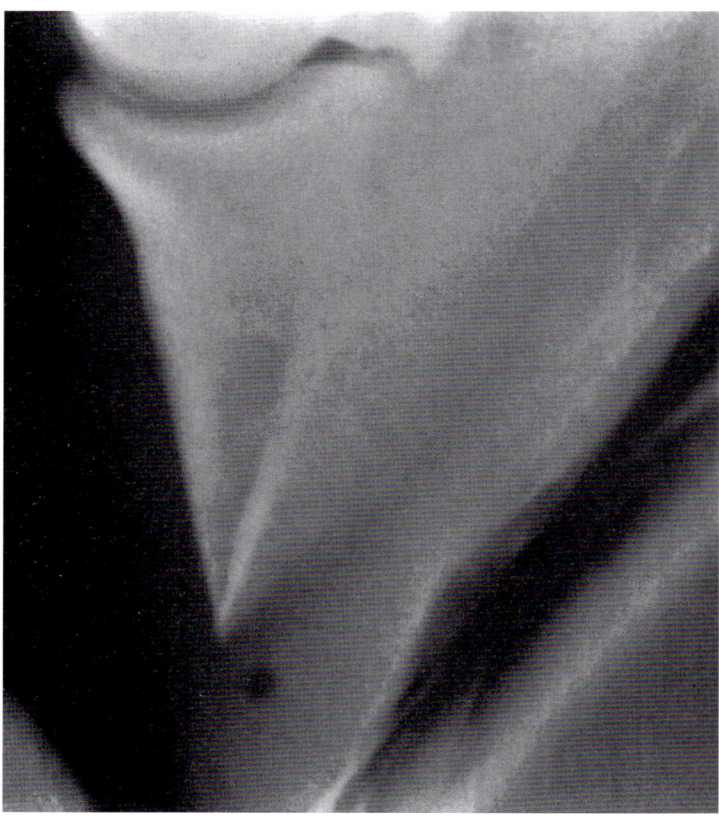

90 Pedal bone, left front, lateromedial view: close-up.
Warmblood, 3 years.

The small, faint, circular, radiolucent area **(1)** in the sole distal to the tip of the pedal bone represents a sole abscess, resulting from nail puncture 1 week prior to examination.

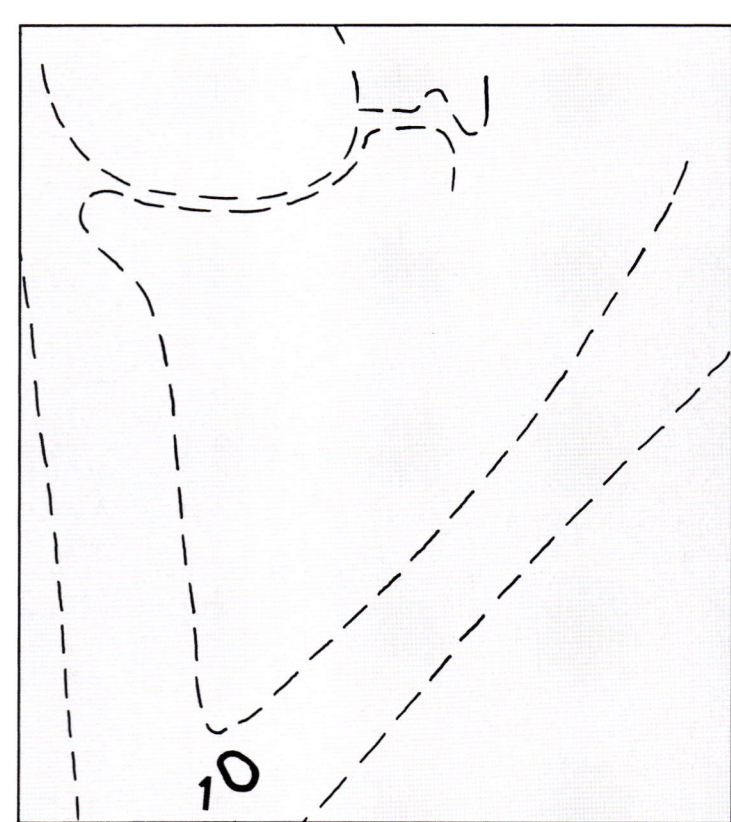

90 a Schematic drawing

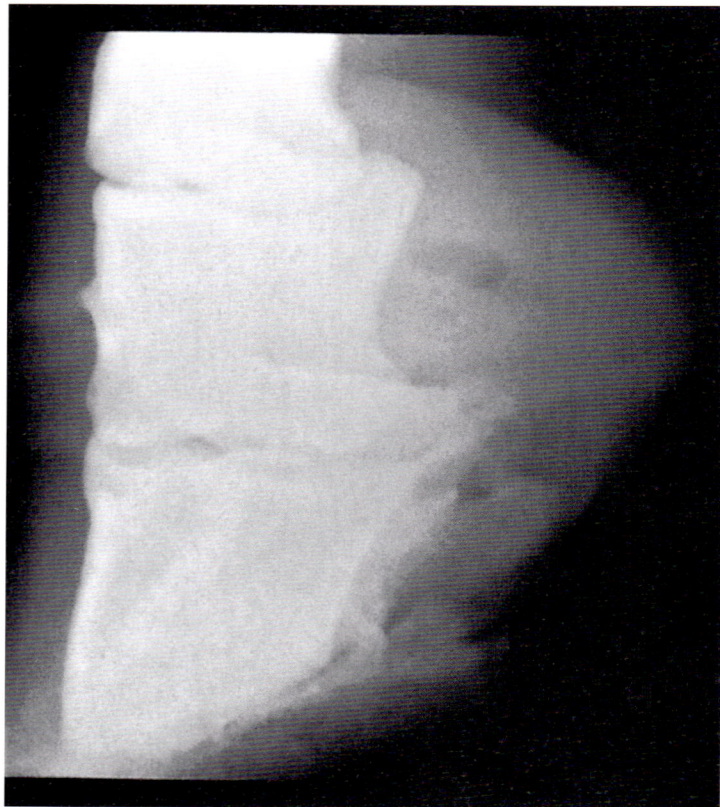

91 Foot, left front, dorsolateral-palmaromedial oblique view.
Warmblood, 8 years.

Palmarolateral to the second phalanx there is soft tissue swelling **(1)** containing a large radiolucent area **(2)** due to abscess formation in the bulb of the heel caused by a puncture wound sustained 1 month previously.

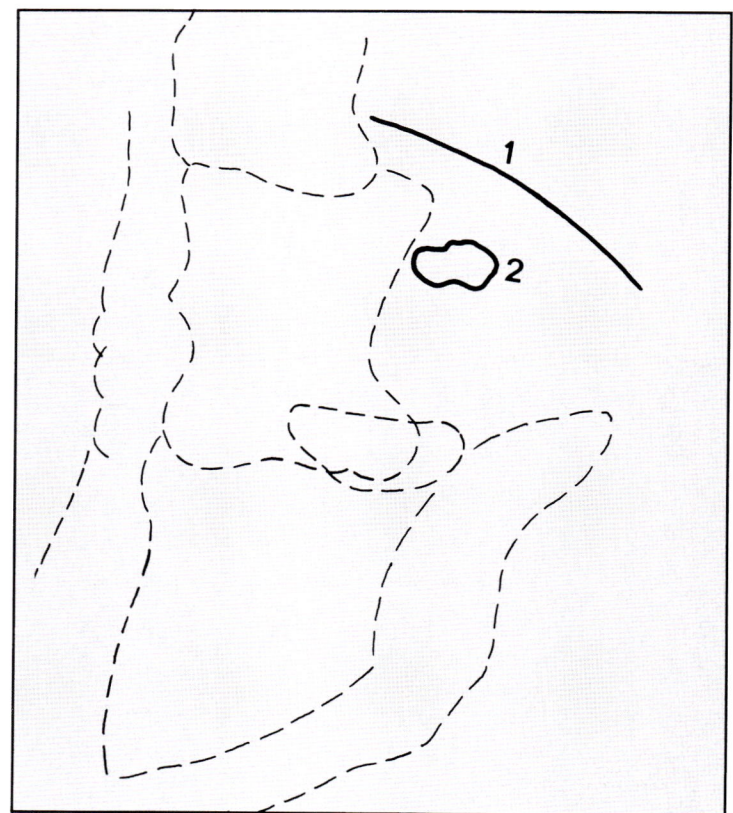

91 a Schematic drawing

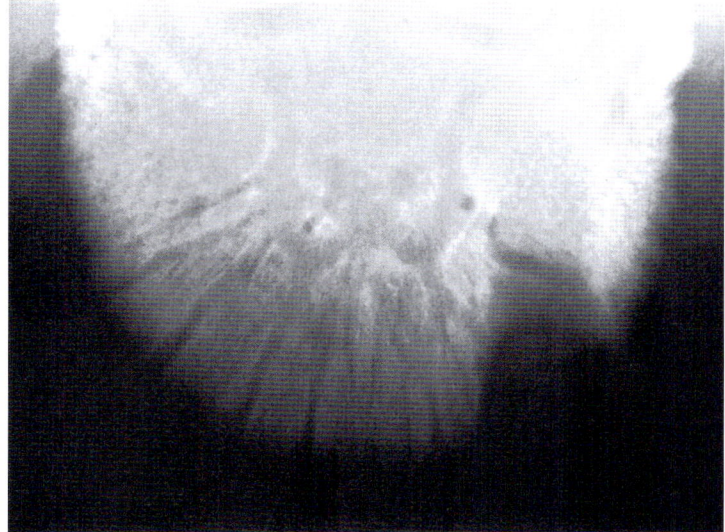

92

92 Pedal bone, left front, upright pedal view (dorsopalmar): close-up of the dorsal aspect of the pedal bone.

Warmblood, 5 years.

A large semicircular radiolucent defect in the distal border of the pedal bone, the result of bone resorption due to a keratoma.

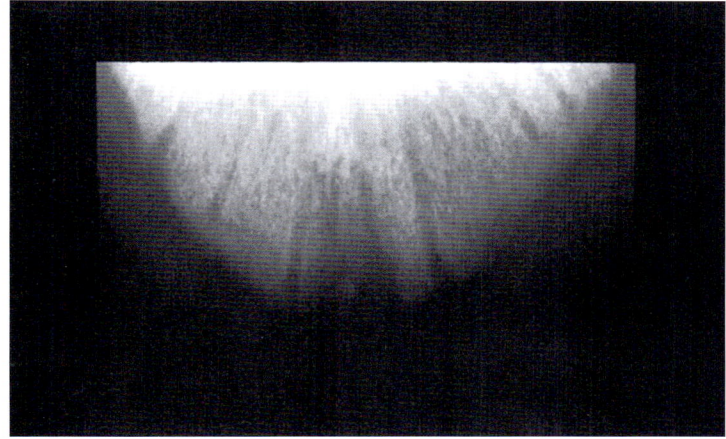

93

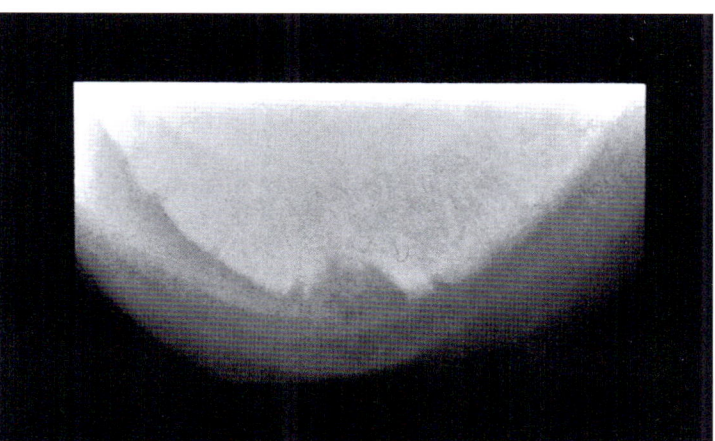

94

93/94 Pedal bone, right front, upright pedal view (dorsopalmar) and dorsoproximal-dorsodistal oblique view: close-ups.

Pony, 12 years.

Fig. 93 upright pedal (dorsopalmar) view, close-up of the dorsal aspect of the pedal bone.

Rarefaction of the tip of the pedal bone.

Fig. 94 dorsoproximal-dorsodistal "skyline" view close-up of the same area, the foot placed on a positioning block with the non-weight-bearing fetlock flexed, the foot in "tiptoe" position, the horizontal beam centred on the coronary band and the cassette in vertical position palmar to the hoof.

The rarefaction of the tip of the pedal bone, appears to be caused by a notch in the distal border of the pedal bone due to a keratoma.

This should not be confused with the normal V-shaped notch often seen in the dorsal aspect of the distal border of the pedal bone.

Ossification of the deep flexor tendon
Calcified neurectomy scar

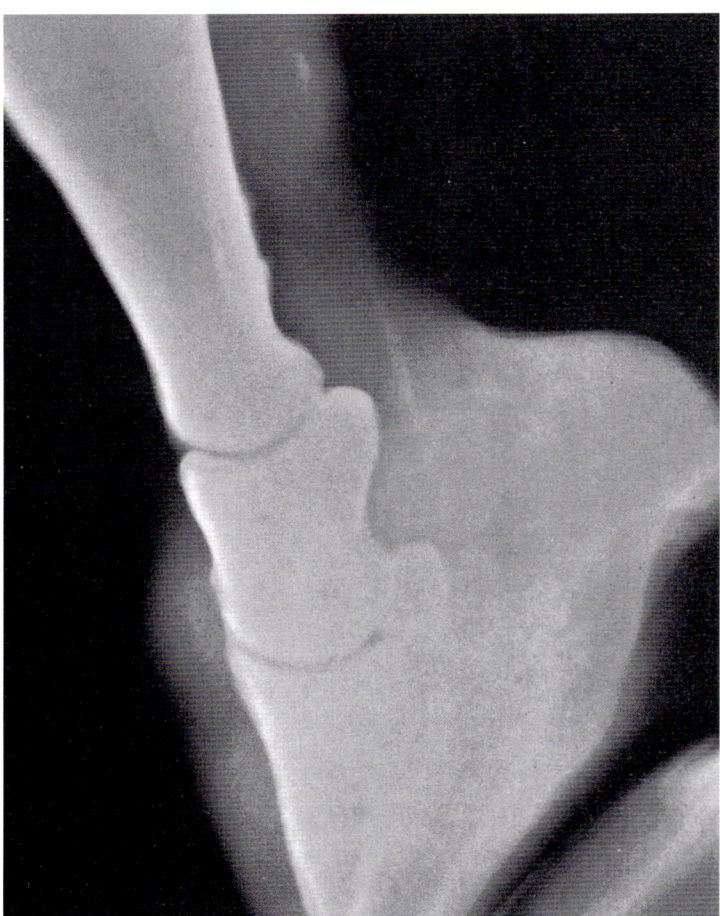

95

95 Foot, left front, lateromedial view.

Warmblood, 11 years.

The radiopaque zone in the soft tissues along the palmar aspect of the first and second phalanx represents ossification of the deep flexor tendon.

Additional finding: ossification of the accessory cartilages.

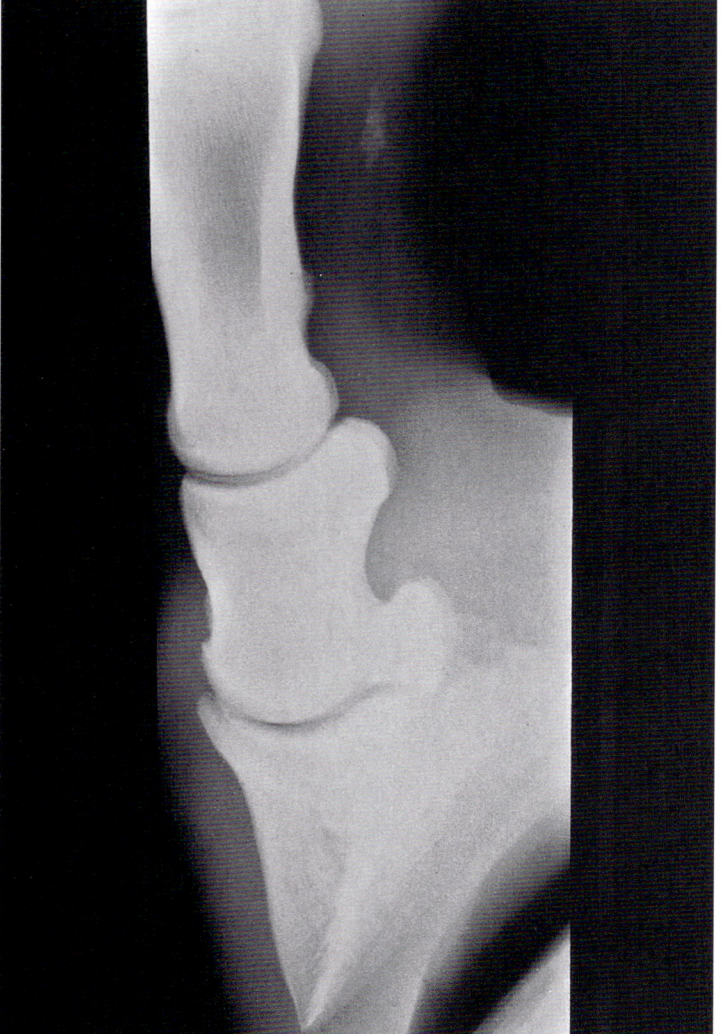

96

96 Foot, right front, lateromedial view.

Warmblood, 9 years.

Local soft tissue calcification in the palmar midpastern region, resulting from palmar digital neurectomy.

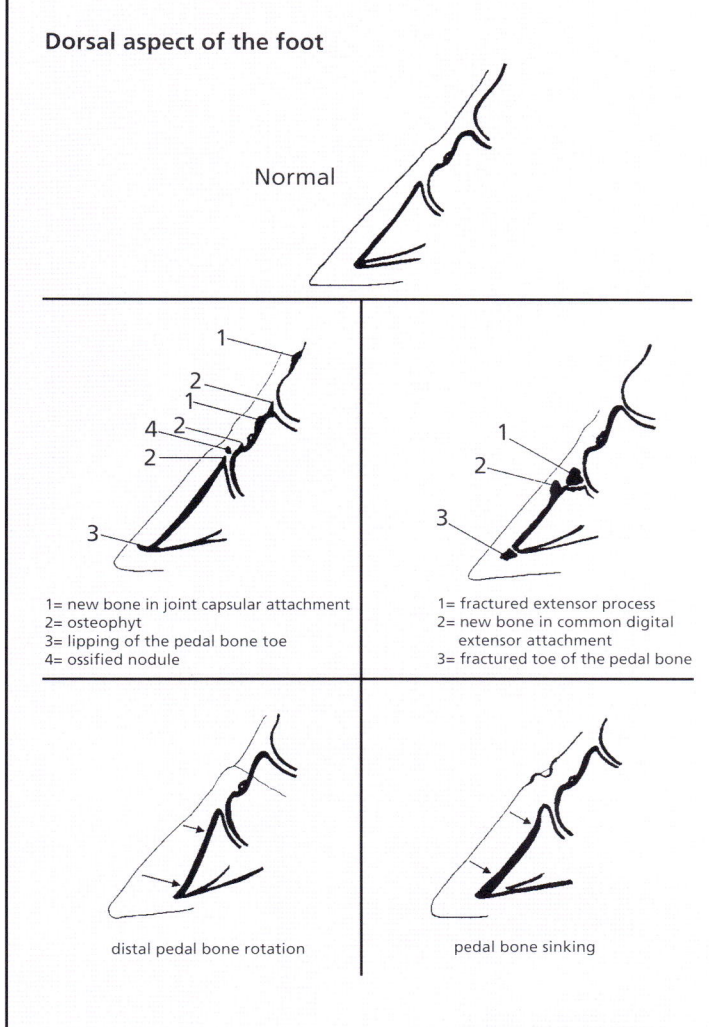

Dorsal aspect of the foot

Normal

1= new bone in joint capsular attachment
2= osteophyt
3= lipping of the pedal bone toe
4= ossified nodule

1= fractured extensor process
2= new bone in common digital extensor attachment
3= fractured toe of the pedal bone

distal pedal bone rotation

pedal bone sinking

97

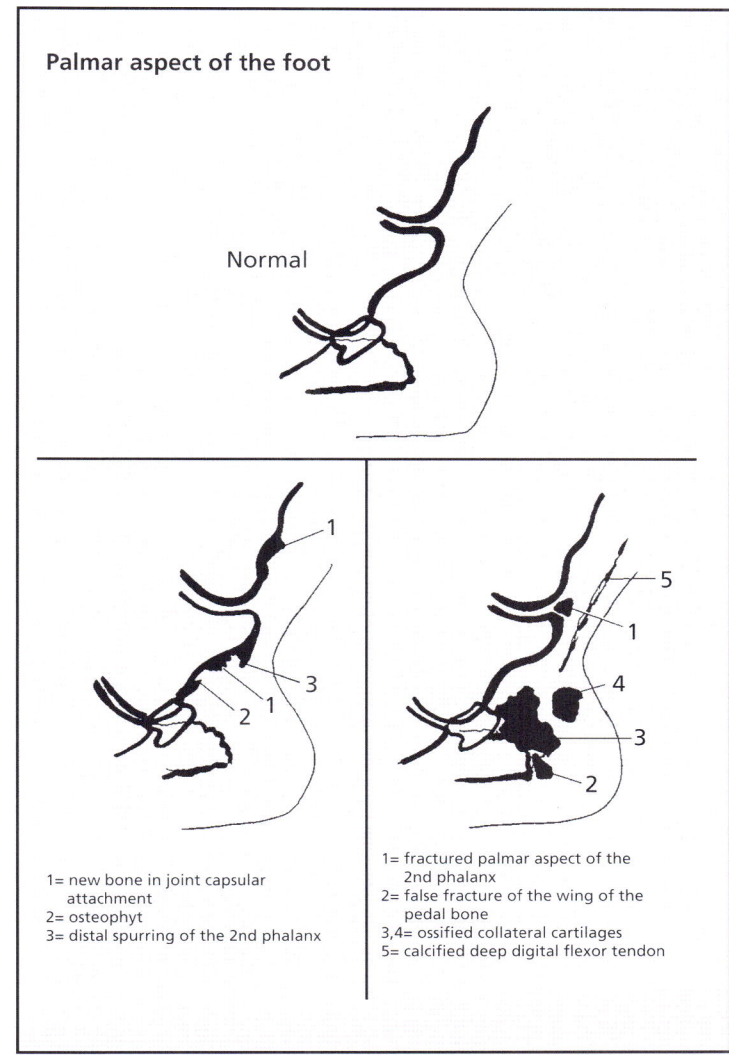

Palmar aspect of the foot

Normal

1= new bone in joint capsular attachment
2= osteophyt
3= distal spurring of the 2nd phalanx

1= fractured palmar aspect of the 2nd phalanx
2= false fracture of the wing of the pedal bone
3,4= ossified collateral cartilages
5= calcified deep digital flexor tendon

98

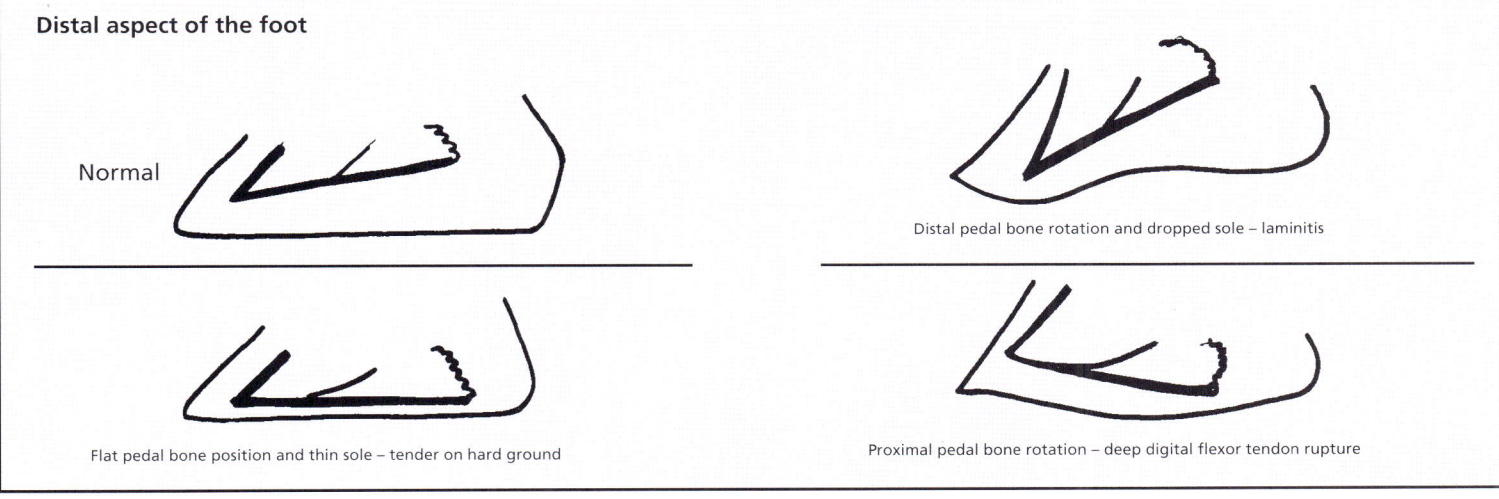

Distal aspect of the foot

Normal

Distal pedal bone rotation and dropped sole – laminitis

Flat pedal bone position and thin sole – tender on hard ground

Proximal pedal bone rotation – deep digital flexor tendon rupture

99

97/98/99 Schematic drawings of the dorsal, palmar and distal aspect of the foot.

The normal dorsal (Fig. 97), palmar (Fig. 98) and distal (Fig. 99) appearance of the foot versus various radiographic abnormalities visible on lateral radiographs of the foot.

Schematic drawings

Dorsal view of the foot

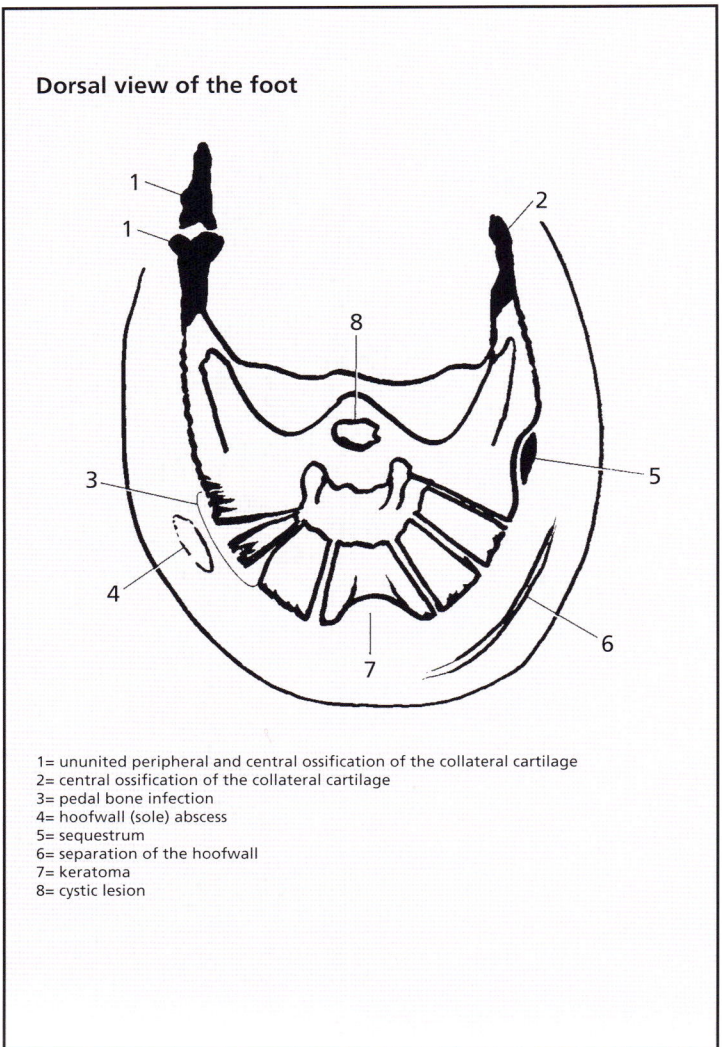

1= ununited peripheral and central ossification of the collateral cartilage
2= central ossification of the collateral cartilage
3= pedal bone infection
4= hoofwall (sole) abscess
5= sequestrum
6= separation of the hoofwall
7= keratoma
8= cystic lesion

Synovial cavities of the distal limb

1= metacarpophalangeal joint cavity
2= prox. interphalangeal joint cavity
3= dist. interphalangeal joint cavity
4= subtendinous bursa
5= navicular bursa
6= digital sheath

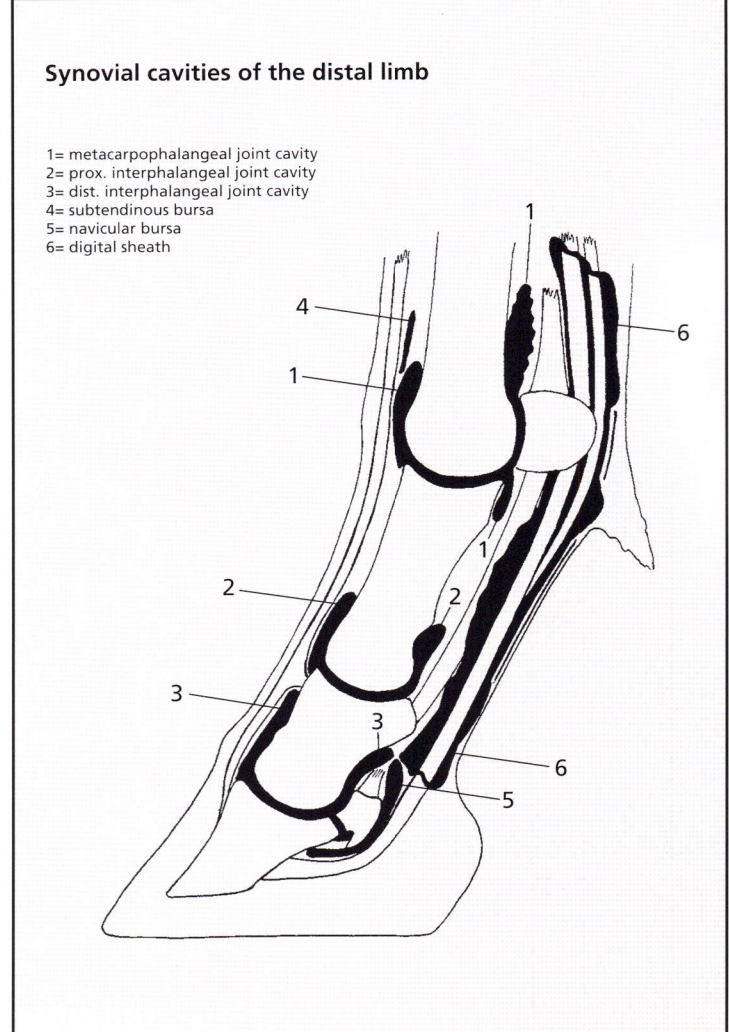

100 Schematic dorsal view of the foot.

A summary of various abnormalities visible on dorsopalmar radiographs of the foot.

101 Schematic lateral appearance of the synovial cavities of the distal limb.

Accurate radiological differentiation between intra-articular and extra-articular lesions requires detailed knowledge of the extent of the dorsal aand palmar joint pouches.

The Pastern Joint

Fracture

Fracture/Luxation

Luxation

Osteoarthrosis

Infectious arthritis

Ischaemic bone necrosis

Bone cyst

Osteomyelitis

Diaphyseal angular deformity

Granuloma

Fracture

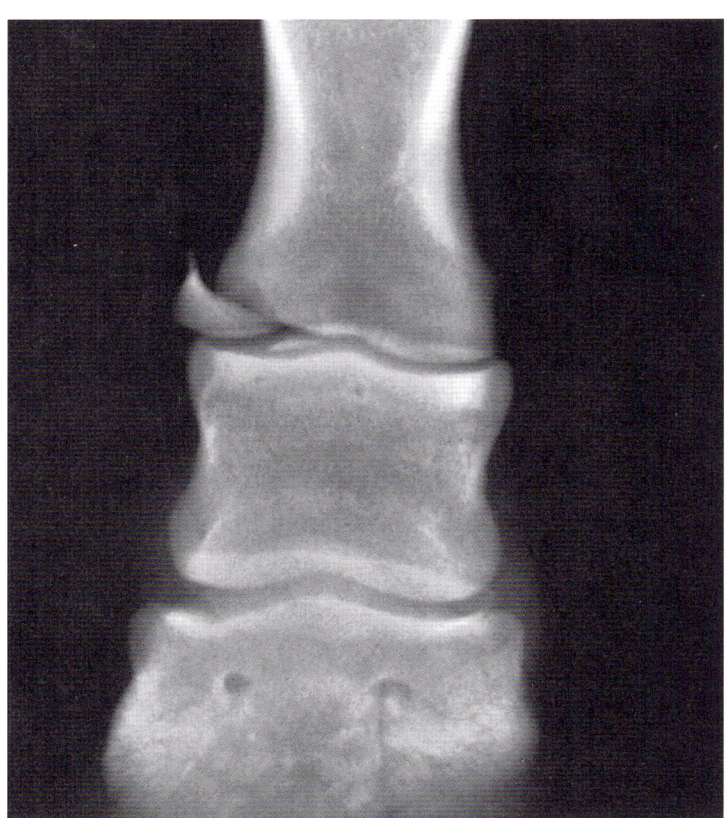

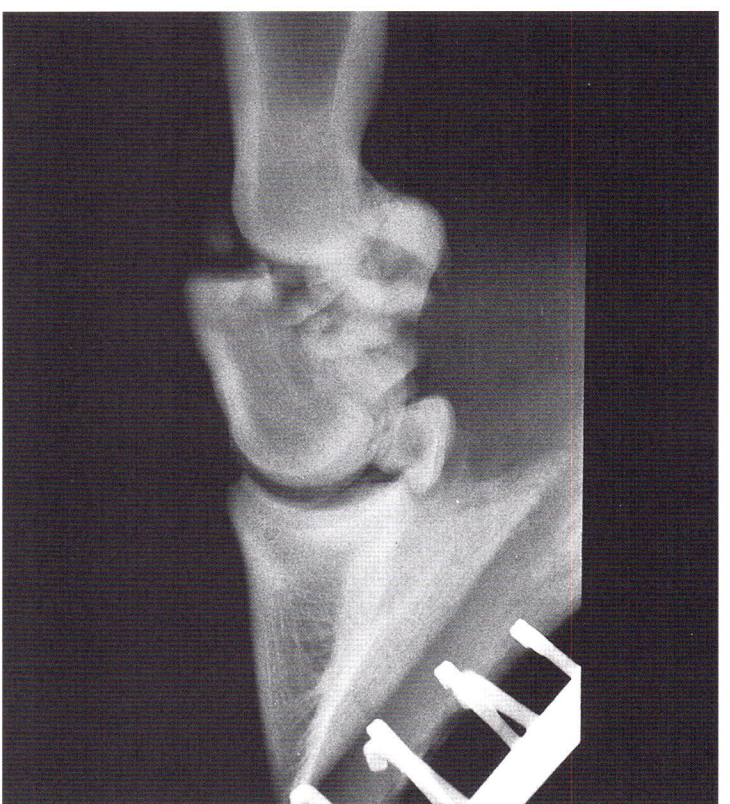

102 Foot, right front, dorsopalmar view.

Warmblood, 1 year.

The isolated, sharply bordered, slightly displaced bone fragment arising from the lateral distal portion of the first phalanx is the result of a recent, simple, oblique, intra-articular fracture.

103 Foot, left hind, lateromedial view.

Warmblood, 13 years.

Multiple poorly defined fragments arising from the proximal and plantar aspect of the second phalanx indicating a recent comminuted fracture.

The pastern joint is obscured by overriding fracture fragments, due to the impaction type of injury. The fracture mainly involves the pastern joint, but also extends into the plantar aspect of the coffin joint; therefore, the prognosis for future athletic soundness is poor.

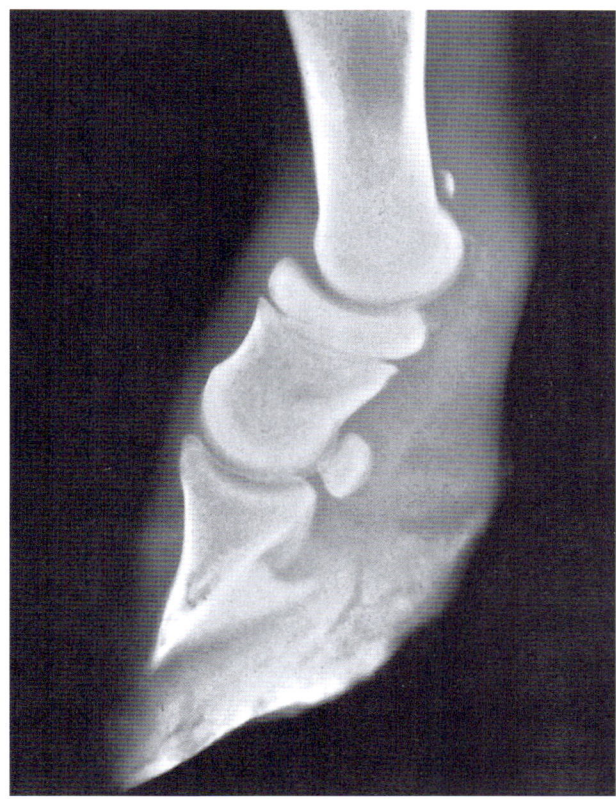

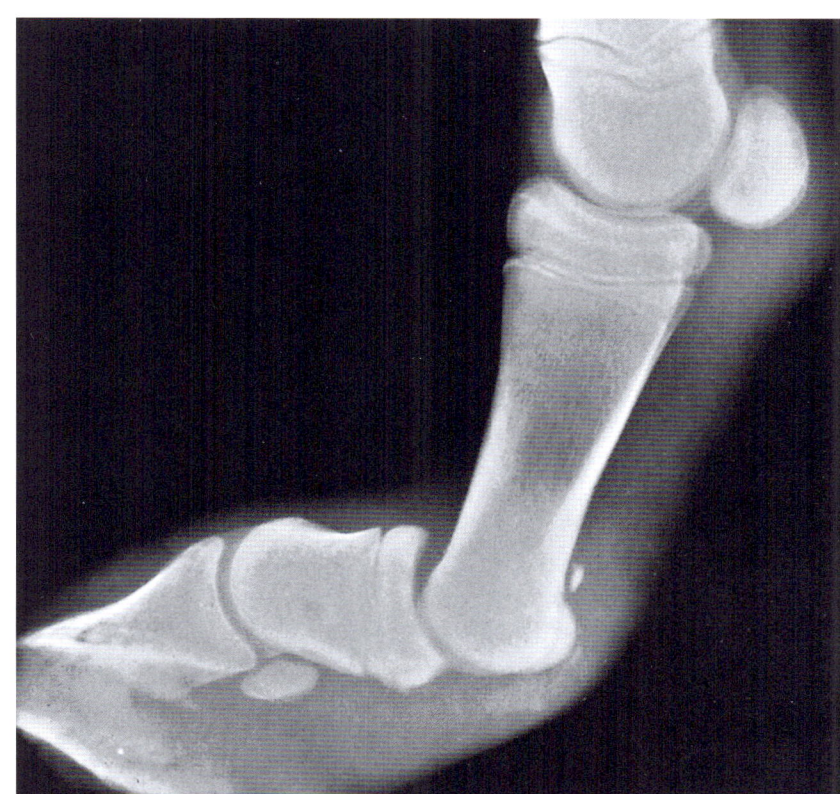

104

105

104/105 Foot, left front, non-weight-bearing (Fig. 104) and weight-bearing (Fig. 105) lateromedial view.

Foal, 2 weeks.

The non-weight-bearing lateromedial view presents dorsal displacement of the proximal articular surface of the second phalanx, indicating subluxation of the pastern joint, more clearly demonstrated by the weight-bearing view. Both views show small isolated bone fragments palmar to the distal end of the first phalanx and the proximal end of the second phalanx, indicating that dislocation occurred with associated fracture.

The origin of the avulsed fragments is not visible.

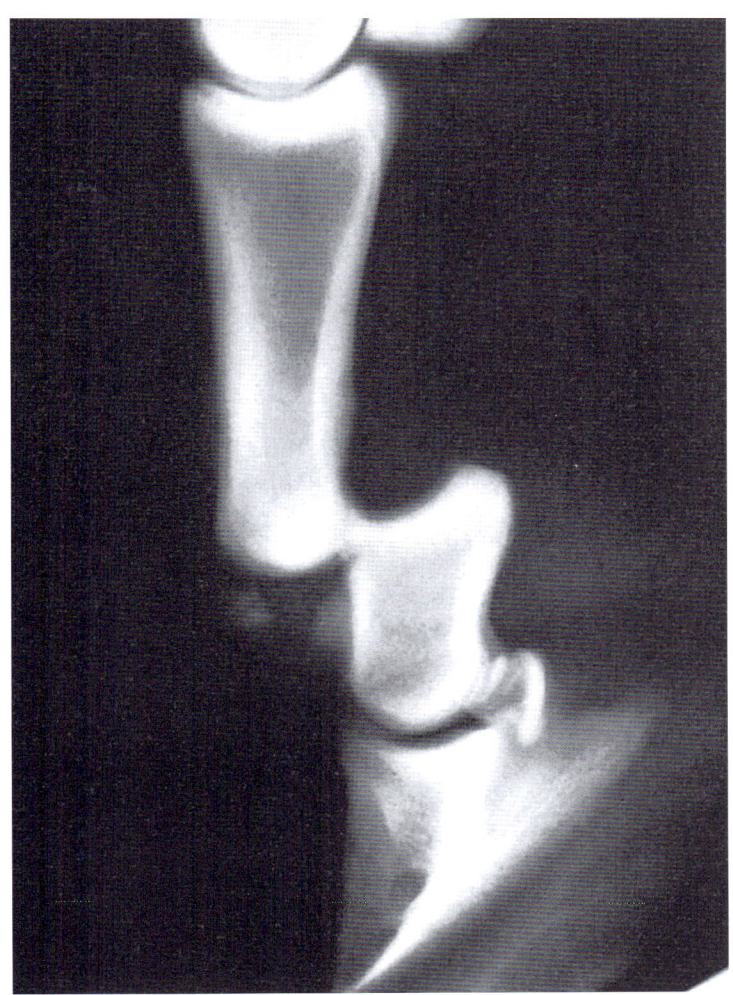

106 Foot, left front, lateromedial view.

Warmblood, 7 years.

Complete luxation of the pastern joint with palmar displacement of the second phalanx and overriding of the distal end of the first phalanx.

The obscure bone fragment distal to the articular surface of the first phalanx suggests that dislocation occurred with associated fracture. The faint, ill bordered periosteal new bone along the dorsal aspect of the second phalanx indicates that the luxation has been present for at least 2 weeks.

106

Subluxation

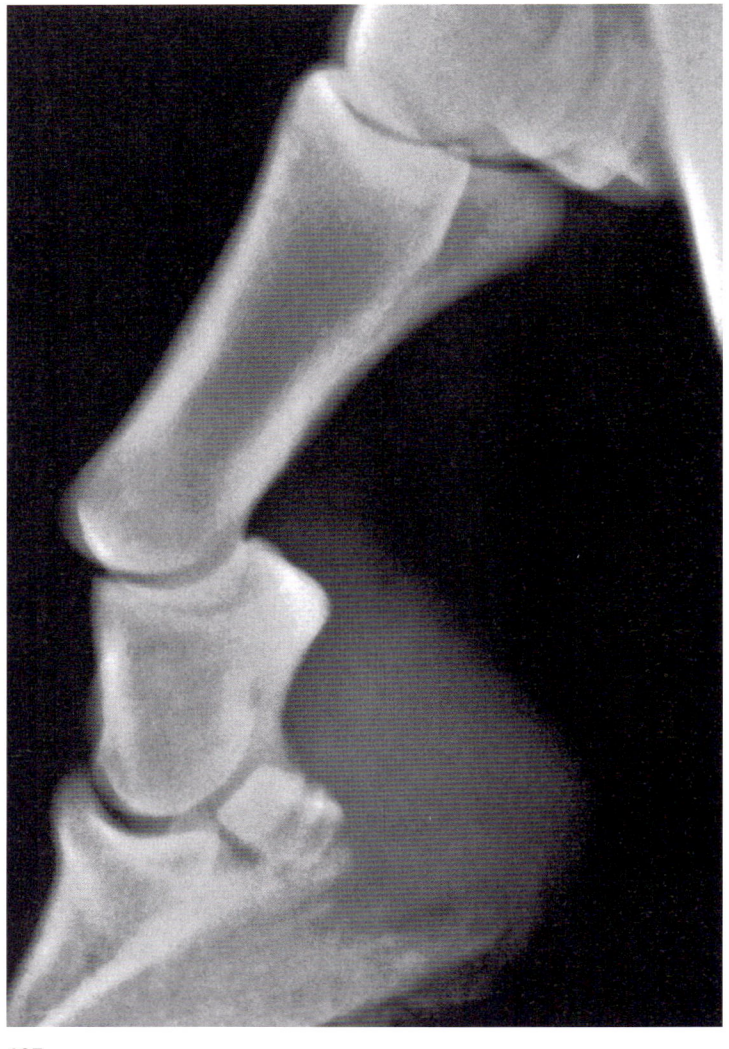

107

107 Foot, right front, lateromedial view.

Warmblood, 2 ½ years.

Palmar displacement of the proximal articular surface of the second phalanx, due to subluxation of the pastern joint without associated fracture.

108/109/110 Foot, left front, dorsopalmar routine and additional stress views.

Warmblood, 6 years.

A dorsopalmar stress view obtained during abduction of the foot (Fig. 109) reveals marked widening of the medial aspect and severe narrowing of the lateral aspect of the pastern joint. A repeat view during adduction of the foot (Fig. 110) only results in mild narrowing of the medial aspect of the pastern joint.

These findings indicate pastern joint instability, due to laxity or rupture of the medial collateral joint ligament, which is not obvious on the routine dorsopalmar view (Fig. 108).

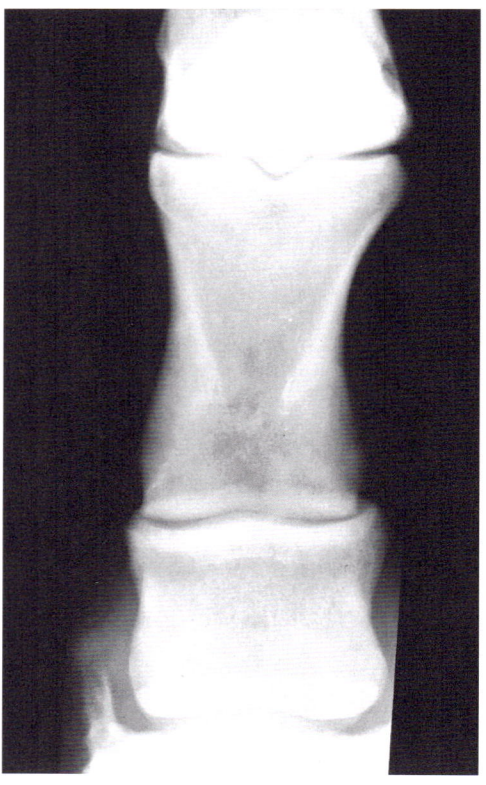

108

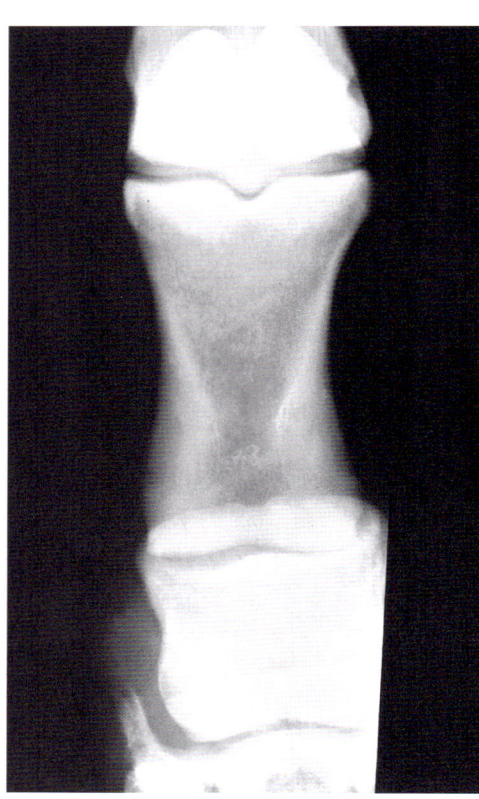

109

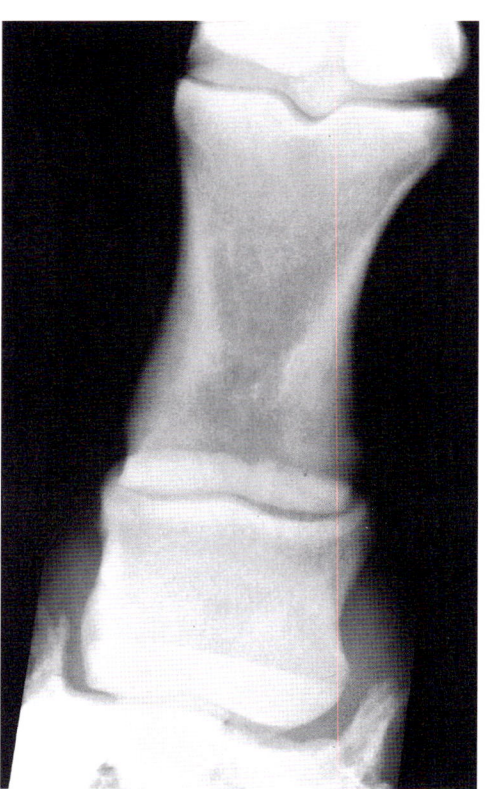

110

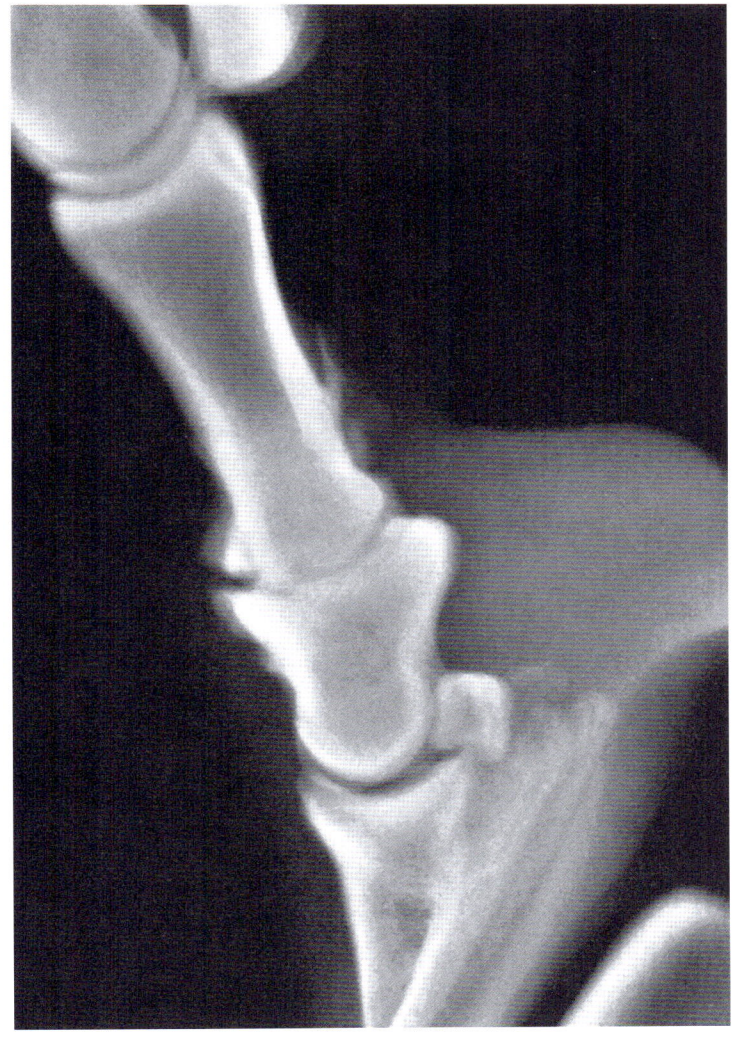

111

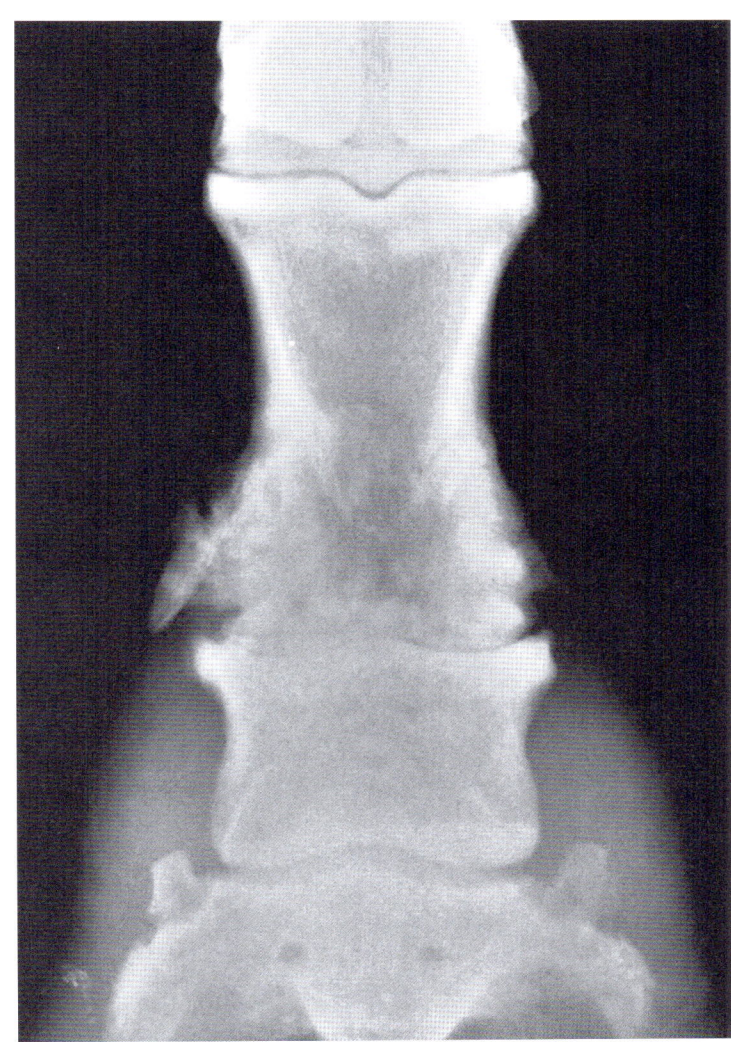

112

111/112 Foot, left front, lateromedial (Fig. 111) and dorsopalmar (Fig. 112) view.

Pony, 8 years.

Marked collapse of the pastern joint, an obscure area of radiolucency in the distal end of the first phalanx (lateromedial view), prominent lipping of the joint margins and extensive new bone formation at the capsular, collateral and distal sesamoidean ligamentous fibro-osseous attachment. These radiographic changes are characteristic of osteoarthrosis (articular as well as peri-articular "High ringbone").

Infectious arthritis

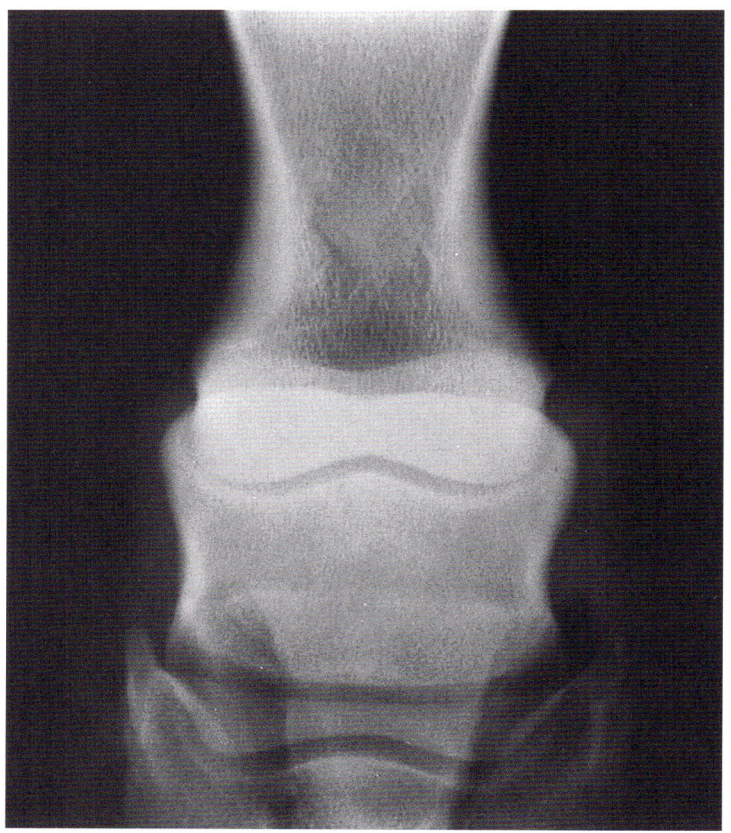

113

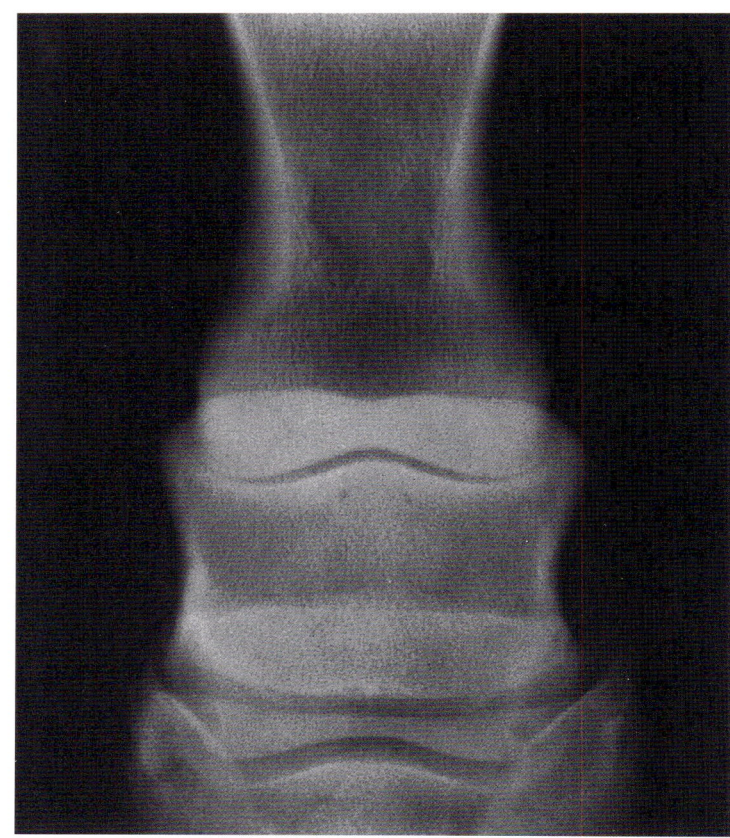

114

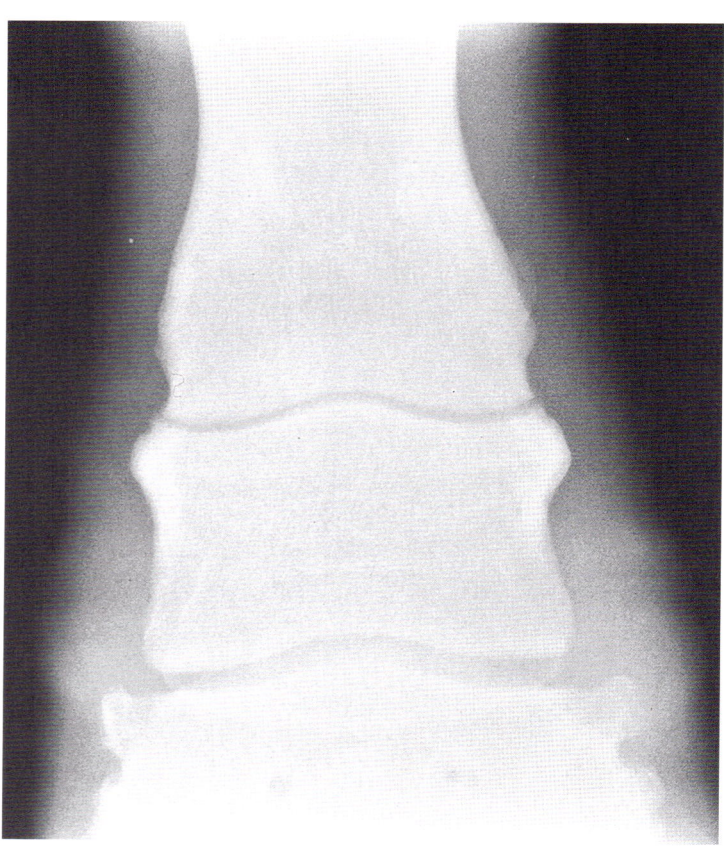

115

113/114/115 Foot, right front, serial dorsopalmar views.

Warmblood, 2 years.

The initial view (Fig. 113), 1 day after the onset of acute severe lameness, reveals slight symmetric widening of the pastern joint. (On dorsopalmar radiographs of normal horses this joint space appears twice as small as the coffin joint).

Ten days later (Fig. 114) marked symmetric narrowing of the pastern joint is obvious.

Ten days later (Fig. 115), i.e. 3 weeks after the onset of lameness, indistinct new bone formation at the distomedial aspect of the first phalanx and roughening of the distolateral contour of this bone indicate early periosteal reaction adjacent to the pastern joint.

These changes represent the earliest and subsequent radiographic features of infectious arthritis.

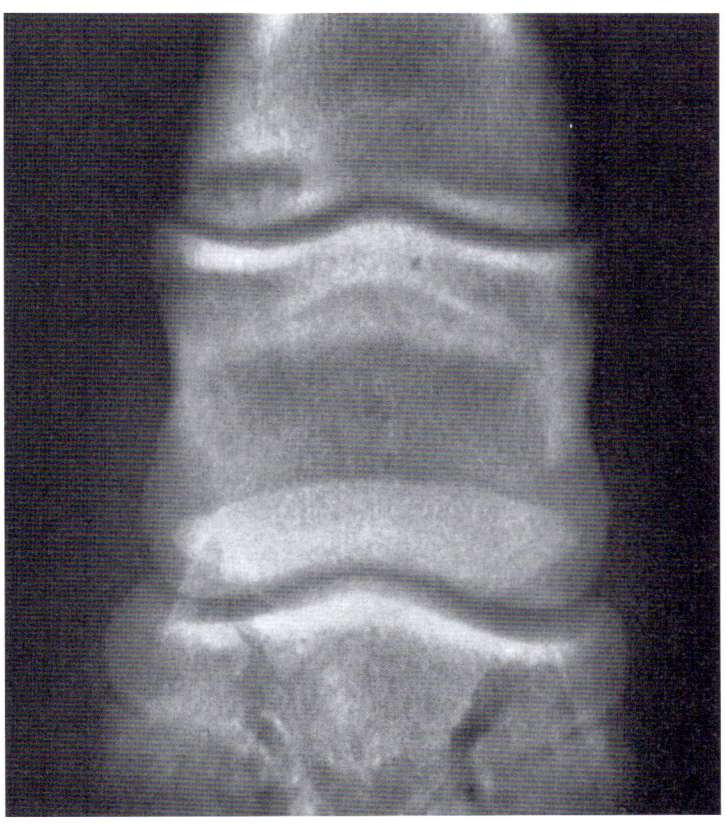

116 Foot, left front, dorsopalmar view: close-up.

Foal, 6 months.

A circumscribed, ellipsoidal area of irregularly decreased bone density in the subchondral bone of the distomedial end of the first phalanx due to ischaemic bone necrosis.

Bone cyst

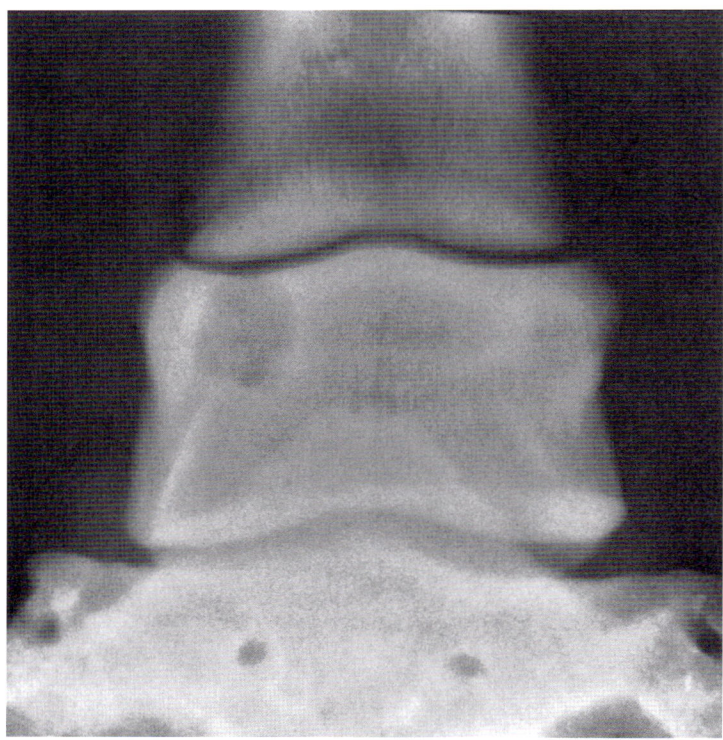

117

117 Second phalanx, left front, dorsopalmar view: close-up.

Warmblood, 7 years.

A solitary, clearly defined, cystic area of diffuse radiolucency within the proximomedial end of the second phalanx, indicating a bone cyst surrounded by a thin sclerotic zone. The subchondral bone in the corresponding area is disrupted suggesting direct communication between the cyst and the joint space, or separation of the lesion from the joint by only a thin layer of articular cartilage.

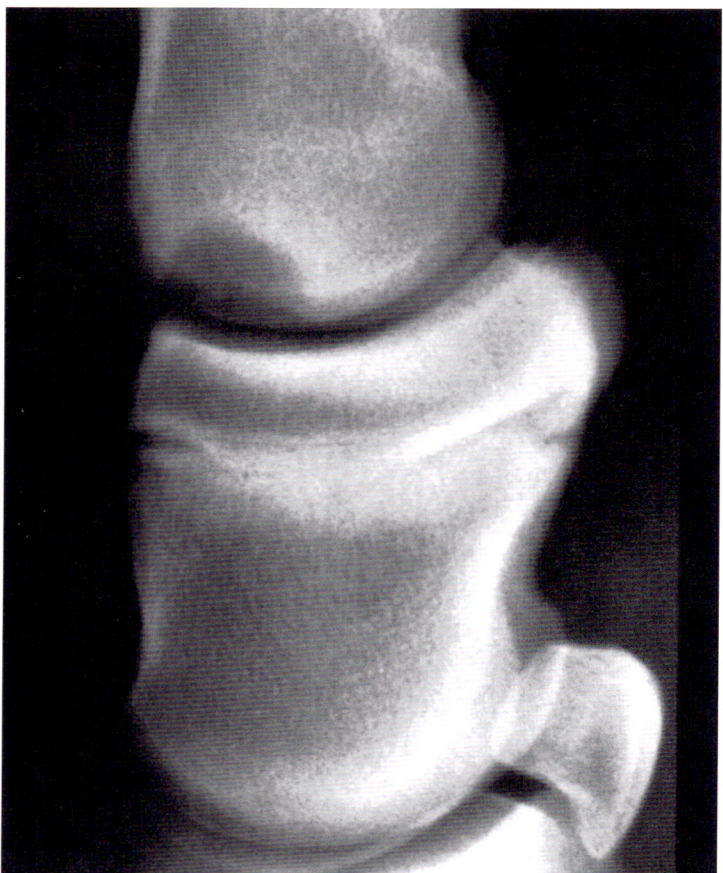

118

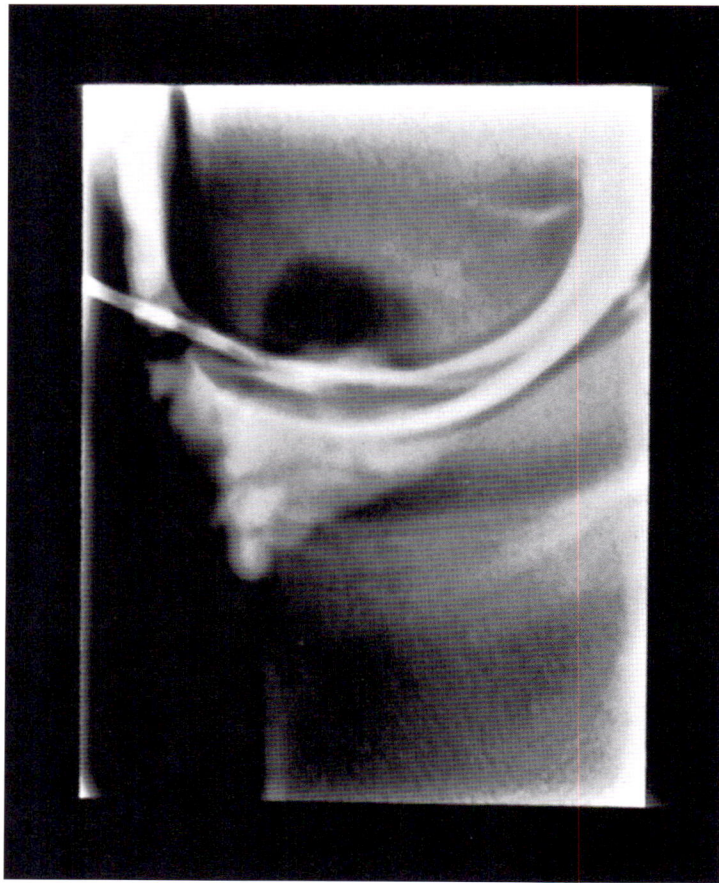

119

118/119 Pastern joint, left hind, lateromedial survey (Fig. 118) and positive contrast study (Fig. 119): close-ups.

Foal, 6 months.

The survey study reveals a solitary, well defined, semicircular area of diffuse radiolucency within the distal end of the first phalanx, indicating the presence of a bone cyst. Five ml positive contrast material injected into the joint does not enter the cyst, although the joint cartilage is eroded.

There is no direct communication between the cyst lumen and the pastern joint, despite the absence of bone tissue between the lesion and the joint.

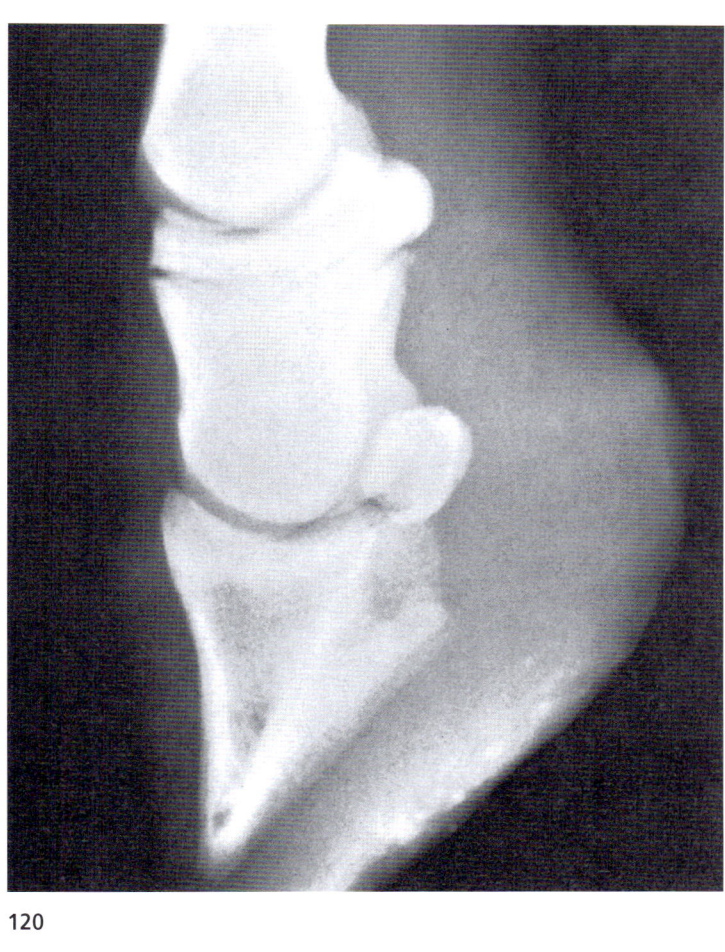

120

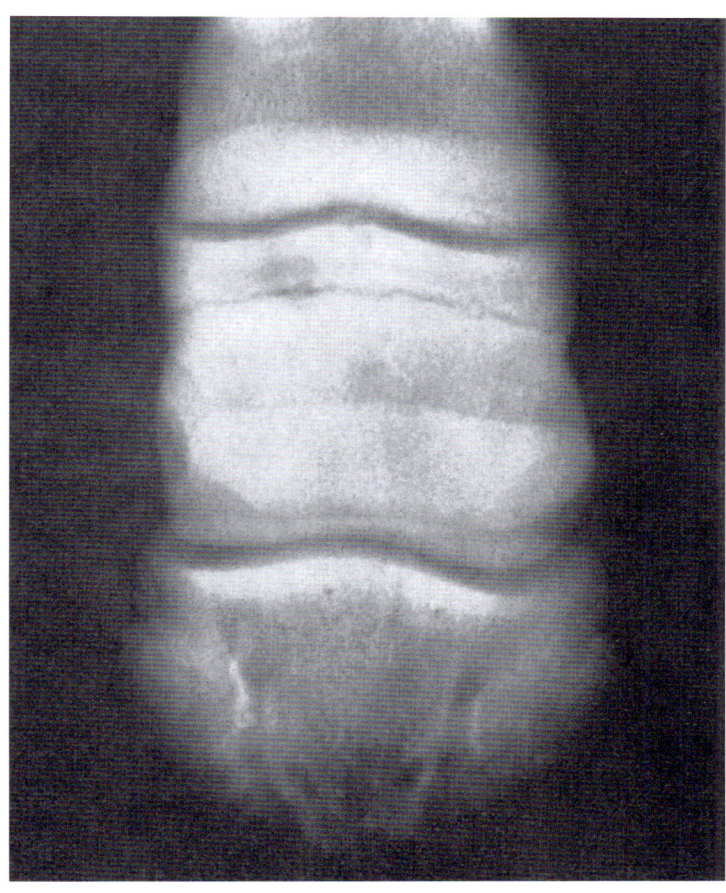

121

122

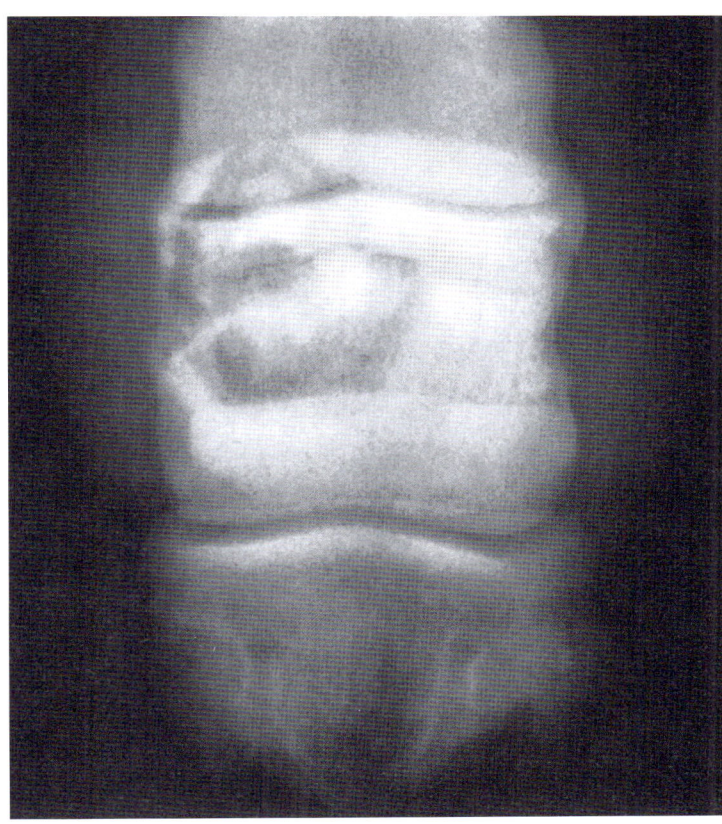

123

120/121/122/123 Foot, left hind, serial lateromedial and dorsoplantar views.

Foal, 3 ½ months.

The initial examination (Fig. 120, 121) 10 days after the onset of lameness, reveals a faint, thin layer of periosteal new bone along the dorsal aspect of the second phalanx and an obscure area of radiolucency in the proximomedial end of the second phalanx adjacent to the physis, indicating hematogenous osteomyelitis of recent onset.

On a second examination 3 weeks later (Fig. 122, 123), soft tissue swelling surrounding the second phalanx is obvious. The periosteal new bone is much more prominent and active, as indicated by its ill defined margin. The radiolucent lesion has spread widely throughout the bone. The irregular radiopaque pattern surrounded by a radiolucent zone suggests the formation of a sequestrum. The medial cortex and the plantaroproximal extremity of the second phalanx are disrupted and calcified soft tissue is visible plantar to the second phalanx, indicating extension of the disease process into the soft tissue.

Diaphyseal angular deformity

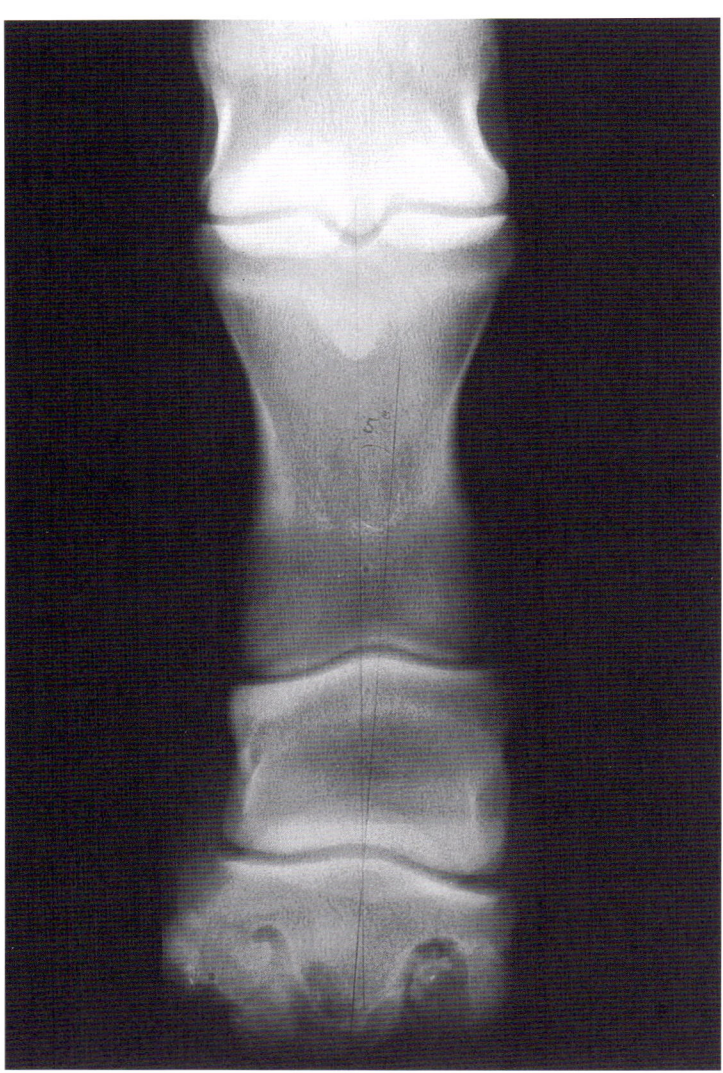

124

124 Foot, left hind, dorsopalmar view.

Foal, 8 months.

Prominent assymetry of the medial and lateral length of the second phalanx, causing angulation of the pastern and coffin joint.

A very seldom occuring varus deformity of unknown origin.

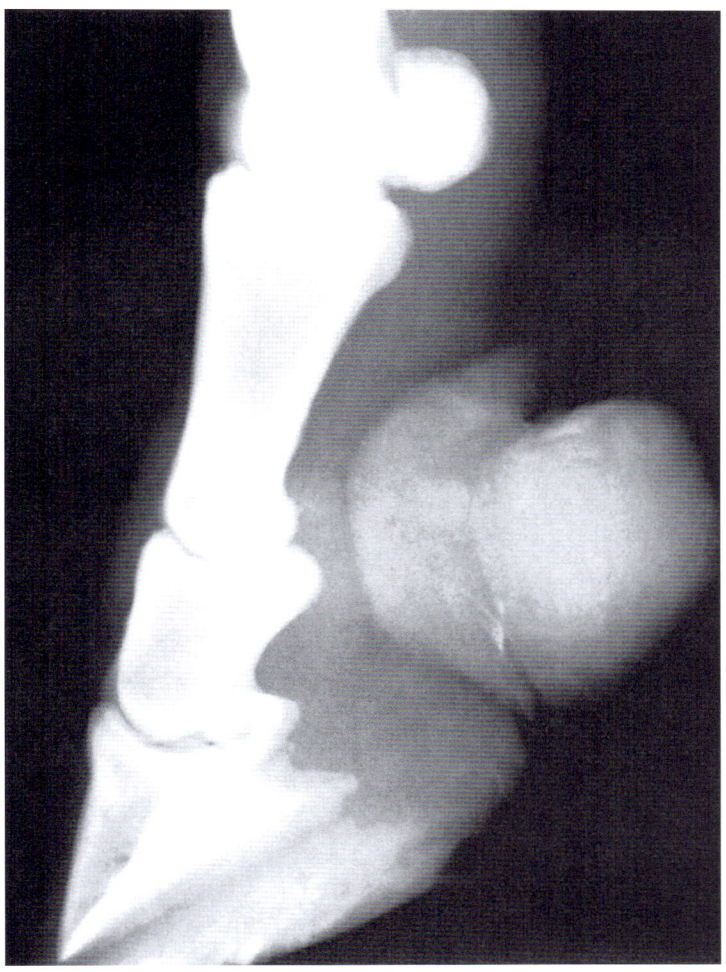

125 Foot, left hind, lateromedial view.

Warmblood, 9 years.

A large, nodular, soft tissue mass granuloma of uniform density plantar to the pastern joint.

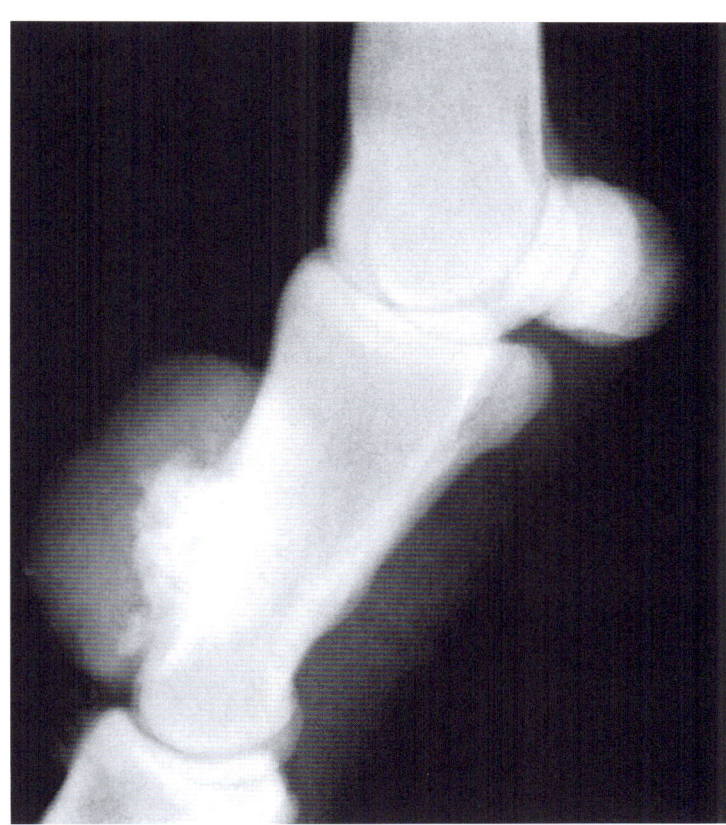

126 First phalanx, left hind, lateromedial view: close-up.

Warmblood, 4 ½ years.

A large, nodular, granuloma dorsal to the first phalanx and periosteal new bone along the dorsal aspect of the first and second phalanx, both resulting from trauma.

The new bone formation is inactive, as indicated by the well defined margin.

The Fetlock Joint

Fracture

Fracture / Luxation

Avulsion injuries of the proximal sesamoid bones

Diseases of the proximal sesamoid bone

Osteoarthrosis

Osteochondrosis

Schematic drawings of fetlock fragments

Villonodular synovitis

Ischaemic bone necrosis

Bone cyst

Osteomyelitis

"Epiphysitis"

Diaphyseal angular deformity

Puncture wound

Osselets

Granuloma

Fracture

Cannon bone

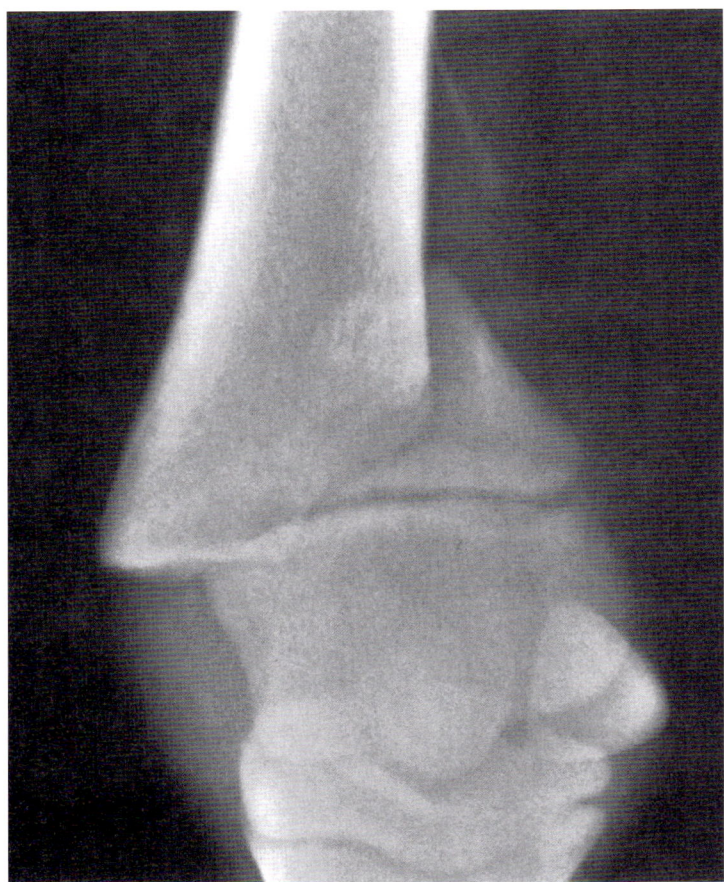

127

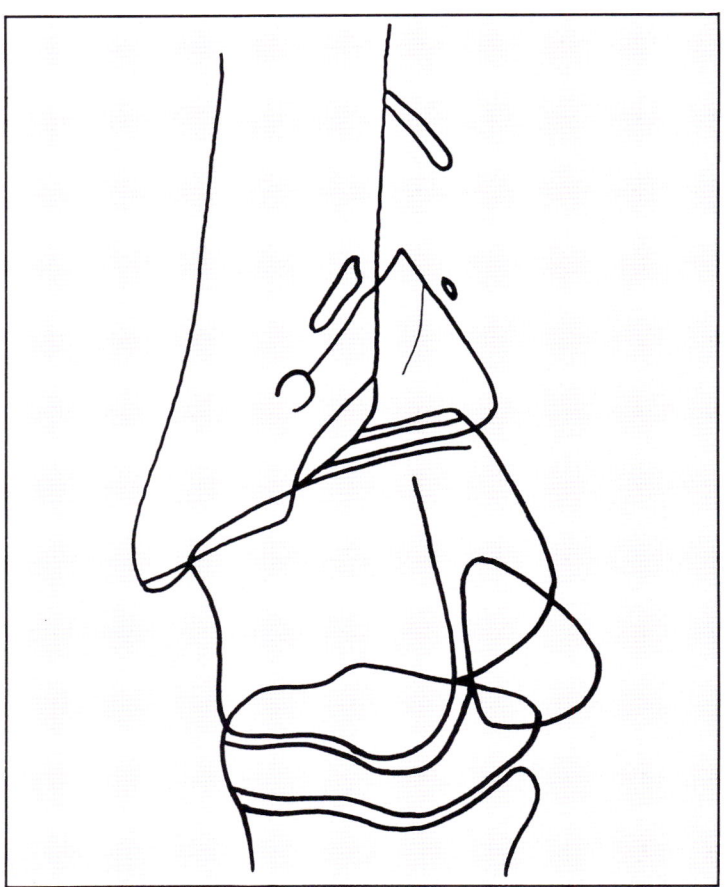

127 a

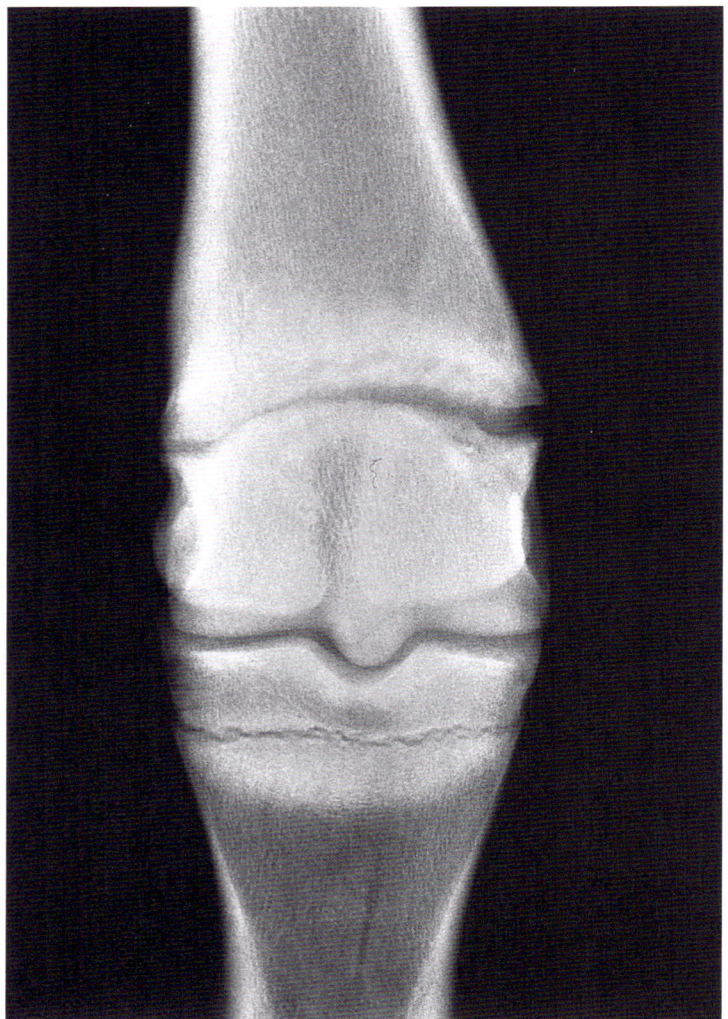

128

127 Fetlock joint, right front, dorsolateral-palmaromedial oblique view: close-up.

Foal, 8 days.

Disruption of the cortex and lateral shifting of the metacarpal epiphysis resulting in a "step" defect between epi- and metaphysis, due to a recent fracture with slight overriding of the fracture fragments. The line of separation extends along the physis before passing through a portion of the metaphysis (Salter-Harris type 2 physeal injury). Small additional fracture fragments are visible lateral and medial to the large triangular shaped metaphyseal fragment, the small medial bone fragments being obscured by the superimposed cannon bone.

Additional finding: angular displacement of the distal end of the lateral splint bone, probably the result of a fracture although the fracture line is not visible.

127 a Schematic drawing

128 Fetlock joint, left hind, dorsopalmar view.

Foal, 1 month.

The assymetry, i.e. widening of the lateral aspect and narrowing of the medial aspect of the metatarsal growth plate, indicates a recent Salter-Harris type 1 physeal fracture.

Cannon bone

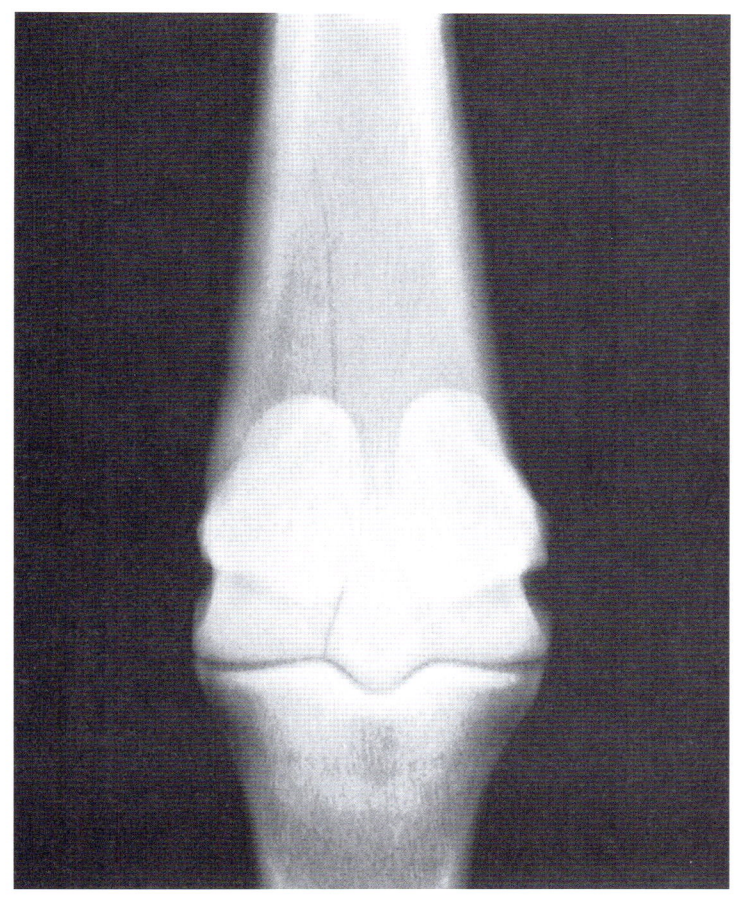

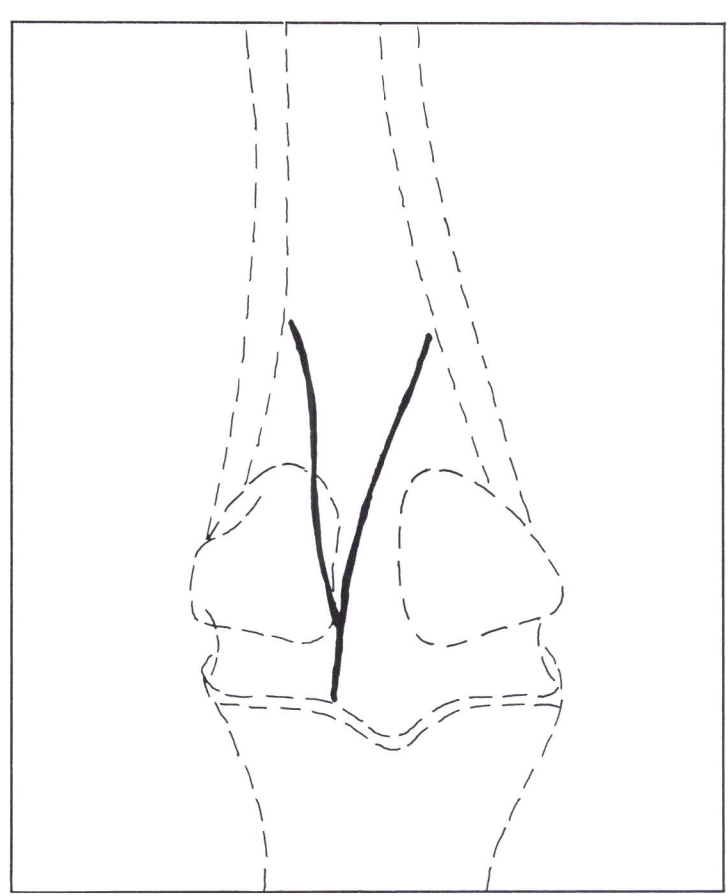

129 Fetlock joint, left front, dorsopalmar view.

Warmblood, 2 years.

Within the medial condyl of the metacarpus a sharply bordered vertical radiolucent line interrupts the distal articular surface close to the sagittal ridge, extends proximally, but does not interrupt the continuity of the proximal cortical bone. This recent incomplete longitudinal intra-articular condylar fissure-fracture of the cannon bone spirals slightly, explaining why the clearly defined radiolucent line at the distal articular surface splits more proximally into two less distinct diverging fracture lines.

129 a Schematic drawing

Fracture

First phalanx

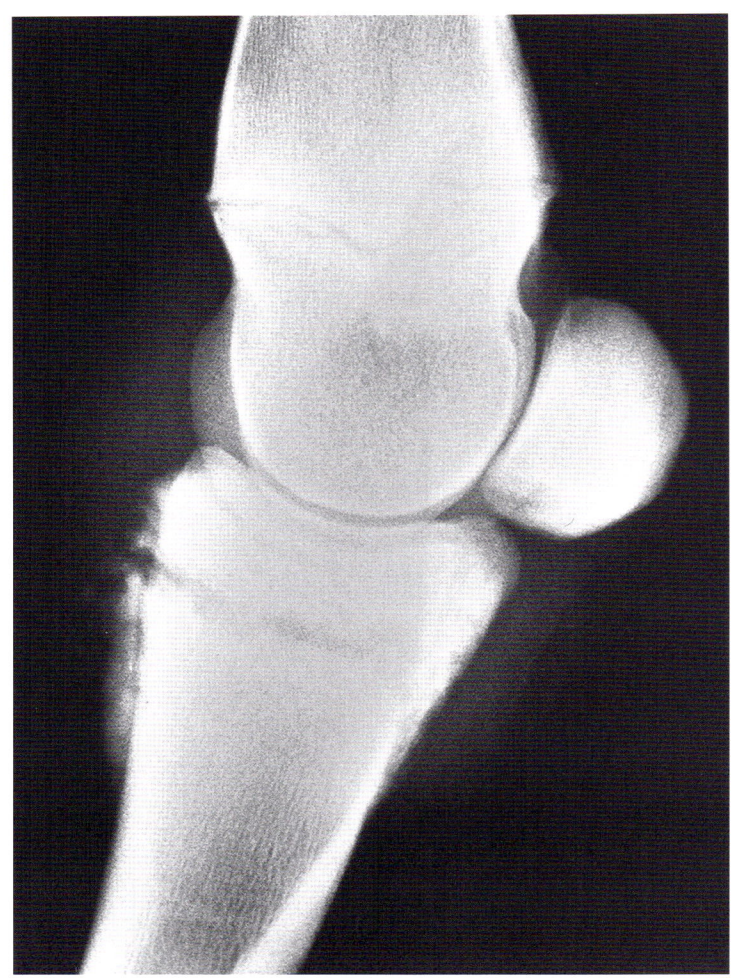

130

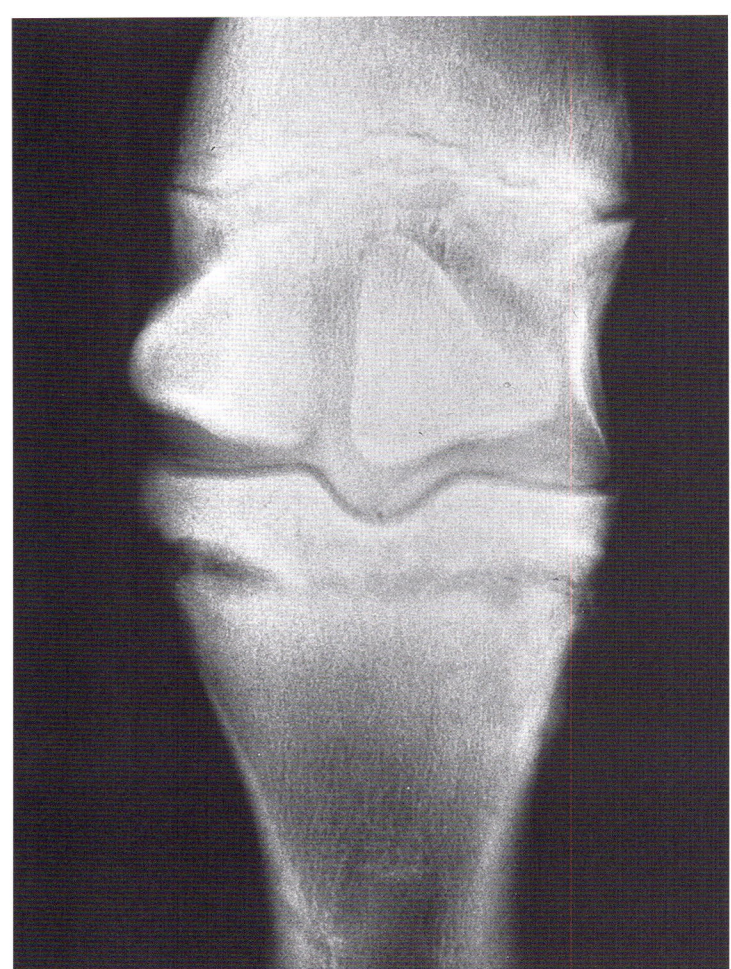

131

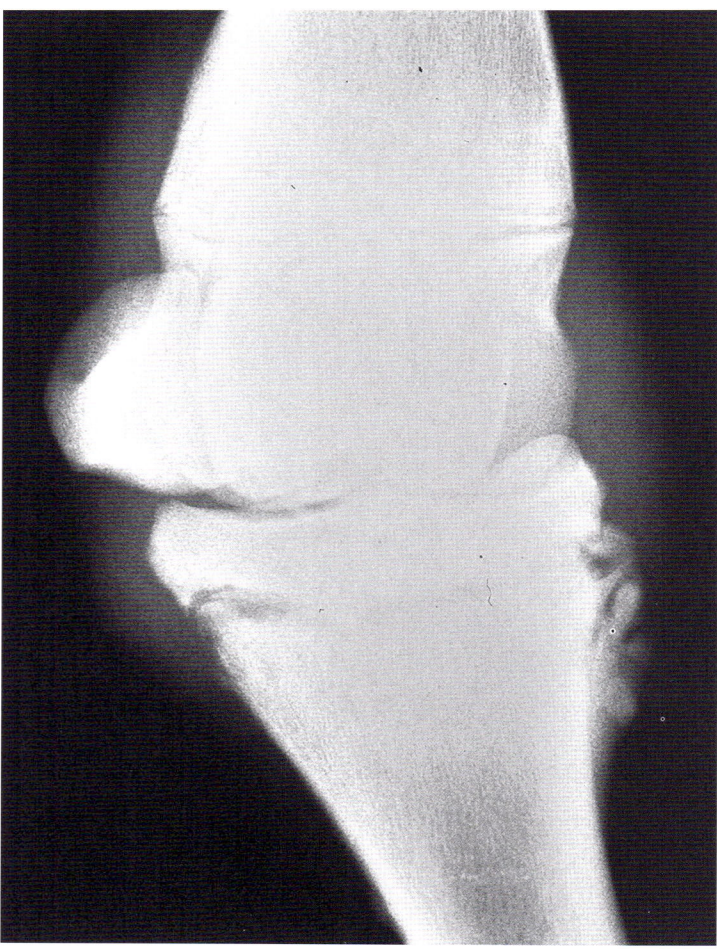

132

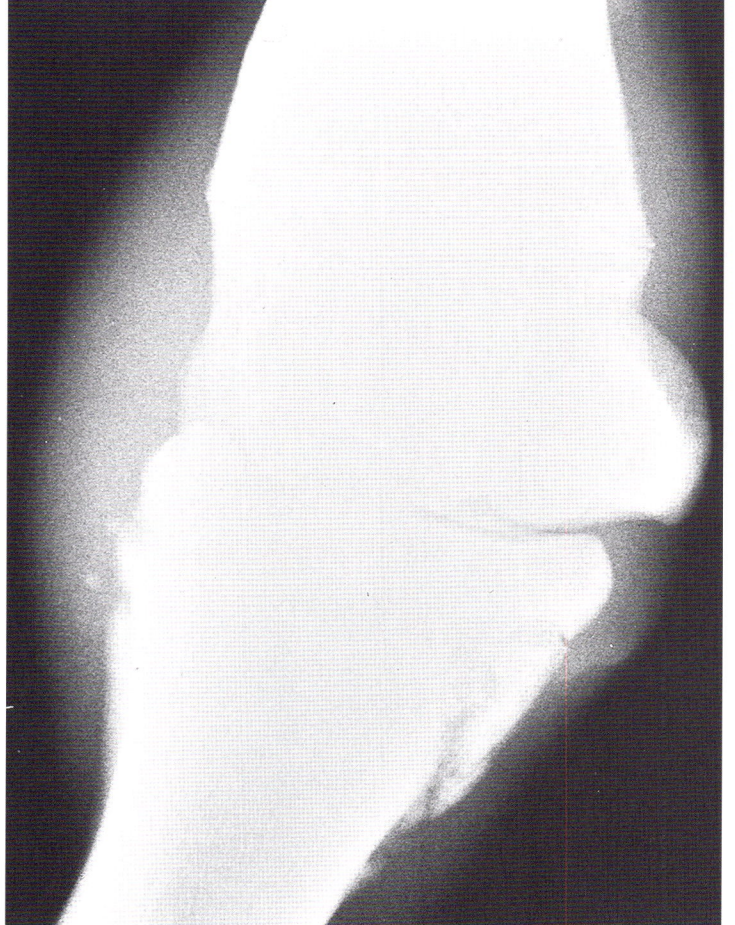

133

First phalanx

130/131/132/133 Fetlock joint, right hind, lateromedial, dorsoplantar, dorsolateral – plantaromedial oblique and dorsomedial – plantarolateral oblique view.

Foal, 5 months.

The lateromedial view (Fig. 130) shows irregularity and blurring of the phalangeal growth plate and rather dense, irregular, ill bordered periosteal new bone formation on the dorsal aspect of the epi- and metaphysis.

The irregular physeal widening and blurring becomes more obvious on the dorsoplantar view (Fig. 131). On the dorsolateral – plantaromedial oblique projection (Fig. 132) the associated irregular dorsal, periosteal metaphyseal new bone appears more prominent. The dorsomedial – plantarolateral oblique radiograph (Fig. 133) visualizes an additional vertical ill bordered radiolucent line through the plantaromedial aspect of the phalangeal metaphysis, which extends to the growth plate and interrupts the plantaromedial cortex.

These changes are consistent with a Salter-Harris type 2 physeal fracture of some duration.

134 Fetlock joint, left front, dorsopalmar view: close-up.

Warmblood, 5 years.

The short, well defined, vertical radiolucent line superimposed on the axial sagittal ridge of the cannon bone and the metacarpo-phalangeal joint space represents a short, incomplete, sagittal, intra-articular fracture of the dorsal aspect of the first phalanx.

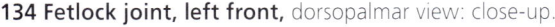

134

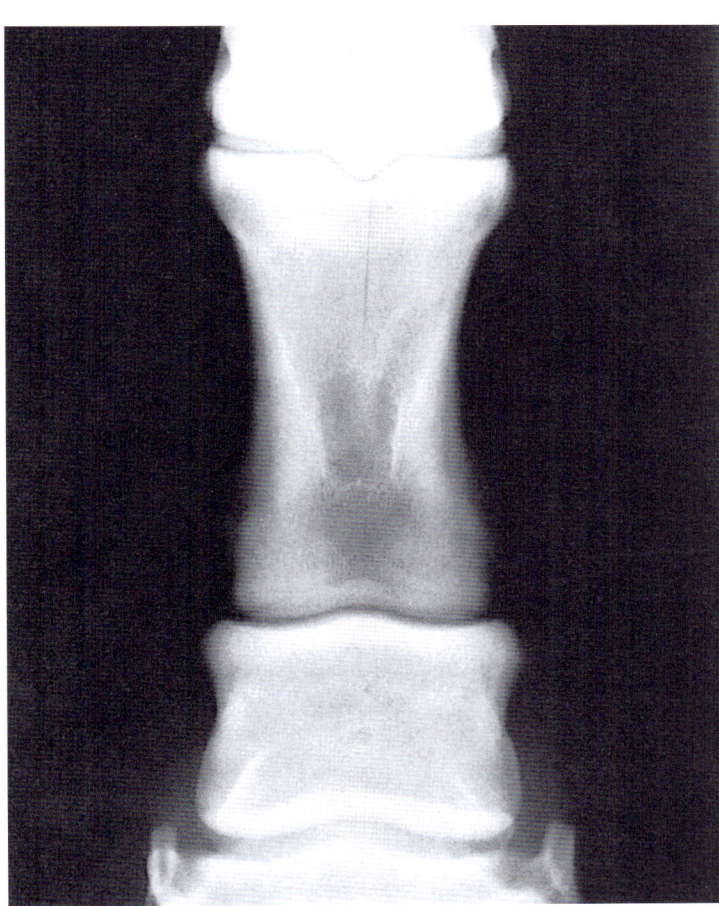

135 Fetlock joint, left front, dorsopalmar view.

Warmblood, 9 years.

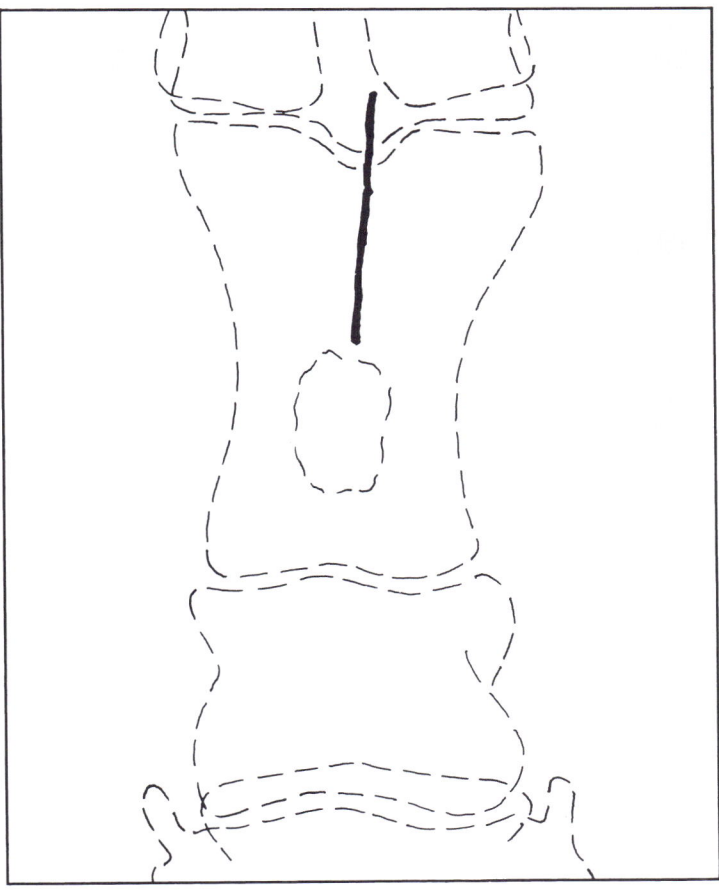

135 a Schematic drawing

A vertical sharply bordered radiolucent line through the proximal half of the first phalanx, the result of a recent incomplete sagittal intra-articular fracture. On a weight-bearing dorsopalmar view centred on the first phalanx the dorsoproximal extremity of the first phalanx is superimposed on the distal end of the cannon bone and the fracture line therefore appears to pass through the metacarpo-phalangeal joint space and into the distal end of the cannon bone.

Fracture

First phalanx

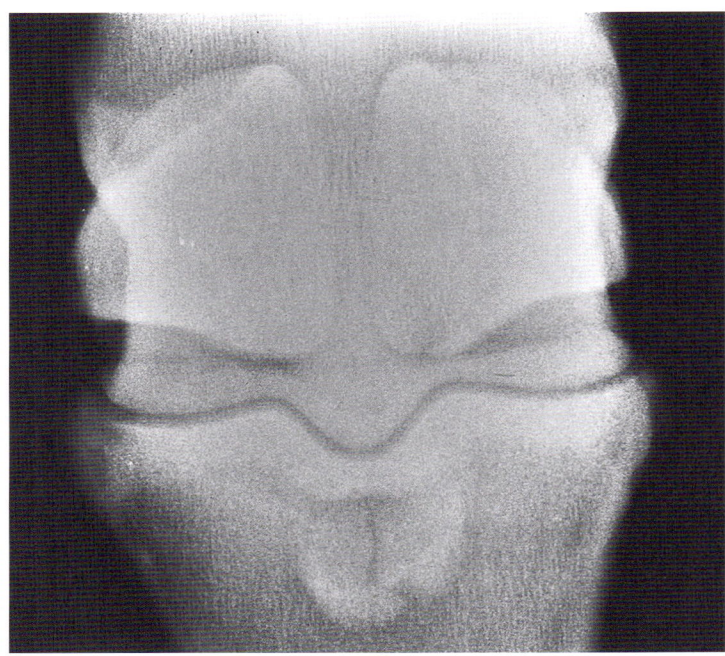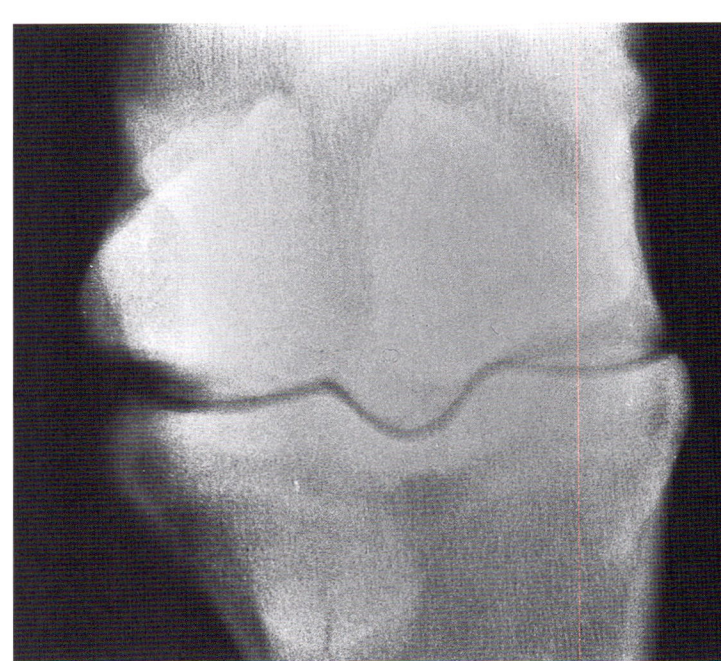

136

137

136/137 Fetlock joint, right hind, dorsoplantar and slightly dorsolateral – plantaromedial oblique view: close-ups.

Warmblood, 7 years.

The dorsoplantar view (Fig. 136) reveals a slightly irregular, vertical radiolucent line surrounded by a circumscribed radiopacity in the proximal region of the first phalanx. On the additional slightly dorsolateral – plantaromedial oblique view (Fig. 137) the radiolucent line and the surrounding opacity shift laterally. These findings indicate a false fracture appearance that resulted from a vertical crack in the radiopaque ergot superimposed on the plantaroproximal aspect of the first phalanx.

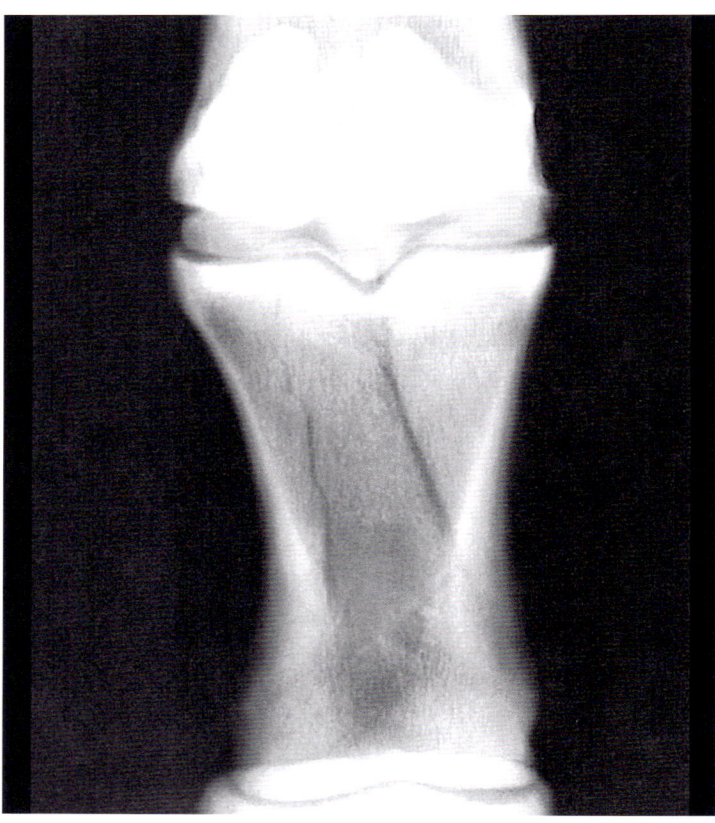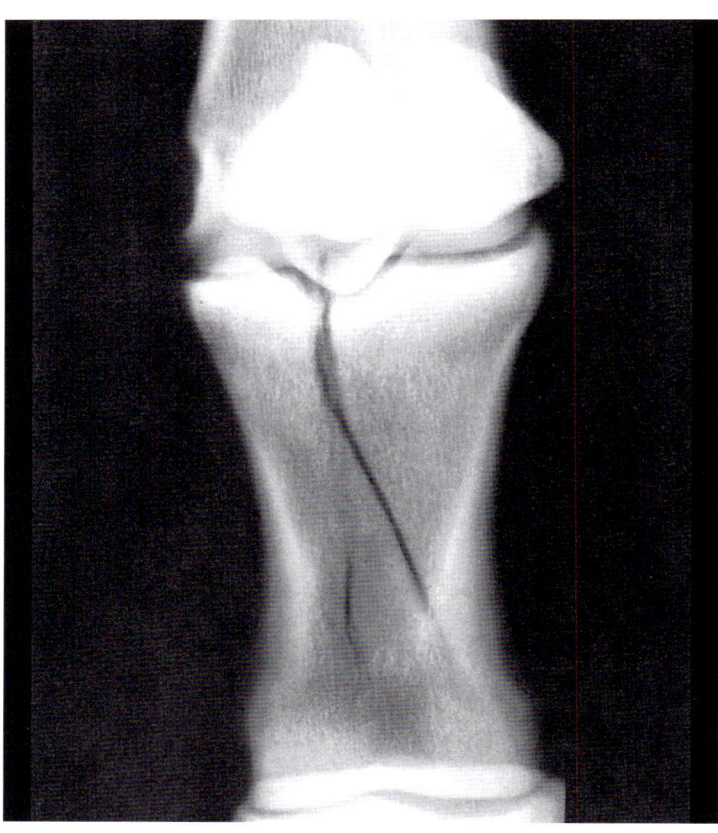

138

139

138/139 Fetlock joint, right front, dorsopalmar and dorsomedial-palmarolateral oblique view: close-ups.

Warmblood, 3 years.

The dorsopalmar view (Fig. 138) reveals a recent incomplete longitudinal intra-articular fracture of the first phalanx. The fracture plane is not parallel to the dorsopalmar directed central beam and therefore two vertical sharply bordered radiolucent lines are visible.

The precise fracture plane is established on a dorsomedial-palmarolateral oblique view the beam shifted 20° medial to the dorsopalmar line (Fig. 139) On this radiograph the radiolucent lines coincide proximally, indicating the fracture line to be parallel to the central beam. Because the fracture spirals slightly the radiolucent line splits into two diverging fracture lines distally.

First phalanx

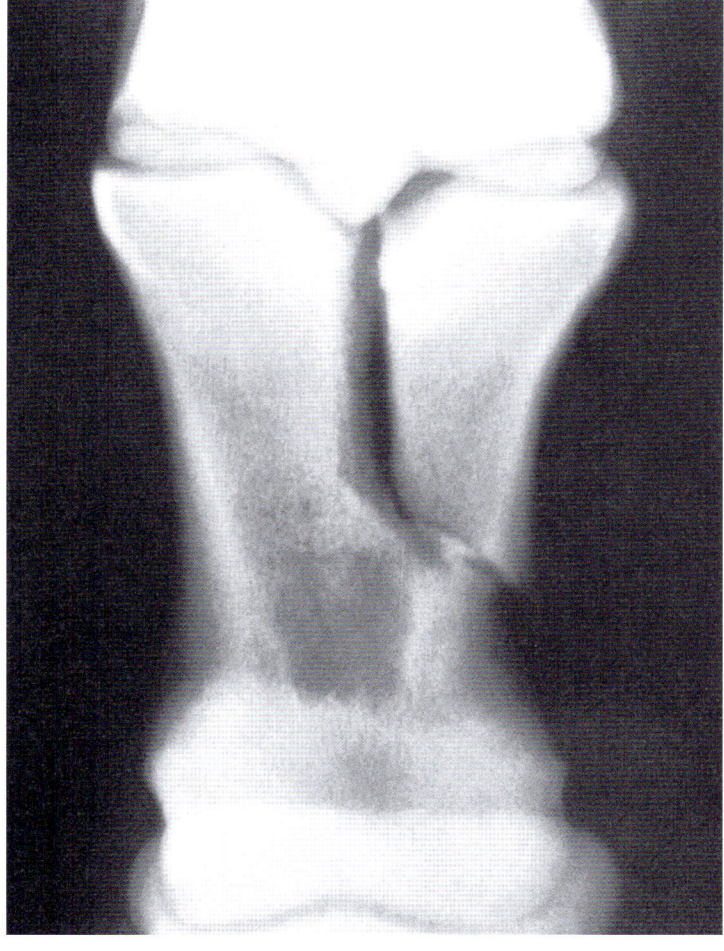

140

140 Fetlock joint, left hind, dorsoplantar view.

Warmblood, 3 years.

A sharply bordered vertical radiolucent zone through the midsagittal portion of the proximal half of the first phalanx interrupting the articular surface and the lateral cortex, indicating a recent, simple, complete, intra-articular fracture. The lateral displacement of the fracture fragment produces a "step" defect halfway along the lateral border of the first phalanx with slight overriding of the fracture fragments.

141/142 Fetlock joint, left front, lateromedial and dorsopalmar view: close-ups.

Warmblood, 6 years.

The lateromedial view (Fig. 141) reveals an irregular zone of periosteal new bone along the dorsal border of the first phalanx which usually indicates the presence of an old longitudinal fracture.

The dorsopalmar view (Fig. 142) shows the longitudinal, intra-articular fracture zone extending through the proximal half of the first phalanx. Proximally the fracture is clearly visible, distally it is ill defined and blurred by callus formation.

Additional finding (lateral view): osteoarthrosis of the fetlock joint, indicated by joint mice dorsal to the distal end of the cannon bone and spur formation on the apex and base of the proximal sesamoid bones and the dorsoproximal extremity of the first phalanx.

N. B. The vertical radiolucent line in the central area of the first phalanx adjacent to the fracture represents the nutrient foramen.

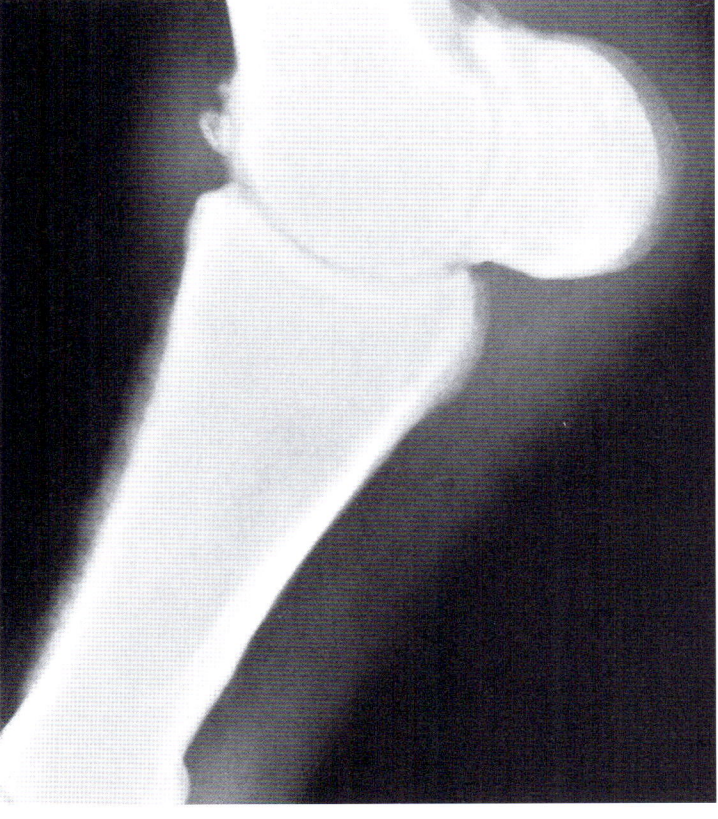

141

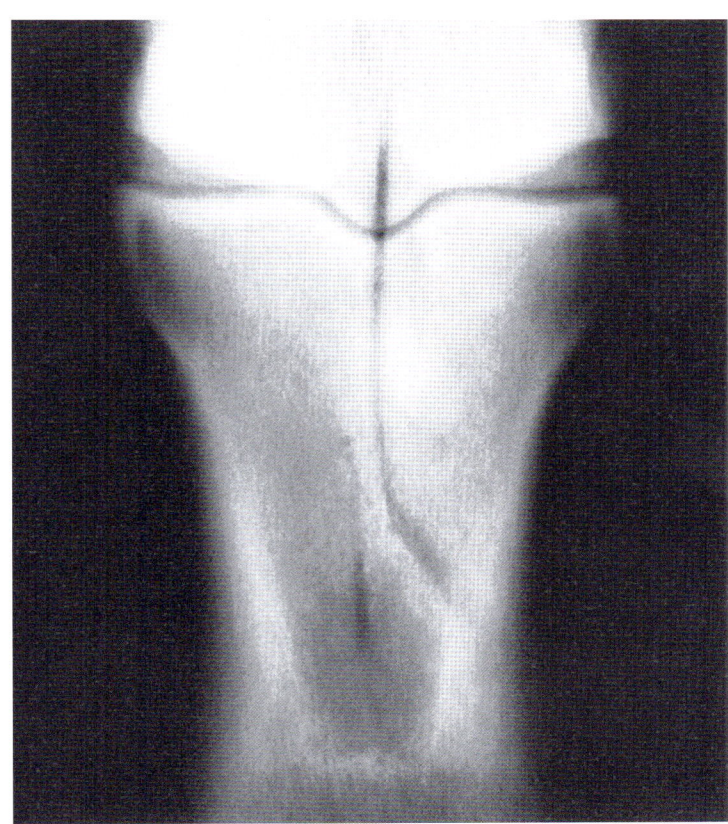

142

Fracture

First phalanx

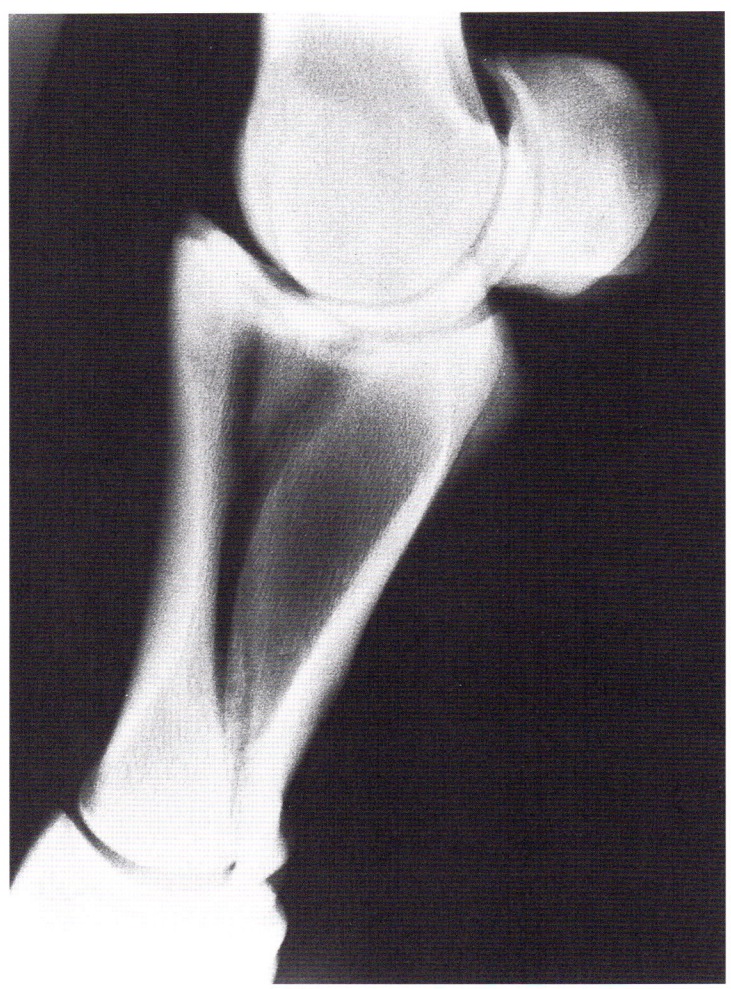

143

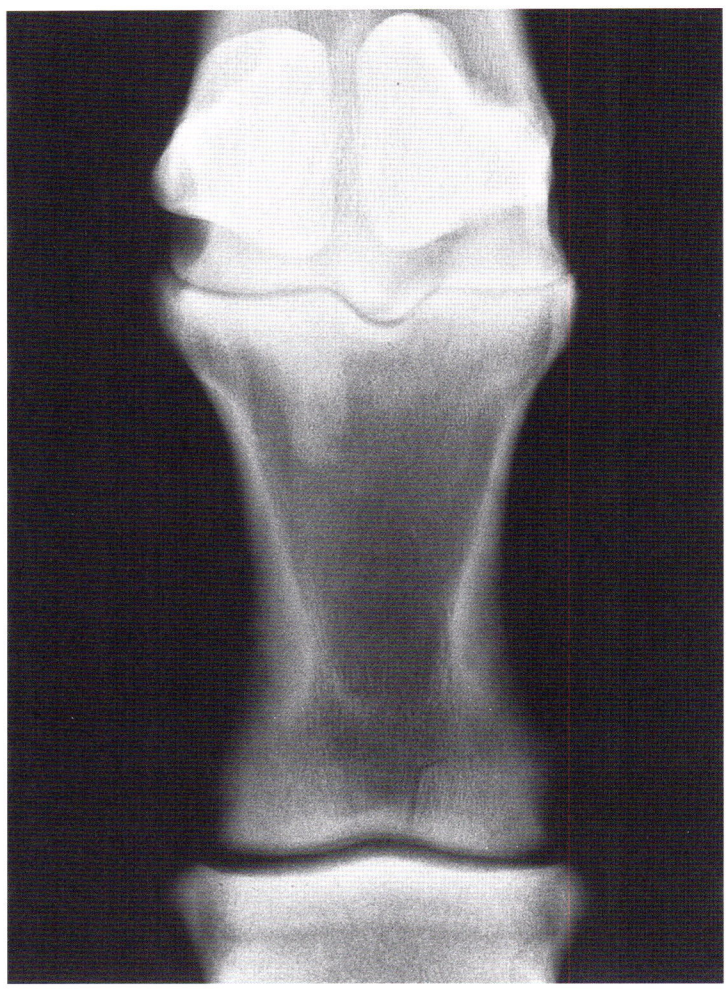

144

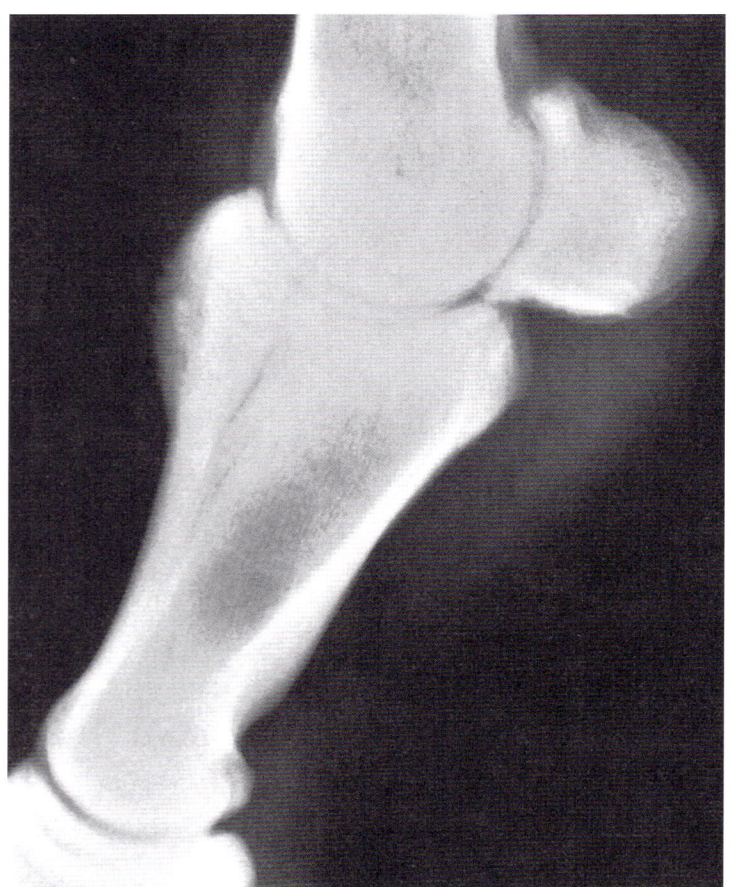

145

143/144 Fetlock joint, left front, lateromedial and dorsopalmar view.

Warmblood, 12 years.

The lateromedial view (Fig. 143) shows a wide, vertical radiolucent zone extending through the first phalanx. Proximally this zone diverges, thus interrupting the dorsal and central aspect of the articular surface.

Distally the radiolucent zone narrows and disrupts the plantar aspect of the articular surface. These findings indicate a recent, complete, transverse fracture, involving the metacarpo-phalangeal and the proximal interphalangeal joint.

On the dorsopalmar radiograph (Fig. 144) the fracture plane is perpendicular to the central beam, therefore the radiolucent fracture zone is not outlined on this view. Only a short vertical radiolucent line through the distolateral aspect of the first phalanx is visible on this projection, probably due to spiraling of the fracture.

145 Fetlock joint, right hind, lateromedial view.

Warmblood, 8 years.

Two obscure diverging radiolucent lines through the proximal half of the first phalanx close to the dorsal cortex interrupting the articular surface and dense sharply bordered periosteal new bone along the dorsoproximal aspect of the first phalanx, the result of a long-standing incomplete transverse intra-articular fracture. Because the fracture plane is not exactly parallel to the lateromedially directed central beam, the radiograph shows two instead of one fracture lines.

Additional finding: osteoarthrosis of the fetlock joint indicated by spur formation on the apex and base of the proximal sesamoid bones and on the dorsoproximal extremity of the first phalanx and irregularity of the dorsal aspect of the distal end of the cannon bone.

First phalanx

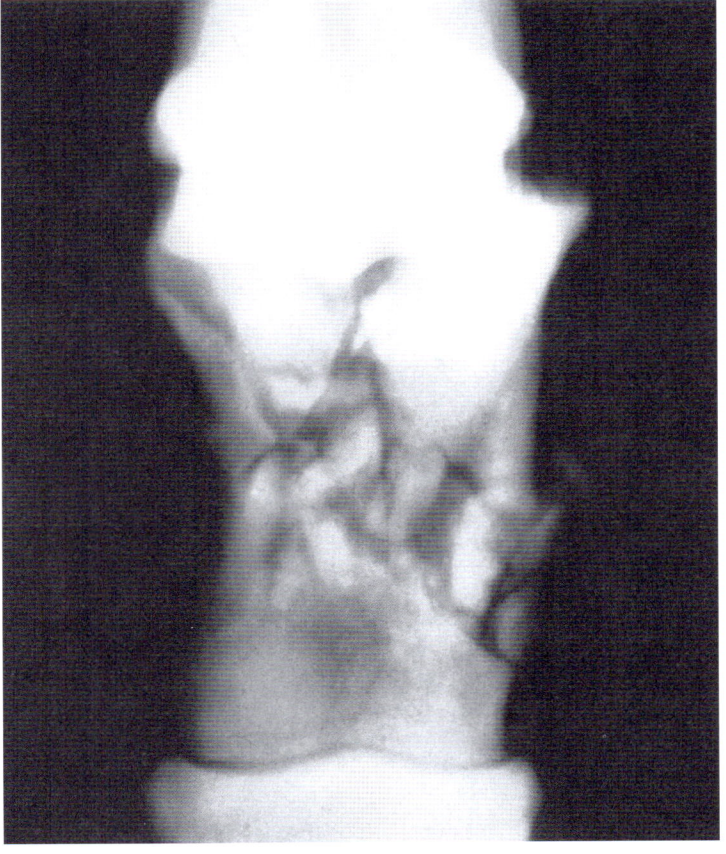

146

146 Fetlock joint, left front, dorsopalmar view.

Warmblood, 4 years.

Radiolucent lines within the first phalanx, some of which interrupt the proximal articular surface. Multiple sharply bordered bone fragments result from a recent comminuted intra-articular fracture.

The fetlock joint is obscured by overriding fracture fragments suggesting an impaction type of injury.

147/148 Fetlock joint, left hind, lateromedial and dorsoplantar view.

Warmblood, 7 years.

Plantar shifting of the distal half of the first phalanx, producing a "step" defect in the dorsal and plantar phalangeal contour, is obvious on the lateromedial view (Fig. 147).

Additional well defined fragmentation of the medial aspect of the first phalanx is visualized on the dorsoplantar view (Fig. 148).

These findings indicate the presence of a recent horizontal multiple fracture.

At both views the horizontal fracture lines are obscured, due to overriding of the fracture fragments.

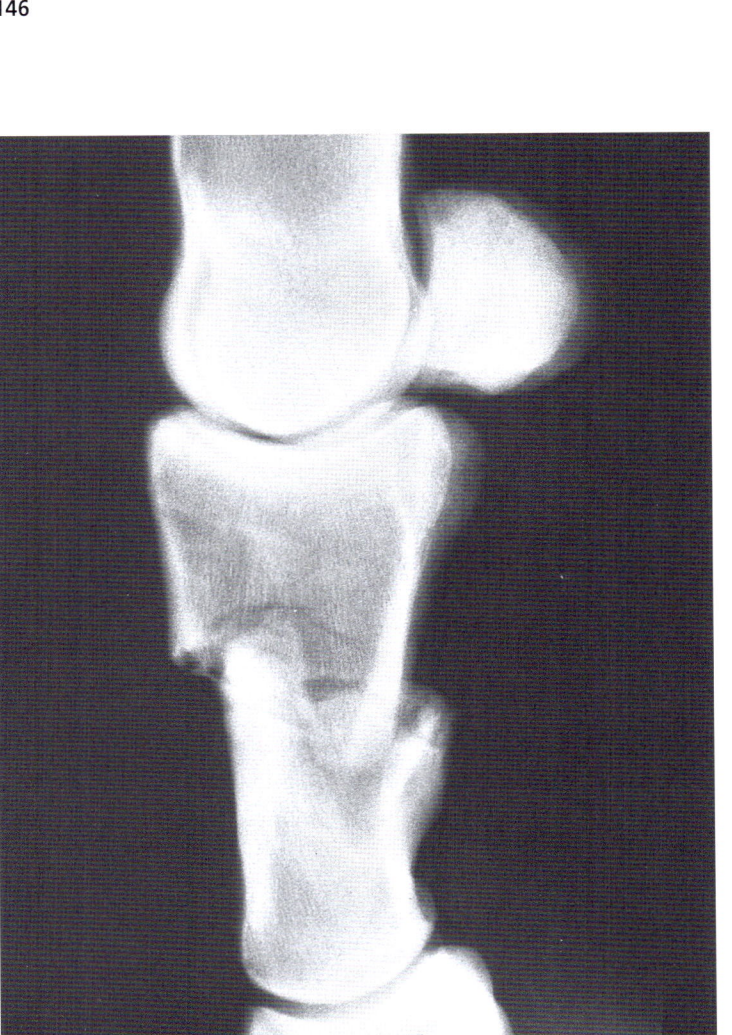

147

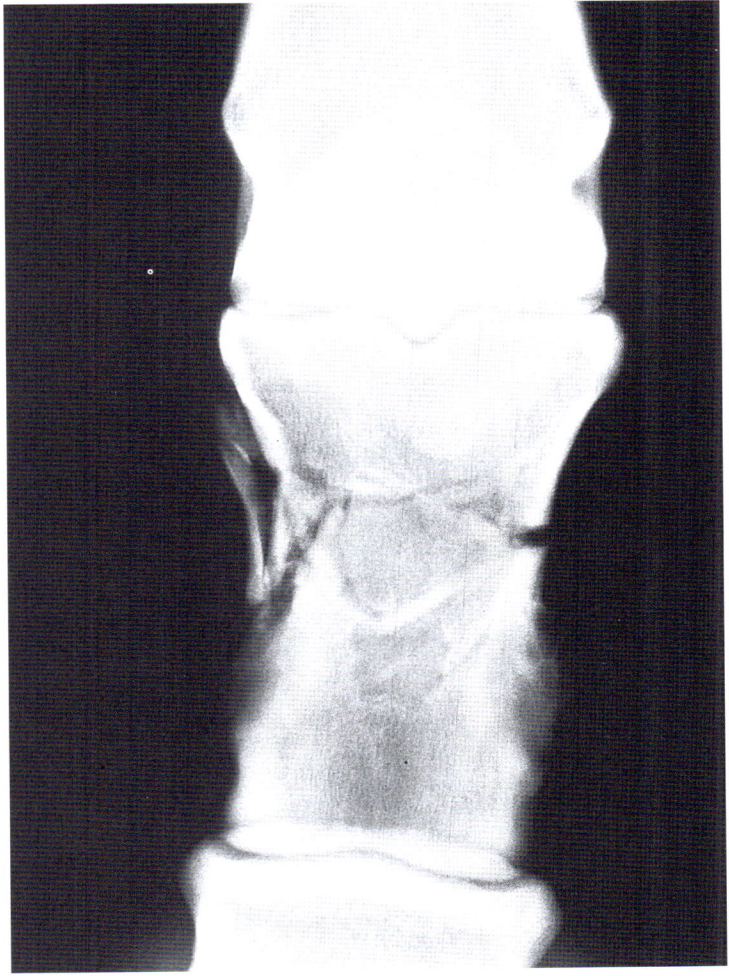

148

Fracture

First phalanx

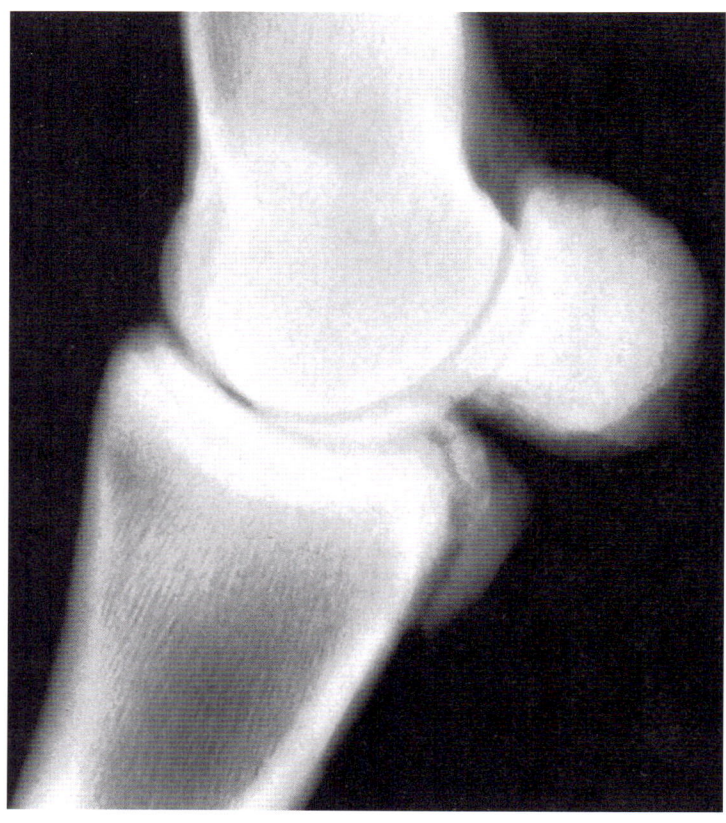

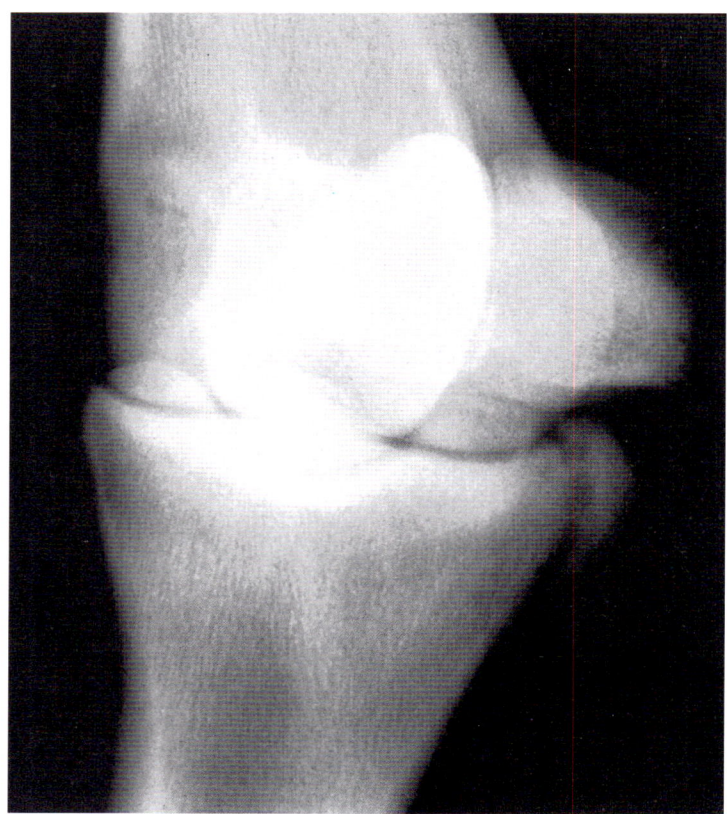

149

150

149/150 Fetlock joint, left hind, lateromedial and dorsomedial-plantarolateral oblique view: close-ups.

Warmblood, 7 years.

The lateromedial view (Fig. 149) shows a large isolated bone fragment plantar to the proximal end of the first phalanx.

The dorsomedial-plantarolateral oblique view indicates that the fragment originated from the medial plantaroproximal extremity of the first phalanx (Fig. 150). The loss of bone density adjacent to the fracture results in irregularity of the fracture zone and indicates a fracture of some duration.

First phalanx

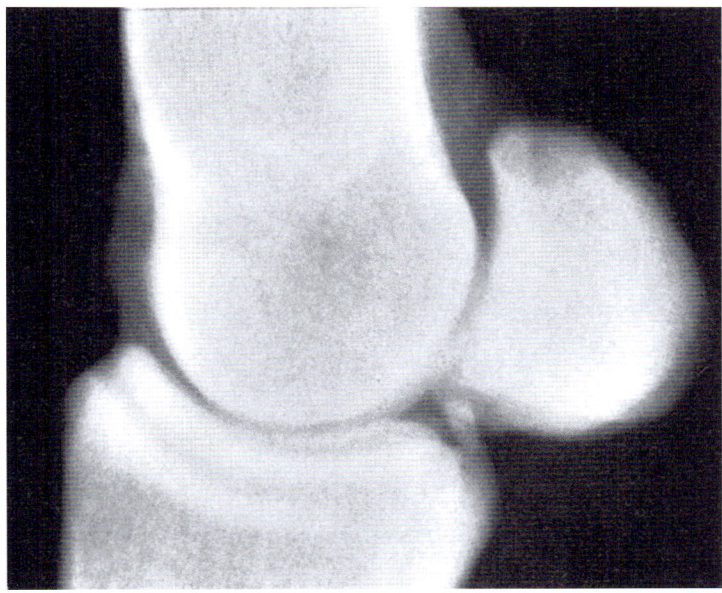

151

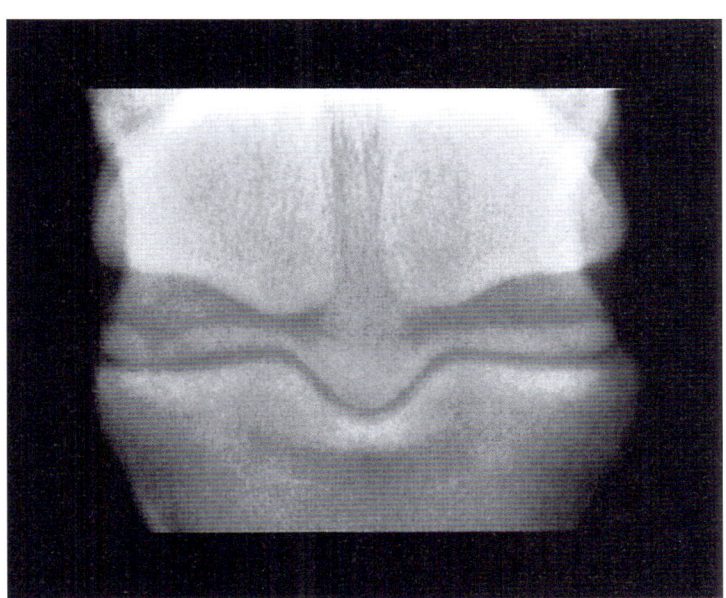

152

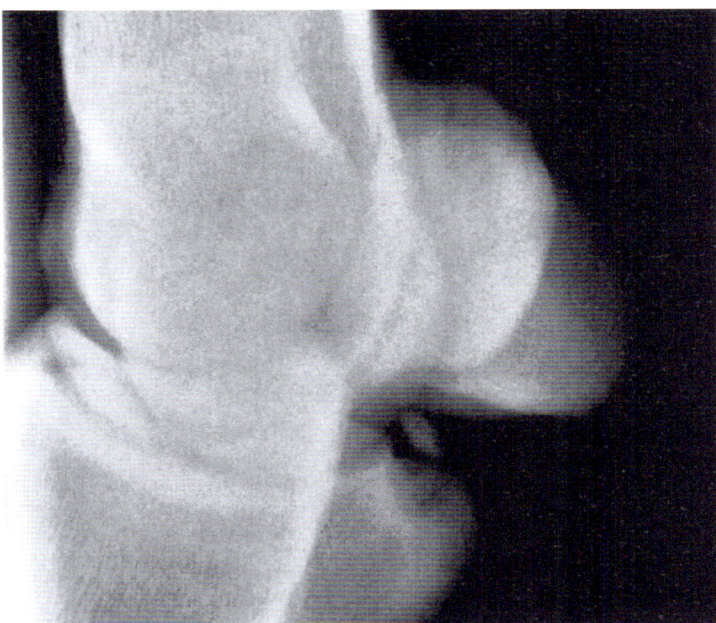

153

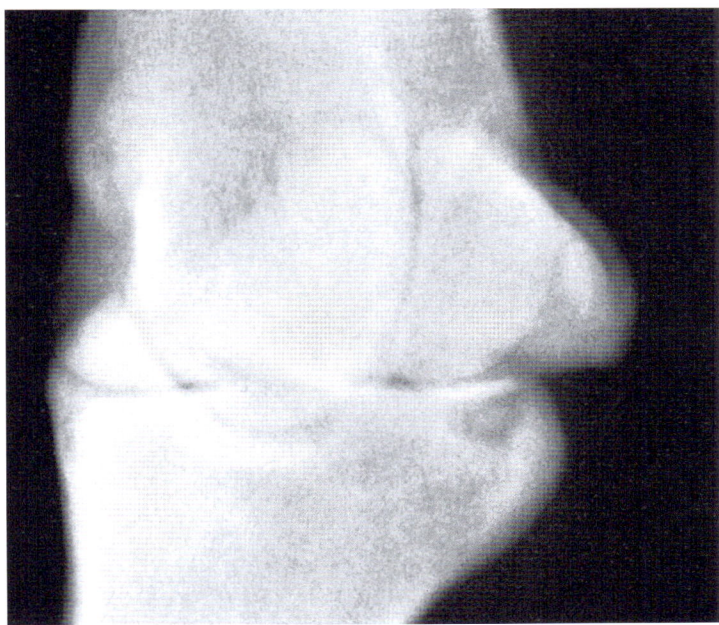

154

151/152/153/154 Fetlock joint, left hind, lateromedial, dorsoplantar, special and dorsomedial-plantarolateral oblique views: close-ups.

Standardbred, 2 years.

The lateromedial view (Fig. 151) shows a well-defined bone fragment between the base of the sesamoid bones and the plantaroproximal extremity of the first phalanx. On a dorsoplantar view (Fig. 152) the bone fragment is obscured almost completely by the superimposed medial condyle of the cannon bone.

A special dorsoproximomedial-plantarodistolateral oblique view made at 20° proximal to the supporting surface and 75° medial to the dorsoplantar line, the beam centred on the medial sesamoid bone (Fig. 153), presents not only the bone fragment but also the fracture "bed" in the medial plantaroproximal extremity of the first phalanx. The usual dorsomedial-plantarolateral oblique view of the medial sesamoid bone reveals only the fracture "bed"; a radiolucent area within the medial plantaroproximal extremity of the first phalanx (Fig. 154).

Additional finding (lateromedial and special view): the slight irregularity of the dorsal aspect of the distal end of the cannon bone and slight spur formation on the dorsoproximal extremity of the first phalanx indicate osteoarthrosis of the fetlock joint.

N. B. Small avulsion fragments of the plantaroproximal extremity of the first phalanx may be a coincidental finding of no clinical significance.

Fracture

First phalanx

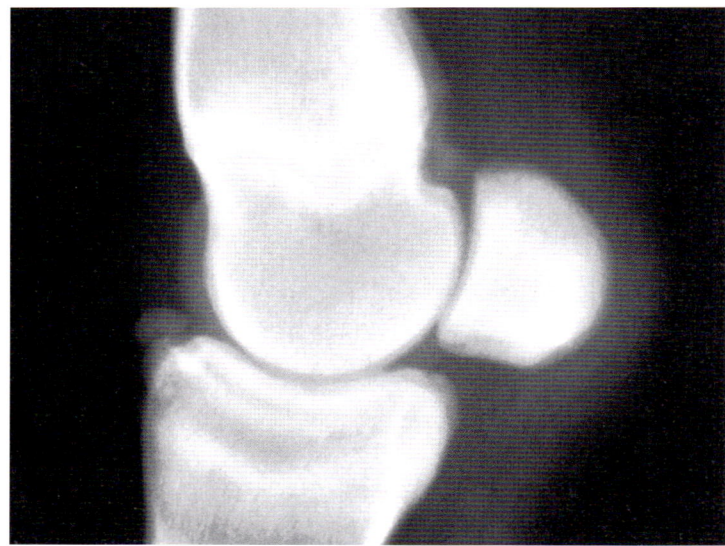

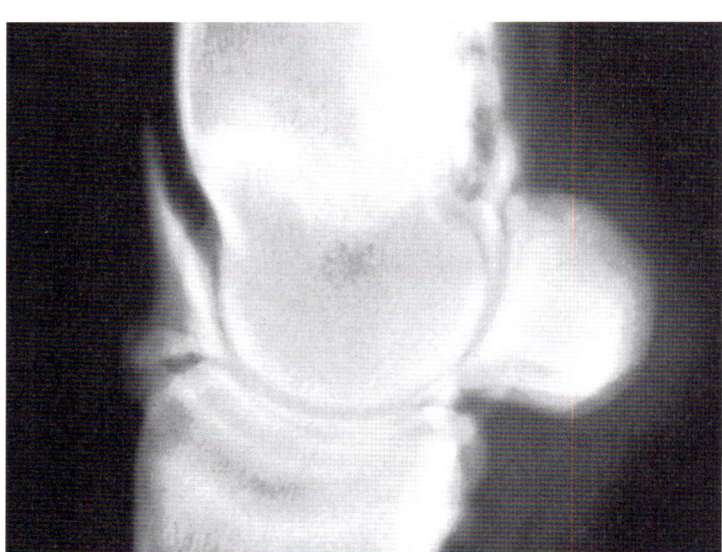

155

156

155/156 Fetlock joint, left hind, lateromedial survey and positive contrast study: close-ups.

Warmblood, 1 ½ years.

The survey study (Fig. 155) reveals a well defined bone fragment close to the dorsoproximal extremity of the first phalanx. The irregularity in the normally smooth cortex indicates that the fragment probably originated from the proximal end of the first phalanx. Four ml positive contrast material (Fig. 156) injected into the joint does not penetrate between the bone fragment and the first phalanx and outlines a thin radiolucent zone covering the bone fragment. These findings indicate that the bone fragment is located intra-articularly, attached to the first phalanx by radiolucent fibrous or cartilaginous tissue and covered by joint cartilage. These bone fragments are relatively common and considered of little or no clinical significance, as long as there is no radiographic or clinical evidence of osteoarthrosis. Mobile intra-articular fragments, either free or attached to the joint capsule, may become trapped between opposing articular surfaces, producing severe acute intermittent lameness.

Proximal sesamoid bone

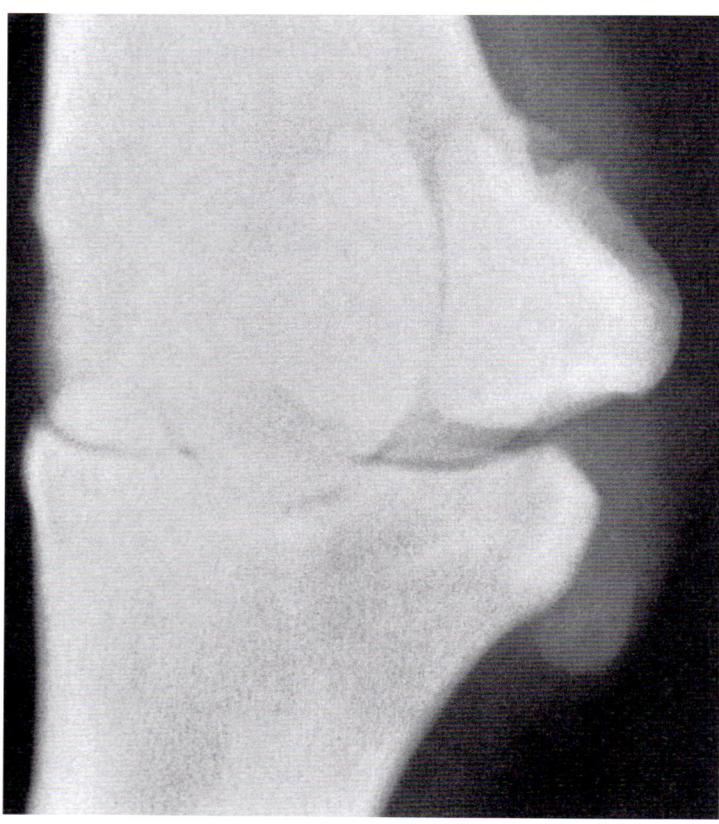

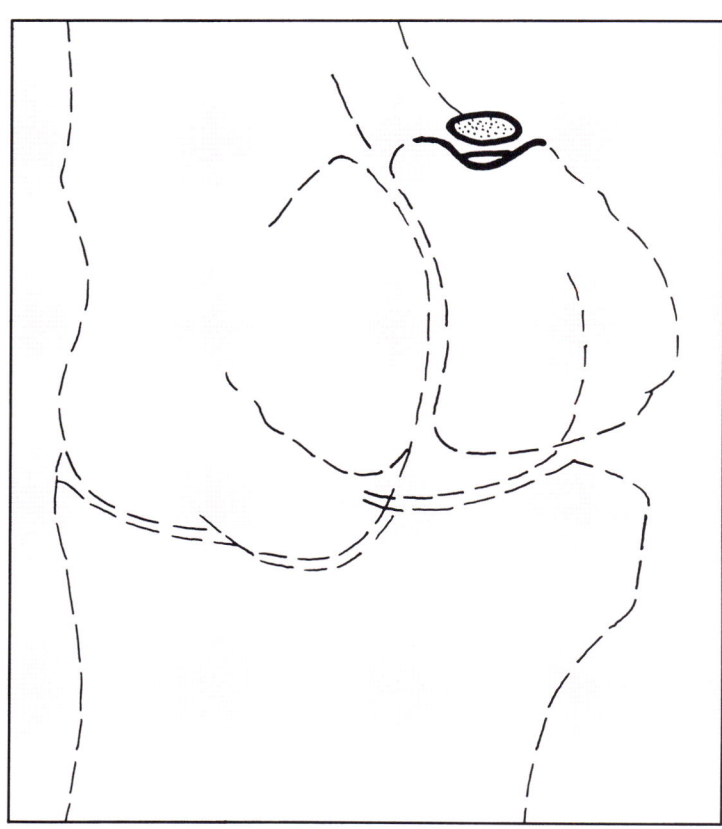

157 Lateral sesamoid bone, left hind, dorsolateral-plantaromedial oblique view: close-up.

Standardbred, 4 years.

A small isolated bone fragment and a corresponding defect in the apical portion of the lateral sesamoid bone, resulting from a simple, extra-articular avulsion fracture.

157 a Schematic drawing

Proximal sesamoid bone

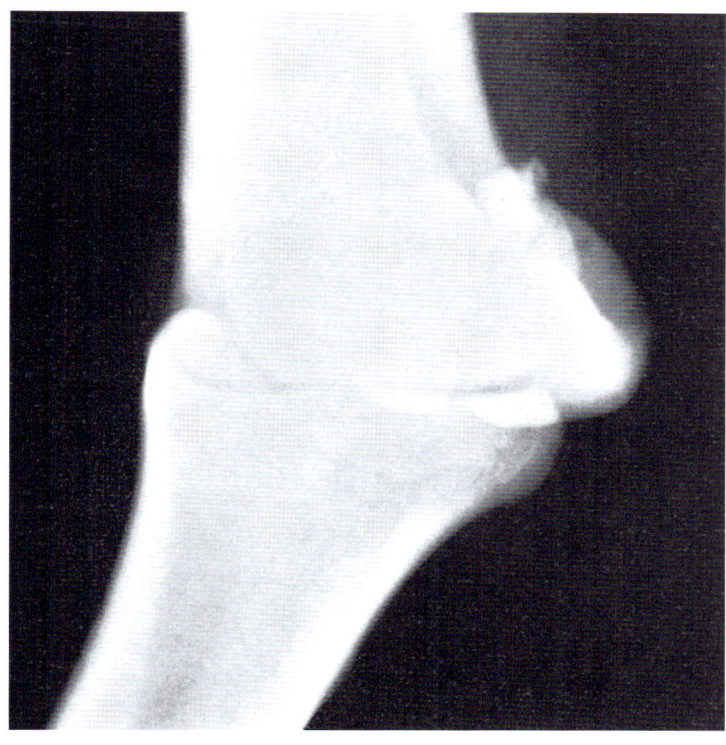

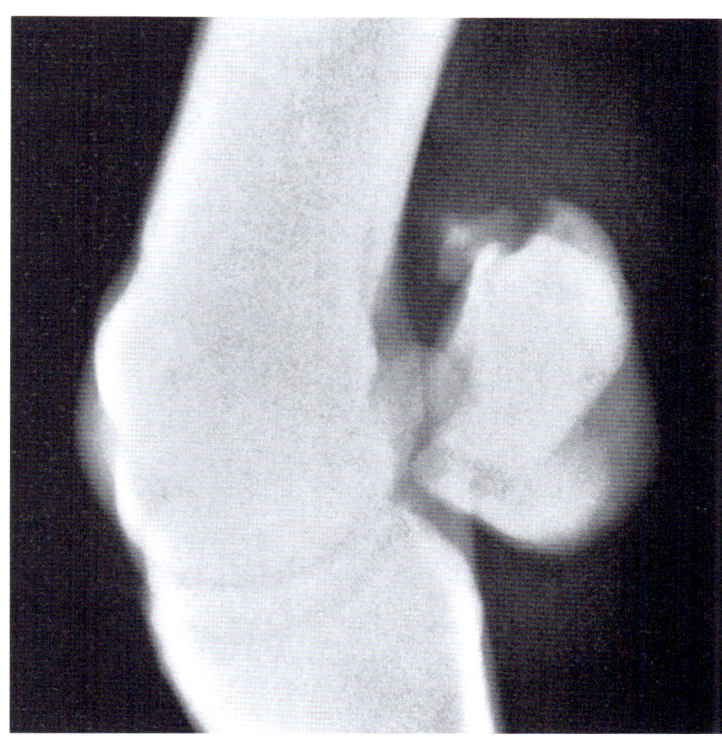

158

159

158/159 Medial sesamoid bone, left front, dorsomedial-palmarolateral oblique and special view.

Warmblood, 4 years.

The usual dorsomedial-palmarolateral oblique view (Fig. 158) presents a remarkable irregular opacity in the apical portion of the medial proximal sesamoid bone, the result of a slightly displaced, overriding, intra-articular, apical fracture fragment, clearly demonstrated by a non-weightbearing, flexed, lateroproximal-mediodistal oblique view made at 20° proximal to the supporting surface, the beam centred on the lateral sesamoid bone (Fig. 159).

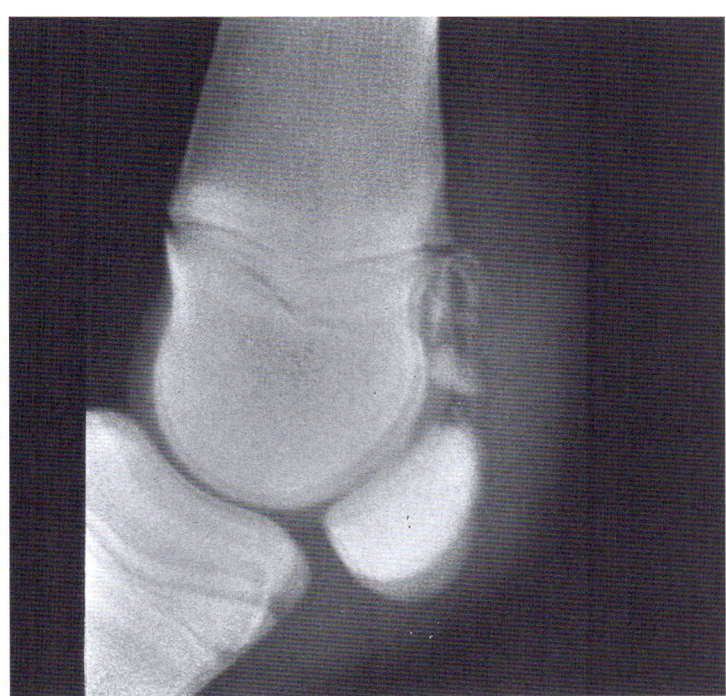

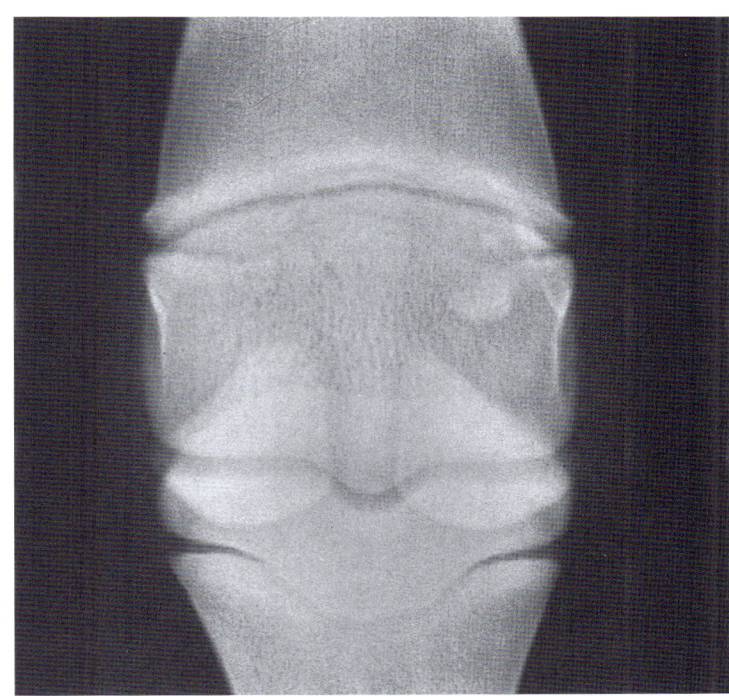

160

161

160/161 Sesamoid bones, left front, lateromedial and dorsopalmar view.

Foal, 1 month.

The lateromedial view (Fig. 160) shows linear and rounded opacities proximal to the sesamoid bones, combined with distal displacement of these bones. The distal displacement of both sesamoid bones is also obvious on the dorsopalmar view (Fig. 161). The crumbly linear opacities are not visible on this projection, the larger rounded opacity appears situated proximal to the lateral sesamoid bone.

These findings indicate apical fragmentation of both sesamoid bones and associated distal displacement of these bones.

In young foals under 2 months of age apical or basilar (Fig. 170, 171) fractures of the proximal sesamoid bones are not uncommon and probably result from galloping to exhaustion while trying to keep up with their dam.

(Pseudo)Fracture

Proximal sesamoid bones

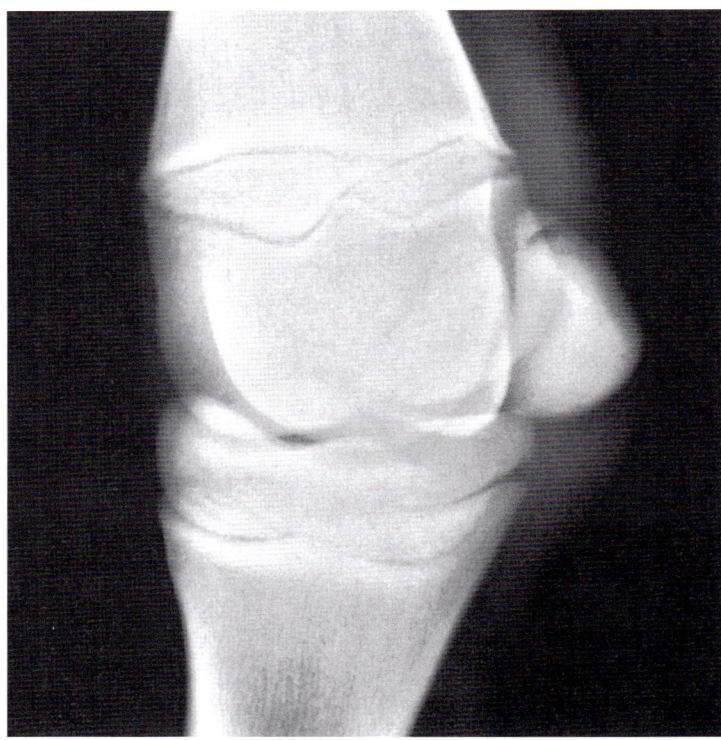

162 Medial sesamoid bone, left front, dorsomedial-palmarolateral oblique view.

Foal, 2 months.

A small isolated non-displaced bone fragment within the apical portion of the medial proximal sesamoid bone. In young foals such as this one either a non-displaced fracture fragment or a separate ossification centre.

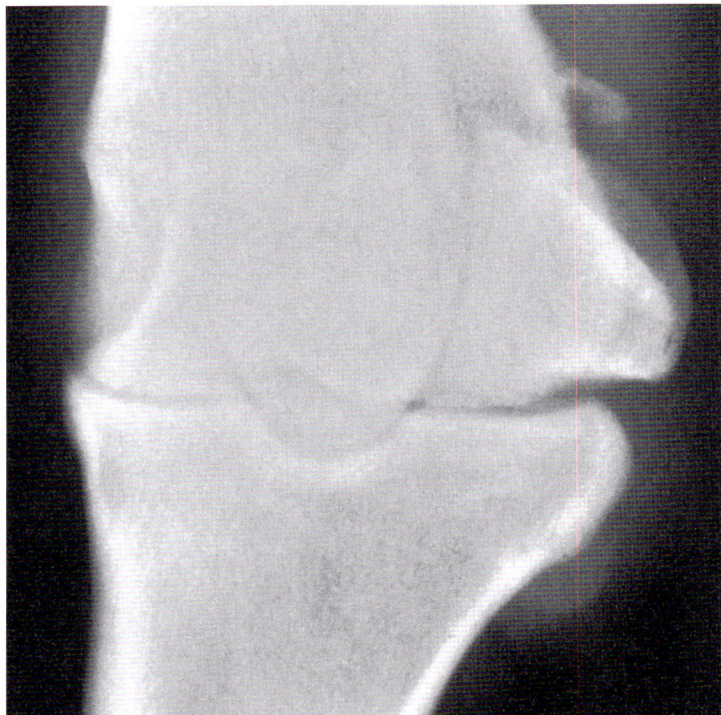

163 Lateral sesamoid bone, left hind, dorsolateral-plantaromedial oblique view.

Warmblood, 6 years.

A well-defined irregular opacity proximal to the apex of the lateral sesamoid bone without a corresponding defect in the abaxial border of the sesamoid bone. The opacity was artefactual, caused by scurf on the skin, demonstrating that the leg should be carefully examined and all debris brushed or washed away before the radiographic examination.

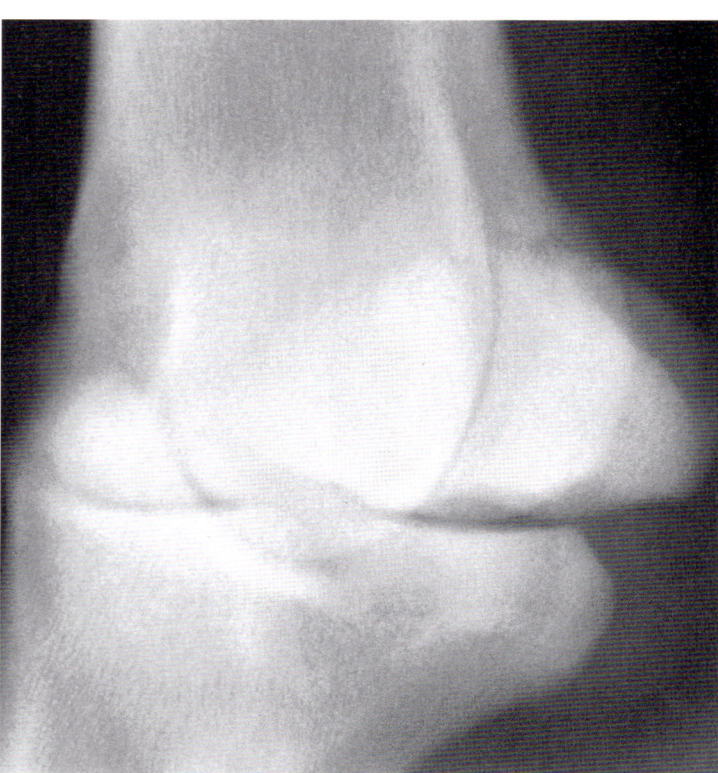

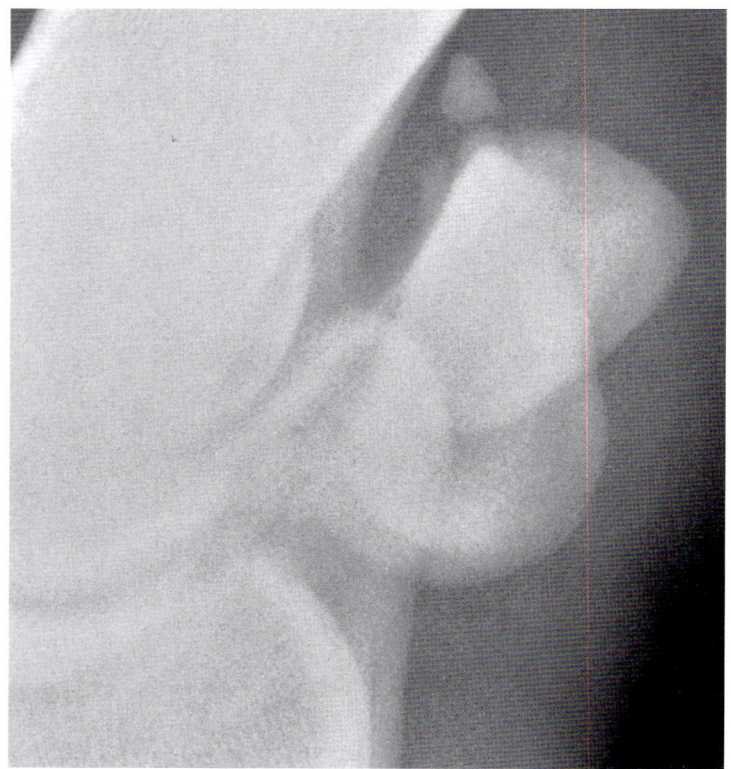

164/165 Lateral sesamoid bone, left front, dorsolateral-palmaromedial oblique and special view: close-ups.

Warmblood, 5 years.

The usual dorsolateral-palmaromedial oblique view (Fig. 164) shows an obscure opacity proximal to the apex of the lateral proximal sesamoid bone without a corresponding defect in the abaxial border. The opacity was an isolated calcified deposit in the apical fibro-osseous junction and not a fracture, clearly demonstrated on a non-weight-bearing flexed medioproximal-laterodistal oblique view made at 20° proximal to the supporting surface, the beam centred on the medial sesamoid bone (Fig. 165).

Proximal sesamoid bones

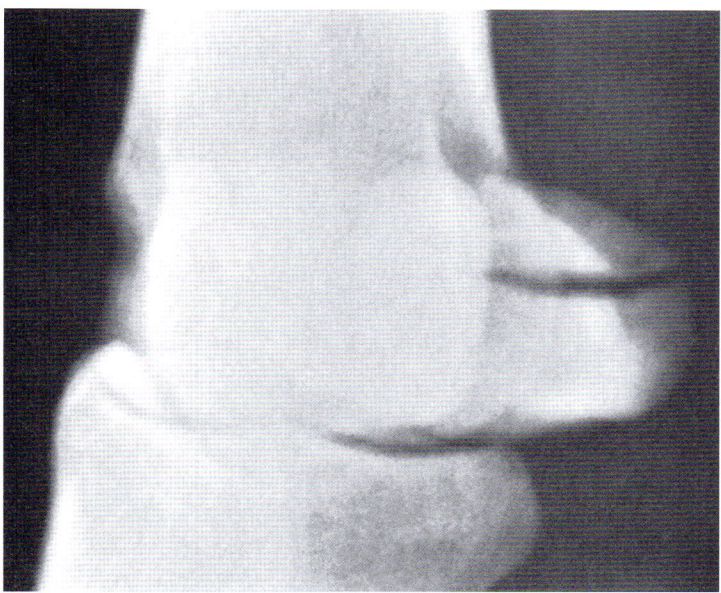

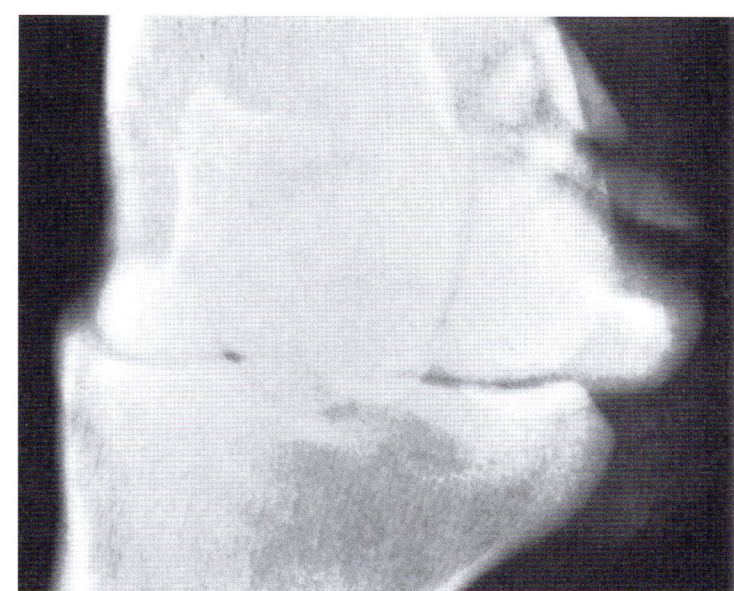

166 Medial sesamoid bone, left hind, dorsomedial-plantarolateral oblique view: close-up.

Standardbred, 4 years.

A horizontal radiolucent zone through the midbody of the medial proximal sesamoid bone due to a simple intra-articular fracture with slight displacement of the proximal fracture fragment. The well defined margins of the fracture zone and uniform density of the bone fragments indicate a recent fracture of traumatic origin.

167 Lateral sesamoid bone, right hind, dorsolateral-plantaromedial oblique view: close-up.

Standardbred, 4 years.

Multiple sharply delineated bone fragments due to a recent intra-articular comminuted fracture of the proximal third of the lateral sesamoid bone.

The fragmentation and gross displacement indicate severe injury of the suspensory attachment.

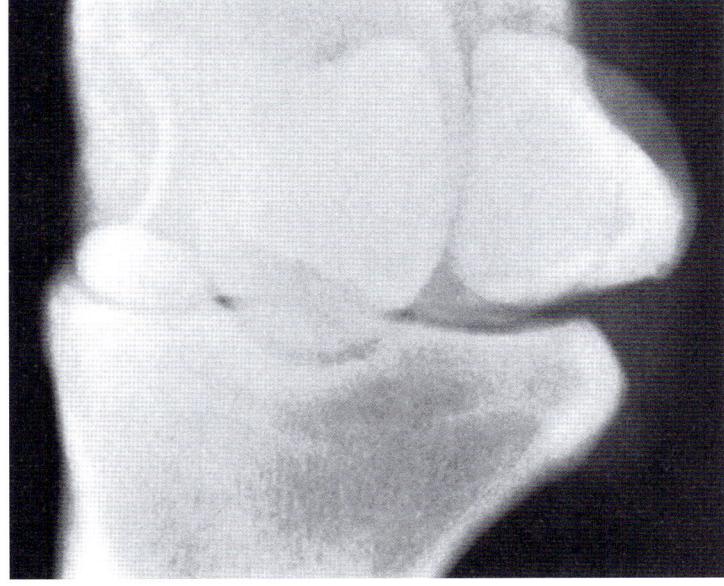

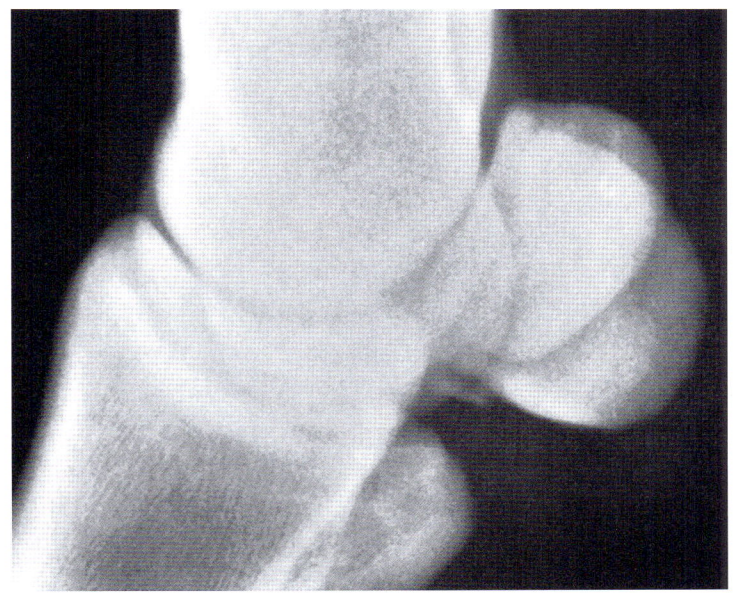

168

169

168/169 Lateral sesamoid bone, right hind, dorsolateral-plantaromedial oblique and special view: close-ups.

Thoroughbred, 12 years.

A special weight-bearing extended dorsoproximolateral-plantarodistomedial oblique view made at 20° proximal to the supporting surface and 75° lateral to the dorsoplantar line, the beam centred on the lateral sesamoid bone (Fig. 169), shows a small isolated bone fragment and a corresponding defect in the basilar surface of the lateral sesamoid bone, indicating a simple intra-articular avulsion fracture. On the usual dorsolateral-plantaromedial oblique projection (Fig. 168) the bone fragment is almost completely obscured by the superimposed sesamoid and cannon bone.

N. B. A small basilar avulsion fragment of the proximal sesamoid bone may be an incidental finding of little or no clinical significance.

Fracture

Proximal sesamoid bone

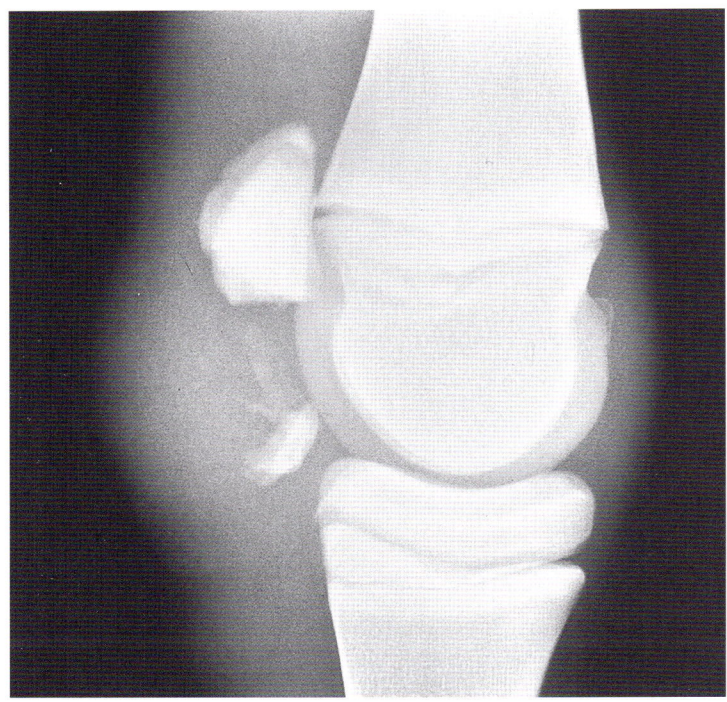

170

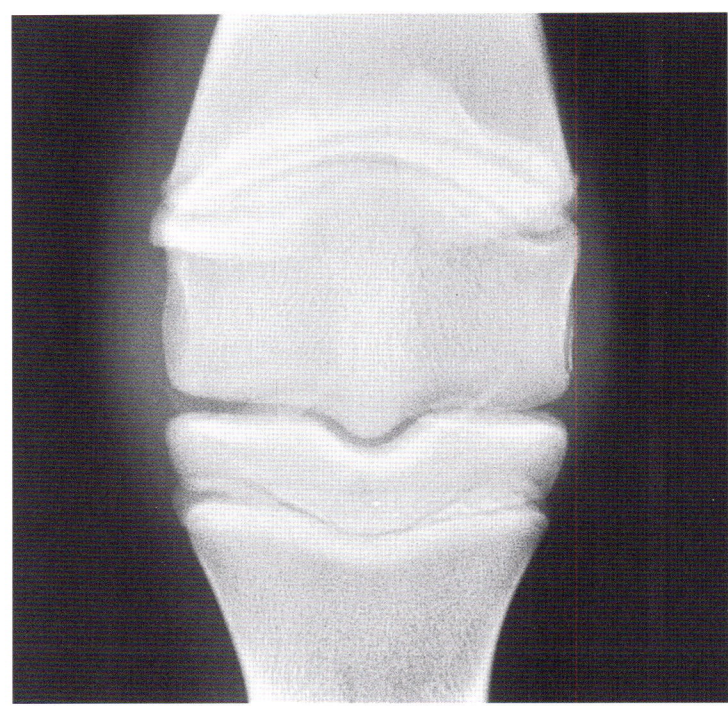

171

170/171 Sesamoid bones, right front, lateromedial and dorsopalmar view

Foal, 10 days.

The lateromedial view shows clear and obscure irregular opacities distal to the sesamoid bones, combined with flattening of the distal sesamoidean contour and proximal displacement of these bones. The proximal displacement of both sesamoid bones is also clearly demonstrated on the dorsopalmar radiograph (Fig. 171), but the basilar opacities are not obvious on this view.

These findings indicate basilar fracture of both sesamoid bones and associated proximal displacement of these bones.

The majority of sesamoidean fractures in young foals are simple basilar fractures of the medial sesamoid bone of the right and/or left front limb. Apical sesamoidean fractures occur less frequently.

Associated sesamoidean displacement occurs if such fractures involve both sesamoid bones. Basilar fractures result in proximal displacement and apical fractures cause distal displacement of both sesamoid bones (Fig. 160, 161).

Fracture/Luxation

Proximal sesamoid bone

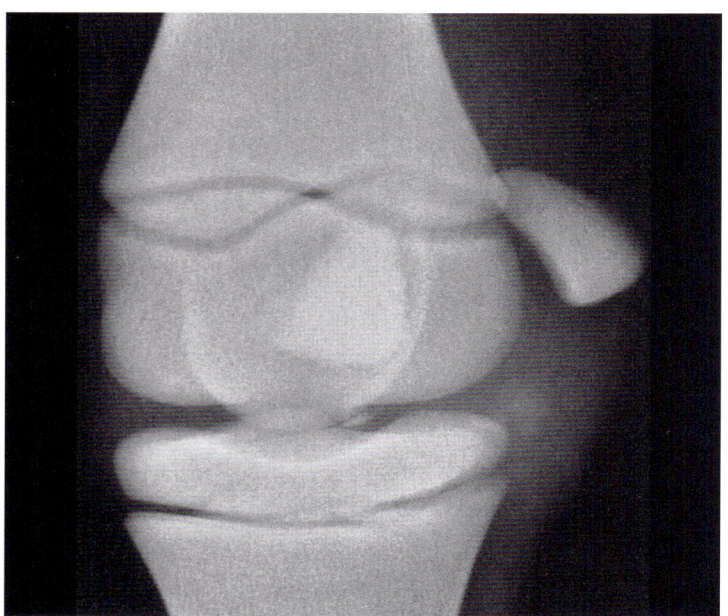

172 Lateral sesamoid bone, right front, dorsolateral-palmaromedial oblique view: close-up.

Foal, 1 month.

Upward rotation and proximal displacement of the lateral proximal sesamoid bone, caused by tearing of the distal ligaments from the sesamoid bone. Small ill defined bone fragments palmar to the medial and lateral palmaroproximal extremity of the first phalanx indicate that rupture of the ligamentous attachment occurred at the time of fracture, although the origin of the avulsed fragments is not visualized.

172

Suspensory ligament avulsion

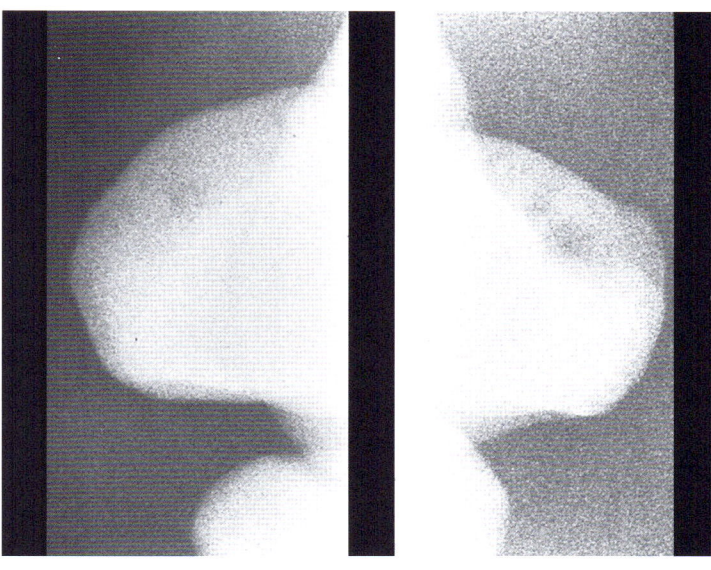

173   174

173/174 Sesamoid bones, right hind, dorsolateral – plantaromedial oblique and dorsomedial-plantarolateral oblique view: close-ups.

Pony, 9 years.

The obscure local textural irregularity in the midproximal region of the lateral sesamoid bone (Fig. 173) and the more obvious rounded lucencies limited to the midproximal region of the medial sesamoid bone (Fig. 174) are suggestive of an insertion injury of both suspensory ligament branches.

A definitive diagnosis requires additional ultrasonographic assessment.

Annular ligament avulsion

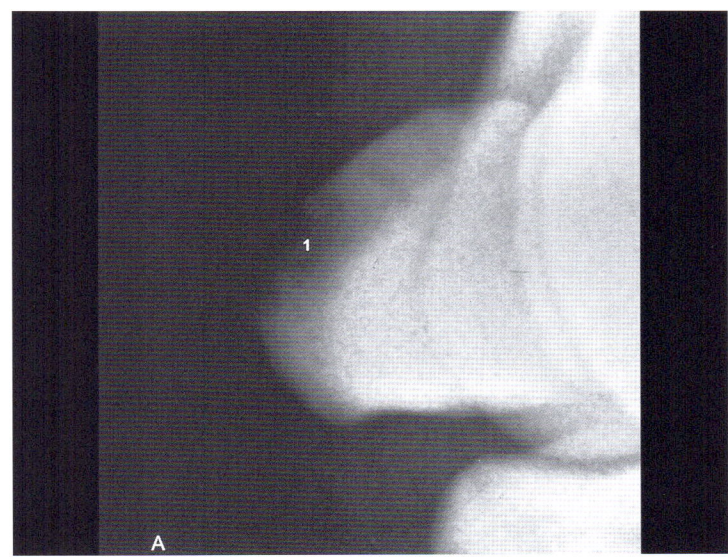

175

175 Lateral sesamoid bone, right hind, dorsolateral – plantaromedial oblique view: close-up.

Quarter horse, 5 years.

Local, ill bordered radiolucency **(1)** in the midabaxial region of the lateral sesamoid bone, suggestive of injury of the attachment of the annular ligament.

Additional imaging with ultrasonography is indicated for a definitive diagnosis.

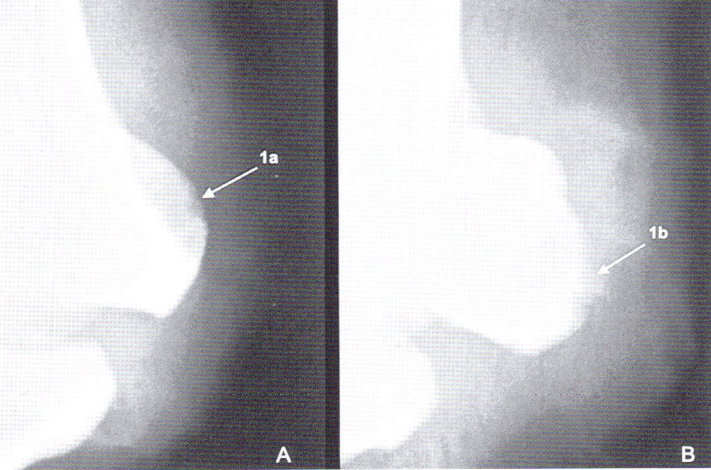

176 a   176 b

176 Lateral sesamoid bone, left hind, dorsolateral-plantaromedial oblique and slightly obliqued lateromedial view: close-ups.

Warmblood, 3 years.

The dorsolateral – plantaromedial oblique view (Fig. 176a) reveals a local ill defined radiolucency **(1a)** in the midabaxial region of the lateral sesamoid bone.

Additional ultrasonography confirmed associated injury of the annular ligament attachment to the abaxial sesamoidean surface.

The slightly obliqued lateromedial radiograph (Fig. 176b) demonstrates that the local midabaxial lucency on the standard oblique radiographic view actually represents the superimposed irregular avulsion defect of the abaxial sesamoidean border **(1b)**.

The differential diagnosis of such a contour defect includes abaxial sesamoid bone lysis due to infection resulting from a puncture wound (Fig. 218).

Avulsion injuries of the proximal sesamoid bones

Annular ligament avulsion

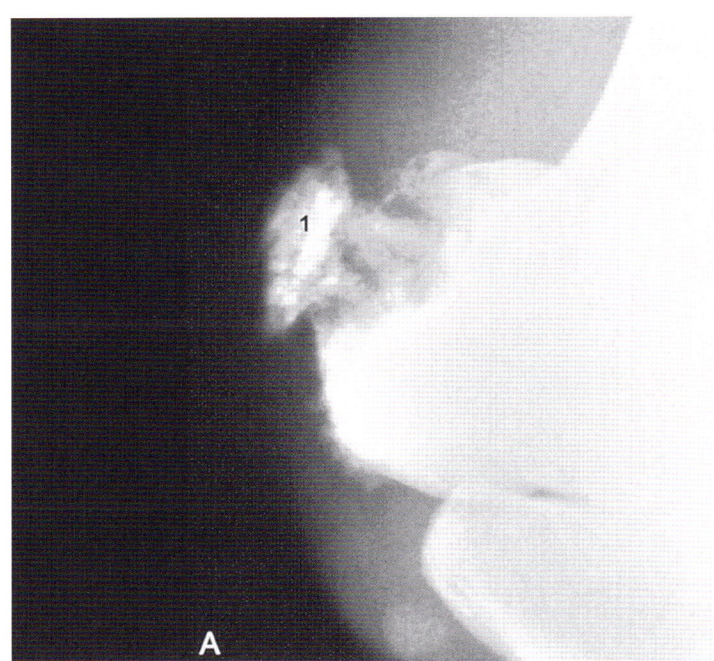
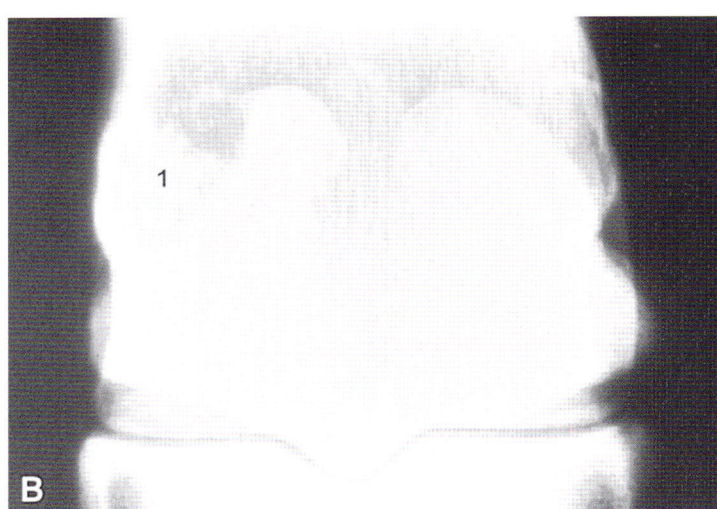

177 a   **177 b**

177 Lateral sesamoid bone, right front, dorsolateral – palmaromedial oblique and dorsopalmar view: close-ups.

Warmblood, 18 years.

A large irregular bone fragment, a corresponding defect in the abaxial sesamoidean contour and associated ill bordered new bone formation along the abaxial border of this bone resulting from an annular ligament avulsion injury of 10 months duration that was confirmed by ultrasonographic examination.

The radiograhic changes are clearly outlined on the standard oblique radiograph (Fig. 177a), but poorly visible on the additional dorsopalmar view (Fig. 177b) and illustrate the variable radiographic appearance of annular ligament insertion injury (see also Fig. 175, 176).

Intersesamoidean ligament avulsion

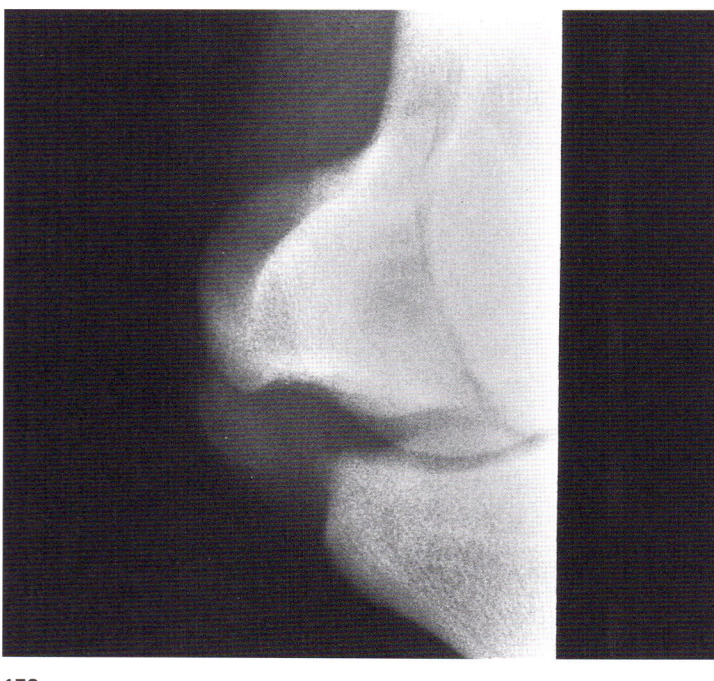
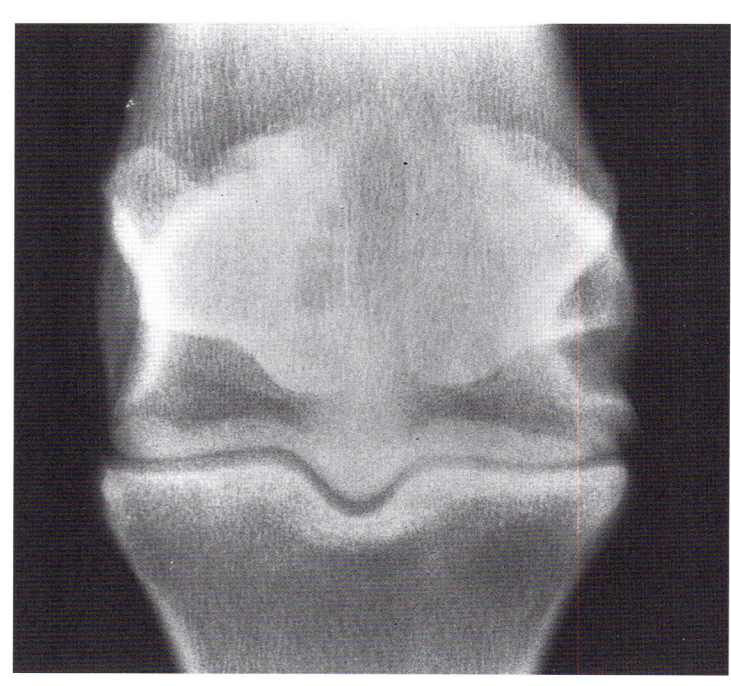

178   **179**

178/179 Lateral sesamoid bone, left hind, dorsolateral – plantaromedial oblique and dorsoplantar view: close-ups.

Warmblood, 2 years.

Local irregular radiolucency in the midaxial region of the lateral sesamoid bone, suggestive of injury of the attachment of the intersesamoidean ligament.

The lesion is most obvious on the dorsoplantar view (Fig. 179) and less apparent on the standard oblique projection (Fig. 178). Additional imaging with ultrasonography is required for a definitive diagnosis.

Schematic drawings

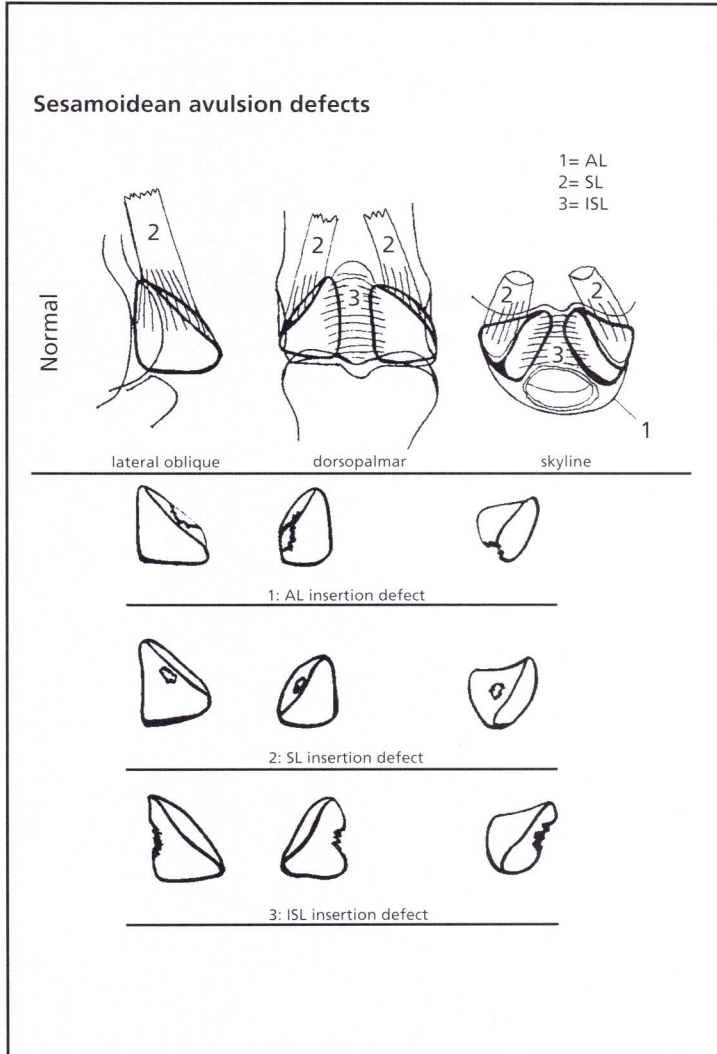

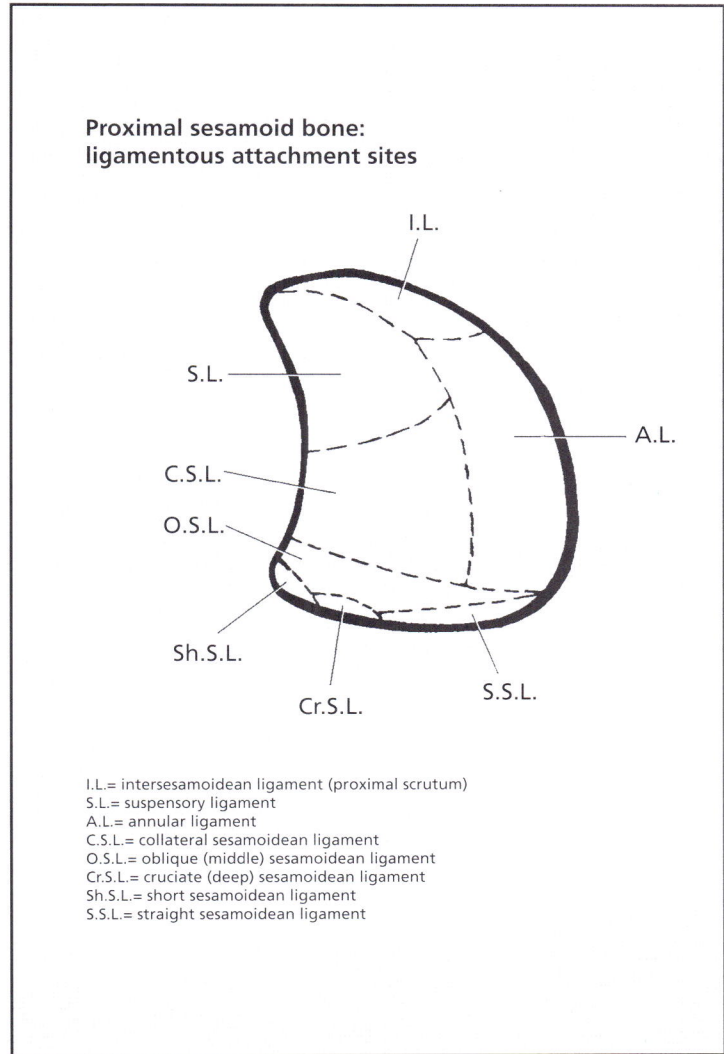

180 Schematic drawing of the location of annular ligament (AL), suspensory ligament (SL) and intersesamoidean ligament (ISL) avulsion defects on the usual oblique and additional dorsopalmar (plantar) or proximodistal skyline radiographs.

181 Schematic drawing demonstrating the various ligamentous attachment sites on the proximal sesamoid bone.

Disease of the proximal sesamoid bone
Dorsolateral-palmaromedial or dorsomedial-palmarolateral oblique views: close-ups.

Extra-articular changes (sesamoiditis)
Vascular channels

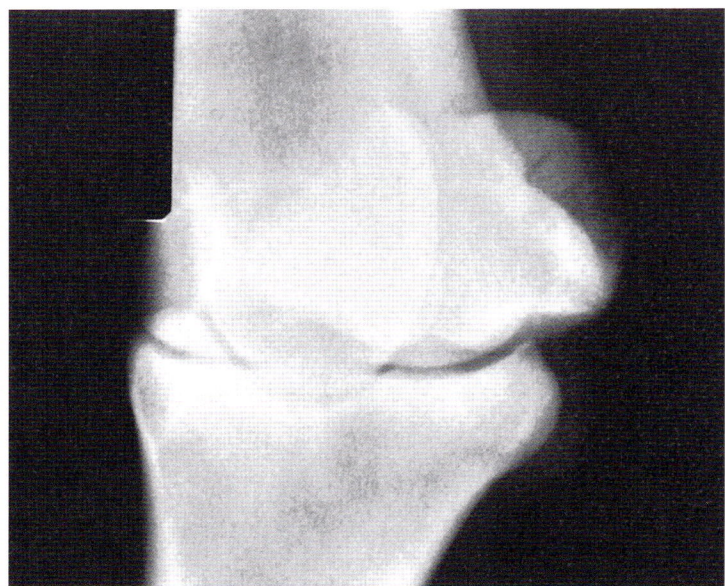

182 Lateral sesamoid bone, left front.

Standardbred, 3 years.

Prominent, slightly widened, sharply bordered vascular channels **(1)**, a slight loss of bone density in the concavity of the abaxial surface and minimal new bone formation **(2)** along the disto-abaxial border of the sesamoid bone.

Sharply bordered vascular channels slightly wider than usual are of variable clinical significance, present in lame as well as sound horses.

Additional finding: a small bony spur **(3)** on the palmar aspect of the proximal margin of the first phalanx.

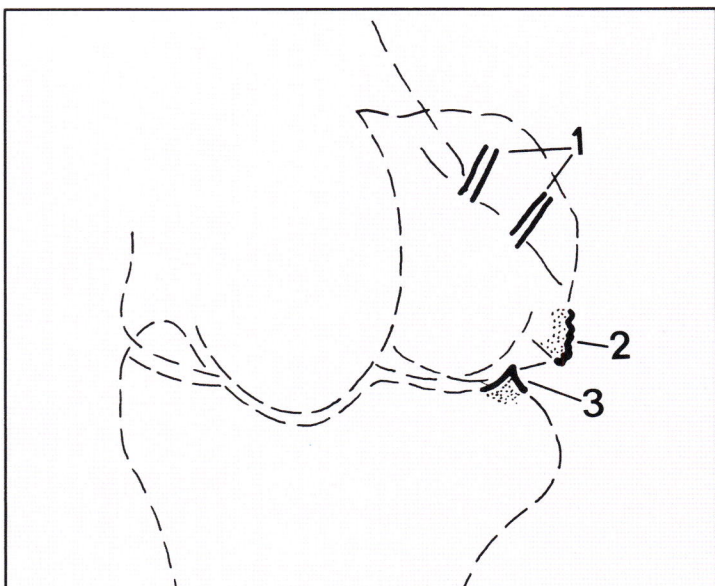

182 a Schematic drawing

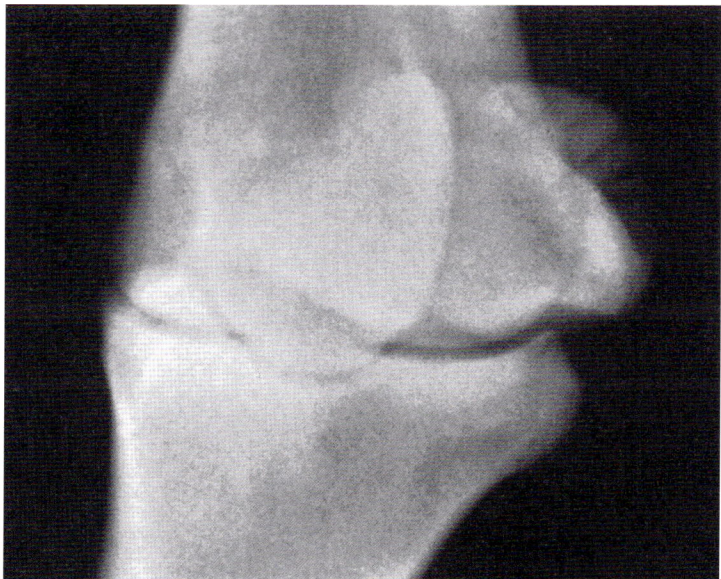

183 Lateral sesamoid bone, right front.

Warmblood, 5 years.

Several small sharply bordered foramina, one widened ill bordered vascular channel **(1)** and slight loss of bone density in the concavity of the abaxial surface.

Three or four narrow vascular channels with definite margins are unimportant changes seen in many sound horses, but widened ill bordered vascular channels are significant changes present mainly in lame horses.

Additional finding: minimal spur formation **(2)** on the dorsal and palmar aspect of the proximal margin of the first phalanx.

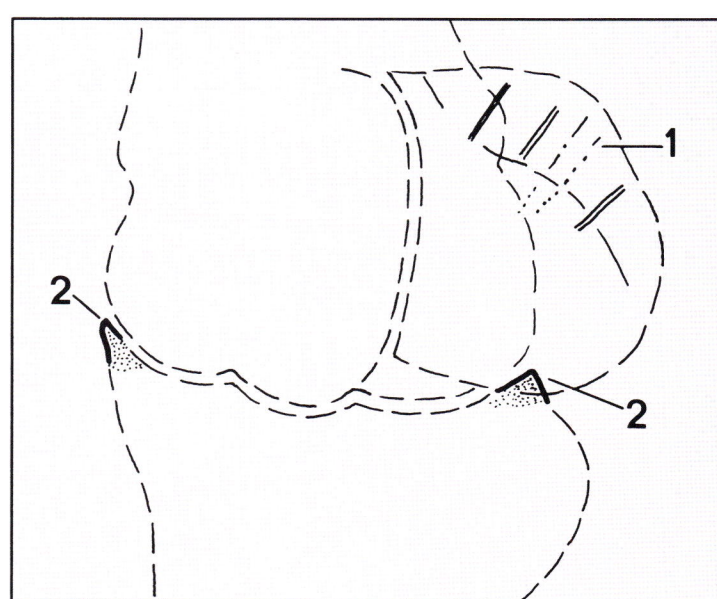

183 a Schematic drawing

Disease of the proximal sesamoid bone
Dorsolateral-palmaromedial or dorsomedial-palmarolateral oblique views: close-ups.

The Fetlock Joint

Extra-articular changes (sesamoiditis)
Vascular changes

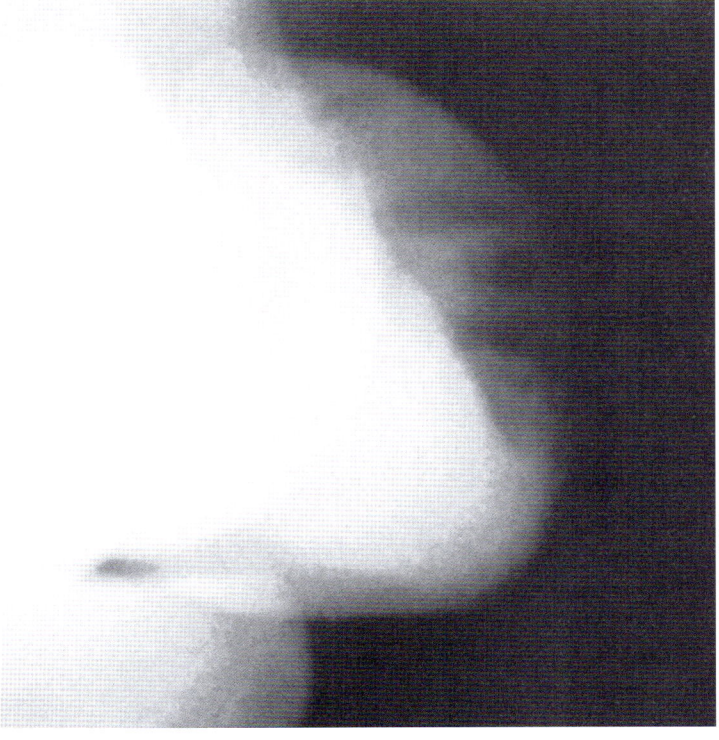

184

184 Medial sesamoid bone, left front.

Standardbred, 3 years.

Extremely widened ill bordered vascular channels, which are present in lame horses and are of definitive clinical significance in confirming sesamoiditis.

Extra-articular changes (sesamoiditis)
Alteration of the trabecular pattern

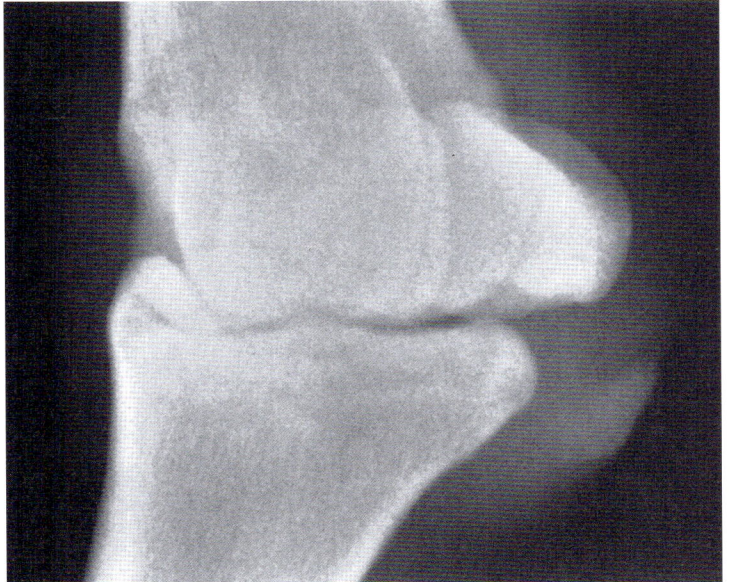

185 Lateral sesamoid bone, left front.

Pony, 2 years.

A coarse trabecular pattern throughout the sesamoid bone, due to slight disuse osteoporosis resulting from 2 months of inactivity (stall rest).

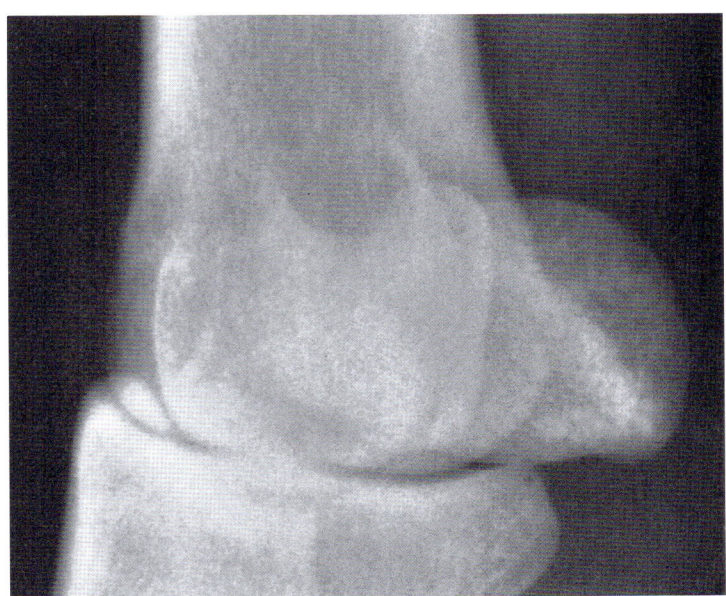

186 Medial sesamoid bone, right front.

Standardbred, 3 years.

A mottled trabecular pattern throughout the sesamoid bone, resulting from severe disuse osteoporosis. Similar radiographic changes are visible within the palmaroproximal extremity of the first phalanx and, less obviously, in the rest of the first phalanx and the cannon bone.

Minimal (disuse) osteoporosis is visible only in thinner (parts of) bones, but severe generalized demineralization is also visible in other parts of the skeleton.

Extra-articular changes (sesamoiditis)
Alteration of the trabecular pattern

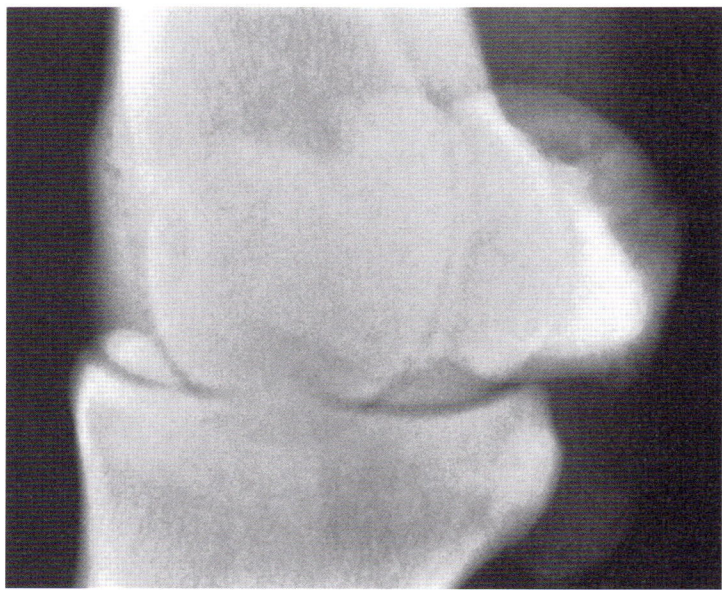

187

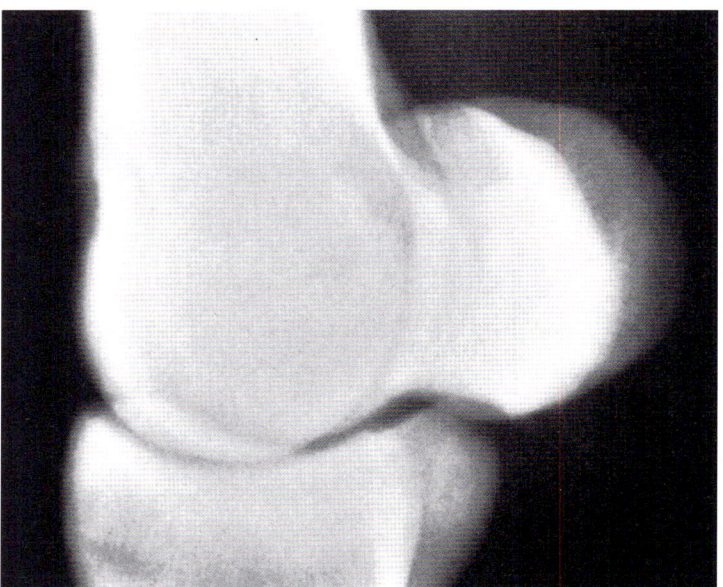

188

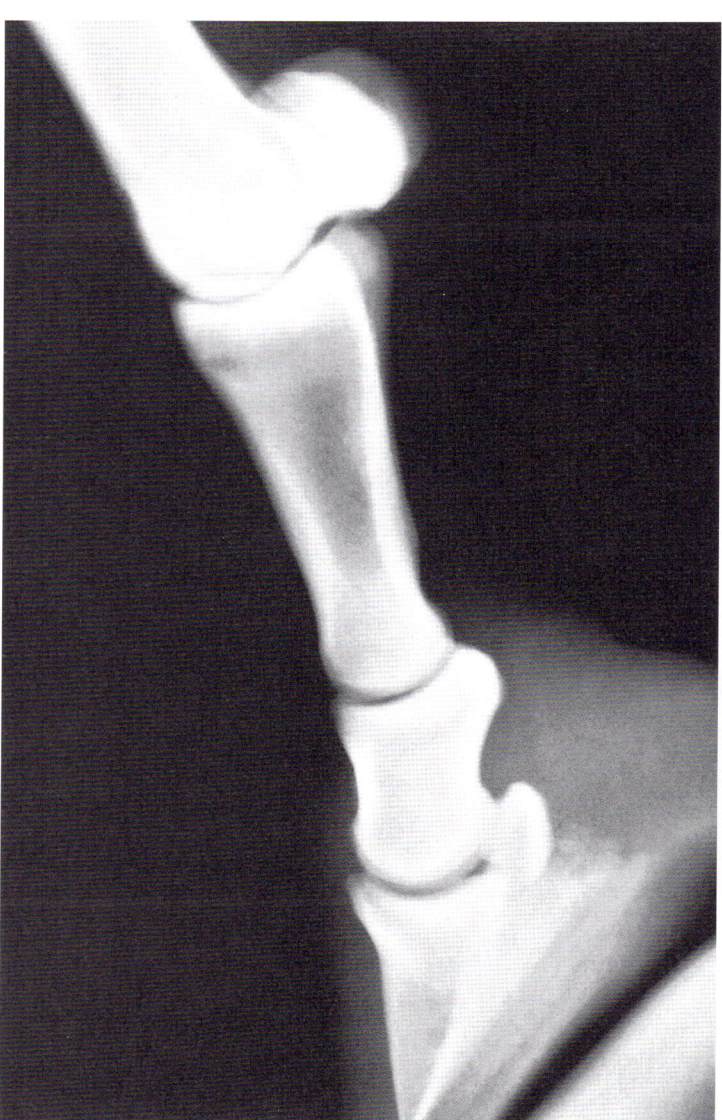

189

187/188/189 Fetlock joint, right front, dorsomedial-palmarolateral oblique view: close-up of the medial sesamoid bone, lateromedial view: close-up of the fetlock joint and lateromedial survey radiograph of the foot including the fetlock.

Warmblood, 6 years.

The dorsomedial-palmarolateral oblique view (Fig. 187) presents a patchy trabecular pattern limited to the concavity of the abaxial surface of the sesamoid bone.

These significant changes are associated with primary disease of the suspensory apparatus and result from local variation in bone production and resorption.

Additional finding: new bone formation at the disto-abaxial border of the sesamoid bone.

On the lateromedial view (Fig. 188) of the fetlock and the lateromedial survey radiograph of the foot (Fig. 189) the irregular patchy trabecular pattern in the sesamoid bone as well as the new bone formation at the disto-abaxial border are obscured by the superimposed lateral sesamoid bone, illustrating the importance of oblique projections for radiographic evaluation of the proximal sesamoid bones.

Disease of the proximal sesamoid bone
Dorsolateral-palmaromedial or dorsomedial-palmarolateral oblique views: close-ups.

The Fetlock Joint

Extra-articular changes (sesamoiditis)
New bone formation – "build up"

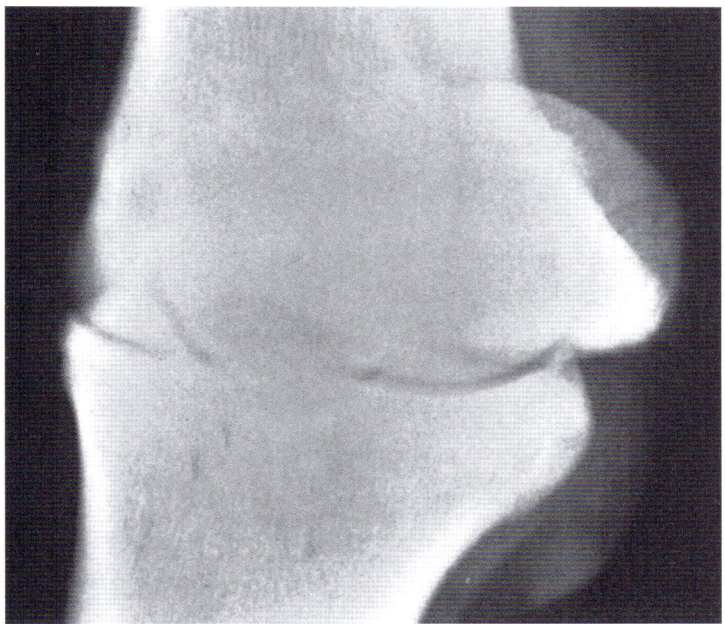

190 Medial sesamoid bone, right front.

Warmblood, 7 years.

Roughening or "sand-paper" appearance **(1)** of the normally smooth outline of the abaxial border and slight irregularity of the trabecular pattern of the sesamoid bone, both resulting from minimal new bone formation along the abaxial surface.

These significant changes are present mainly in lame horses.

Additional finding: a small bony spur **(2)** on the dorsal and palmar aspect of the proximal margin of the first phalanx.

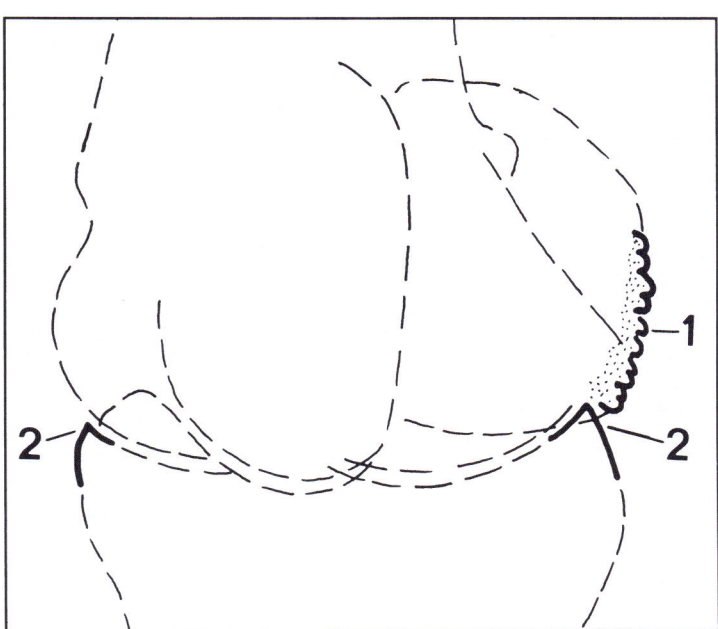

190 a Schematic drawing

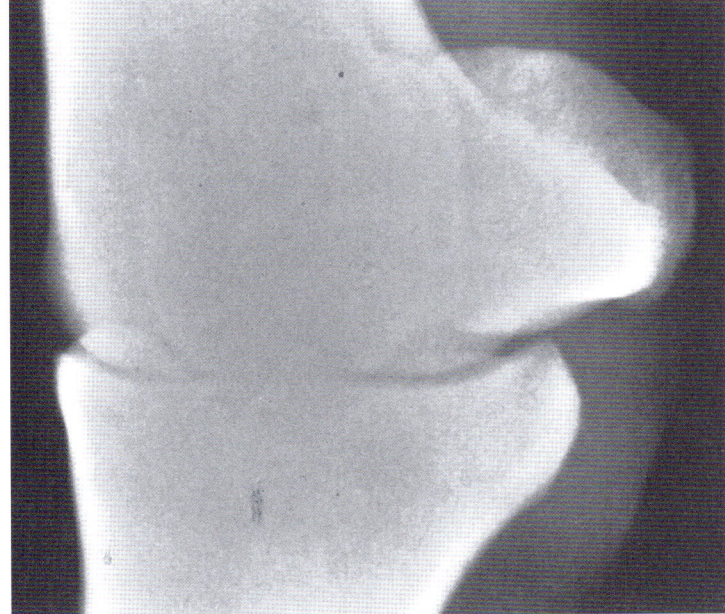

191 Medial sesamoid bone, left front.

Warmblood, 8 years.

More extensive new bone formation along the abaxial border of the sesamoid bone. The sharply delineated outline and density of the bone deposits indicates that the productive response is not recent.

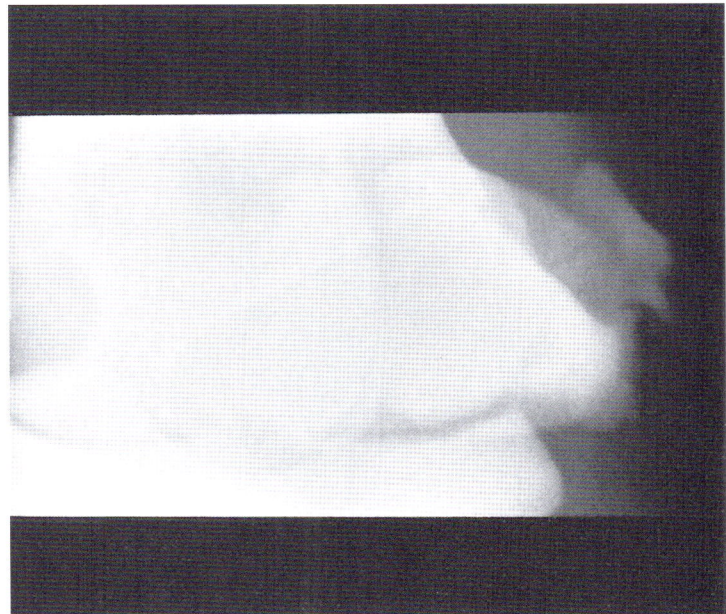

192 Lateral sesamoid bone, left front.

Standardbred, 7 years.

Excessive bone growth at the abaxial border of the sesamoid bone. The enormous build up results in deformation of the affected bone. The changes are of definitive clinical significance in confirming sesamoiditis.

Additional finding: spur formation on the dorsal aspect of the proximal margin of the first phalanx.

Disease of the proximal sesamoid bone
Dorsolateral-palmaromedial or dorsomedial-palmarolateral oblique views: close-ups.

Extra-articular changes
Soft tissue calcification

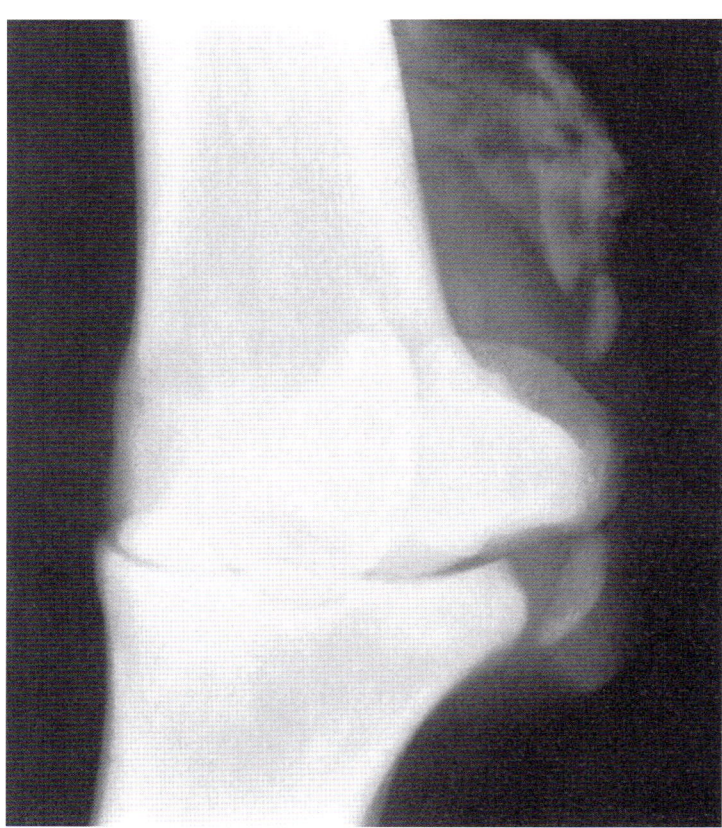

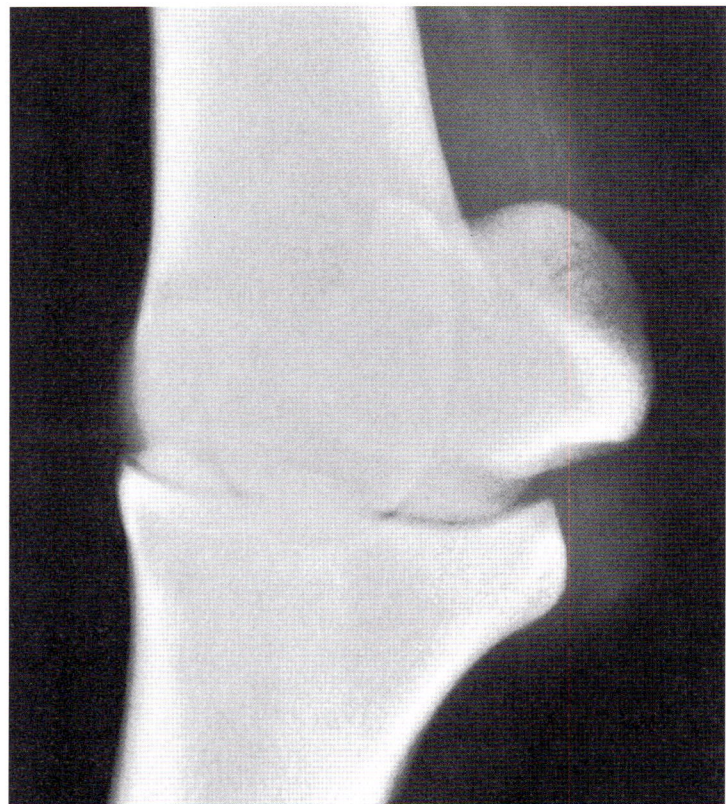

193 Lateral sesamoid bone, left front.

Warmblood, 7 years.

Large clearly defined radiopaque areas proximal and distal to the sesamoid bone, representing calcification of the sesamoidean sheath. Significant changes present mainly in lame horses.

Additional finding: smooth consolidated build up along the abaxial border of the sesamoid bone.

194 Lateral sesamoid bone, right front.

Warmblood, 5 years.

A faint ill bordered linear radiopaque pattern proximal to the sesamoid bone, due to calcification of the ligamentous structures and probably arising from haemorrhage.

These changes are present mainly in lame horses.

N. B. Identical opacities may be artefactual, caused by dirt on the skin.

Additional finding: a widened and ill bordered vascular channel, a coarse trabecular pattern in the sesamoid bone and slight spur formation on the dorsal and palmar aspect of the proximal margin of the first phalanx are indicative of sesamoiditis and osteoarthrosis of the fetlock joint.

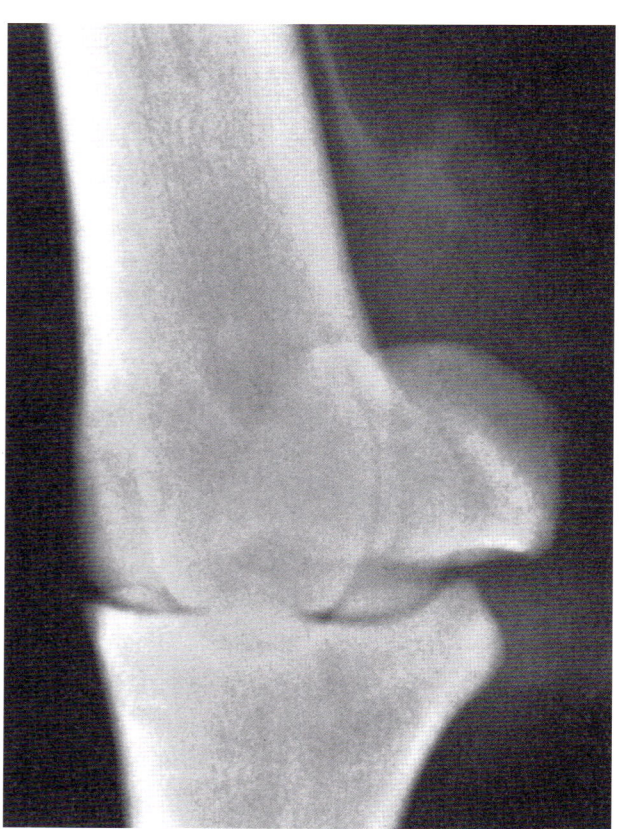

195

195 Medial sesamoid bone, left front.

Standardbred, 6 ¹/₂ years.

A clearly defined soft tissue opacity proximal to the sesamoid bone, representing calcification of the ligamentous structures following local injection of corticosteroids.

Disease of the proximal sesamoid bone
Dorsolateral-palmaromedial or dorsomedial-palmarolateral oblique views: close-ups.

The Fetlock Joint

Extra-articular changes
Soft tissue calcification

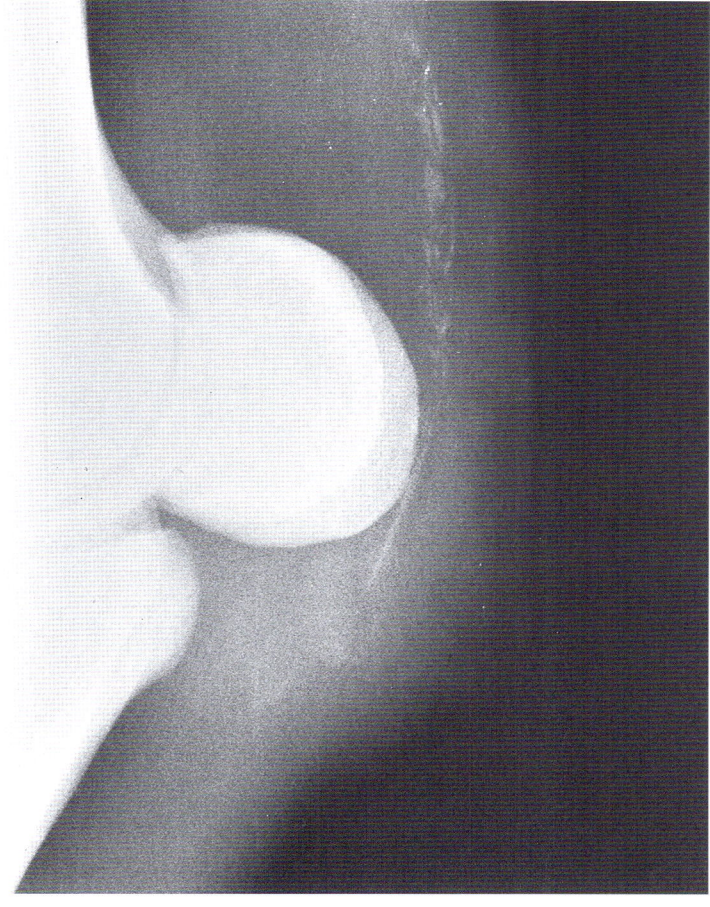

196

196 Sesamoid bones, right front, lateromedial view: close-up.

Warmblood, 10 years,

A vertical zone of clearly defined linear soft tissue radiopacities along the palmar aspect of the sesamoid bones is suggestive of calcification of the deep and/or superficial digital flexor tendon.

Additional imaging with ultrasonography is required for a definitive diagnosis and showed a calcifying core lesion in the deep digital flexor tendon.

Articular changes (osteoarthrosis)
Spur formation

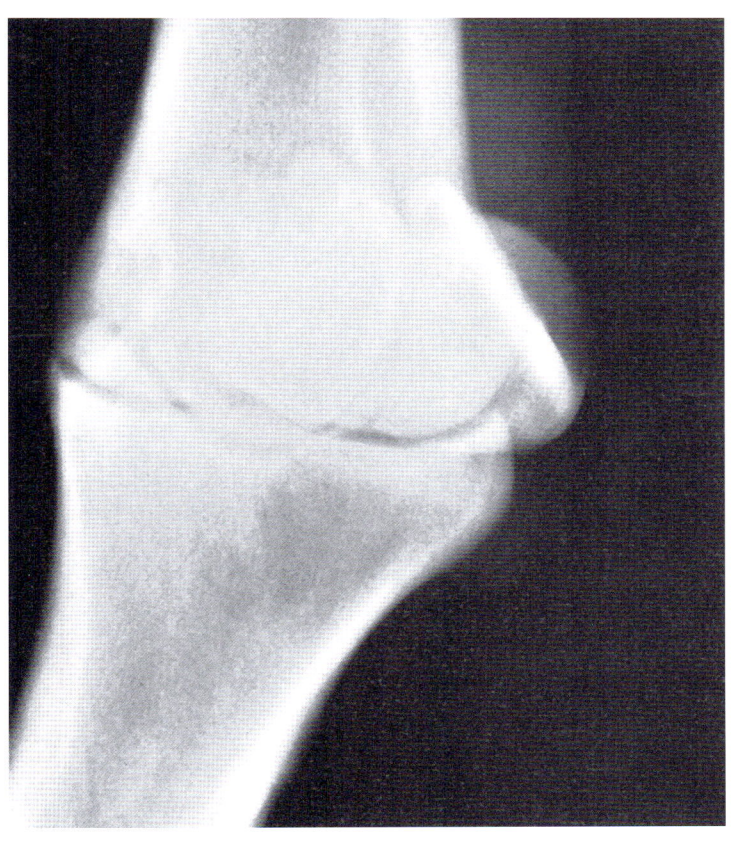

197

197 Lateral sesamoid bone, right front.

Warmblood, 9 years.

Enlargement of the apical portion of the sesamoid bone due to osteophyte formation secondary to osteoarthrosis of the fetlock joint. Similar bony spurs are present on the dorsal and palmar aspect of the proximal margin of the first phalanx.

(Peri)articular osteophytes are changes of variable significance, the larger the spurs the more likely are clinical signs to be present.

Osteoarthrosis

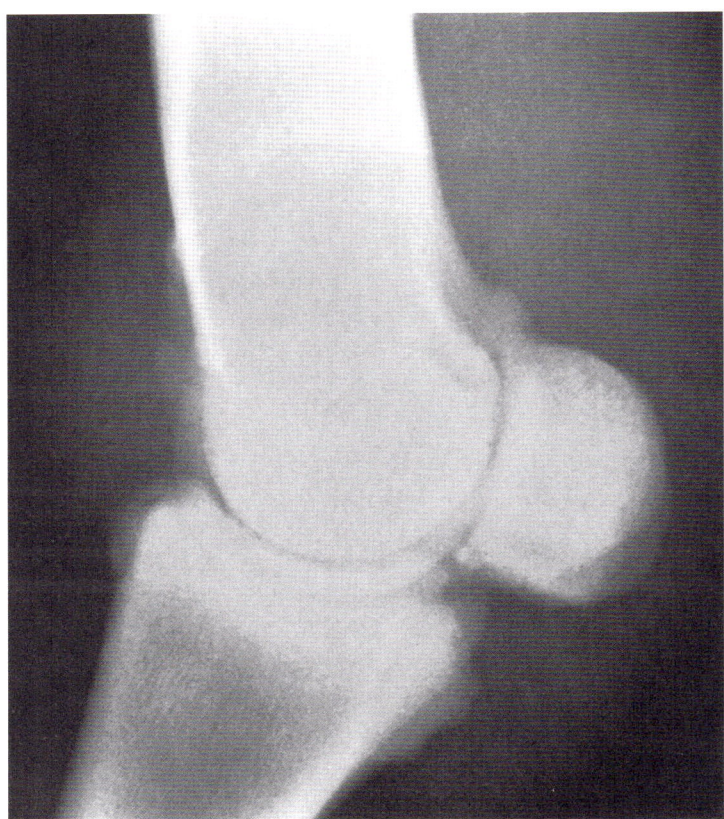

198 Fetlock joint, left hind, lateromedial view.

Warmblood, 7 years.

Distension of the fetlock joint and peri- and intra-articular new bone formation on the dorsal aspect and the plantar aspect of the distal end of the cannon bone, and the proximal end of the first phalanx. These changes result in irregularity of the normally smooth joint margins and indicate the presence of severe osteoarthrosis.

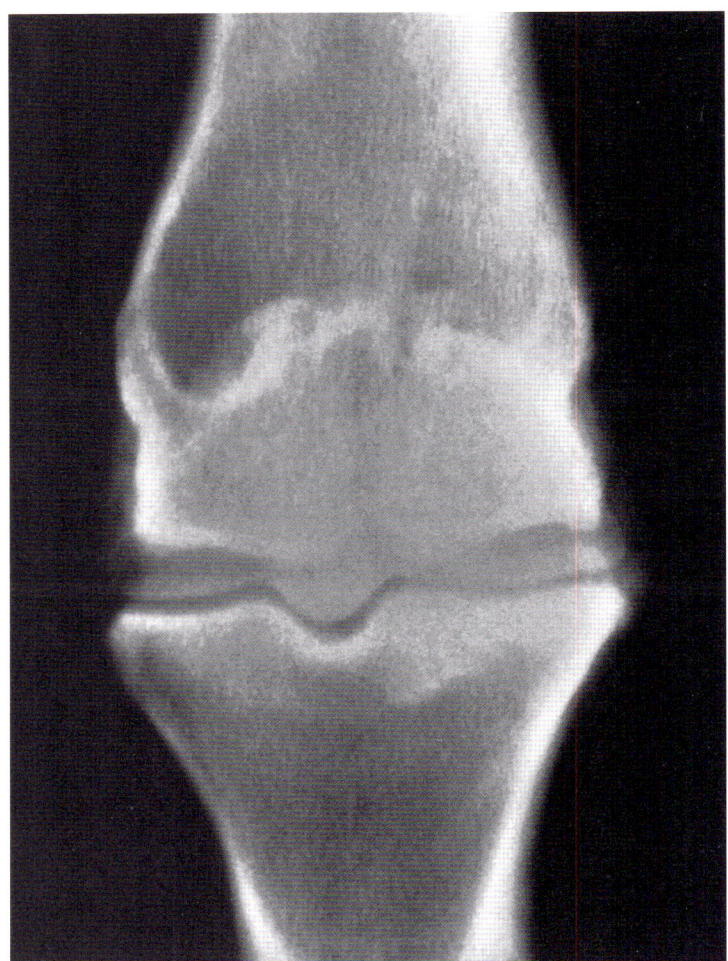

199 Fetlock joint, right hind, dorsoplantar view: close-up.

Warmblood, 2 years.

Narrowing of the medial part of the joint space, subchondral sclerosis in the corresponding portion of the first phalanx, and minimal new bone formation on the corresponding medial aspect of the proximal margin of the first phalanx, indicating osteoarthrosis. The localized subchondral sclerosis (eburnation) results from increased stress due to angulation at the joint space, which also results in unilateral increase in cortical density and thickness of the cannon bone.

Additional finding: extensive deposition of bone along the abaxial border of the sesamoid bones, partly obscured by the superimposed cannon bone.

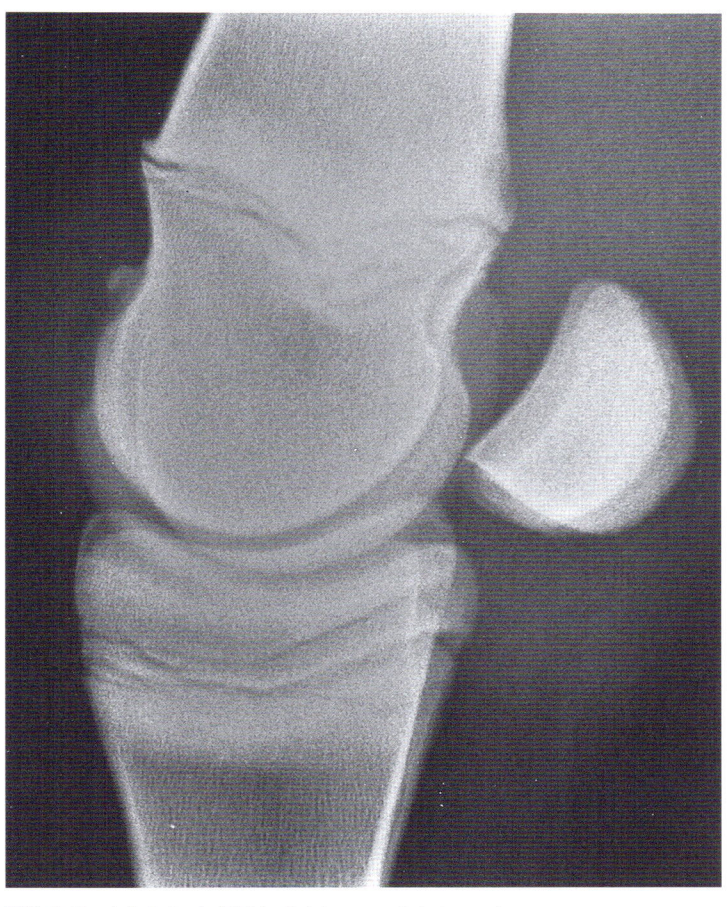

200 Fetlock joint, right hind, lateromedial view: close-up.

Foal, 2 months.

The irregular flattening of the dorsoproximal contour of the sagittal ridge of the cannon bone indicates osteochondrosis.

This condition is a disease of ossifying cartilage and therefore is detectable very early in life. The individual development is variable and unpredictable. The majority of early lesions resolve spontaneously. However, progression is also possible.

Therefore, the radiographic appearance in foals can not be regarded as being definitively abnormal.

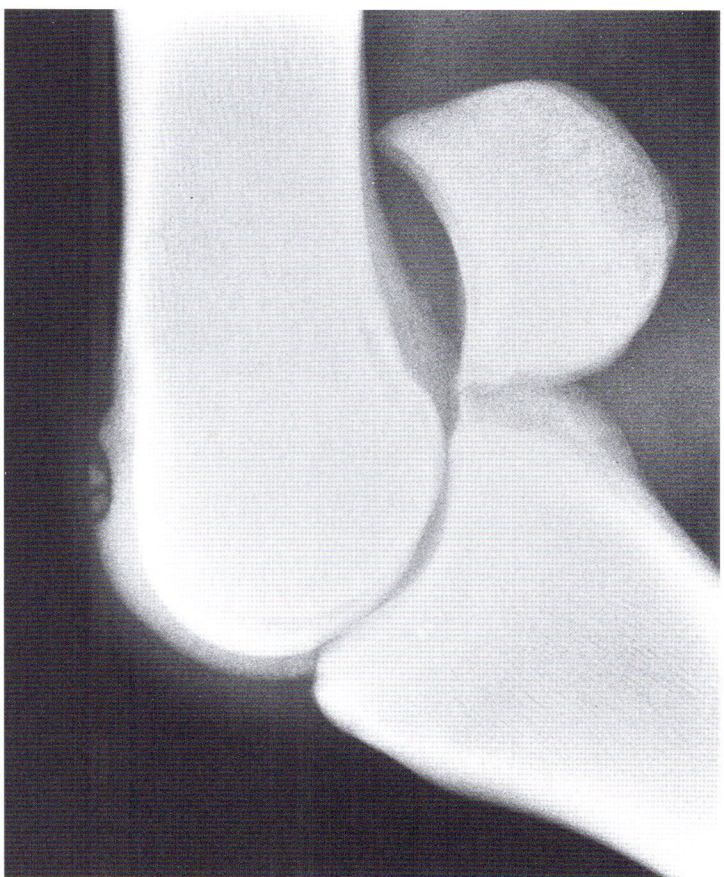

201 Fetlock joint, right front, flexed lateromedial view: close-up.

Warmblood, 4 years.

The rounded concavity and corresponding fragments in the dorsoproximal region of the sagittal ridge of the cannon bone represent the most familiar manifestation of osteochondrosis.

202 Fetlock joint, left hind, lateromedial view.

Warmblood, 4 years.

The obvious rounded concavity in the dorsoproximal contour of the sagittal ridge of the cannon bone, combined with obscure bony fragments situated dorsoproximal to the first phalanx, indicate separation and displacement of osteochondral fragments from the sagittal ridge.

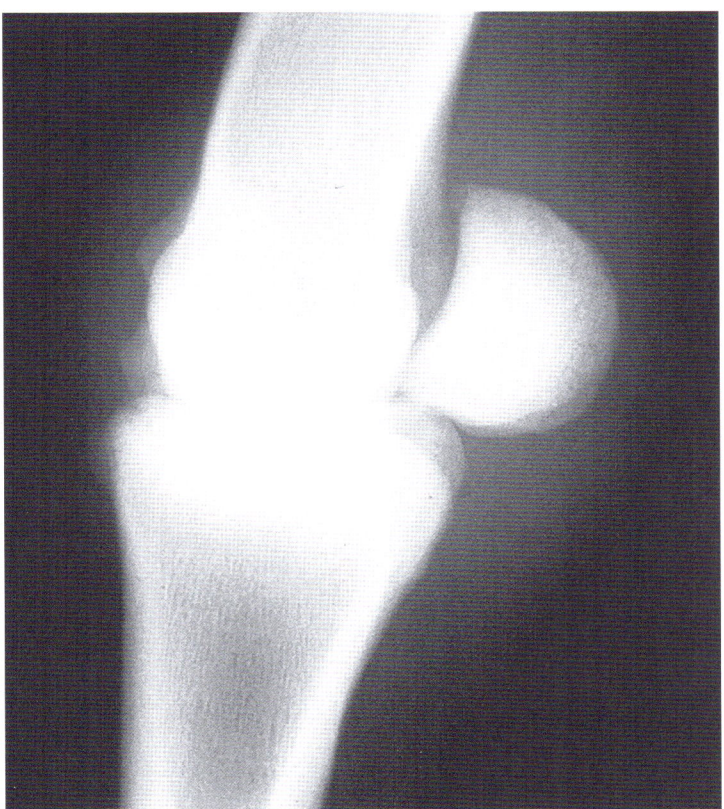

Schematic drawings of fetlock "fragments"

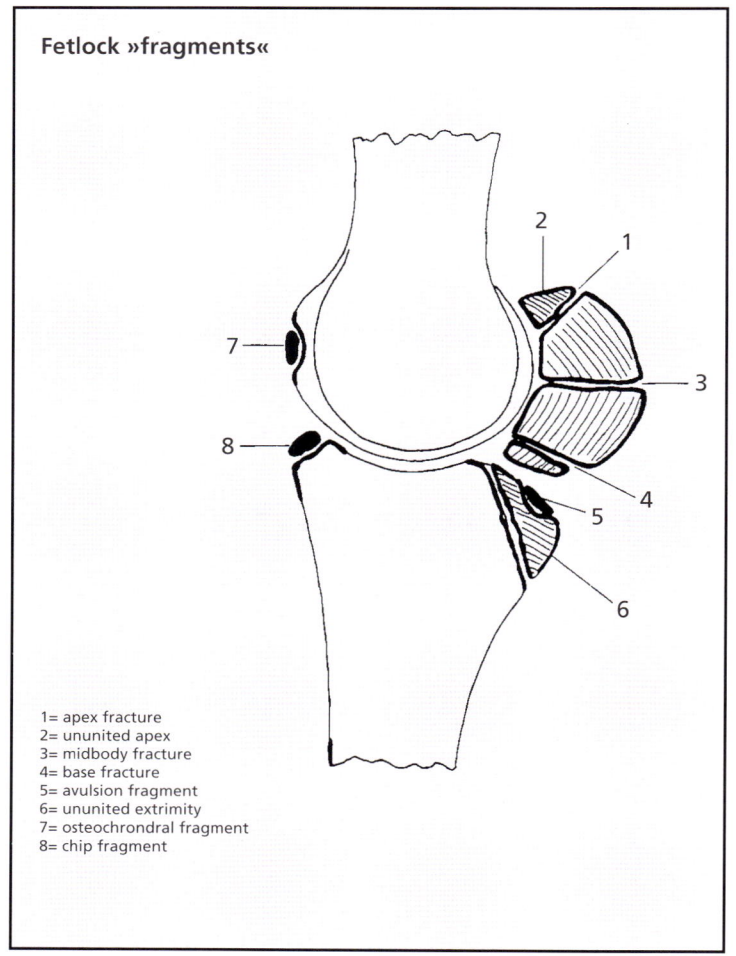

Fetlock »fragments«

1= apex fracture
2= ununited apex
3= midbody fracture
4= base fracture
5= avulsion fragment
6= ununited extrimity
7= osteochrondral fragment
8= chip fragment

203

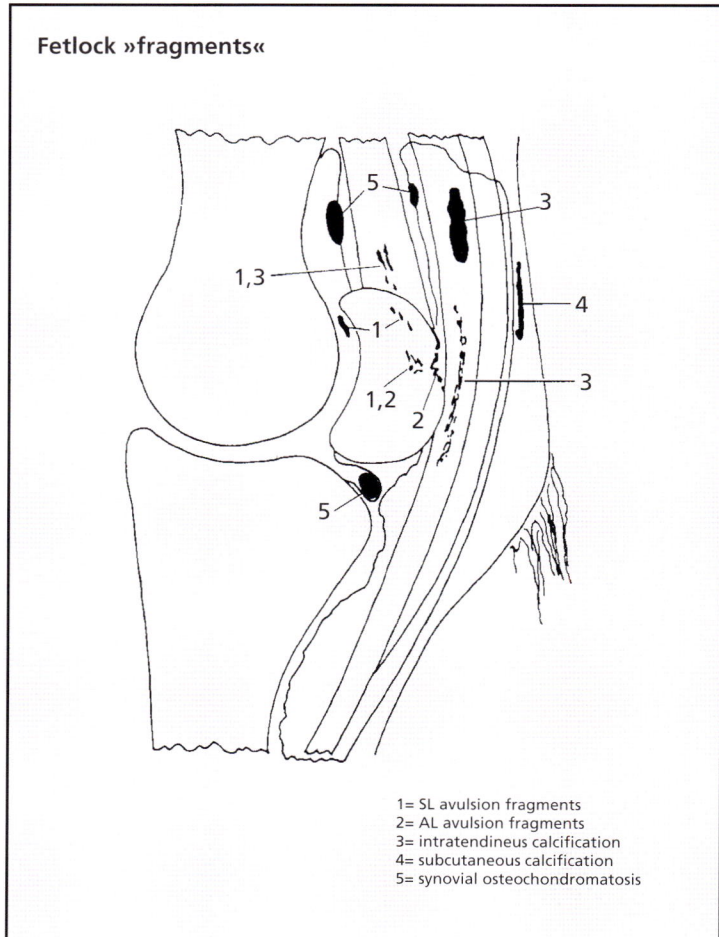

Fetlock »fragments«

1= SL avulsion fragments
2= AL avulsion fragments
3= intratendineus calcification
4= subcutaneous calcification
5= synovial osteochondromatosis

204

203/204 Schematic drawings summarizing the origin and location of various true and false fetlock "fragments".

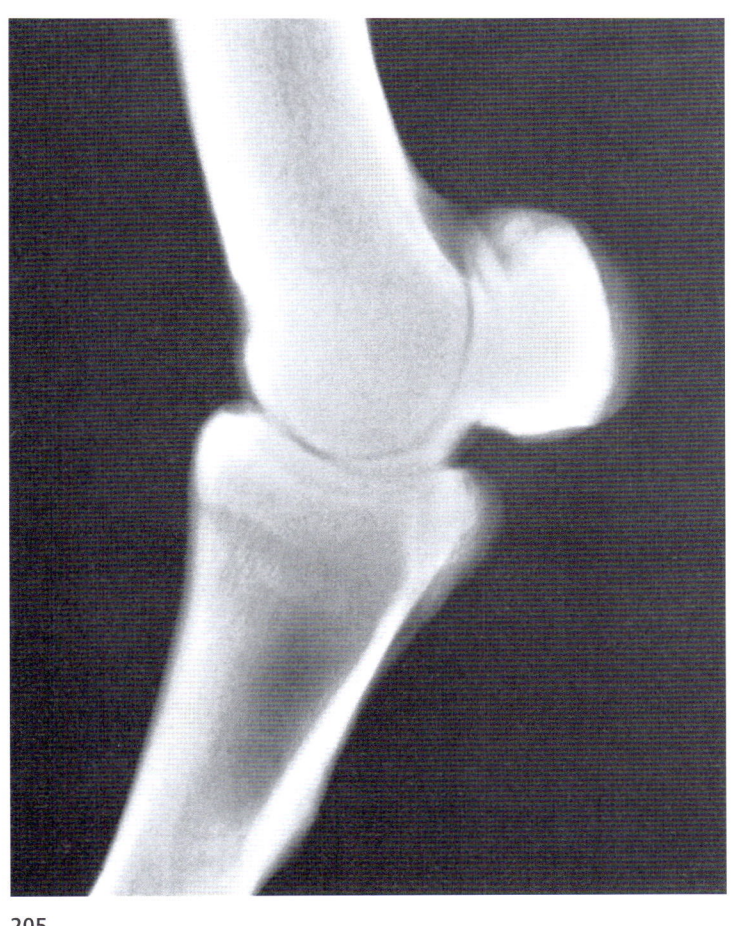

205

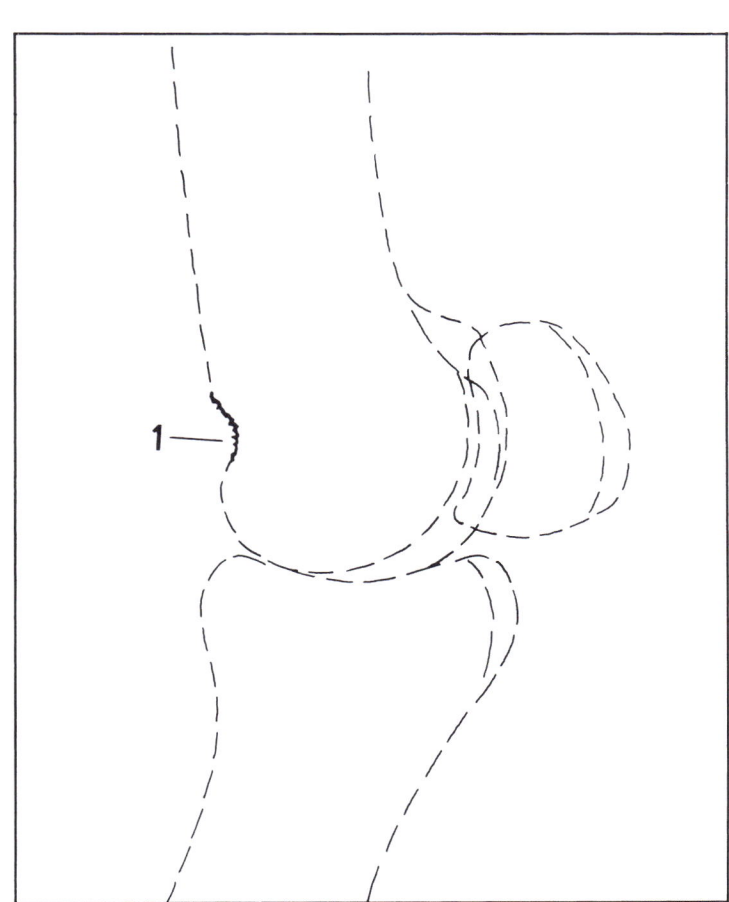

205 a

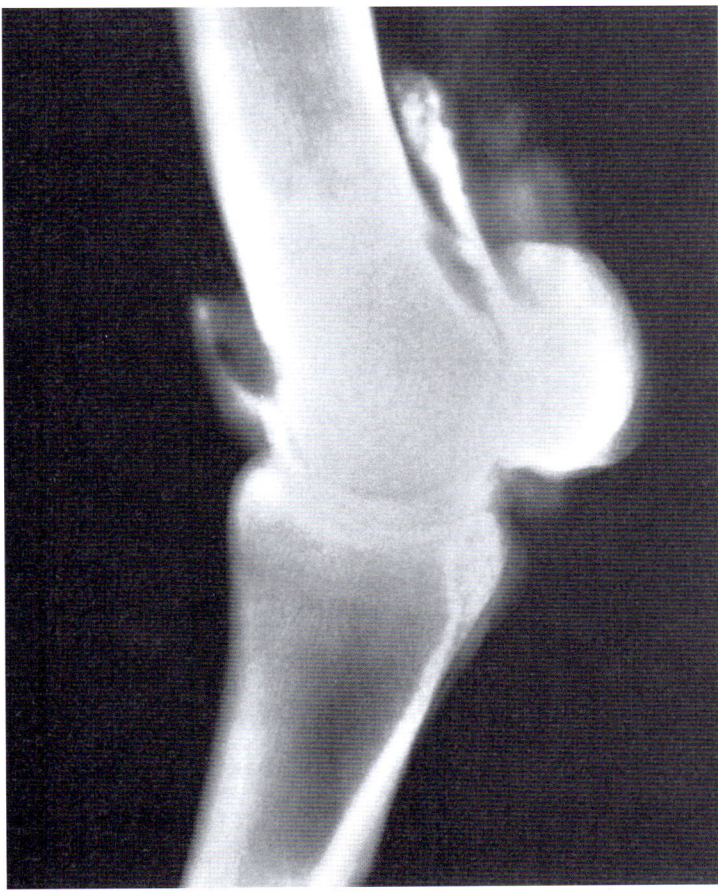

206

206 a

205/206 Fetlock joint, right front, lateromedial survey (Fig. 205) and positive contrast study (Fig. 206).

Warmblood, 5 years.

The lateral survey radiograph reveals a small area of reduced radiographic density **(1)** on the dorsal aspect of the dorsal end of the cannon bone near the chondro-osseous junction. Six ml positive contrast material injected into the joint outlines a nodular "filling defect" **(2)** at the level of the bone erosion which is probably caused by localized increased pressure induced by the villonodular synovial mass.

205 a/206 a Schematic drawings

Ischaemic bone necrosis

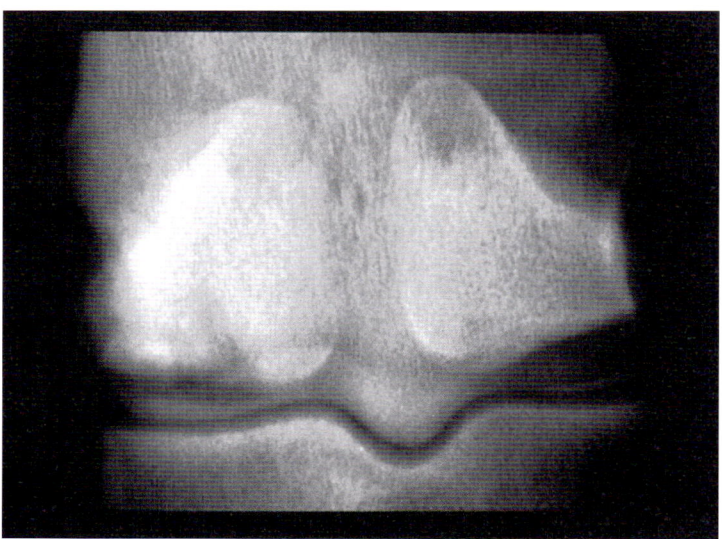 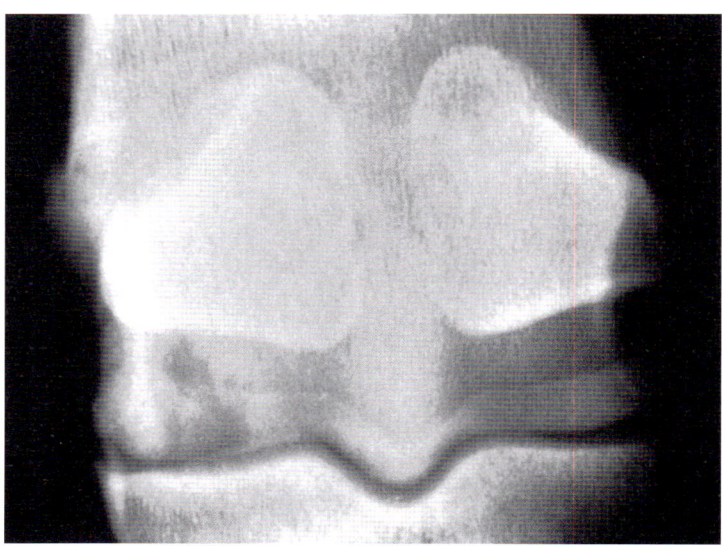

207   208

207/208 Fetlock joint, left front, dorsopalmar view and special dorsoproximal-palmarodistal oblique projection: close-ups.

Foal, 10 months.

The dorsopalmar view (Fig. 207) reveals an obscure area of radiolucency within the subchondral bone of the distomedial end of the cannon bone and irregular new bone formation on the corresponding aspect of the bone.

On an additional dorsoproximal-palmarodistal oblique view made at 40° proximal to the supporting surface, the beam centred on the fetlock joint (Fig. 208), the projection of the sesamoid bones is shifted proximally and results in clearer visualization.

The radiolucent area is irregularly shaped, non-homogeneous and is surrounded by an ill defined sclerotic zone, suggestive of sequestration and demarcation between diseased and normal bone. Differential diagnosis includes ischaemic necrosis as well as infection.

The final diagnosis based on clinical and laboratory data was ischaemic bone necrosis, the bone deposition along the medial aspect of the cannon bone probably having been induced by the same traumatic injury.

Bone cyst

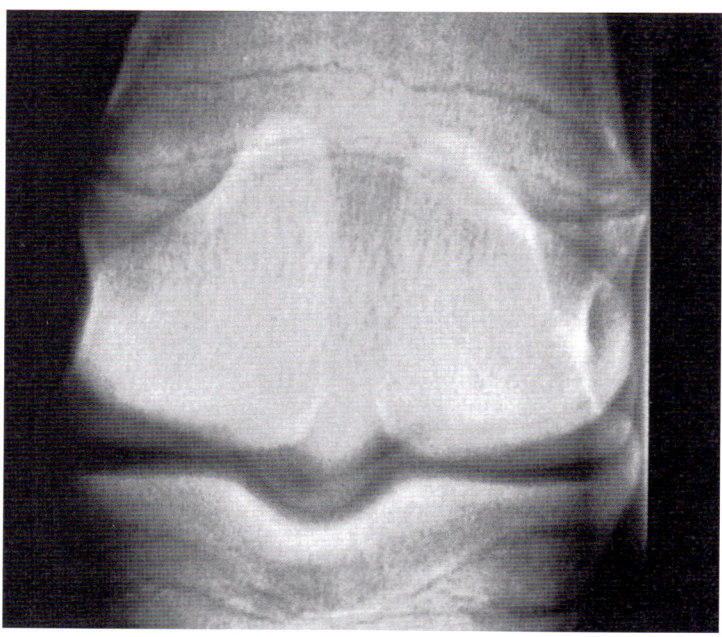 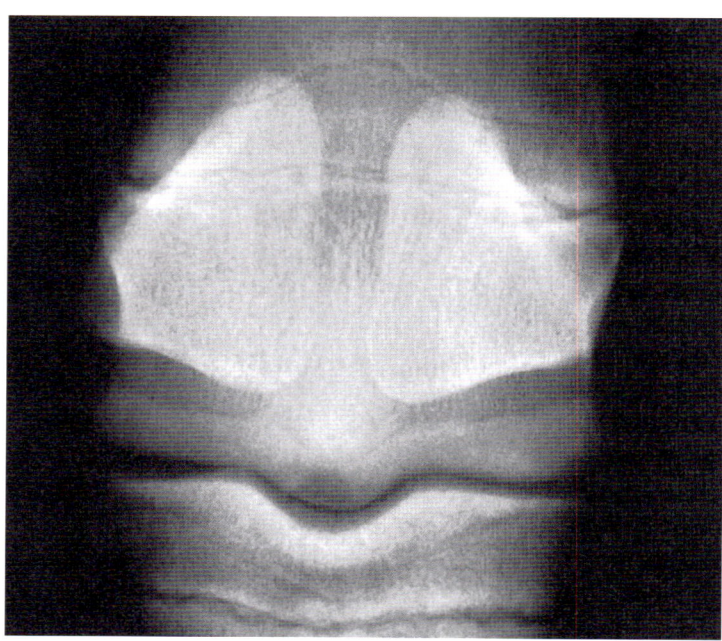

209   210

209/210 Fetlock joint, right front, dorsopalmar view and special dorsoproximal-palmarodistal oblique view: close-ups.

Foal, 3 months.

The dorsopalmar view (Fig. 209) 3 weeks after the onset of lameness reveals an indistinct cystic area of radiolucency in the subchondral bone of the sagittal ridge of the cannon bone, more clearly demonstrated on the additional dorsoproximal-palmarodistal oblique view made at 40° proximal to the supporting surface, the beam centred on the fetlock joint (Fig. 210). The cystic bone lesion is not surrounded by a sclerotic rim, suggesting a recent development of the lesion. The corresponding articular surface of the cannon bone is slightly irregular but not disrupted, consequently there is no radiographic evidence of a direct communication between the cystic lesion and the joint cavity.

Bone cyst

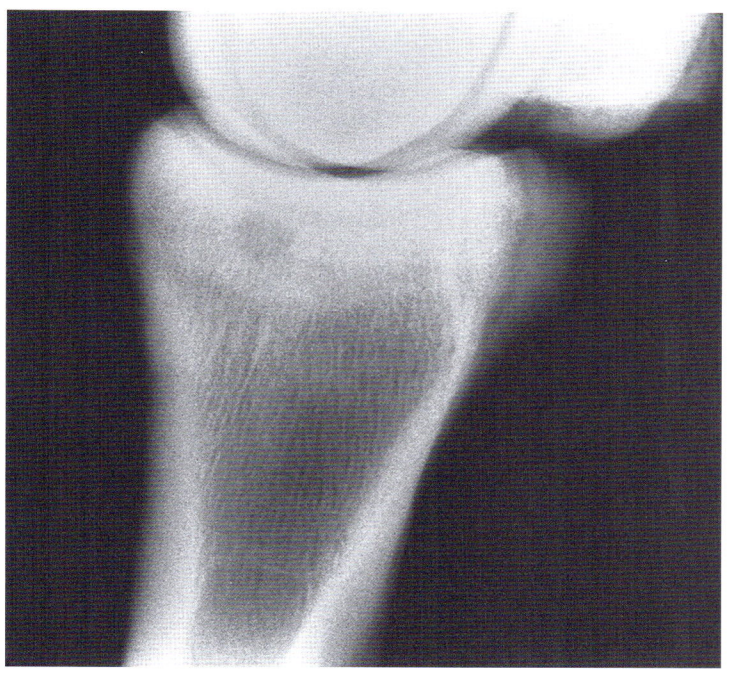

211

211 Fetlock joint, left hind, lateromedial view: close-up.

Warmblood, 5 years.

The rounded area of radiolucency within the proximal end of the first phalanx represents a bone cyst situated near the articular surface.

Cystic lesions in the proximal end of the first phalanx are most commonly encountered in adult horses and probably result fromt trauma to the articular surface and subchondral bone.

Bone cysts within the distal end of the first phalanx (Fig. 118/119) are most common in foals and associated with osteochondrosis.

This illustrates the variable origin of subchondral bone cysts.

Osteomyelitis

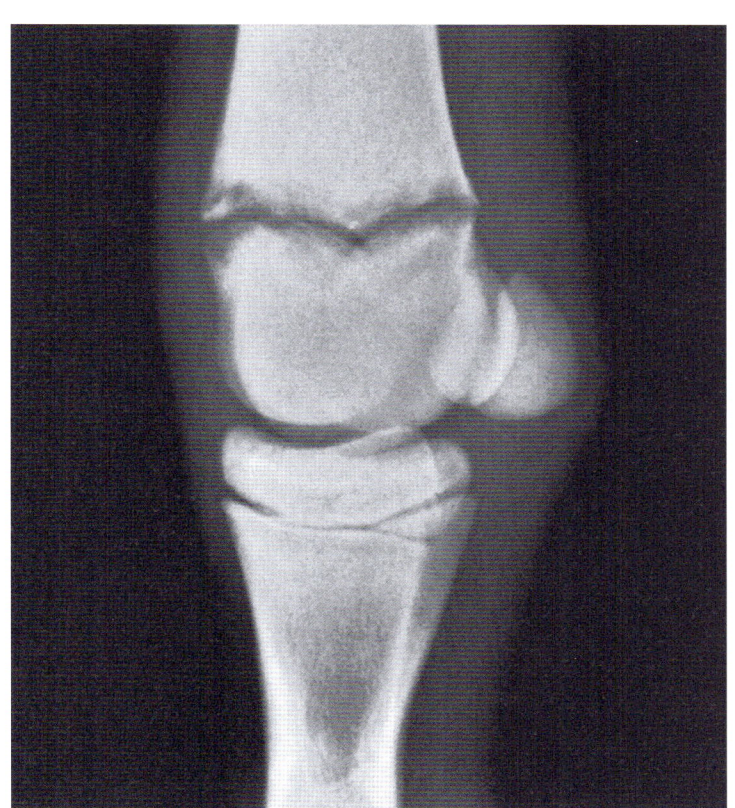

212 Fetlock joint, left hind, lateromedial view.

Foal, 2 weeks.

A zone of irregular radiolucency in the epi- and metaphysis of the cannon bone extending along the entire physis, characteristic of (haematogenous) osteomyelitis type P in young foals. The absence of soft tissue swelling indicates that the inflammation is restricted to the bone.

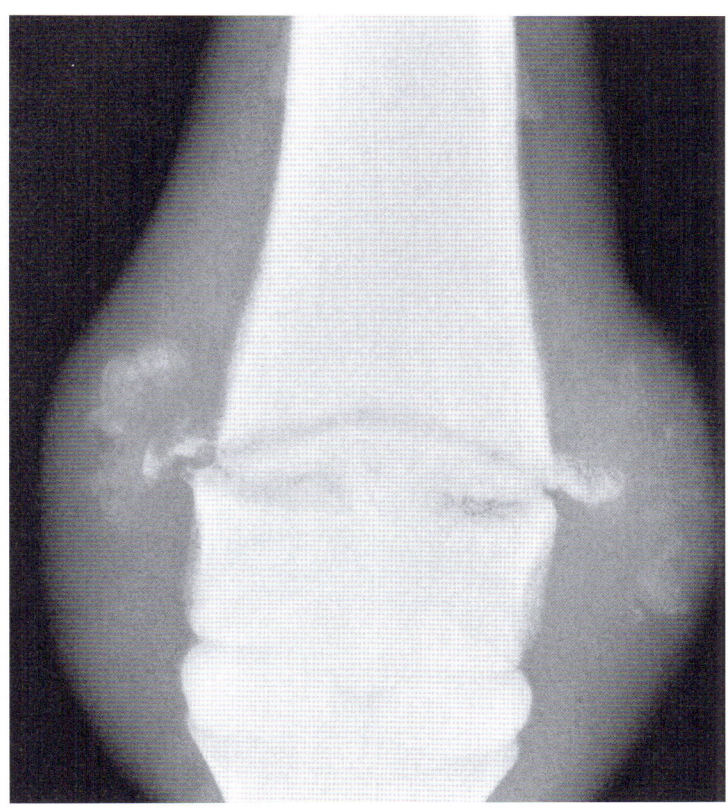

213 Fetlock joint, left hind, dorsoplantar view.

Foal, 3 weeks.

Extensive soft tissue swelling and calcification most prominent over the physis of the cannon bone, a zone of irregular radiolucency extending along the entire physis, minimal subperiosteal new bone along the medial and lateral aspect of the metaphysis and minimal medial displacement of the epiphysis of the cannon bone. A more advanced case of osteomyelitis type P with extension of the disease into the periarticular soft tissue and slipping of the epiphysis induced by destruction of the growth plate.

"Epiphysitis"

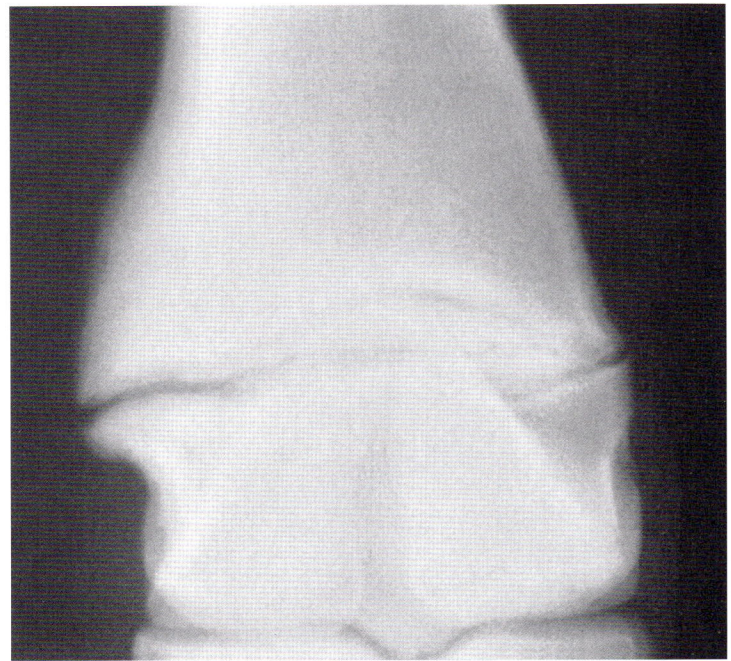

214 Fetlock joint, left front, dorsopalmar view, close-up.

Foal, 4 months.

Asymmetrical widening of the growth plate, tipping, widening and sclerosis of the corresponding portion of meta- and epiphysis and slight wedging of the epiphysis. These radiographic changes are characteristic of "epiphysitis".

214

Diaphyseal angular deformity

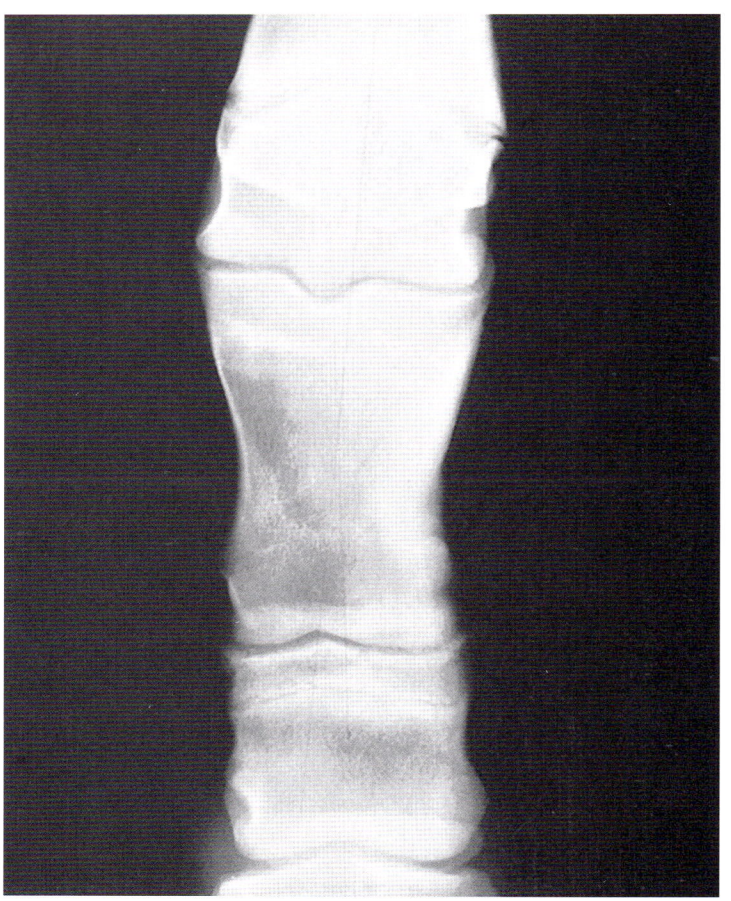

215 Fetlock joint, right hind, dorsoplantar view.

Foal, 5 months.

Angulation (8°) originating in the diaphyseal region of the first phalanx, marked increase in cortical density and thickness on the concave aspect and premature closure of the growth plate.

This syndrome is poorly understood and occurs rarely.

215

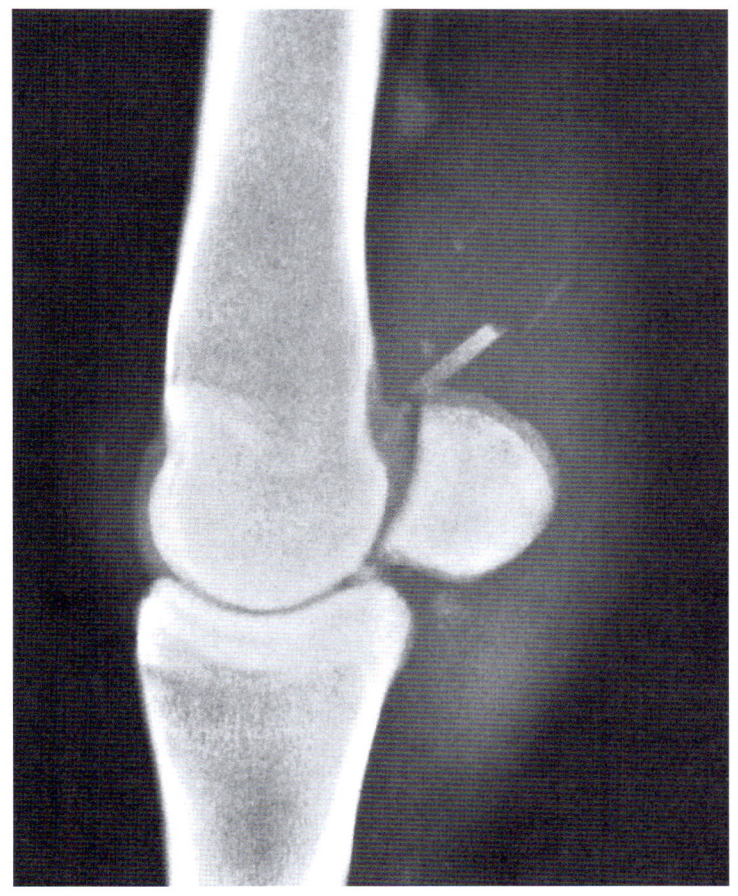

216 Fetlock joint, left hind, lateromedial view: close-up.

Pony, 11 months.

Marked effusion of the fetlock joint and sesamoidean sheath, variable sized ill or sharply defined soft tissue opacities represent pieces of glass, which perforated the joint and tendon sheath 3 weeks prior to examination.

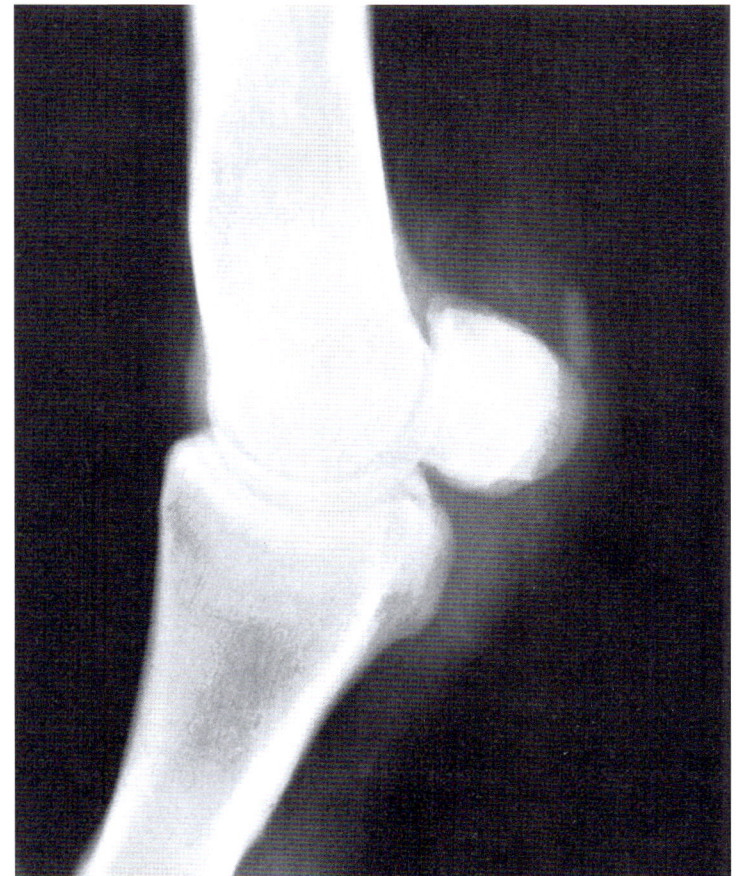

217 Fetlock joint, right hind, lateromedial view.

Pony, 5 years.

Many soft tissue opacities of variable size and definition proximal and distal to the sesamoid bones, with slight effusion of the sesamoidean sheath. These opacities were artefactual, created by the dirty tail in the primary beam.

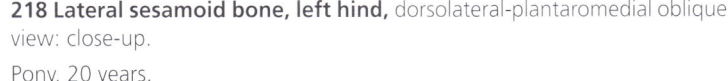

218 Lateral sesamoid bone, left hind, dorsolateral-plantaromedial oblique view: close-up.

Pony, 20 years.

Local bone destruction and new bone formation at the abaxial border of the sesamoid bone, resulting from a puncture wound 1 month prior to the examination.

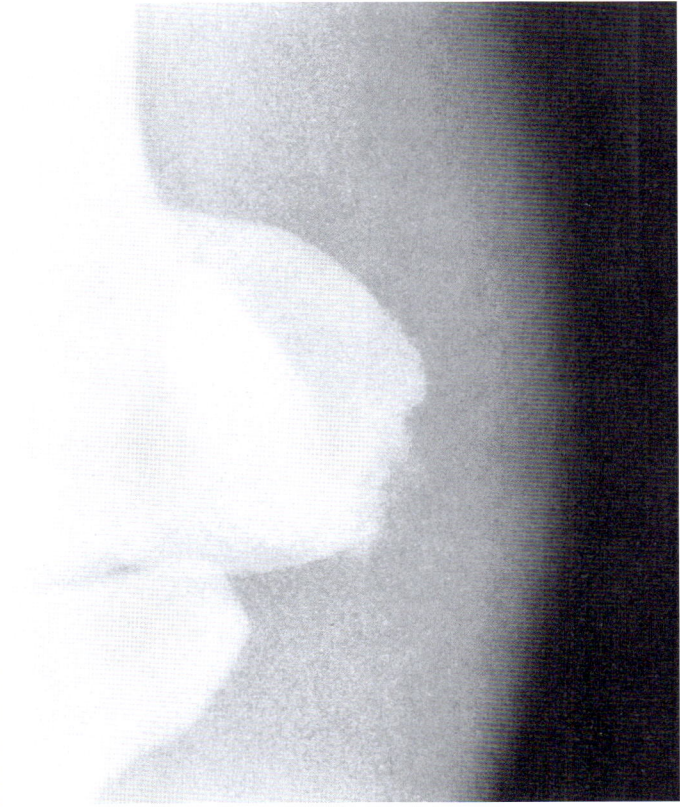

218

Puncture wound

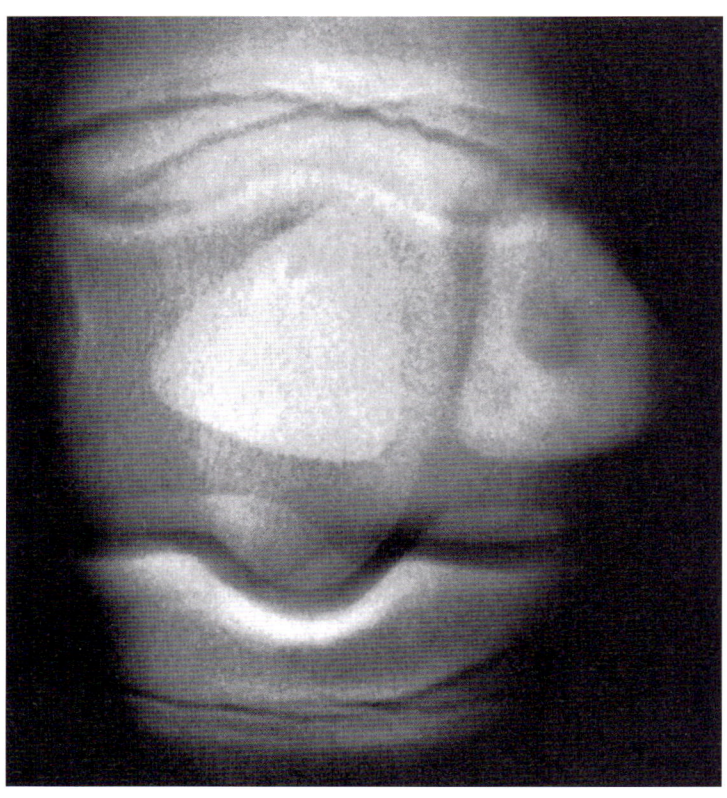

219

219 Lateral sesamoid bone, left hind, dorsolateral-plantaromedial oblique view: close-up.

Foal, 3 weeks.

A well defined cystic radiolucent defect within the midbody of the lateral sesamoid bone, resulting from a bone abscess introduced by a puncture wound (or from haematogenous infection).

N. B. Usually the earliest radiographic changes of infectious bone destruction will not occur until 7–10 days after the onset of clinical symptoms.

In young foals like this one well defined sharply marginated lytic areas with a diffuse radiolucent pattern, representing the more advanced infectious bone lesions, may present within 1 or 2 days after the first apparent loco-motor signs.

Osselets

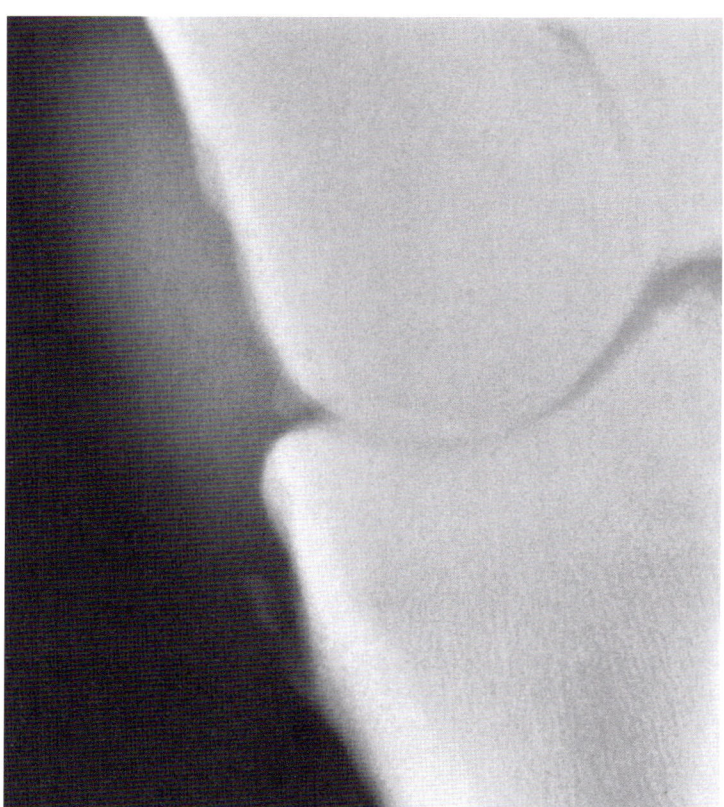

220 Fetlock joint, left front, lateromedial view: close-up.
Warmblood, 6 years.

220 a Schematic drawing

New bone formation on the dorsal aspect of the proximal end of the first phalanx **(1)**, resulting from excessive stress upon the attachment of the lateral digital extensor. Additional finding: distension of the dorsal pouch of the fetlock joint **(2)** and an isolated bone fragment **(3)** close to the dorsoproximal extremity of the first phalanx, probably the result of fracture.

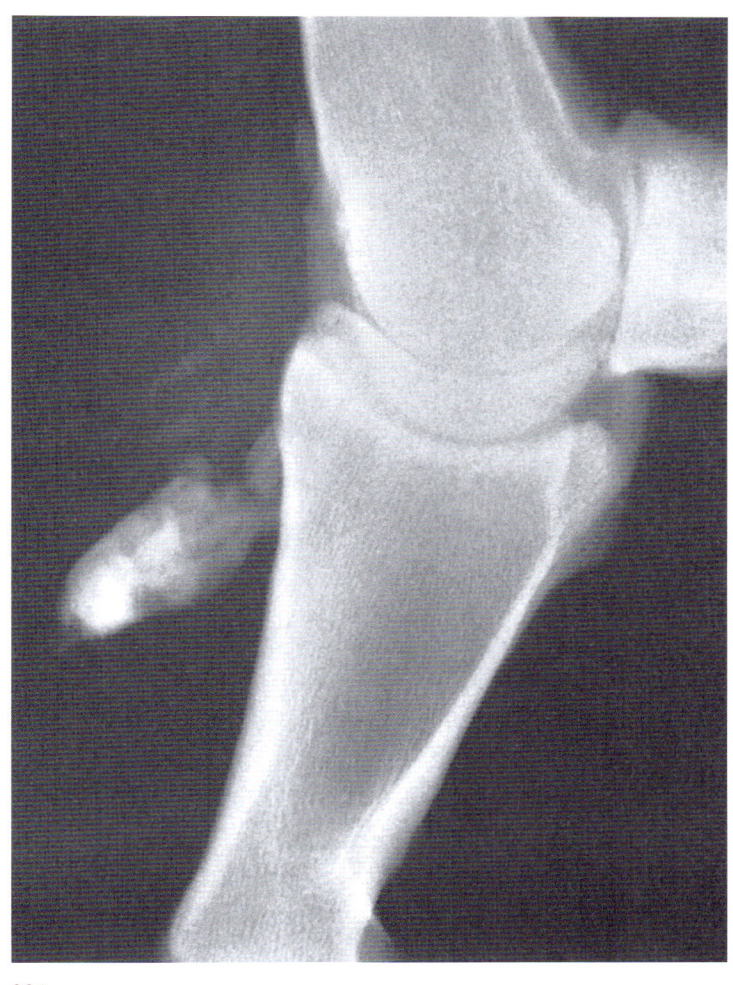

221

221 Fetlock joint, left hind, lateromedial view.

Warmblood, 3 years.

A large well defined soft tissue opacity close to and partly superimposed by the dorsal aspect of the proximal end of the first phalanx, resulting from a calcified granuloma.

Cannon and Splint Bones

Fracture

Bone sequestration

Traumatic periostitis

Diaphyseal angular deformity

Osteomyelitis

Cannon bone

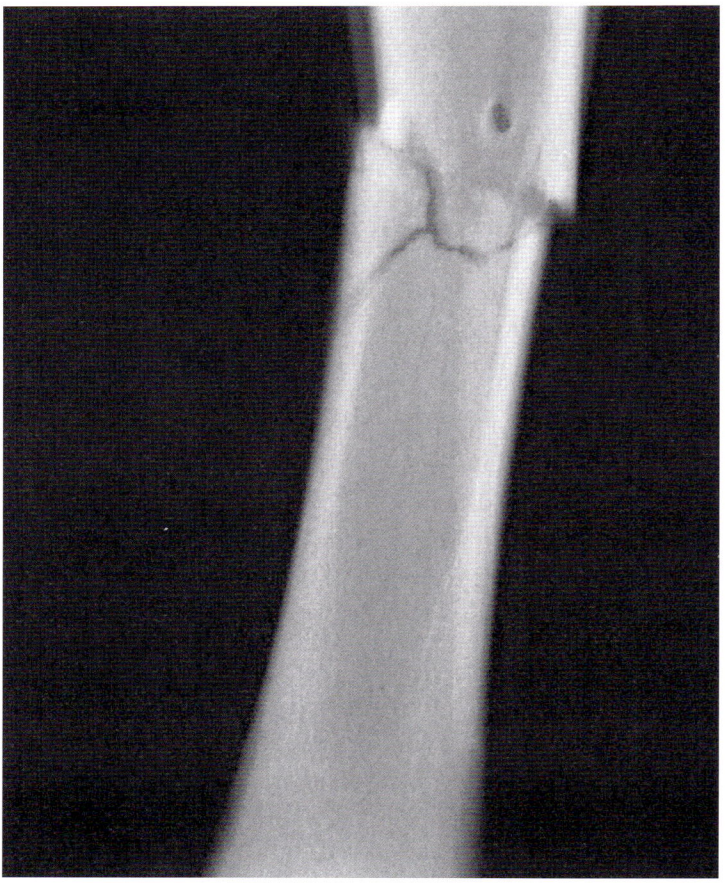

222

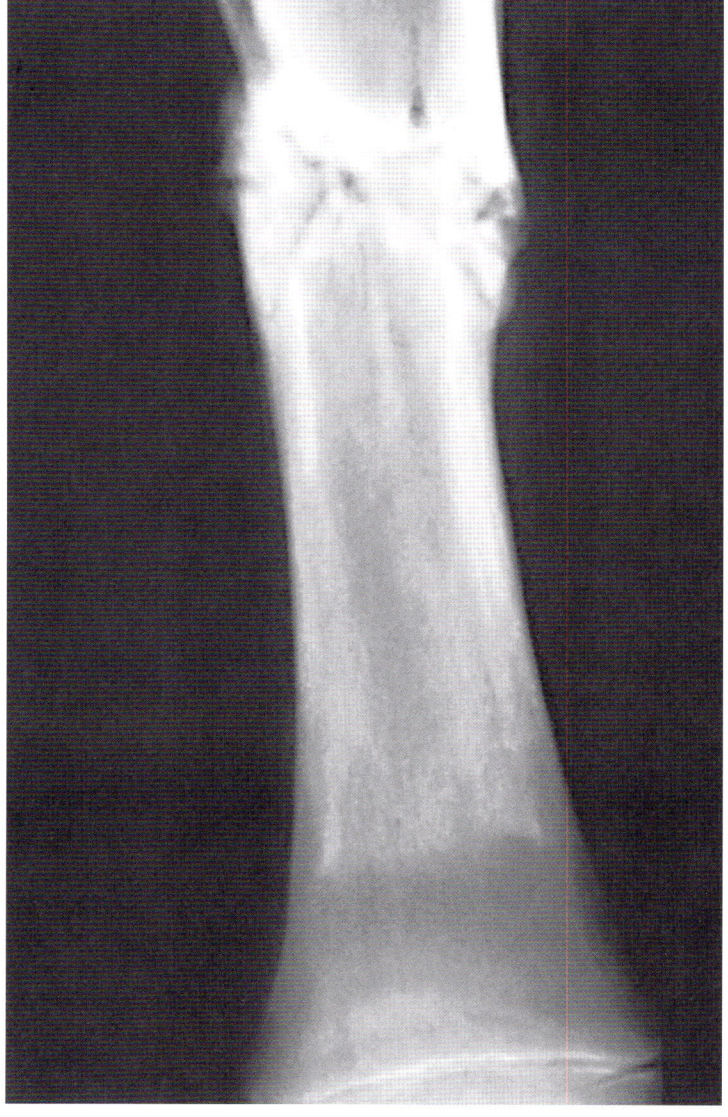

223

222/223 Right metacarpus, serial dorsopalmar views: close-ups.

Foal, 5 days.

The initial examination (Fig. 222) reveals multiple sharp radiolucent lines through the cannon bone distal to the nutrient foramen, indicating the presence of a recent comminuted fracture. The horizontal and oblique fracture lines are complete, resulting in several well defined fracture fragments and slight angular displacement. The vertical fracture lines are less obvious and incomplete.

On a follow-up radiograph (Fig. 223) one month after anatomical reduction and immobilization, the fracture lines are blurred by both callus formation adjacent to and overlying the fracture site and increased ossification in the diaphyseal region of the cannon bone. The band of radiolucency restricted to the metaphyseal region represents a less common form of disuse osteoporosis subsequent to fracture and immobilization.

Cannon bone

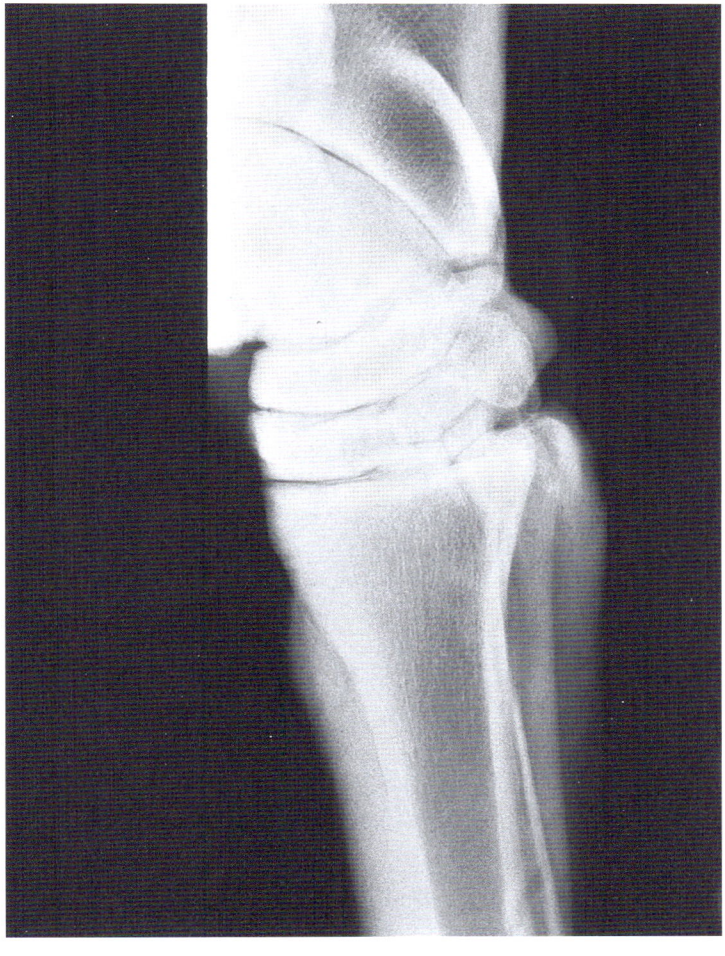

224

224 Left metatarsus, lateromedial view.

Standardbred, 4 years.

The oblique radiolucent line extending proximodistally through the dorso-proximal cortex of the cannon bone and the dense overlying subperiosteal callus represent a (relatively seldom occuring) dorsal metatarsal cortical stress fracture of some duration.

Dorsal cortical stress fractures are predominantly encountered in the dorso-lateral aspect of the middle third of the metacarpus, the linear radiolucency traversing distoproximally at a 30 – 45° angle to the dorsal cortex.

The different location and direction of metacarpal and metatarsal cortical stress fractures may result from dorsopalmar metacarpal bending versus plantarodorsal metatarsal bending during loading.

Due to the relatively slow healing of these fractures the density of the periosteal callus is not a good criteria of fracture duration.

225/226 Left metacarpus, dorsopalmar and dorsolateral – palmaromedial oblique view.

Standardbred, 4 years.

The dorsolateral – palmaromedial oblique view (Fig. 226) reveals a vertical radiolucent line within the dorsoproximomedial aspect of the cannon bone.

This line superimposes the medial splint bone and extends to the articular surface of the carpometacarpal joint. These findings indicate a recent incomplete dorsomedial intra-articular fracture of the proximal aspect of the third metacarpal bone. Contrary to the majority of these cases, concurrent chronic periosteal new bone formation at the extensor carpi radialis attachment site is not obvious.

On the dorsopalmar radiograph (Fig. 225) the fracture plane is not parallel with the central beam and therefore completely invisible.

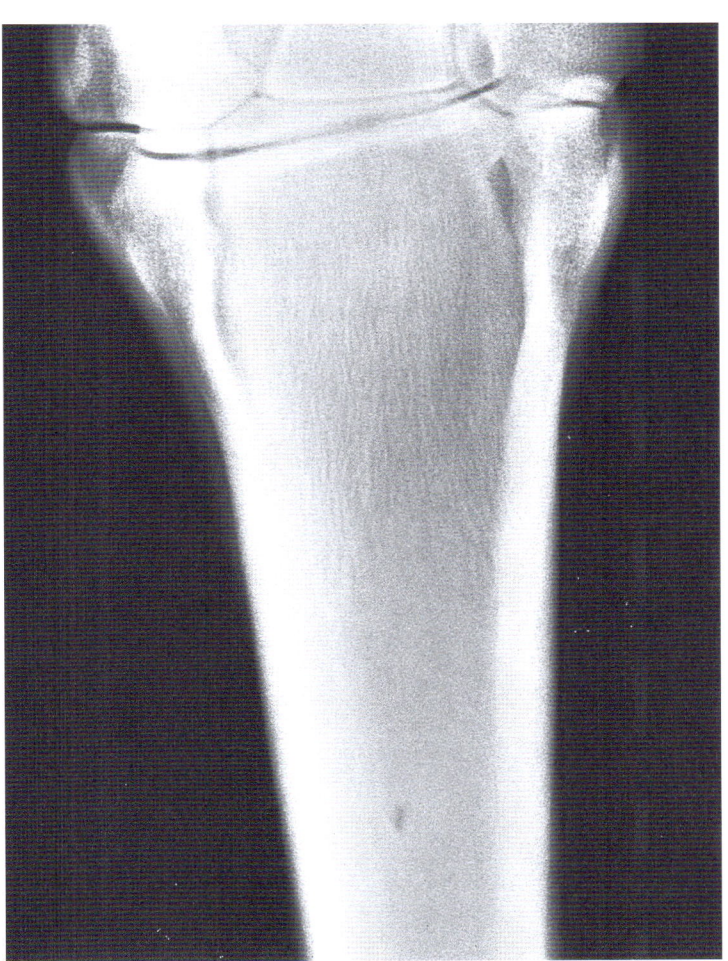

225

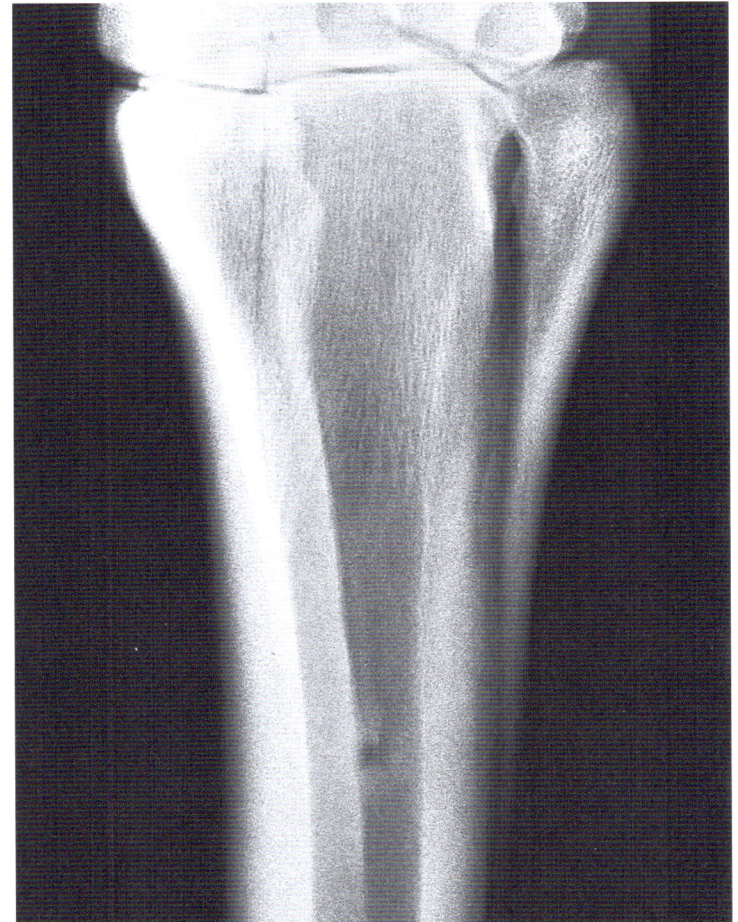

226

Fracture

Splint bone

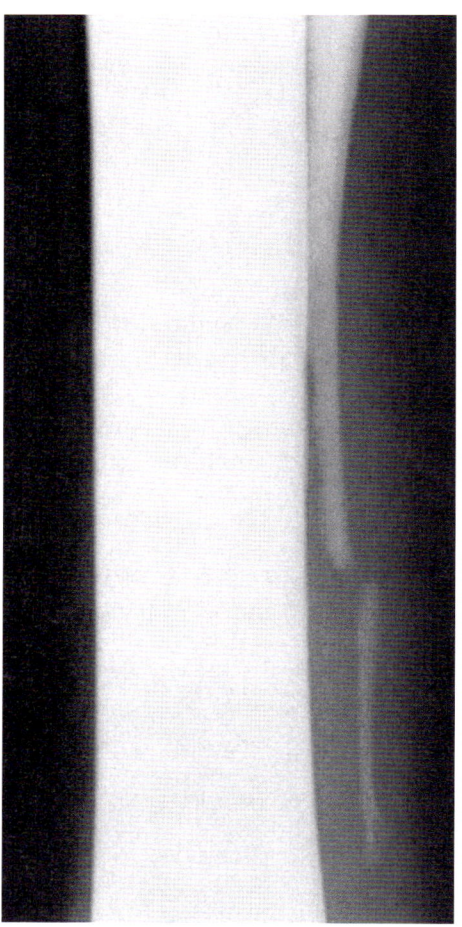 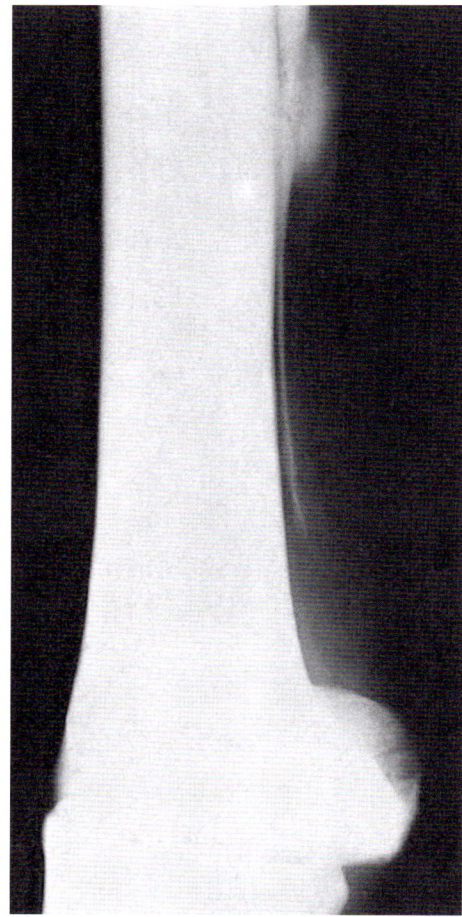 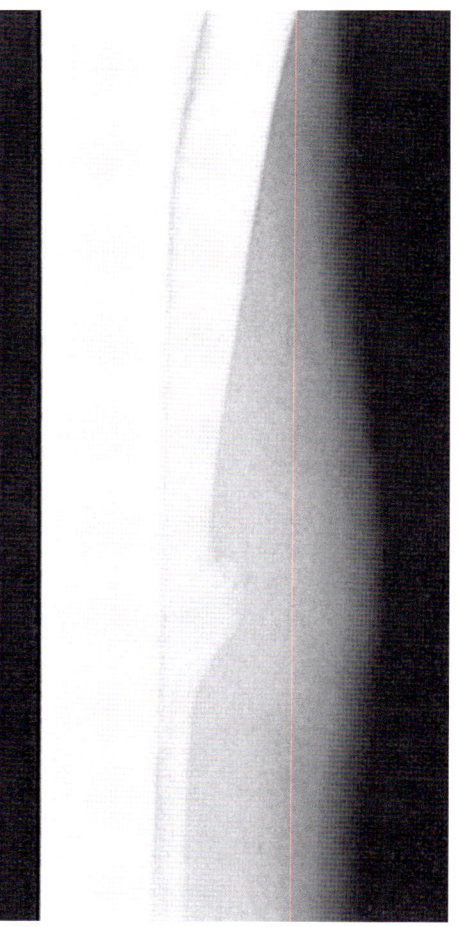

227 Medial splint bone, left front, dorso-medial-palmarolateral oblique view: close-up.

Standardbred, 4 years.

Palmar displacement of the distal portion of the medial splint bone due to a simple complete transverse fracture. The minimal periosteal new bone formation on both fragments adjacent to the fracture site suggest a fracture of some duration.

228 Medial splint bone, right front, dorso-medial-palmarolateral oblique view: close-up.

Warmblood, 5 years.

An obscure, slightly oblique radiolucent line through the mid-portion of the medial splint bone, due to a simple, oblique, complete, non-displaced fracture.

The fracture line is blurred by callus formation adjacent to and overlying the fracture site. The periosteal callus is immature, as indicated by its ill defined border.

Additional finding: marked loss of bone density in the concavity of the abaxial surface of the proximal sesamoid bone, indicative of sesamoiditis.

N. B. The presence of a fracture line avoids confusion with the disease called "splints" (which results from damage to the interosseous ligament) or ordinary traumatic periostitis.

229 Lateral splint bone, right hind, dorso-lateral-plantaromedial oblique view: close-up.

Warmblood, 6 years.

A simple, transverse, non-displaced fracture through the mid-portion of the lateral splint bone and soft tissue swelling in the corresponding region of the flexor tendons. It is extremely difficult to identify the radiolucent fracture line, due to the dense overlying callus.

The callus formation is mature, as indicated by its sharp margin.

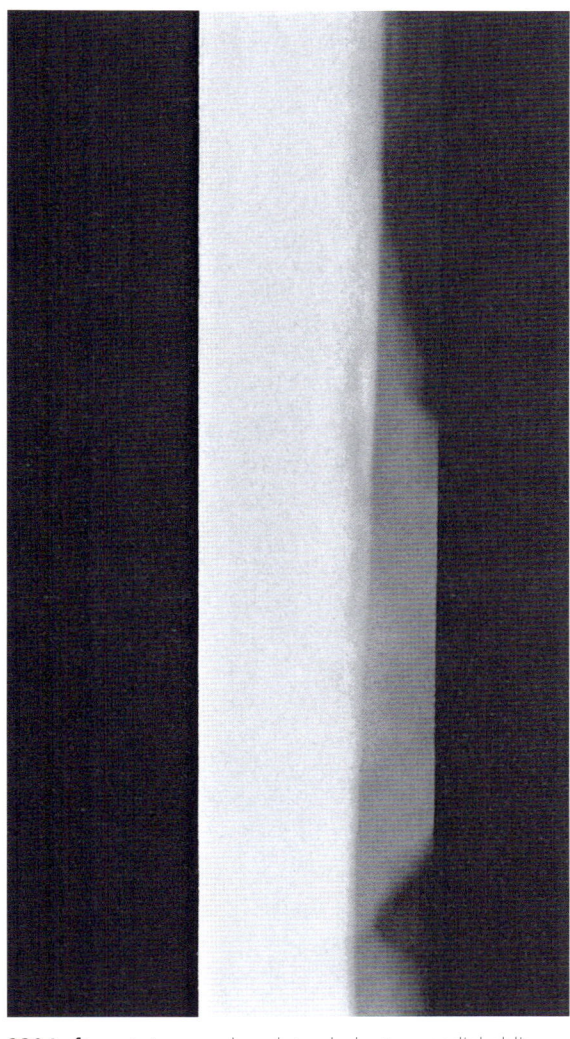

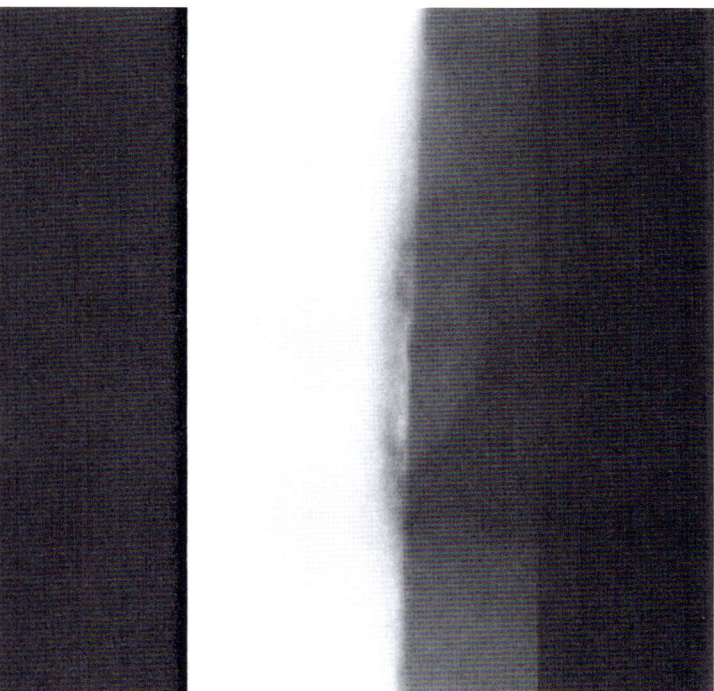

231 Right metatarsus, dorsomedial-plantarolateral oblique view: close-up of the dorsolateral area of the cannon bone.

Warmblood, 6 years.

A radiolucent band beneath the outer cortex of the cannon bone is separating a thin superficial layer of bone from the cortex, 21 days after a traumatic injury. An indistinct soft tissue swelling is present dorsal to the bone lesion. The radiographic changes represent an intermediate stage of bone sequestration, the sequestrum not yet being completely separate from the cortex.

230 Left metatarsus, dorsolateral-plantaromedial oblique view: close-up of the dorsomedial area of the cannon bone.

Warmblood, 4 ½ years.

Regional soft tissue swelling and a poorly demarcated vertical radiolucent line in the outer cortex of the corresponding portion of the cannon bone 21 days after a traumatic injury.

The radiographic changes represent the earliest stage of bone sequestration.

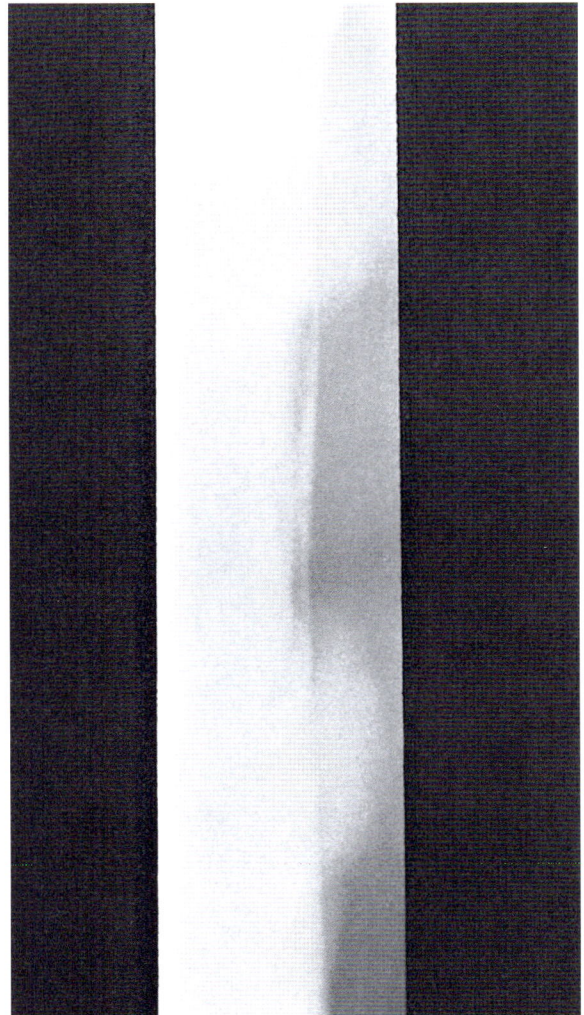

232 Right metatarsus, lateromedial view: close-up of the dorsal area of the cannon bone.

Warmblood, 1 year.

A radiolucent band beneath the outer cortex of the cannon bone incompletely separating a superficial layer of bone from the cortex 19 days after a traumatic injury, representing an intermediate stage of sequestration. Periosteal new bone formation is visible proximal and distal to the sequestrum. The new bone formation is immature, as indicated by its ill defined margin.

232

Bone sequestration

233

234

233/234 Left metatarsus, dorsomedial-plantarolateral oblique and lateromedial view: close-ups of the dorsolateral and dorsal area of the cannon bone.

Warmblood, 2 years.

The dorsomedial-plantarolateral oblique view (Fig. 233) shows ill bordered periosteal new bone formation proximal and distal to a superficial cortical defect. The immature periosteal reaction encloses a sharply delineated dense bone fragment completely separated from the cortex, which represents a mature sequestrum, 23 days after a wire cut injury.

The semicircular bone defect adjacent to the distal new bone formation results directly from the wire cut.

Irregular soft tissue swelling superimposes the bony changes. The periosteal new bone formation forms a wall (involucrum) around the dead bone and is superimposed over the sequestrum on the lateromedial view (Fig. 234).

Superimposition obscures the bone fragment and may mimic embedding of the sequestrum in the periosteal new bone. Multiple projections are required to evaluate the full extent of the sequestration process.

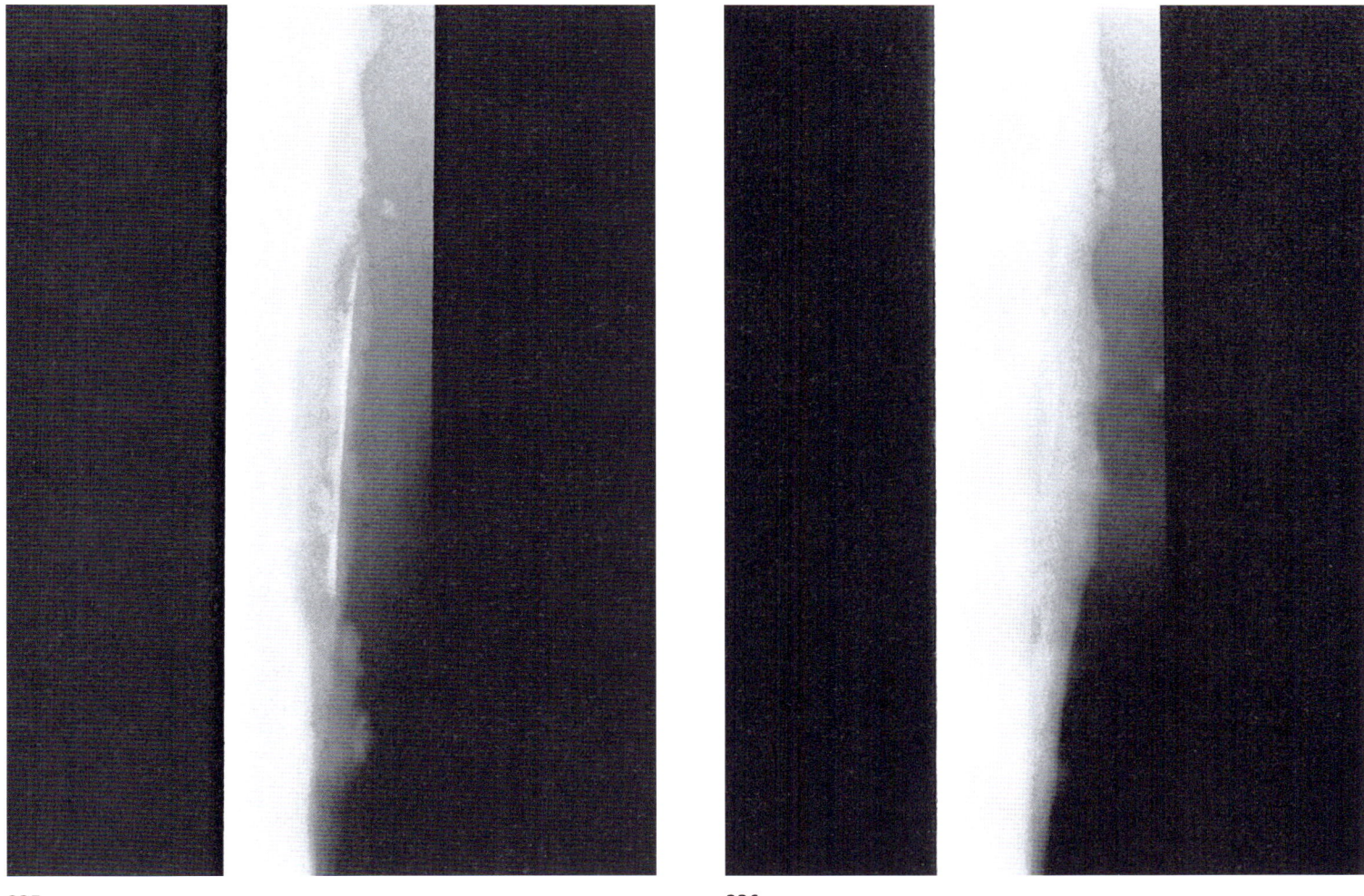

235   236

235/236 Right metatarsus, dorsomedial-plantarolateral oblique and lateromedial view: close-ups of the dorsolateral and dorsal area of the cannon bone.

Warmblood, 6 years.

The dorsomedial-plantarolateral oblique view (Fig. 235) presents a long thin dense clearly defined bone fragment adjacent to a superficial cortical defect 4 weeks after a traumatic injury. The bone fragment results from sequestration.

On the lateromedial projection (Fig. 236) the beam does not strike the edge of the sequestrum and its shadow is thus obscured. On both views the periosteal new bone is superimposed on the sequestrum, suggesting the avascular bone chip really is embedded in the involucrum. The periosteal new bone is mature, as indicated by its distinct margin.

Bone sequestration

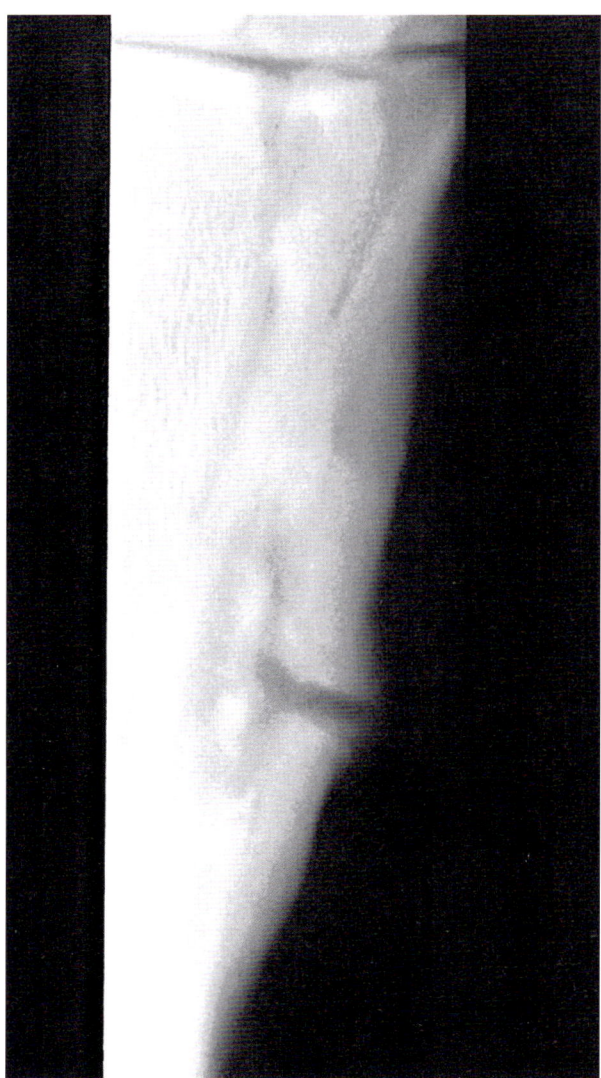

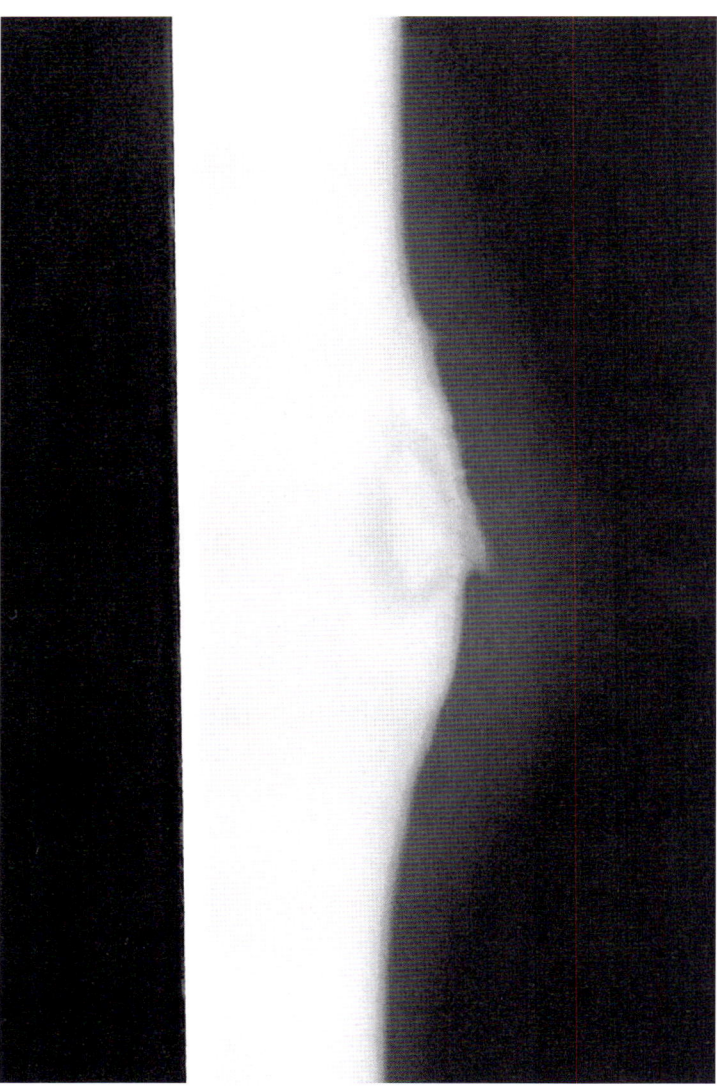

237 Medial splint bone, left front, dorsomedial-palmarolateral oblique view: close-up of the proximal end of the medial splint bone.

Foal, 10 months.

A sharply delineated thick bone fragment originating from the splint bone in a radiolucent pocket, covered by an interrupted wall of sharply bordered periosteal new bone, 1 month after a traumatic injury. The radiographic changes are characteristic of a mature, completely separated bone sequestrum bathed in a pocket of pus and communicating with a fistulous tract by a small opening (cloaca) in the involucrum.

238 Left metacarpus, dorsopalmar view: close-up of the lateral area of the cannon bone.

Foal, 1 year.

A sharply delineated thick dense bone fragment surrounded by a radiolucent zone, covered by a continuous wall of periosteal new bone represents a bone sequestrum completely enveloped in a thick bony shell 3 months after a traumatic injury.

Traumatic periostitis

239/240/241/242 Left metatarsus, serial dorsoplantar views: close-ups of the lateral area of the cannon bone.

Warmblood, 2 years.

The initial examination (Fig. 239) 3 weeks after a traumatic injury reveals a faint ill bordered layer of periosteal new bone on the lateral aspect of the cannon bone, indicating recently developed, active, immature, traumatic periosteal new bone formation. The periosteal new bone is superimposed by irregular soft tissue opacities resulting from the same trauma.

Three weeks later (Fig. 240), the periosteal new bone is thicker, denser and less active, as indicated by its more clearly defined margin.

Ten weeks after the original trauma (Fig. 241) the sharp margin of the periosteal bone shows that the growth has stopped.

The density of the mature inactive periosteal new bone is the same as that of the underlying cortex.

Soft tissue swelling is less obvious.

Four months (Fig. 242) after the traumatic injury the exostosis has become flattened and rather smooth, indicating remodelling of the periosteal new bone.

N. B. The density of the traumatic periosteal new bone formation in relation to the underlying cortex determines its duration and the delineation of the periosteal new bone determines its maturity (activity).

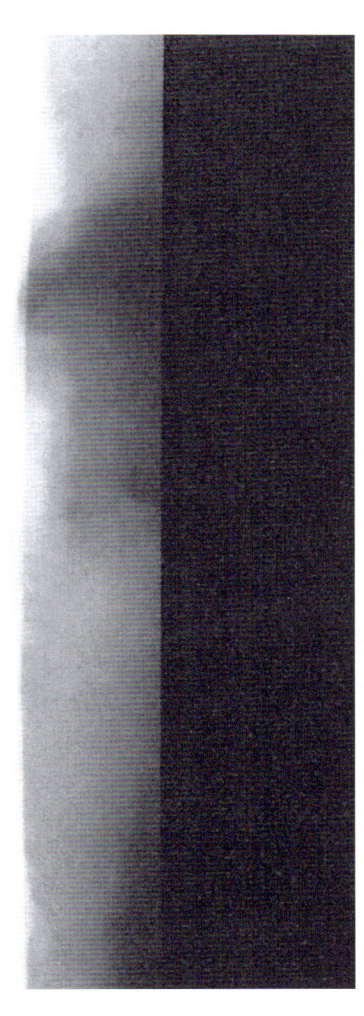

239

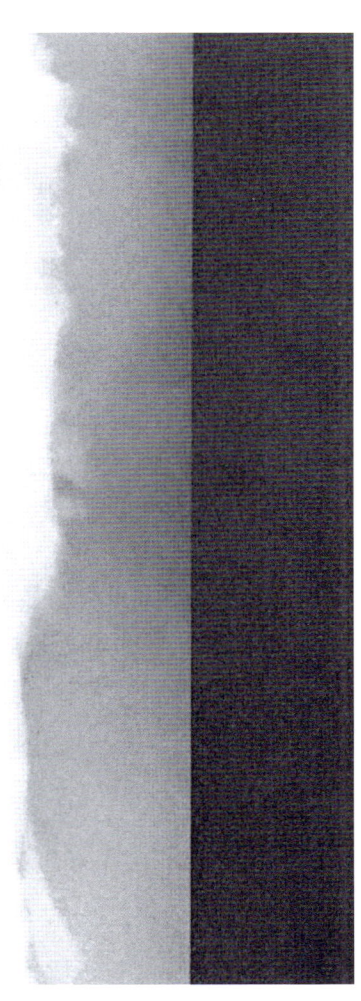

240

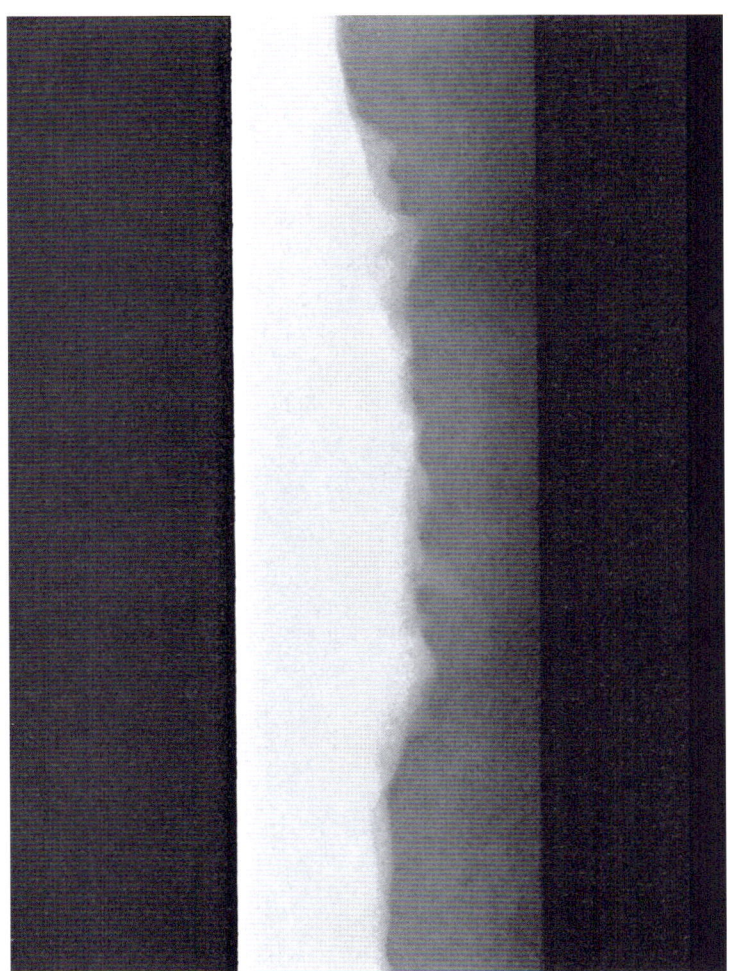

241

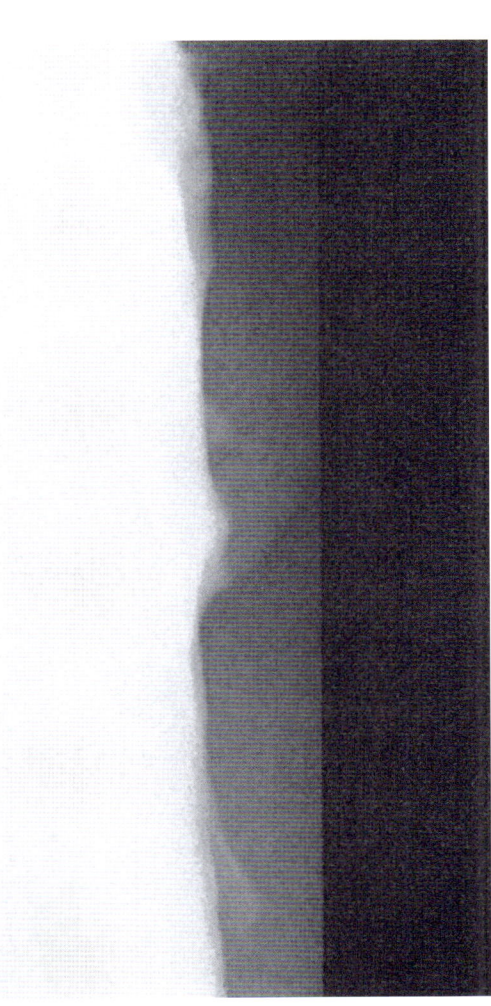

242

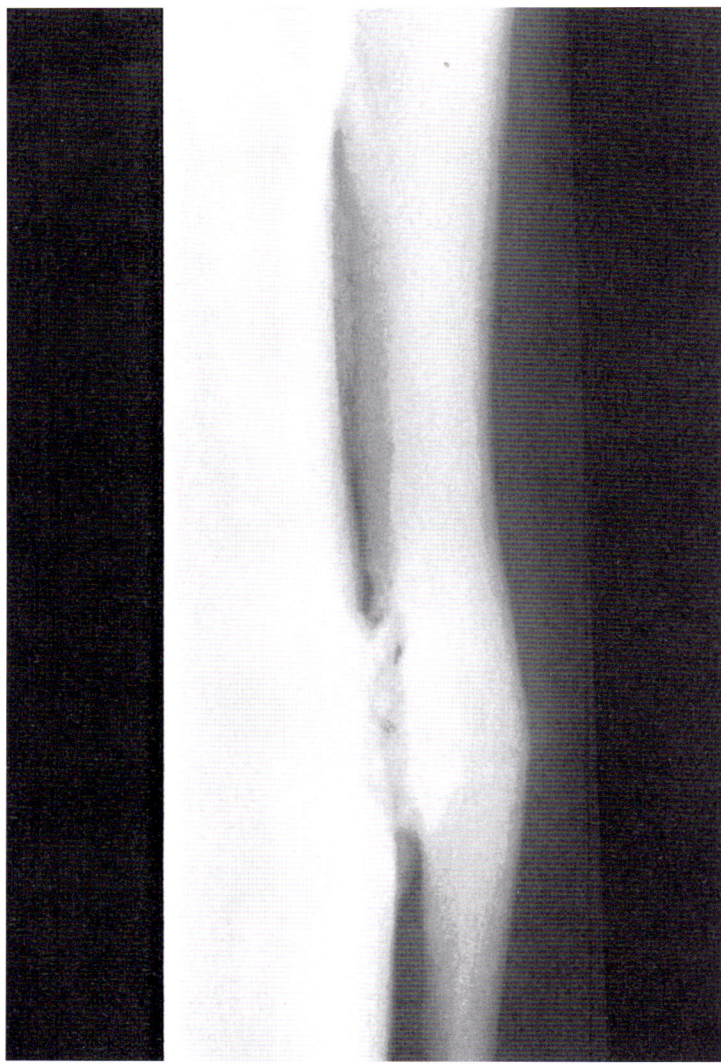

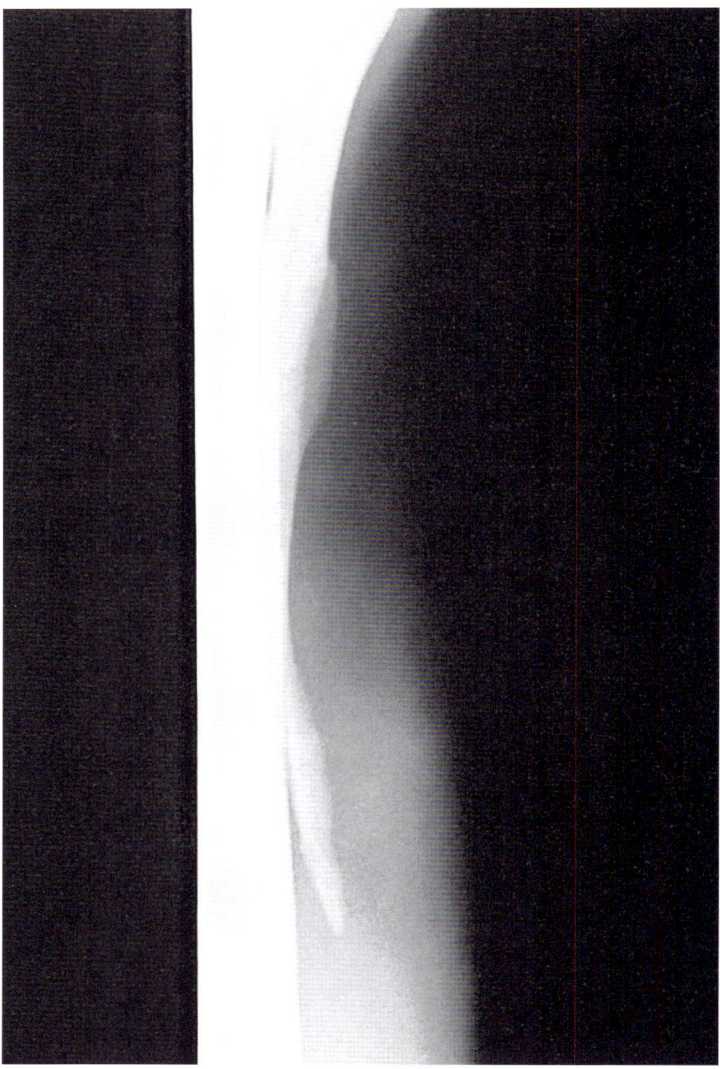

243 Lateral splint bone, left hind, dorsolateral-plantaromedial oblique view: close-up of the middle portion of the lateral splint bone.

Foal, 1 year.

Clearly defined local new bone formation bridging the splint bone and cannon bone, resulting from damage to the interosseous ligament, characteristic of the disease called "splints".

244 Medial splint bone, right front, dorsomedial-palmarolateral oblique view: close-up of the medial splint bone.

Warmblood, 8 years.

Periosteal new bone formation at the proximal and distal portion of the splint bone. The proximal exostosis is flat, smooth and sharply bordered, indicating long-standing mature new bone growth. The distal new bone formation is immature, as indicated by its indistinct border; the corresponding soft tissue swelling suggests simultaneous soft tissue damage.

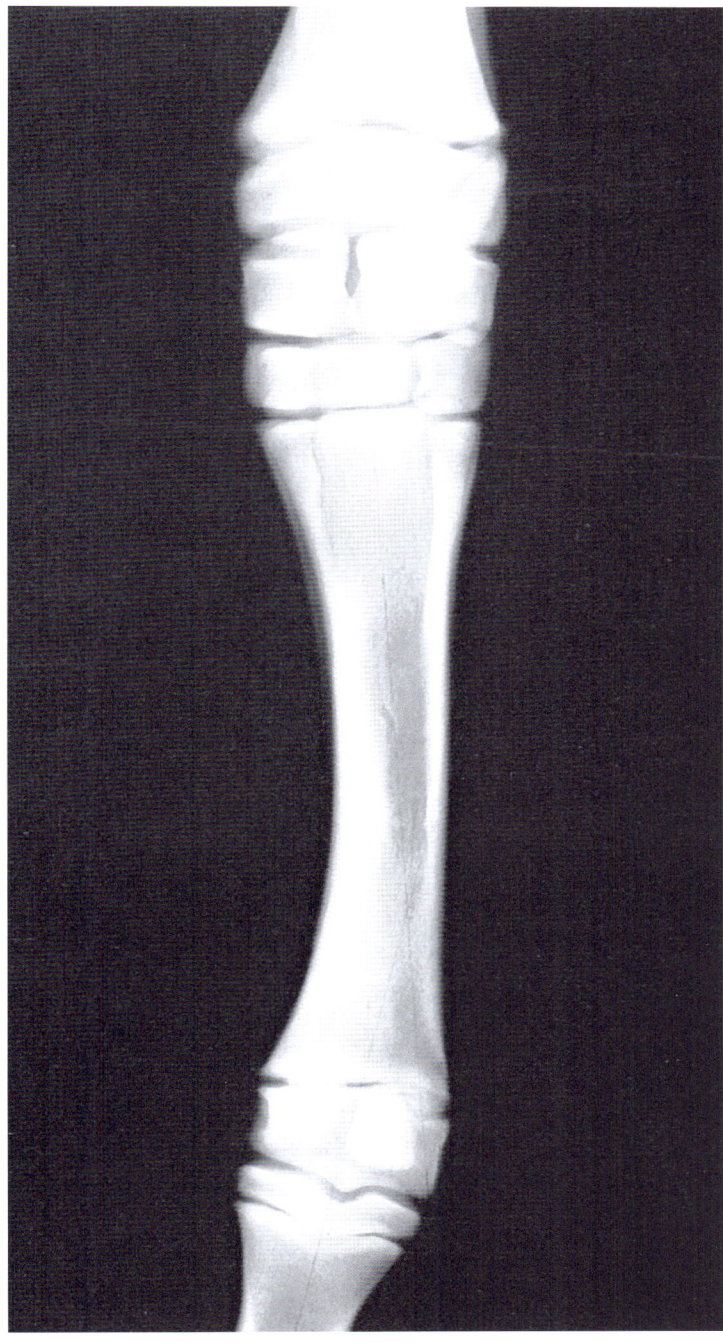

245

245 Left metacarpus, dorsopalmar view.

Foal, 3 weeks.

Angulation of 18° originating in the diaphyseal region of the cannon bone distal to the nutrient foramen, marked increase in cortical density and thickening on the concave aspect of the curvature and wedging of the metacarpal epiphysis.

This is a seldom occurring and ill defined syndrome of unknown origin in foals.

Cannon- and Splint Bones

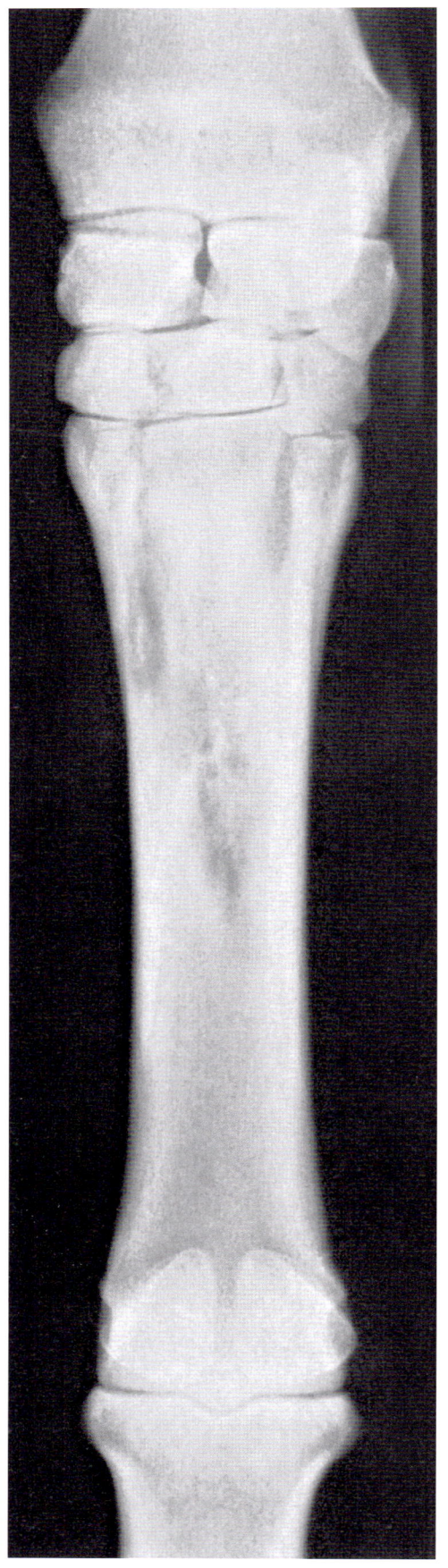

246

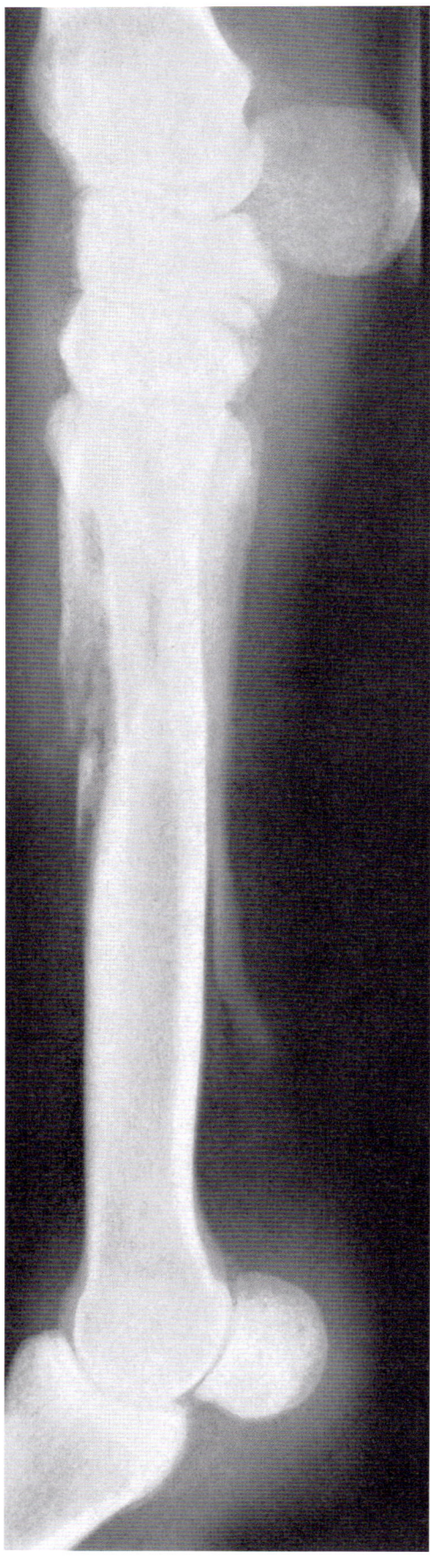

247

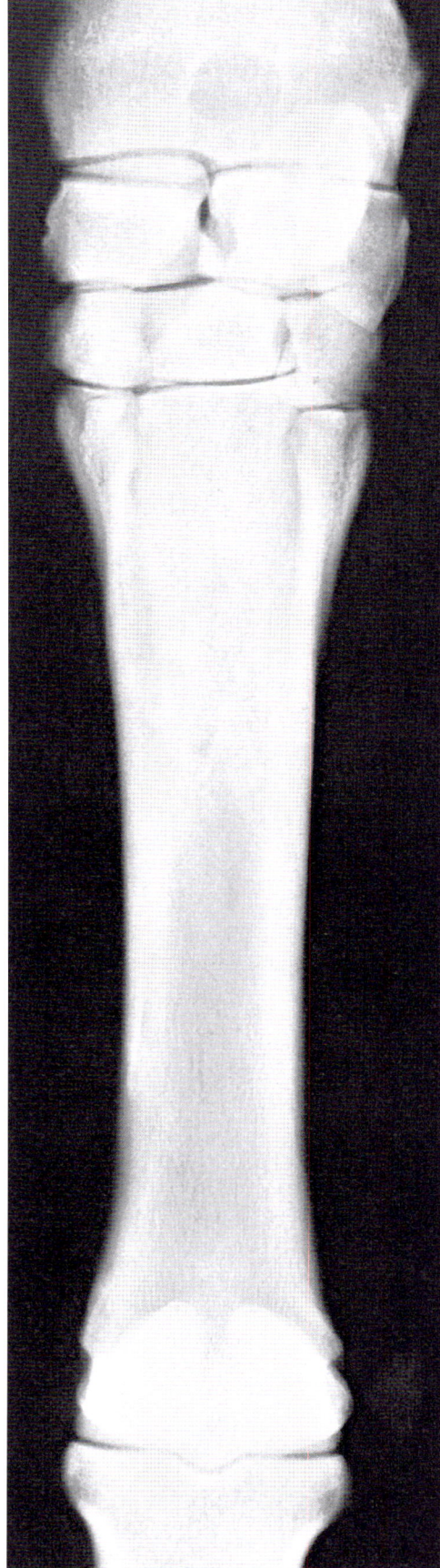

248

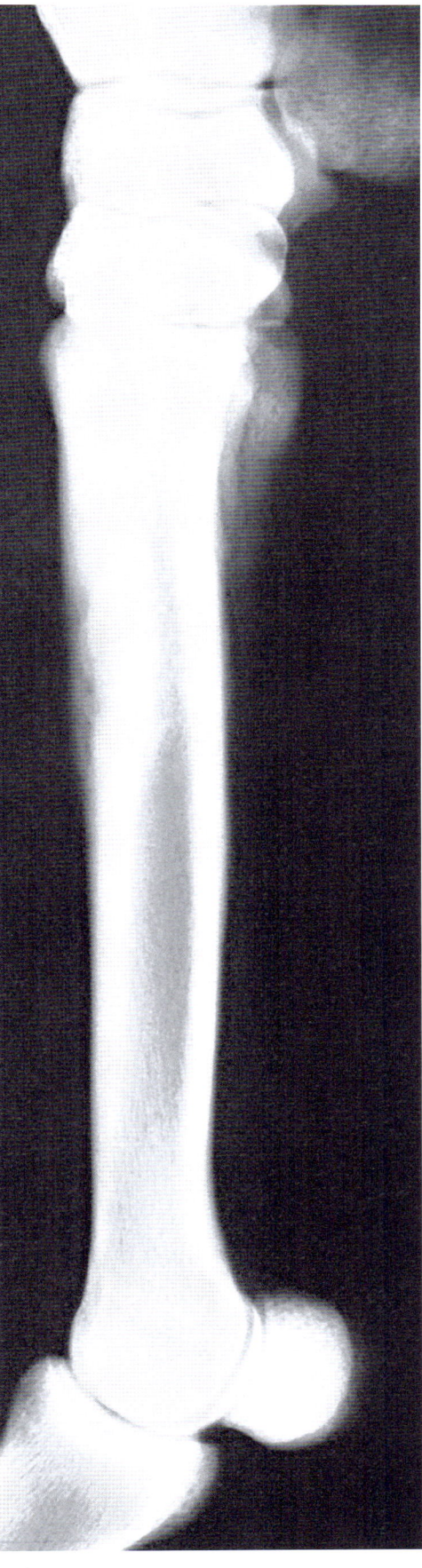

246/247/248/249 Left metacarpus, serial dorsopalmar and lateromedial views.

Pony, 2 ½ years.

The initial dorsopalmar view (Fig. 245) 6 weeks after the onset of lameness shows a capricious area of ill defined radiolucency in the proximal half of the cannon bone superimposing the nutrient foramen.

The corresponding lateromedial view (Fig. 246) reveals soft tissue swelling dorsal to the proximal part of the cannon bone and an area of radiolucency and fragmentation involving the whole thickness of the dorsal metacarpal cortex.

The radiographic changes represent osteolysis and sequestration resulting from (haematogenous) osteomyelitis. Three months later (Fig. 247, 248) healing has occurred. The lytic bone lesion is now filled with heavy sclerotic bone tissue.

A slight irregularity remains in the outer dorsal cortical surface of the cannon bone.

249

The Carpus

Fracture

Fracture/Luxation

Avulsion injury of the palmar intercarpal ligaments

Herniation of the joint capsule

Traumatic periostitis

Osteoarthrosis

Infectious arthritis

Osteomyelitis

Bone cyst

Bone sequestration

"Epiphysitis"

Angular limb deformities

Puncture wound

Hygroma

Osteochondroma

Osteoblastoma

Synovial sarcoma

Fracture

Radius

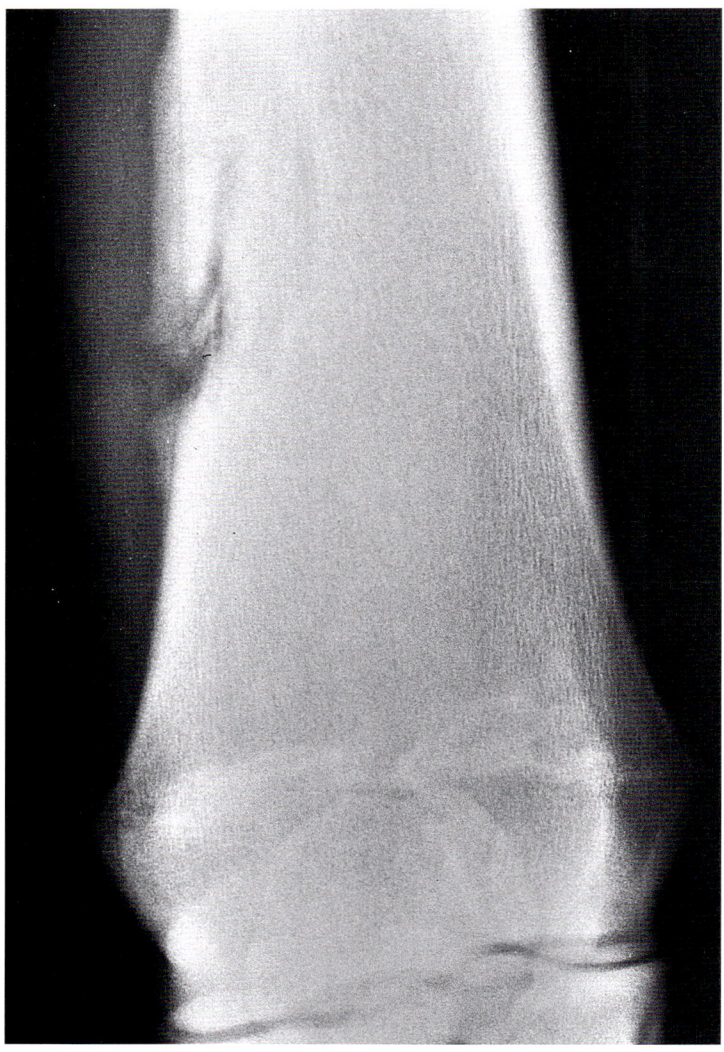

250

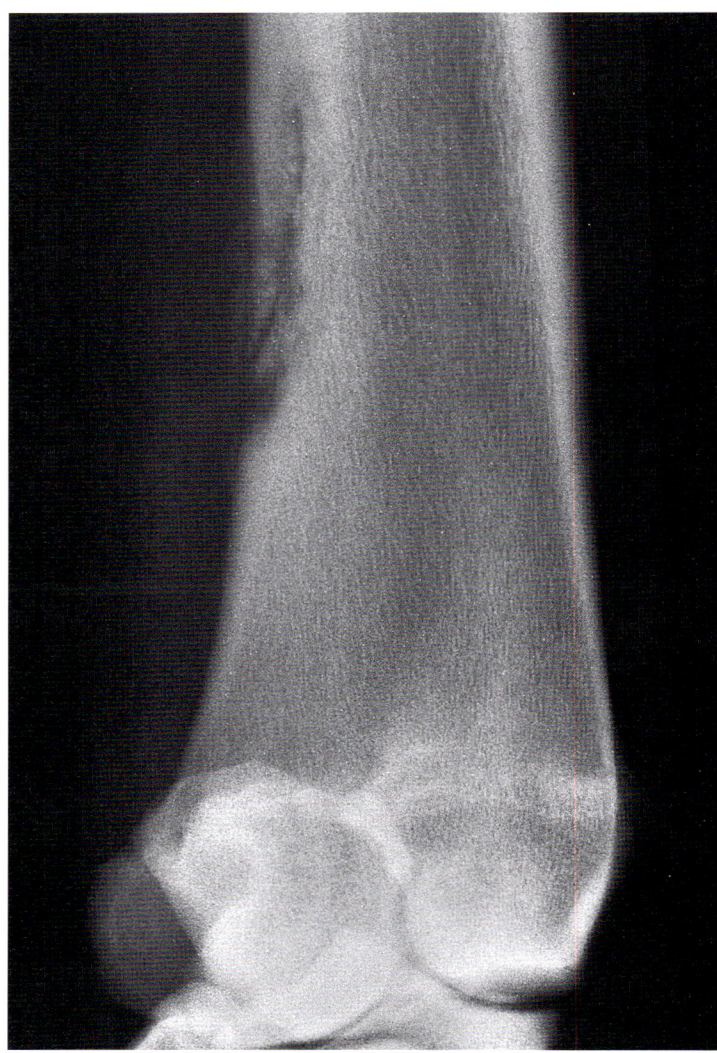

251

250/251 Left radius, craniocaudal and craniomedial – caudolateral oblique view.

Pony, 3 years.

A short oblique radiolucent line extending distoproximally through the medial cortex at the junction of the middle and distal third of the radius representing an incomplete medial cortical fracture.

The density and delineation of the overlying periosteal callus indicate a fracture of 3 – 4 weeks duration.

252/253/254/255 Right radius, serial craniocaudal and craniomedial – caudolateral oblique views.

Arabian, 11 years.

The initial craniocaudal (Fig. 252) and craniomedial – caudolateral oblique view (Fig. 253), 1 day after the onset of acute severe lameness, show a long oblique clearly defined radiolucent line extending proximodistally through the mid and distal radial diaphysis that represents a recent incomplete oblique diaphyseal fracture. Two months later, the fracture is almost invisible on the craniocaudal view (Fig. 254) and blurred on the craniomedial – caudolateral oblique radiograph (Fig. 255) due to callus formation bridging the fracture site.

Radius

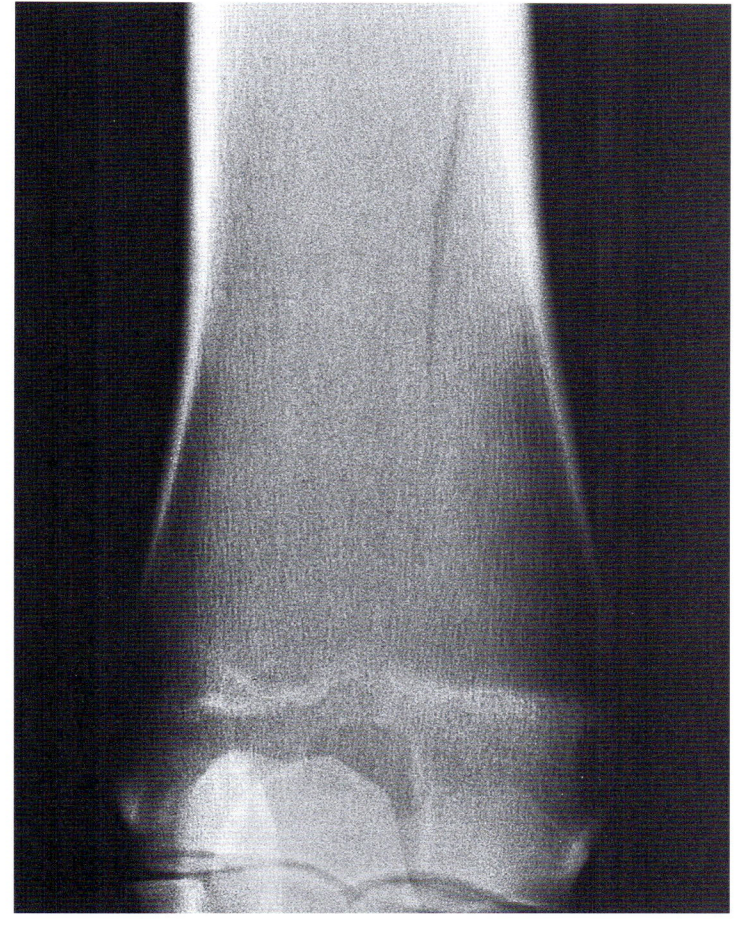

252

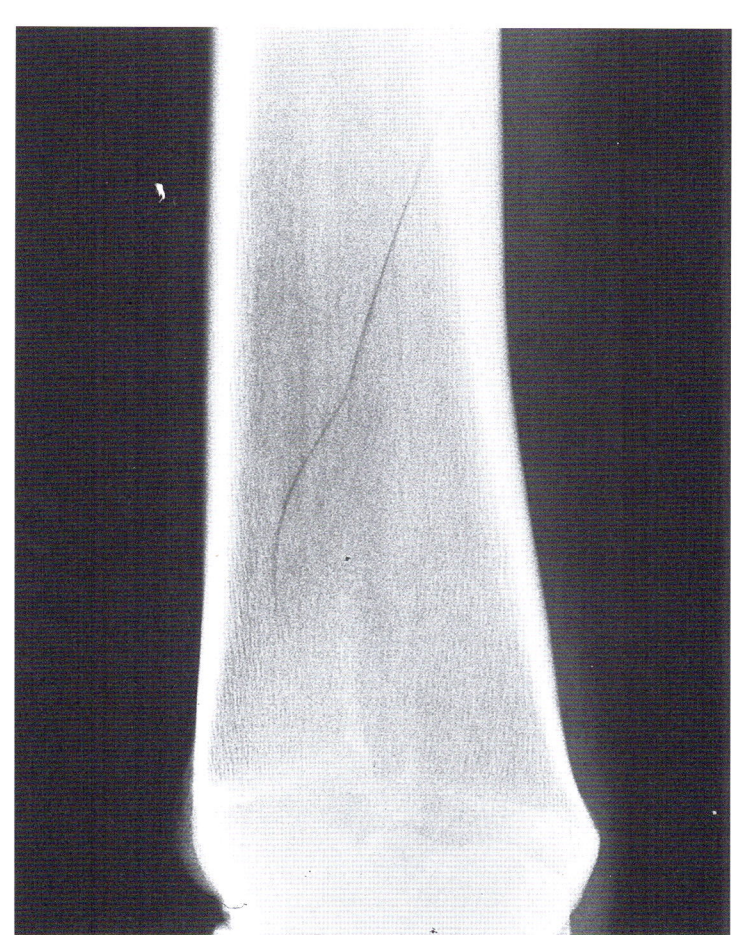

253

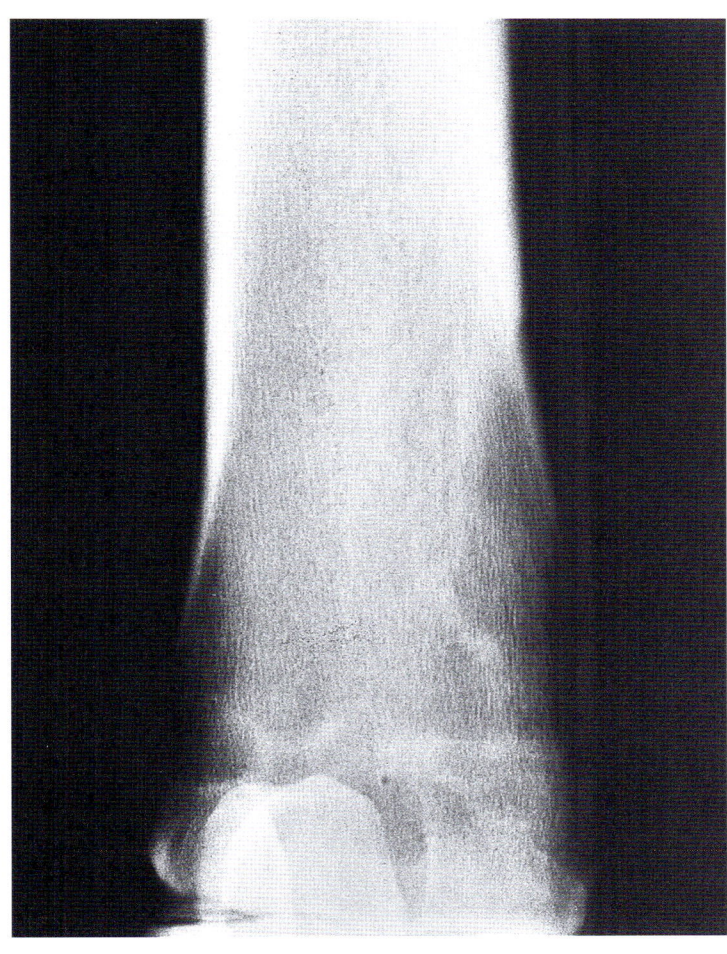

254

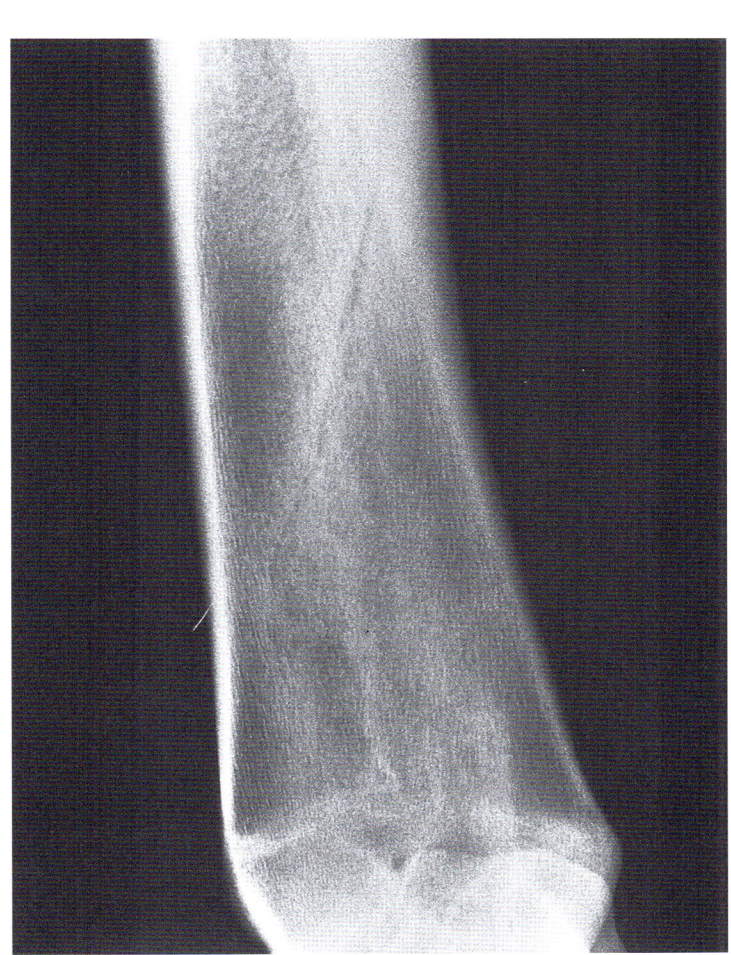

255

Fracture

Radius

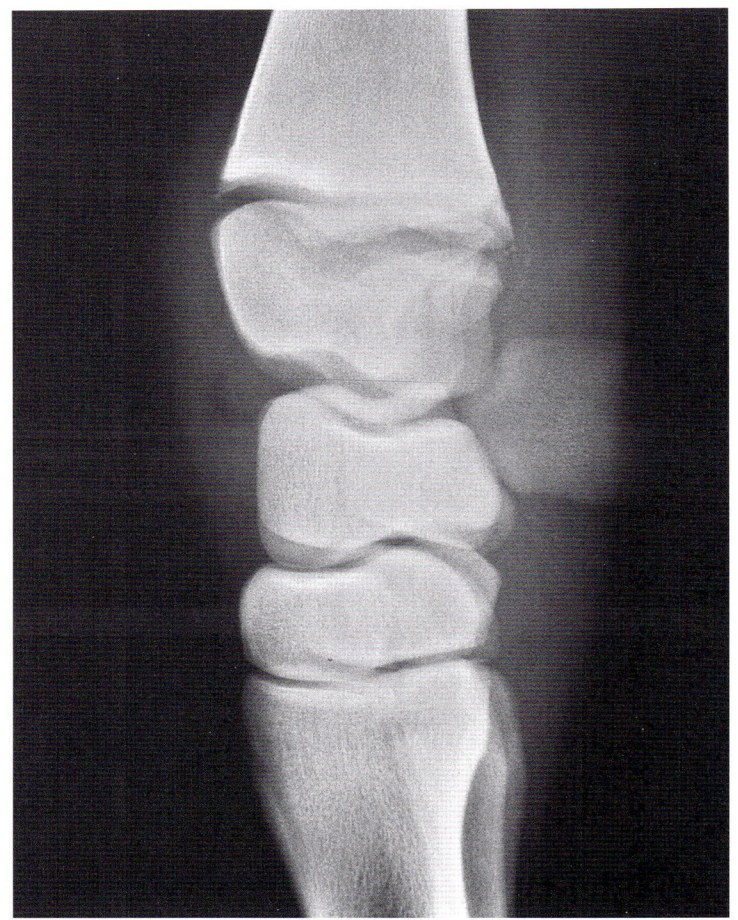

256

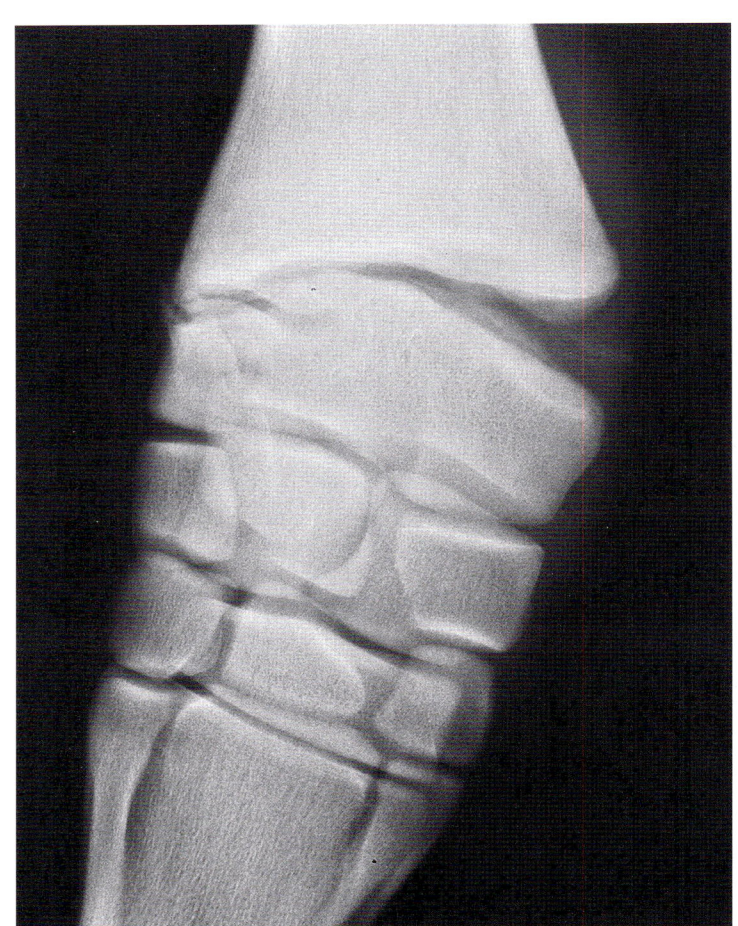

257

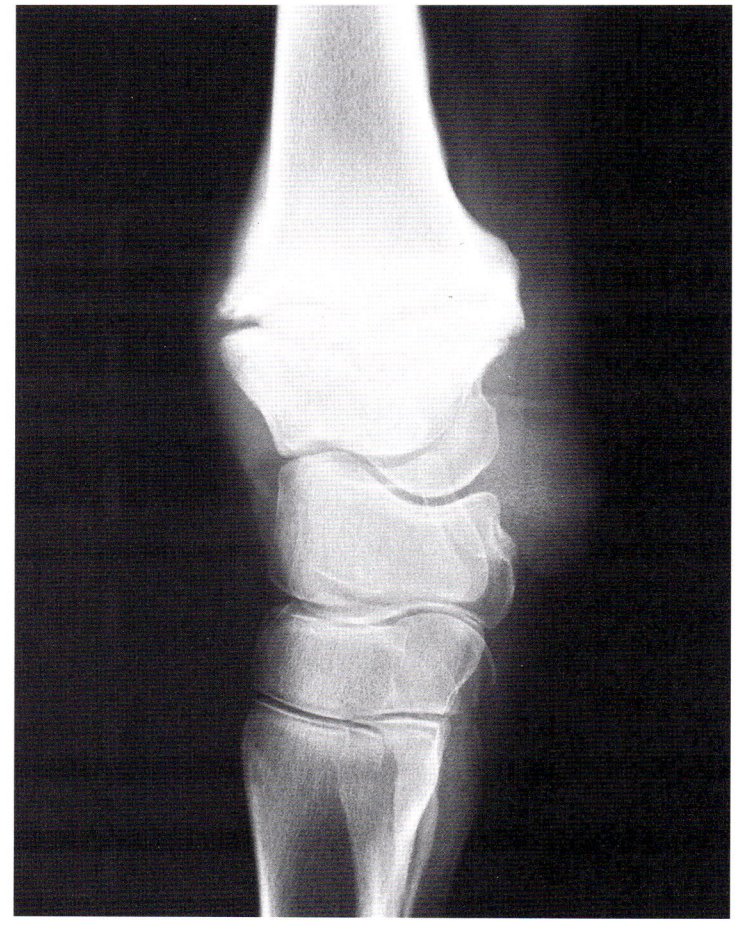

258

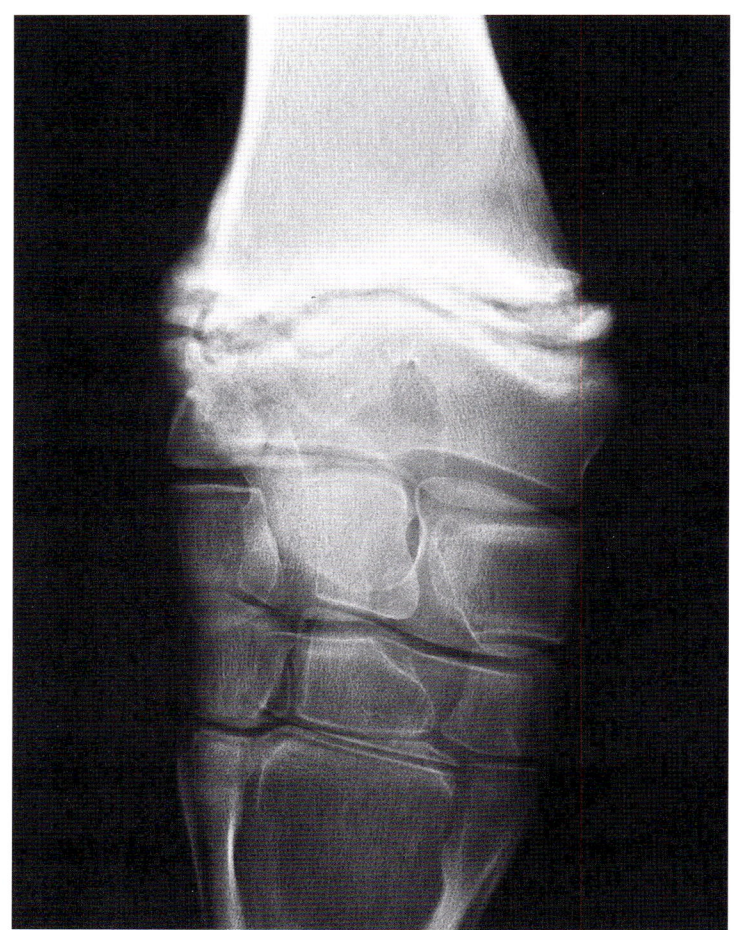

259

Radius

256/257/258/259 Right carpus, serial lateromedial and dorsopalmar views.

Foal, 2 weeks.

The initial dorsopalmar view (Fig. 257), 1 day after the onset of acute severe lameness, reveals prominent widening of the medial aspect of the distal radial physis, with linear opacities in the widened medial physeal region and a very small triangular bony fragment at the lateral physeal border. A very small dorsal metaphyseal fragment and obscure crumbly fragmentation in the palmar physeal region are visible on the corresponding lateromedial radiograph (Fig. 256).

These findings are consistent with a recent physeal fracture with minimal metaphyseal fragmentation.

Six weeks later (Fig. 258, 259) dense periosteal new bone formation is obvious along the cranial, caudal and lateral metaphyseal border.

Mild carpal and metacarpal radiolucency indicates disuse osteoporosis subsequent to fracture and immobilization.

Salter-Harris type 1 or 2 physeal fractures usually do not result in premature physeal closure, but the irregular contour of the lateral physeal region outlined on the dorsopalmar follow-up radiograph (Fig. 259) indicates secondary "epiphysitis", i.e. delayed ossification, probably resulting from lateral metaphyseal compression injury.

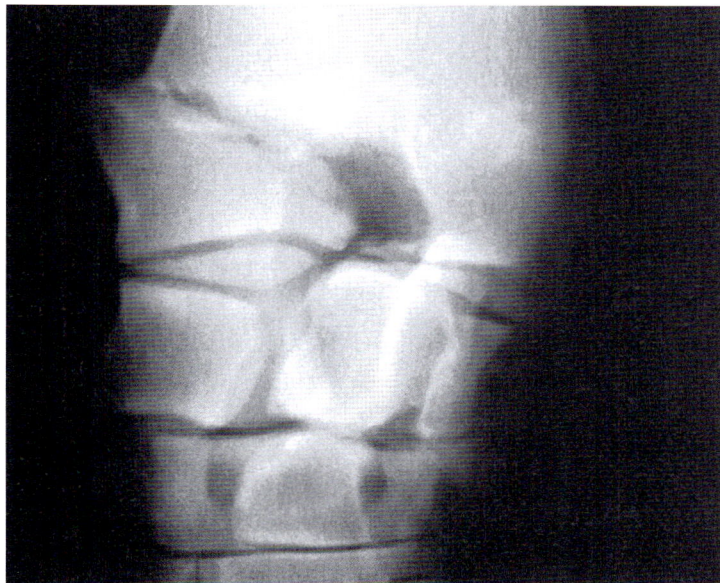

260

260 Left carpus, dorsopalmar view: close-up

Standardbred, 2 years.

Medial shifting of the medial half of the trochlea radii interrupting the continuity of the articular surface and producing a "step" defect in the medial aspect of the distal radius. This was due to a recent, simple, complete, intra-articular trochlear fracture. The fracture line is obscured by slight overriding of the fracture fragments.

Fracture

Accessory carpal bone

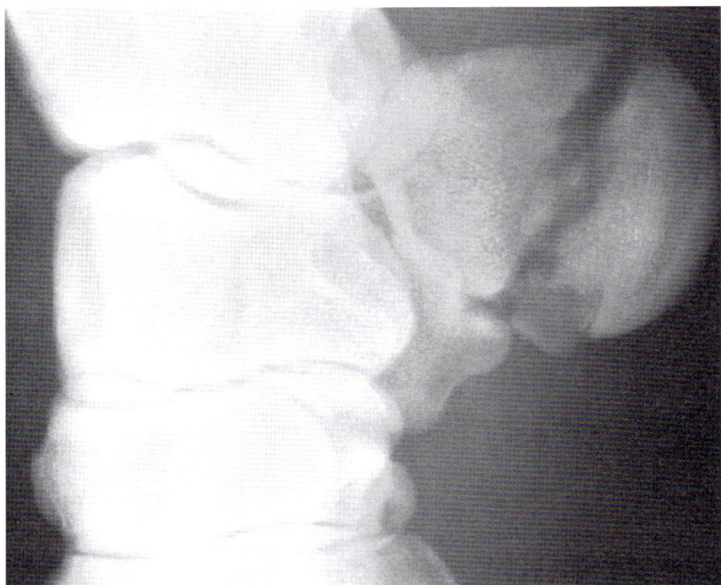

261

261 Left carpus, lateromedial view: close-up.

Standardbred, 9 years.

A sharply bordered, slightly oblique radiolucent zone through the palmar portion of the accessory carpal bone due to a recent simple fracture.

The palmar displacement of the fracture fragment makes the diagnosis quite simple.

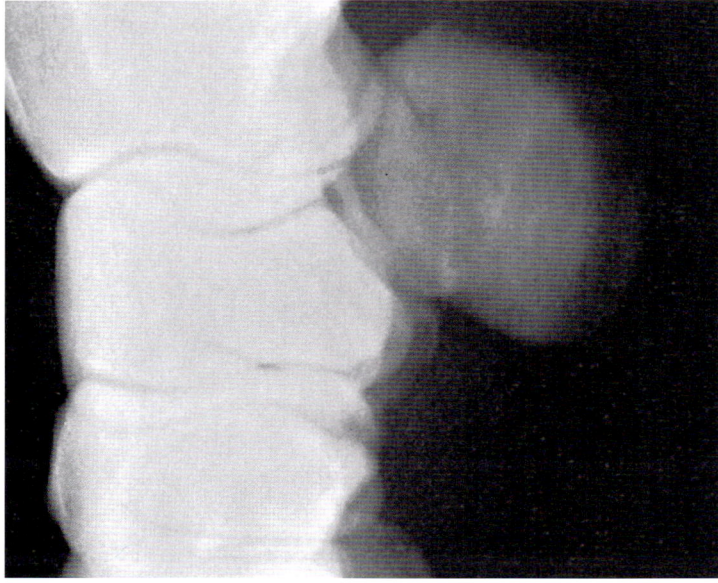

262

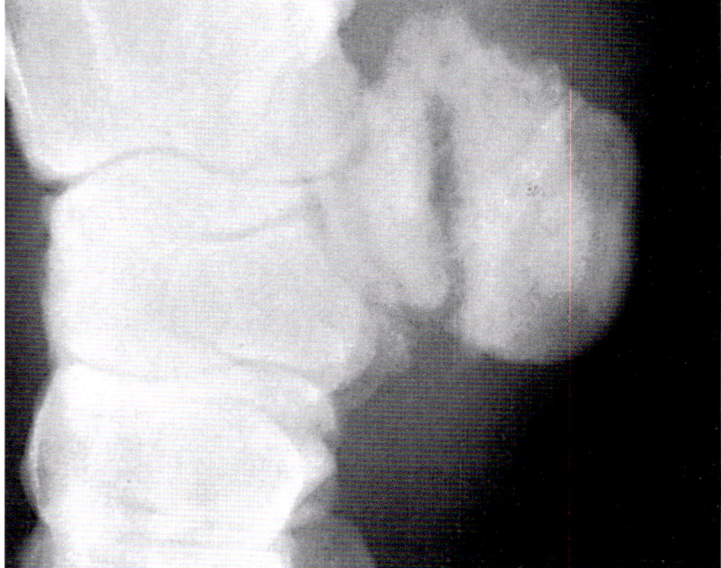

263

262/263 Right carpus, serial lateromedial views: close-ups.

Warmblood, 5 years.

The initial examination (Fig. 262) reveals a narrow, slightly oblique radiolucent line through the dorsal portion of the accessory carpal bone, due to a recent simple fracture. The fracture fragments are not displaced and the fracture line is therefore difficult to identify.

Five months later (Fig. 263) the fracture zone is widened and ill bordered and although periosteal callus is present at the proximal and distal border of the accessory carpal bone, it fails to bridge the fracture site. These radiological findings indicate non-union.

Radial carpal bone

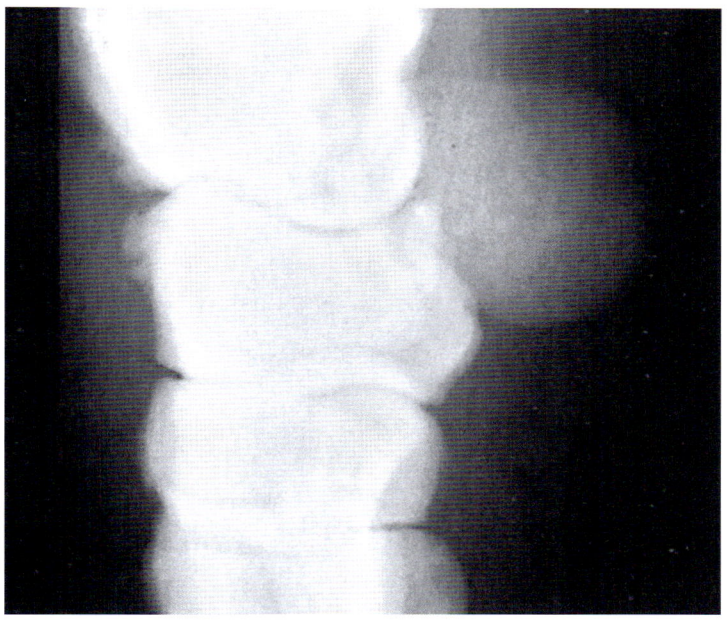

264

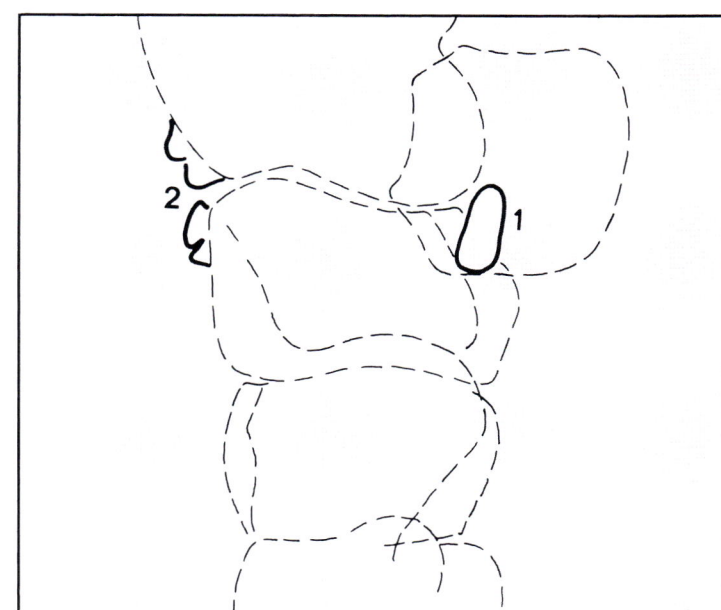

264 a

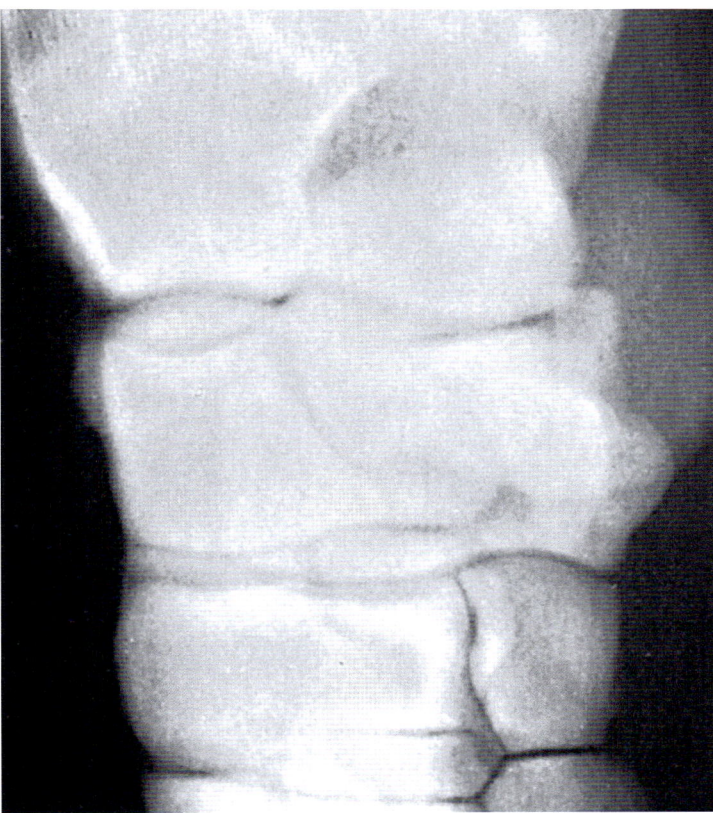

265

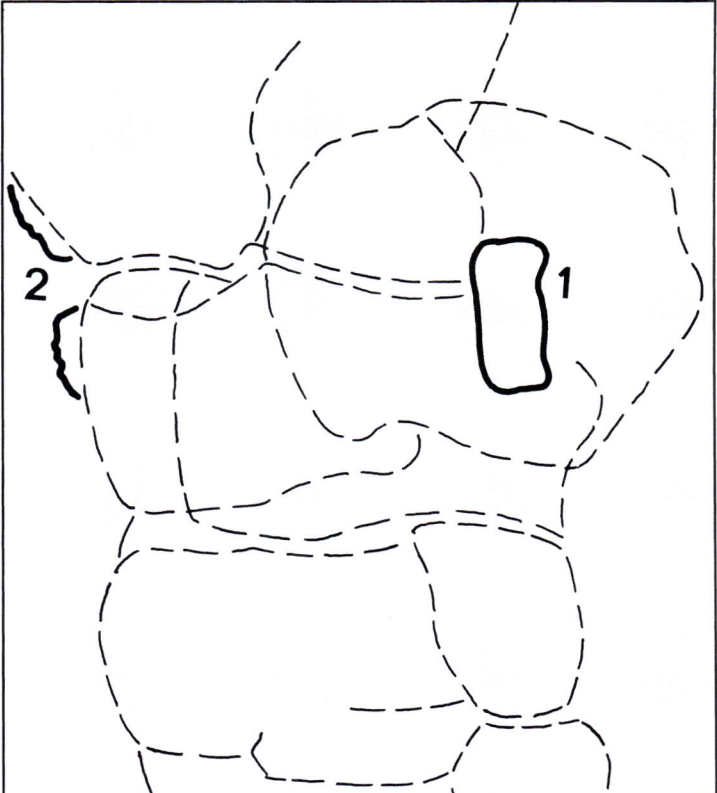

265 a

264/265 Right carpus, lateromedial and dorsomedial-palmarolateral oblique view: close-ups.

Pony, 5 years.

The lateromedial view (Fig. 264) presents an obscure isolated rectangular bone fragment **(1)** palmar to the radiocarpal joint, due to a slightly displaced chip fracture originating from the mediopalmar aspect of the radial carpal bone demonstrated by the dorsomedial-palmarolateral oblique view (Fig. 265), the fracture "bed" is not visible.

Additional finding: osteoarthrosis of the radiocarpal joint indicated by the peri- and intra-articular new bone formation **(2)** on the dorsal and dorso-lateral aspect of the distal end of the radius and the proximal end of the ulnar carpal bone.

The new bone growth is mature, as indicated by its density and sharp border, but the dense, sharply bordered fracture fragment suggests recent fracture. Consequently the two phenomena do not necessarily result from the same traumatic injury.

264 a/265 a Schematic drawings

Fracture

Radial carpal bone

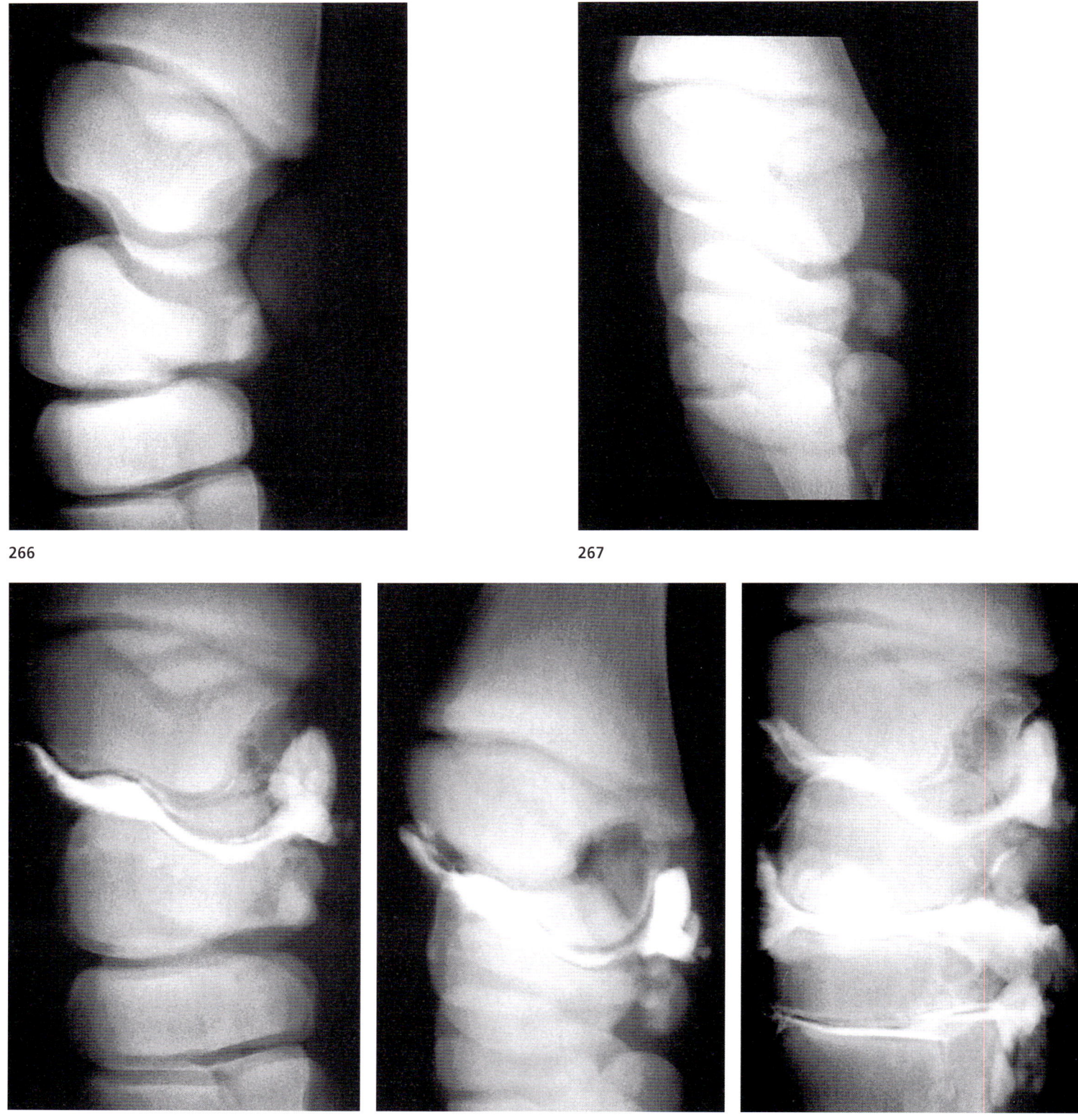

266

267

268

269

270

266/267/268/269/270 Right carpus, lateromedial and dorsomedial-palmarolateral oblique survey and positive contrast study: close-ups.

Foal, 2 weeks.

A lateromedial survey radiograph (Fig. 266) several hours after the onset of lameness reveals an isolated capricious opacity with an irregular mottled appearance in the palmar region of the proximal row of carpal bones, belonging to the mediopalmar portion of the radial carpal bone, demonstrated by a dorsomedial-palmarolateral oblique view (Fig. 267). The differential diagnosis is a separate ossification centre or a fracture fragment. Radiographic examination of the left (sound) carpus revealed similar "abnormalities". Two ml positive contrast material injected into the radiocarpal joint (Fig. 268 — lateromedial view, Fig. 269 — dorsomedial-palmarolateral oblique view) reveals no abnormalities. Four ml positive contrast material injected into the intercarpal joint (Fig. 270 — dorsomedial-palmarolateral oblique view) penetrates between the isolated opacity and the remaining portion of the radial carpal bone. Lameness had therefore resulted from a vertical intra-articular fracture through an incompletely ossified portion of the radial carpal bone.

Ulnar carpal bone

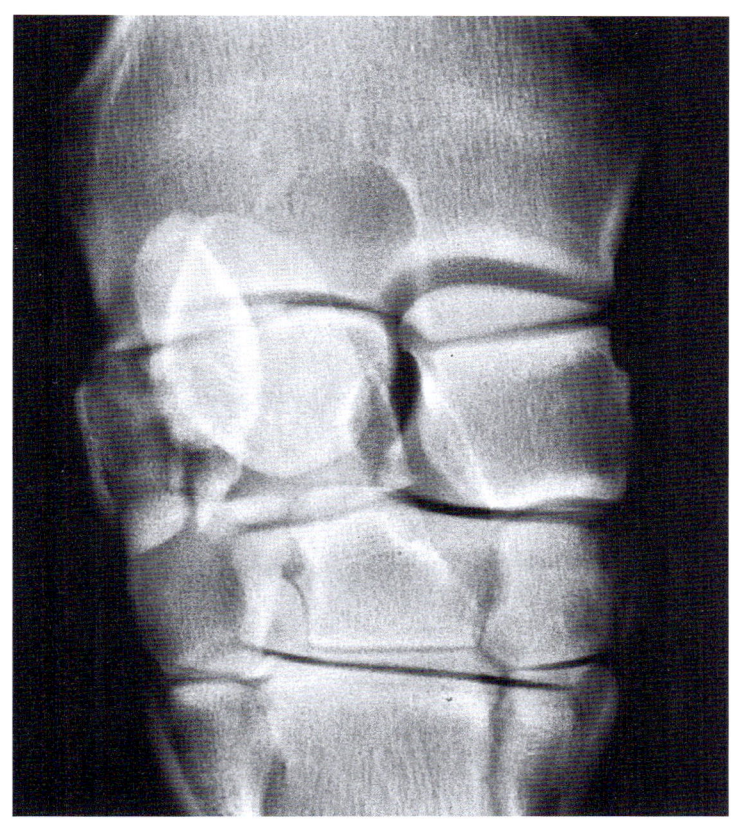

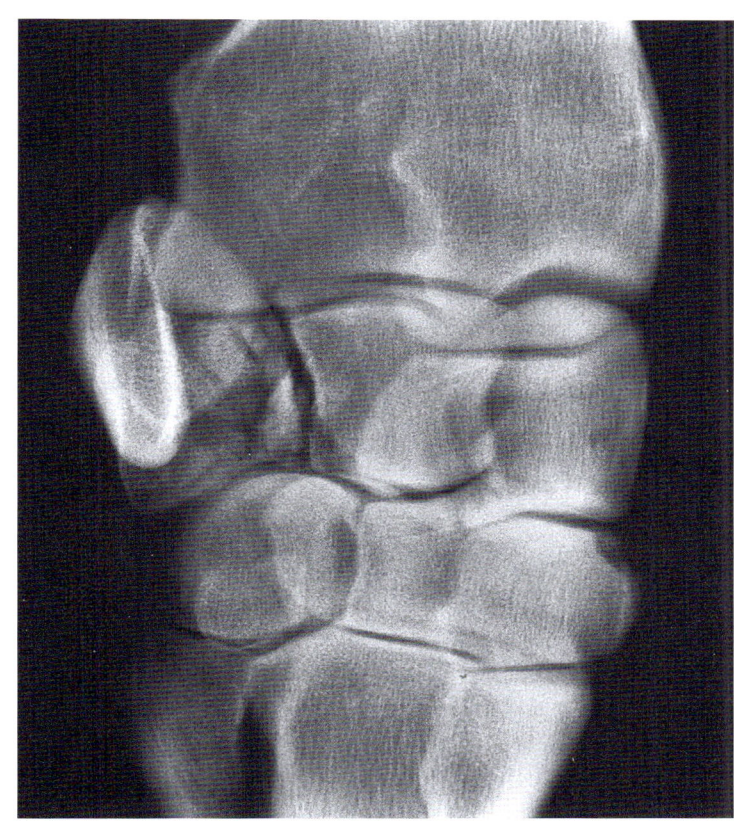

271

272

271/272 Right carpus, dorsopalmar and dorsolateral – palmaromedial oblique view: close-ups.

Arabian, 11 years.

The dorsopalmar view (Fig. 271) reveals a vertical radiolucent zone through the mid region of the ulnar carpal interrupting the articular surface of the radiocarpal and intercarpal joint. This indicates the presence of a recent sagittal fracture. On the dorsolateral – palmaromedial oblique view (Fig. 272) the fracture plane is not parallel to the central beam, therefore two vertical oblique radiolucent lines extending from the radiocarpal joint into the proximal half of the ulnar carpal bone are visible.

Third carpal bone

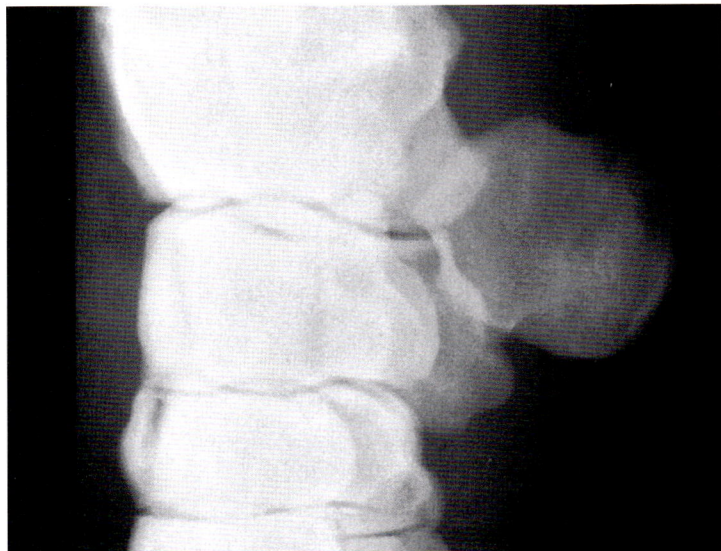

273

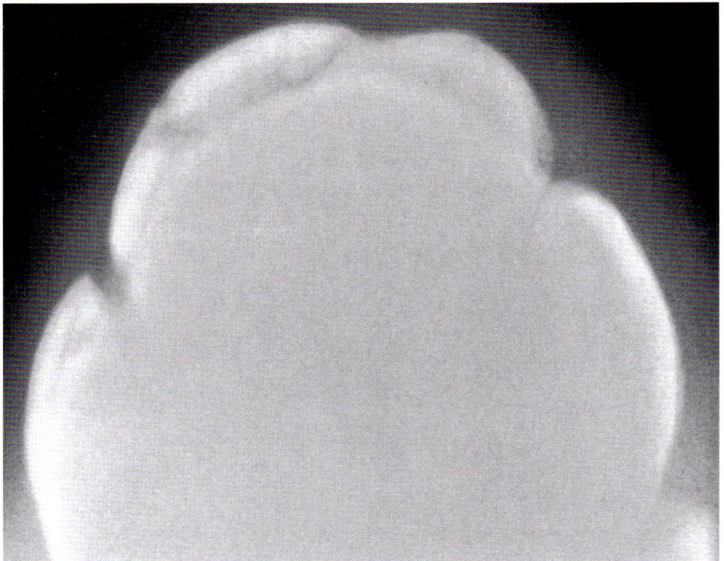

274

273/274 Right carpus, lateromedial and dorsoproximal-dorsodistal oblique "skyline" view: close-ups.

Standardbred, 3 years.

The lateromedial view (Fig. 273) reveals a vertical radiolucent zone through the dorsal portion of the distal row of carpal bones, extending from the intercarpal joint to the carpometacarpal joint.

This indicates the presence of a recent slab fracture originating from the third carpal bone, as demonstrated in the dorsoproximal-dorsodistal oblique "skyline" view (Fig. 274) of the distal carpal row, which shows a rather large fragment **(2)** and a narrow irregular obscure fracture line **(1)** through the mediodorsal aspect of the third carpal bone.

274 a Schematic drawing

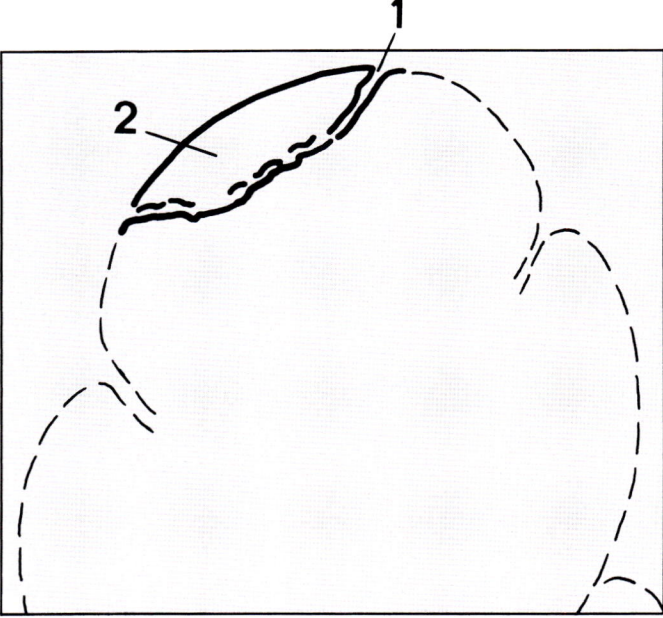

274 a

Third carpal bone

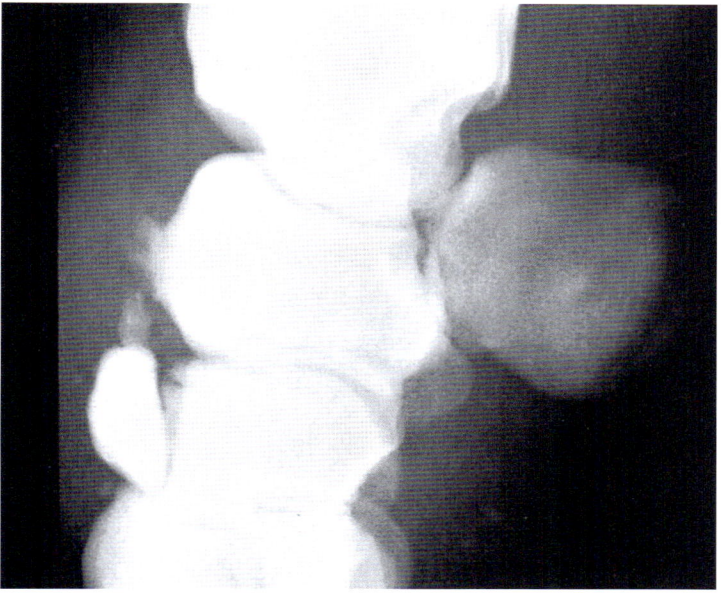

275 Left carpus, lateromedial view: close-up.

Thoroughbred, 4 years.

A large, dense, sharply bordered bone fragment separated from the dorsal aspect of the distal row of carpal bones, indicates the presence of a slab fracture.

The displacement of the fracture fragment makes the diagnosis relatively simple. The ill defined opacities proximal and distal to the large slab fragment represent additional fracture fragments.

Additional finding: extensive ill bordered new bone growth on the dorsal surface of the proximal row of carpal bones. The sharply bordered fracture zone and density of the bone fragment suggest a recent fracture. The density of the periosteal new bone indicates a longer duration, consequently the two phenomena do not necessarily result from the same traumatic injury.

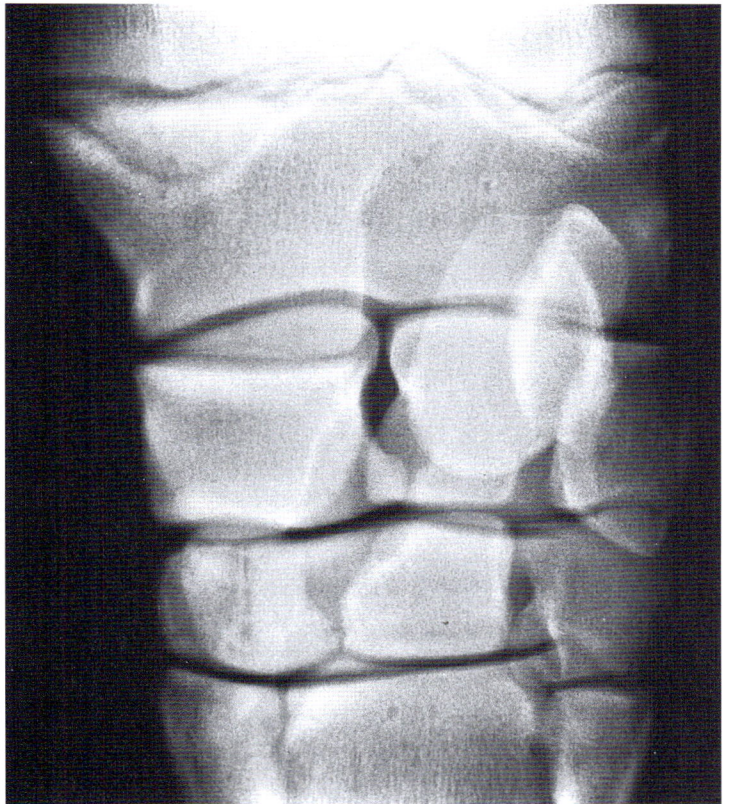

276

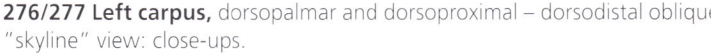

277

276/277 Left carpus, dorsopalmar and dorsoproximal – dorsodistal oblique "skyline" view: close-ups.

Standardbred, 1 year.

The dorsopalmar view (Fig. 276) visualizes a vertical radiolucent line extending from the intercarpal joint through the medial portion of the third carpal bone.

On the dorsoproximal – dorsodistal "skyline" view (Fig. 277) this line is also visible and extends in dorsopalmar direction.

These findings are consistent with a recent sagittal fracture that is a less common type of third carpal bone fracture. These fractures are easily missed on standard lateromedial, and dorsopalmar views, more obvious on oblique projections and clearly detectable on additional dorsoproximal – dorsodistal oblique skyline views, probably due to the dorsomedial – palmarolateral oblique direction of the fracture zone. In this case the fracture extended in dorsopalmar direction and, therefore, was also visible on the dorsopalmar radiograph.

Fracture

Third carpal bone

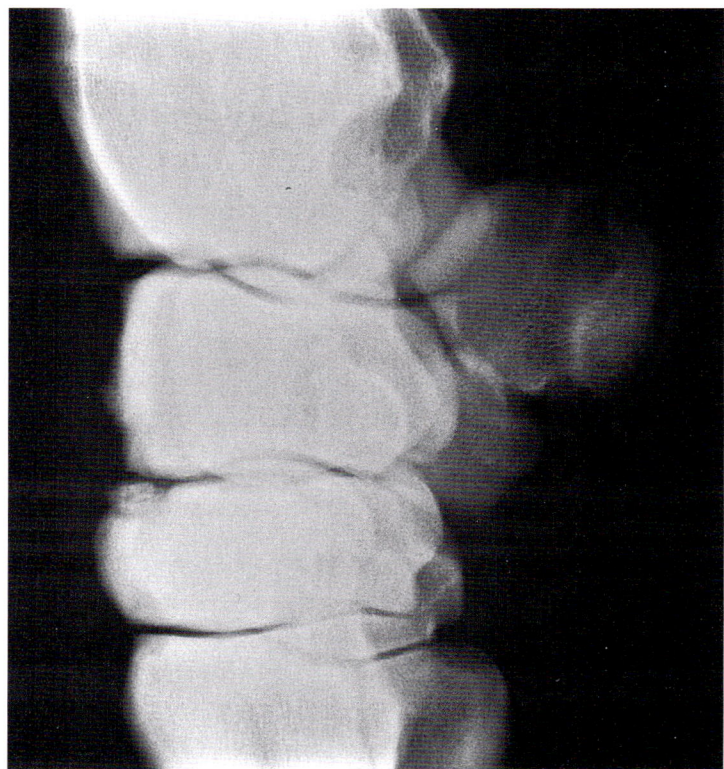

278

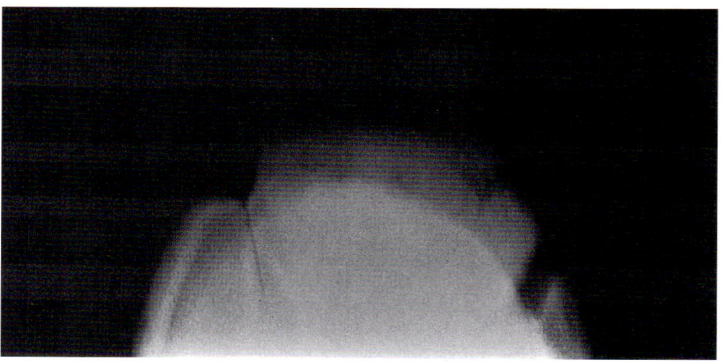

280

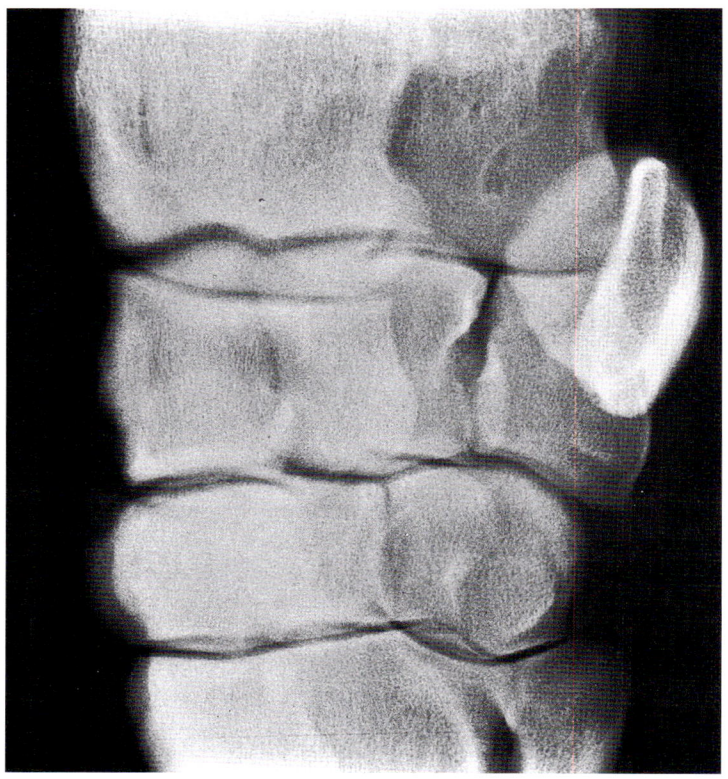

279

278/279/280 Left carpus, lateromedial, dorsolateral – palmaromedial oblique and dorso-proximal – dorsodistal oblique "skyline" view: close-ups.

Thoroughbred, 3 years.

The well defined bony fragment and corresponding defect in the dorso-proximal contour of the distal row of carpal bones is characteristic of a chip fracture of the third carpal bone. The periosteal new bone on the dorsal surface of the proximal row of carpal bones suggests a fracture of some duration. The dorsomedial location of the chip fragment is poorly demonstrated on the dorsolateral – palmaromedial oblique view (Fig. 279), but more obvious on the dorsoproximal – dorsodistal oblique "skyline" radiograph (Fig. 280).

Radial and third carpal bone

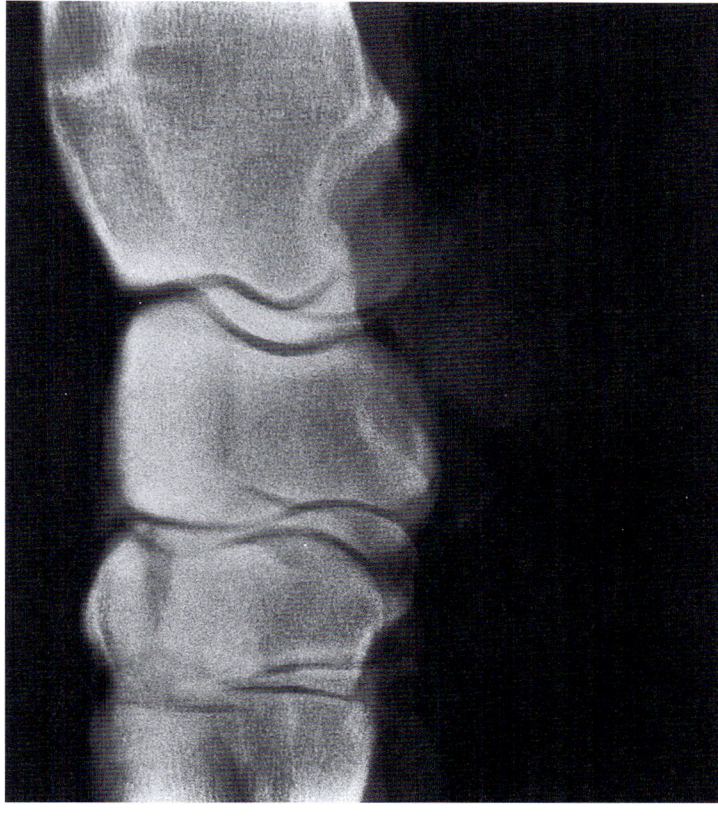

281

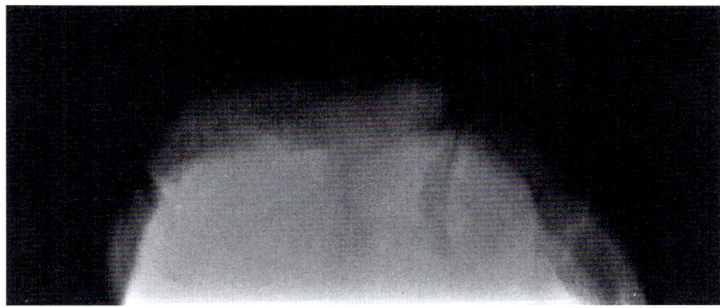

283

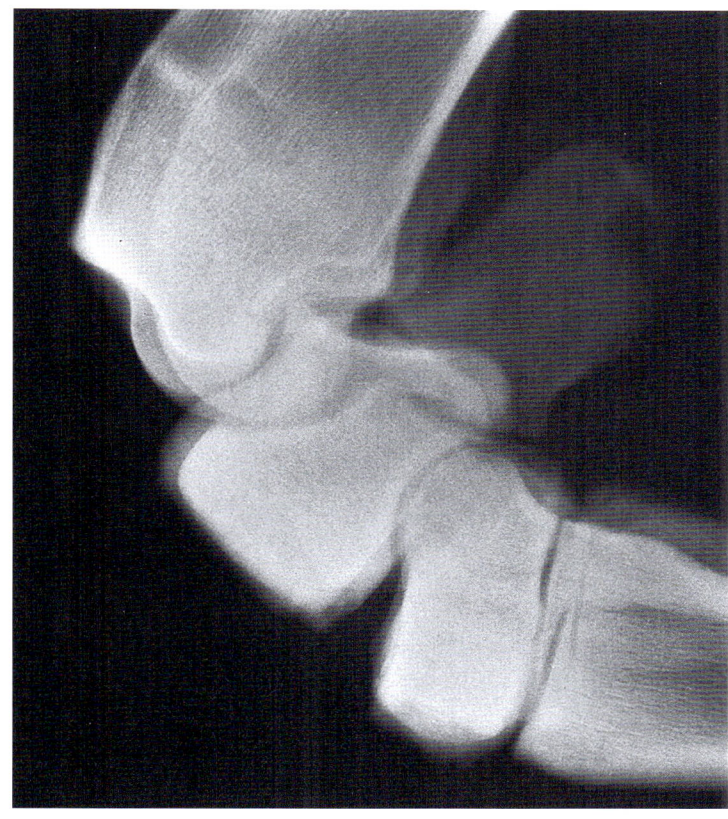

282

281/282/283 Right carpus, lateromedial, flexed lateromedial and dorso-proximal-dorsodistal oblique "skyline" view; close-ups.

Thoroughbred, 3 years.

The standard lateromedial view (Fig. 281) shows an ill defined fragment in the dorsal aspect of the intercarpal joint and a vertical radiolucent zone through the dorsal portion of the distal row of carpal bones.

These features represent the combination of a recent radial chip fracture and a third carpal slab fracture.

The chip fragment originating from the dorsodistal aspect of the radial carpal bone becomes more obvious on the flexed lateromedial view (Fig. 282).

The slab fragment separated from the dorsal aspect of the third carpal bone is ascertained by the dorsoproximal-dorsodistal "skyline" view (Fig. 283).

Fracture

Fourth carpal bone

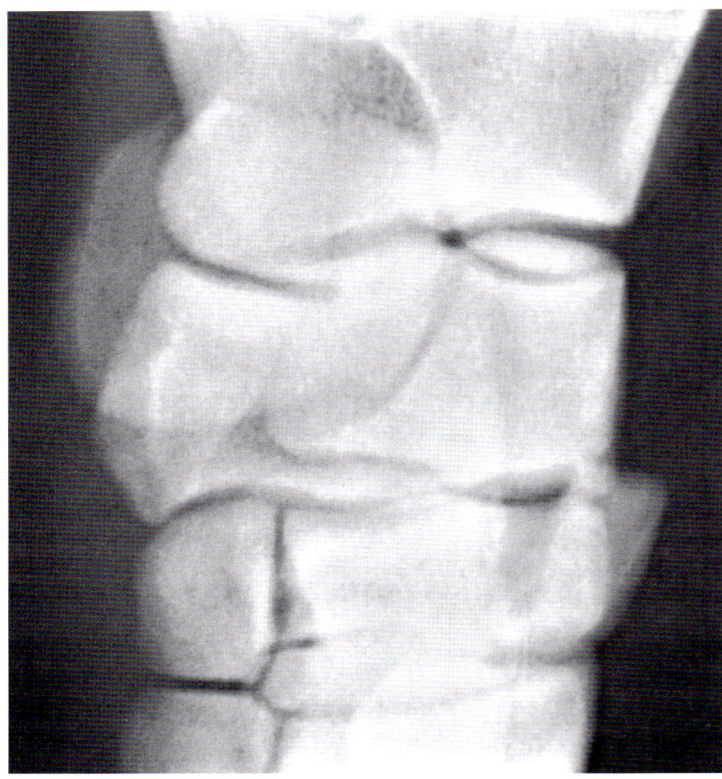

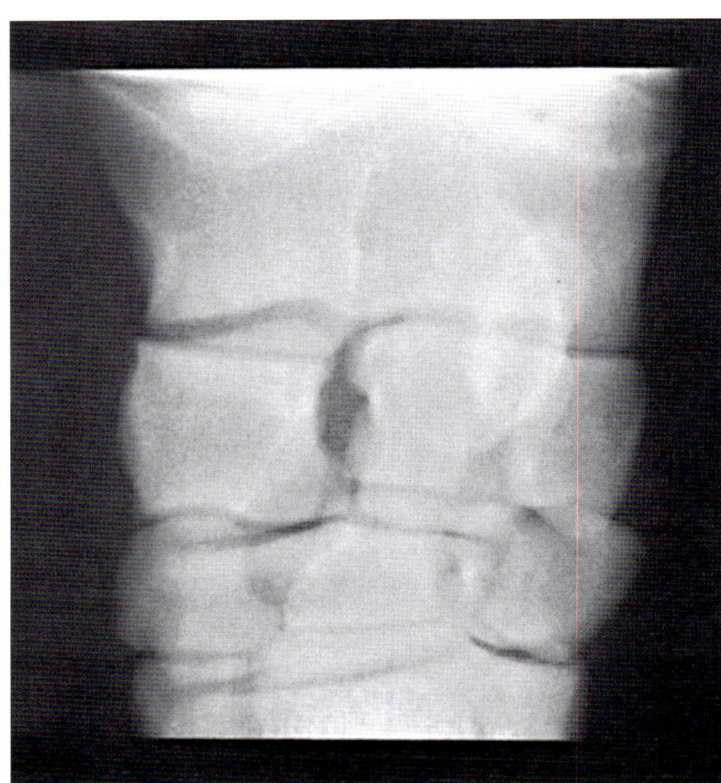

284

285

284/285 Left carpus, dorsomedial-palmarolateral oblique and dorsopalmar view: close-ups.

Pony, 2 years.

The dorsomedial-palmarolateral oblique view (Fig. 284) reveals a "step" defect laterally between the ulnar carpal bone and the fourth carpal bone and a vertical, wide, V-shaped, sharply bordered radiolucent zone through the fourth carpal bone, extending from the intercarpal joint to the carpometacarpal joint. These signs are consistent with a recent slab fracture of the fourth carpal bone. The "step" defect is created by rotation of the fracture fragment.

The fracture zone and rotation are less obvious on the dorsopalmar view (Fig. 285).

Fourth and intermediate carpal bone

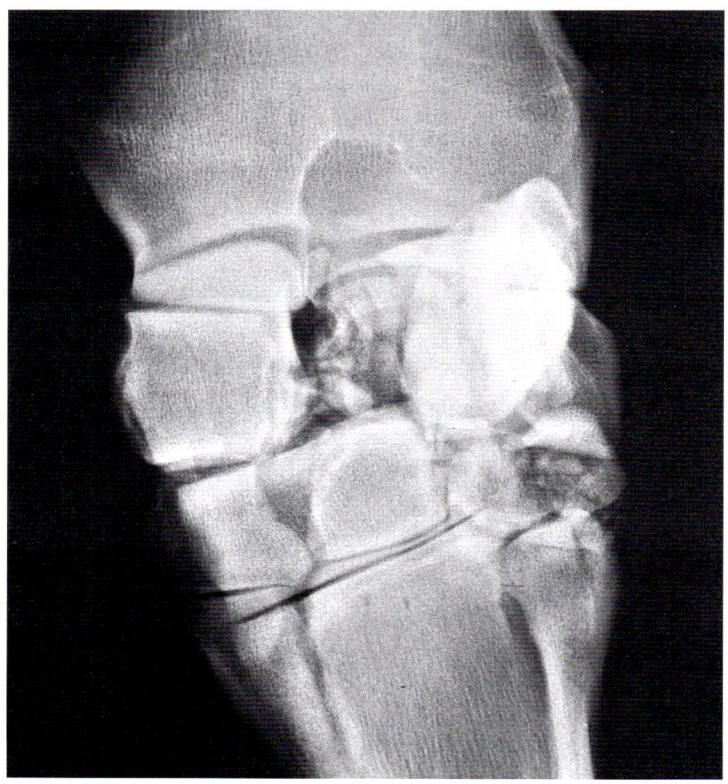

286

286 Left carpus, dorsopalmar view: close-up.

Warmblood, 13 years.

Multiple clearly defined bone fragments and radiolucent lines involving the entire intermediate carpal bone and the lateral half of the fourth carpal bone, due to a recent comminuted fracture of these bones, resulting in mild valgus deformity.

Contrary to foals, in adult horses (sudden occuring) carpal angular deformity usually has a traumatic origin.

Cannon bone

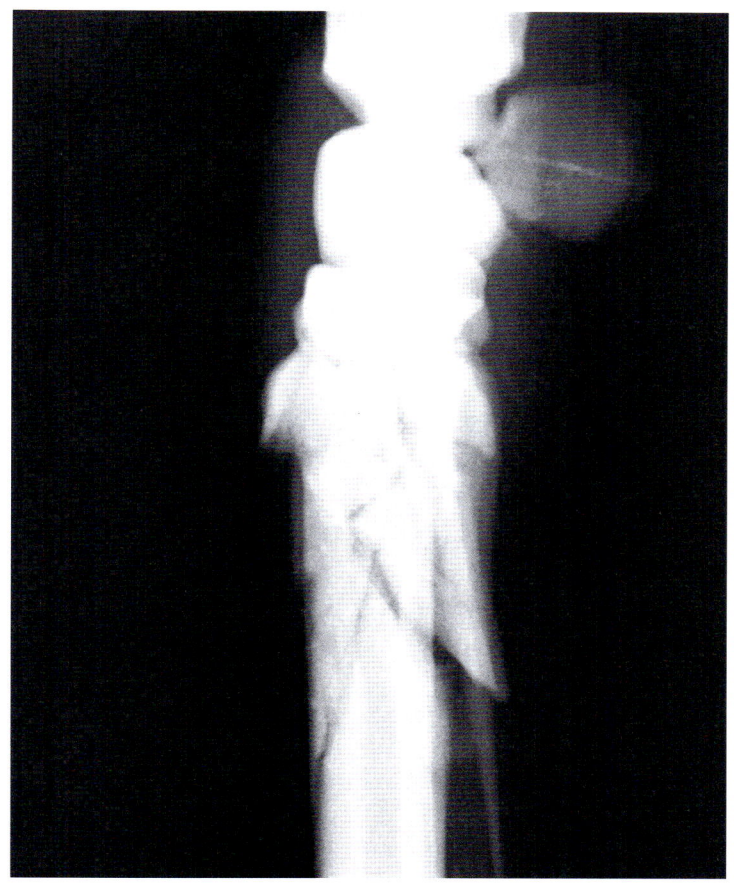

287

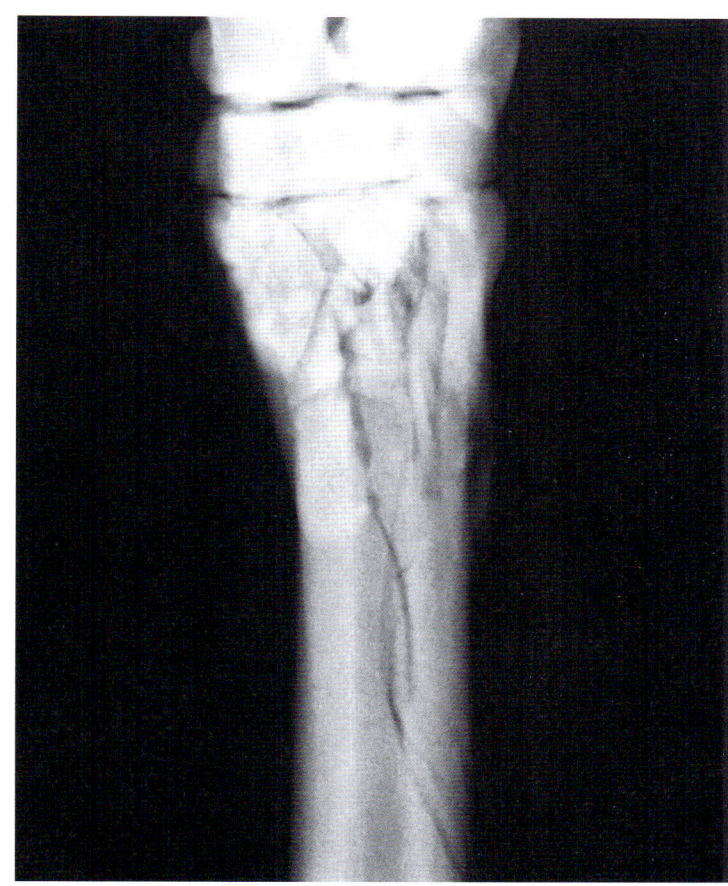

288

287/288 Left carpus, lateromedial and dorsopalmar view.

Pony, 6 years.

Multiple sharply bordered bone fragments and radiolucent lines in the proximal half of the cannon bone, interrupting the articular surface as well as the continuity of the metacarpal cortex, indicating a recent comminuted intra-articular fracture of the cannon bone.

Splint bone

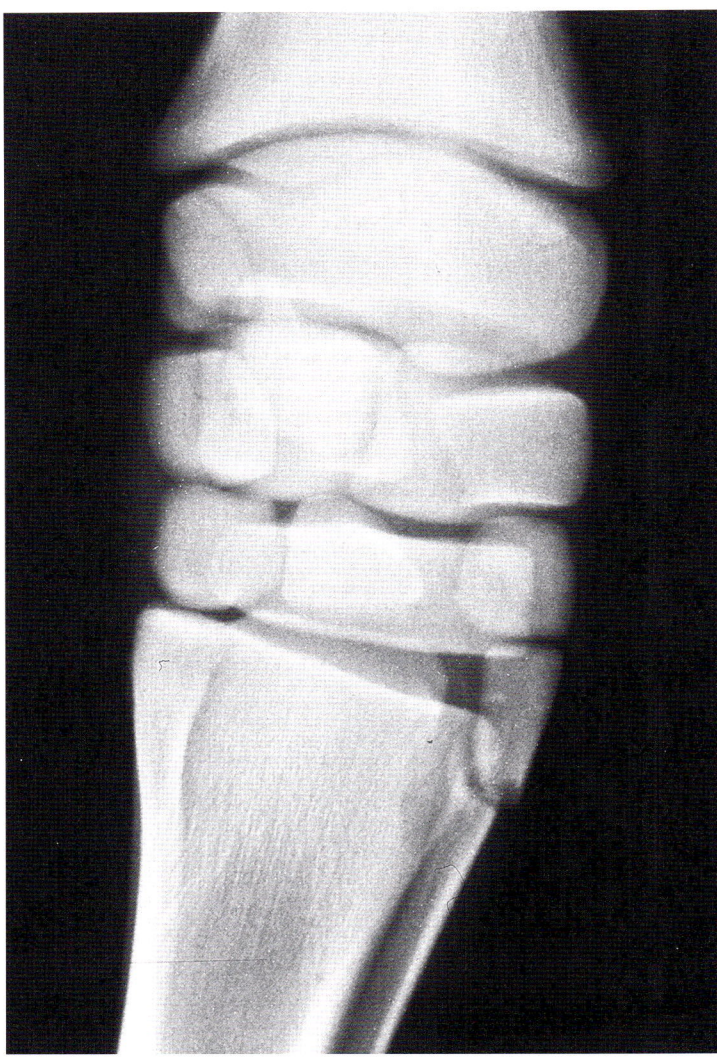 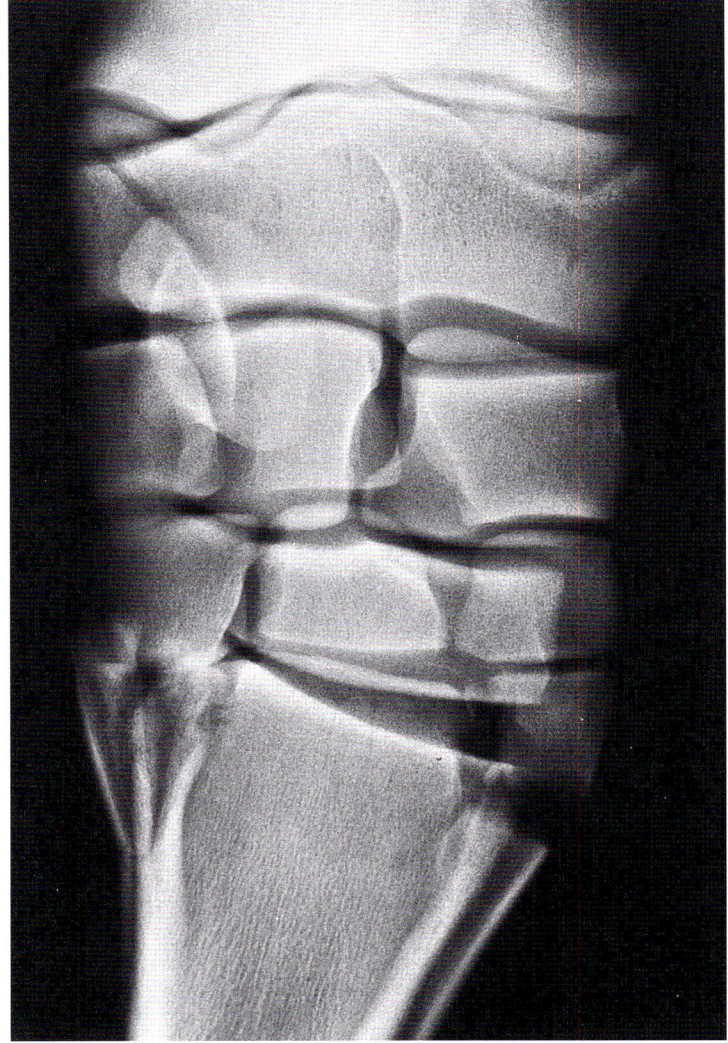

289 Right carpus, dorsopalmar view: close-up.

Foal, 1 day.

Marked widening of the medial aspect of the carpometacarpal joint, discontinuity and a corresponding step defect of the proximal portion of the medial splint bone and a small intra-articular bone fragment superimposed on the proximal end of the medial splint bone.

These changes indicate a traumatic valgus deformity due to a recent fracture of the medial splint bone and associated subluxation of the carpometacarpal joint.

290 Right carpus, dorsopalmar view: close-up.

Foal, 2 months.

Prominent widening of the medial aspect of the carpometacarpal joint, obvious discontinuity of the proximal portion of the medial splint bone and obscure fragmentation of the head of the lateral splint bone.

These features indicate fracture of the proximal extremity of both splint bones and associated carpometacarpal subluxation.

Contrary to adult horses, in foals traumatic carpal angular deformity occurs relatively seldom.

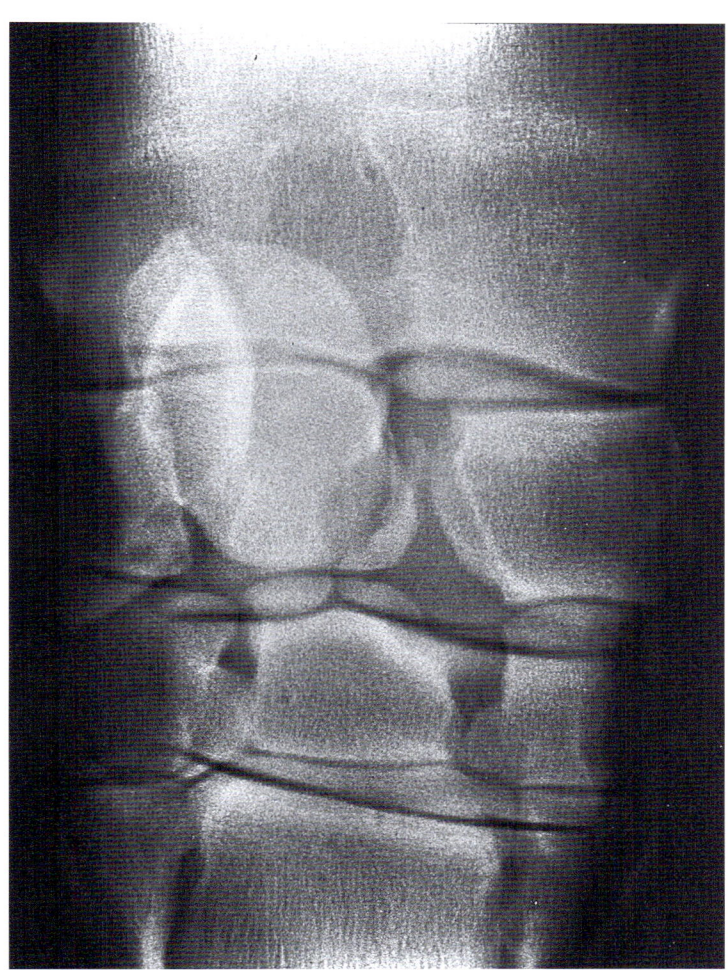

291 Right carpus, dorsopalmar view: close-up.

Standardbred, 3 years.

The small rounded radiolucencies within the distomedial aspect of the ulnar carpal bone are suggestive of tearing of the proximal insertion of the lateral palmar intercarpal ligament. Tearing of the medial and/or lateral palmar intercarpal ligament seldom results in radiographic avulsion defects. Therefore, additional assessment with arthroscopy is required for a definitive diagnosis.

291

Herniation of the joint capsule

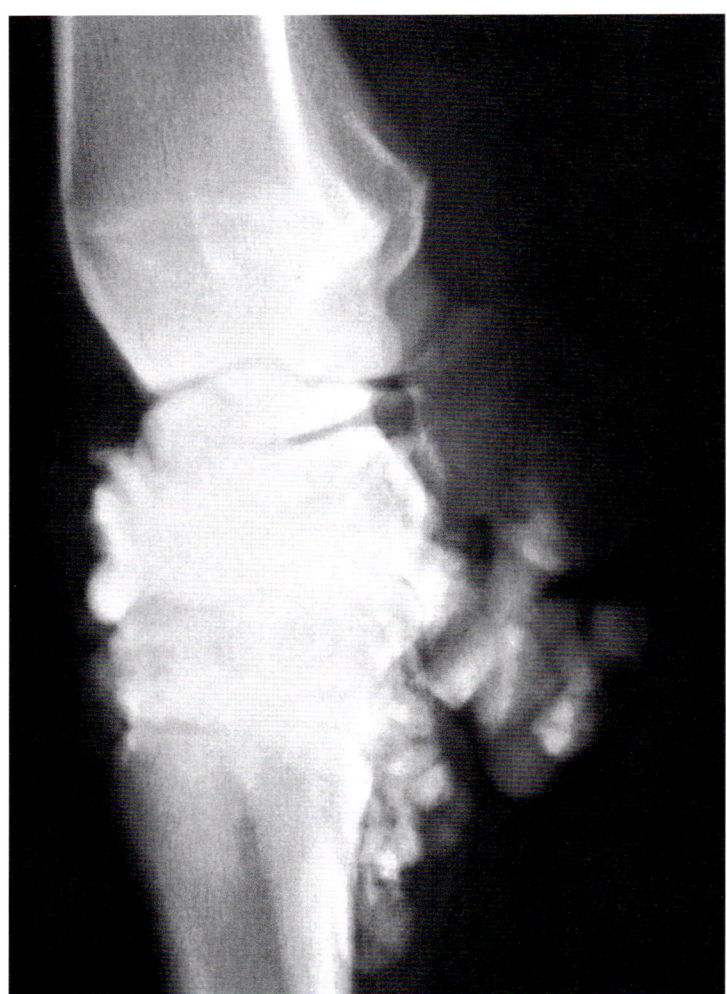

293

292

292/293 Left carpus, lateromedial contrast studies of an abnormal and a normal carpus: close-ups.

Standardbred, 4 years (abnormal carpus).

Several hours after the onset of lameness, the horse having been caught by a fence, 10 ml positive contrast material injected into the intercarpal joint (Fig. 292) shows severe distension of the palmar surface of the joint capsule. The distension was caused by herniation, which was confirmed by surgery.

The usual palmar extension of the intercarpal joint capsule is demonstrated by a double contrast arthrogram of a normal intercarpal joint (Fig. 293).

Traumatic periostitis

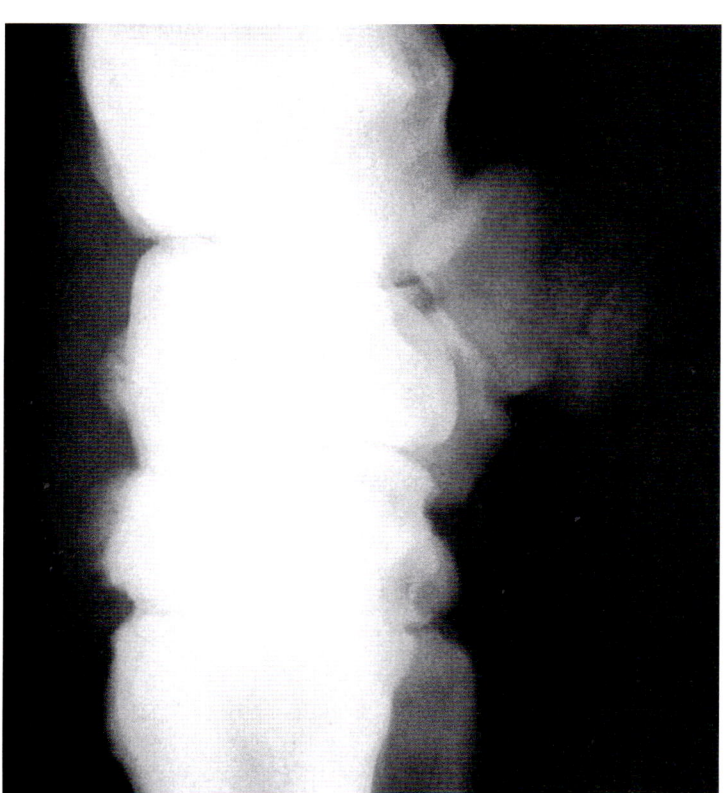

294

294 Right carpus, lateromedial view: close-up.

Warmblood, 9 years.

Periosteal new bone formation on the dorsal surface of the proximal and distal row of carpal bones, resulting from percutaneous trauma or following tearing of the joint capsule attachments. The periosteal reaction on the distal row of carpal bones involves the joint surfaces. The periosteal new bone on the proximal row of carpal bones involves the joint capsule attachment of the radiocarpal and intercarpal joint. The ill defined border of the periosteal new bone indicates that the lesion is active.

N. B. The vertical radiolucent line in the accessory carpal bone is a normal anatomical feature and should not be confused with fracture.

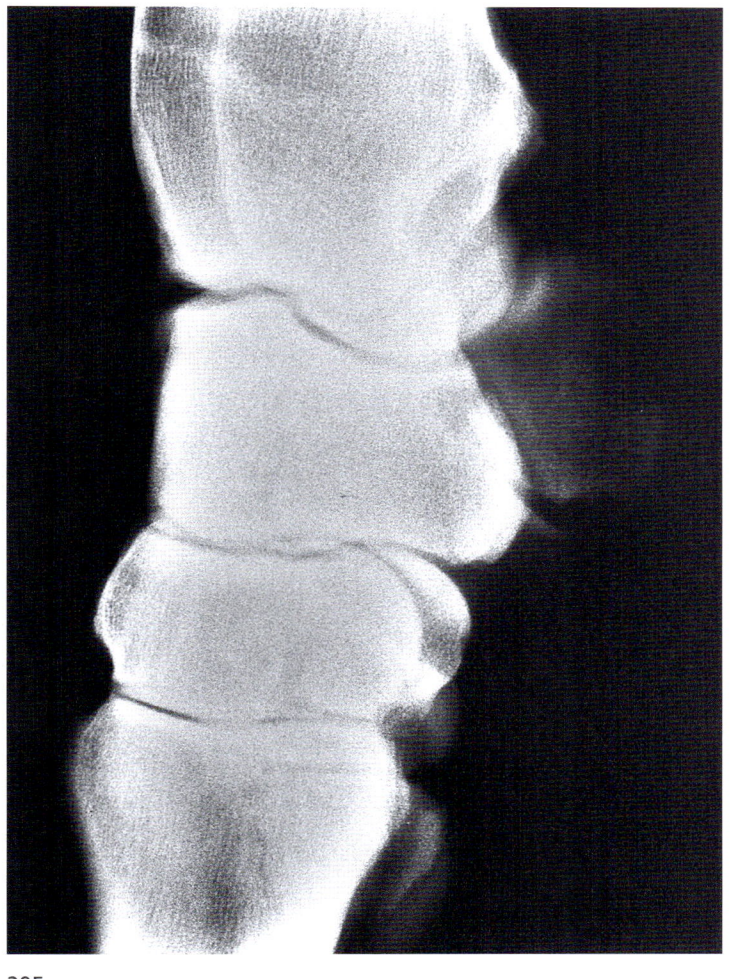

295

296

295/296/297 Right carpus, lateromedial, dorsopalmar and dorsolateral-palmaromedial oblique view: close-ups.

Warmblood, 13 years.

The dorsolateral-palmaromedial oblique view (Fig. 297) clearly shows marginal spurring on the dorsoproximomedial aspect of the radial carpal bone, thus indicating mild osteoarthrosis of the radiocarpal joint.

On the dorsopalmar radiograph (Fig. 296) the marginal spurring of the radial carpal bone appears less prominent, but this view also demonstrates mild spurring of the opposite distomedial border of the radial epiphysis.

The lateromedial view (Fig. 295) only reveals rounding of the normally right-angled shape of the dorsoproximal contour of the radial carpal bone. As demonstrated by this case marginal spurring may involve only part of the joint. Therefore, examinations for (carpal) osteoarthrosis should not be limited to lateromedial and dorsopalmar views, but also include oblique projections.

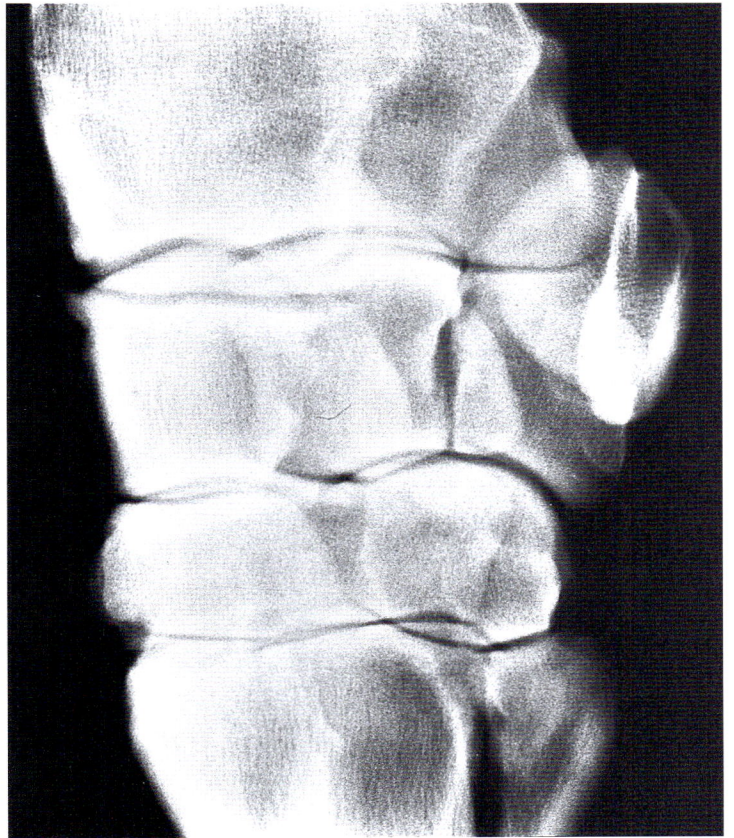

297

Osteoarthrosis

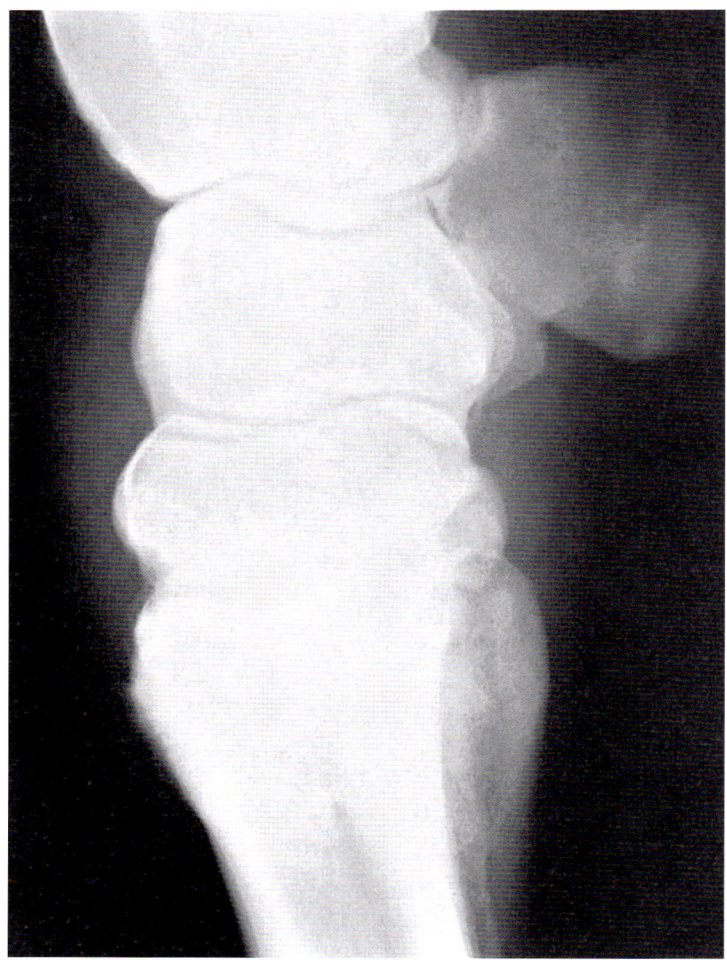

298

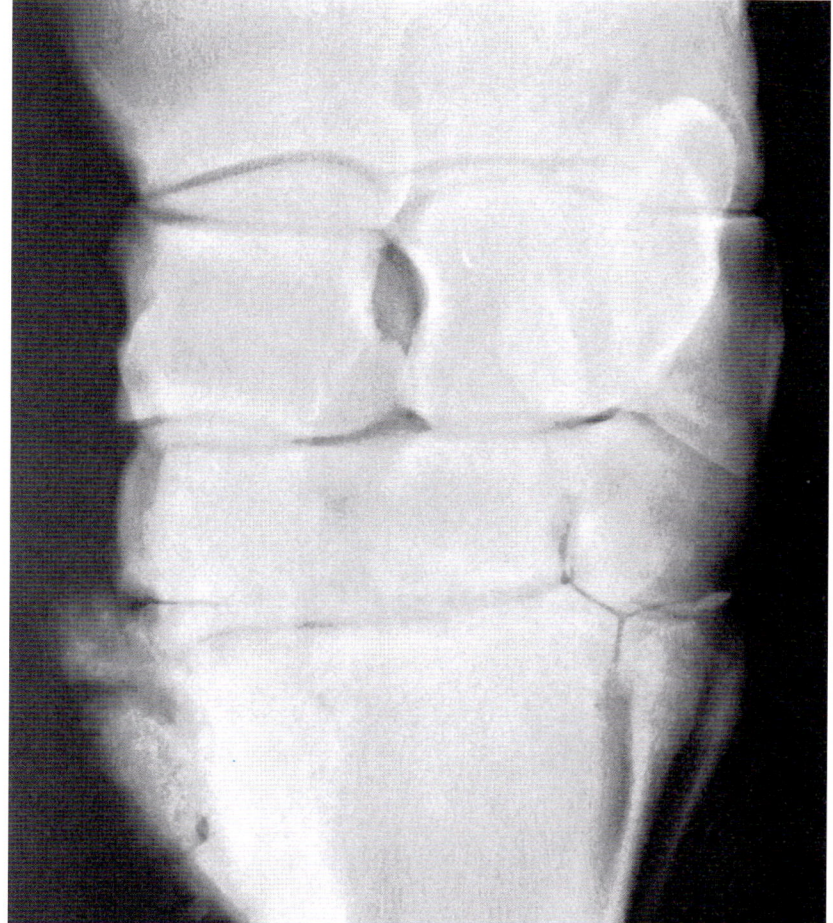

299

298/299 Left carpus, lateromedial and dorsopalmar view: close-ups. Warmblood, 4 years.

Collapse of the carpometacarpal joint, obscure subchondral radiolucent areas in the third carpal bone and extensive articular and periarticular new bone formation on the medioproximal aspect of the cannon bone, indicative of osteoarthrosis.

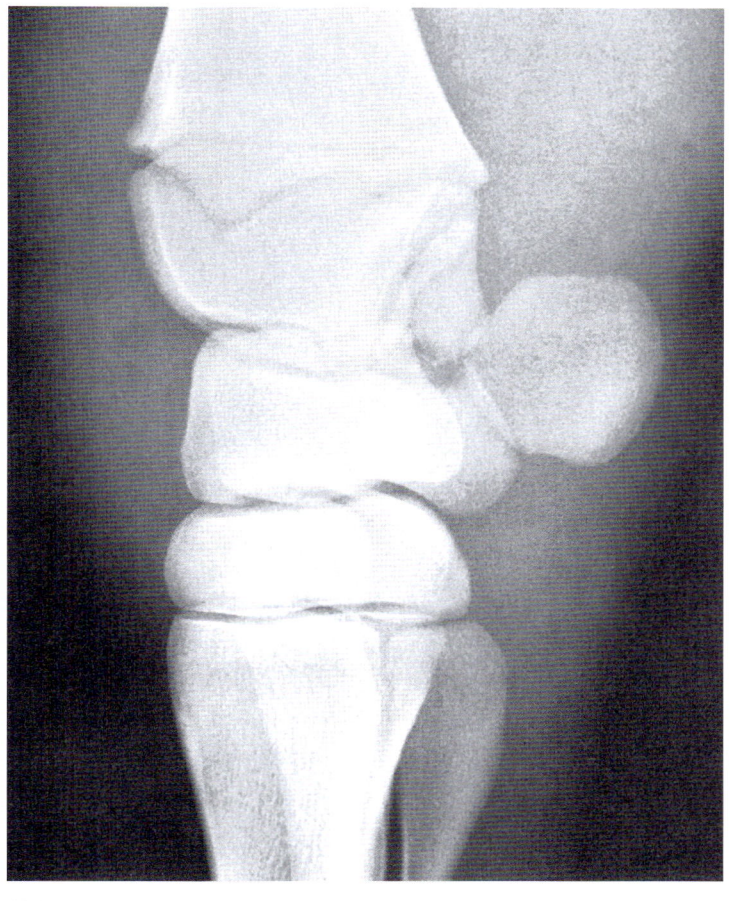

300

301

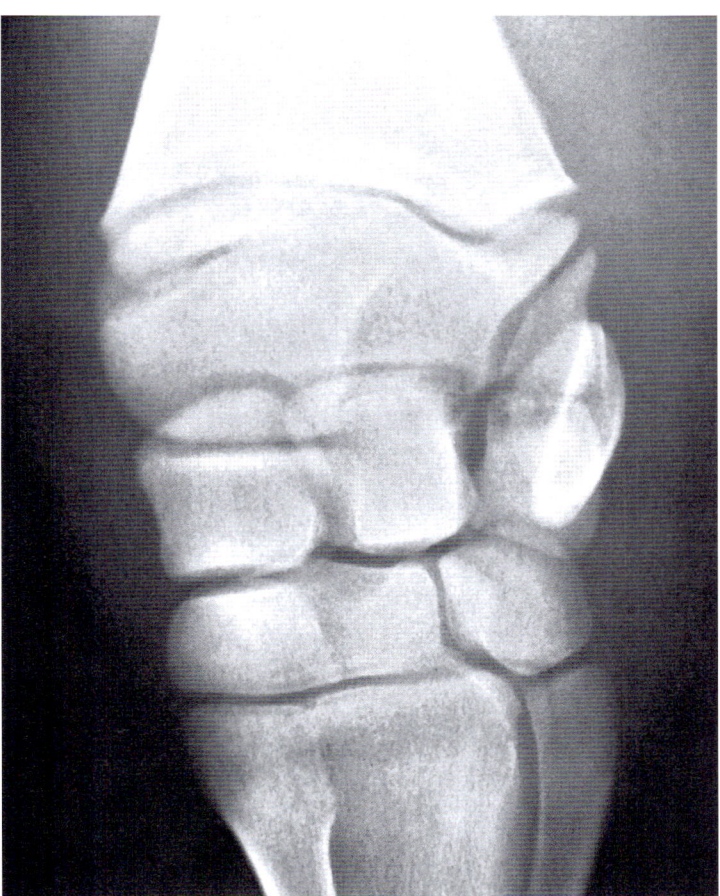

302

300/301/302 Left carpus, lateromedial (Fig. 300), dorsopalmar (Fig. 301) and dorsolateral-palmaromedial oblique (Fig. 302) view.

Foal, 4 weeks.

The soft tissue swelling palmar and lateral to the distal radius and the proximal row of carpal bones and the subchondral radiolucent areas in both the lateral styloid process and intermediate and ulnar carpal bones are a consequence of haematogenous subchondral osteomyelitis type E in a young foal, resulting in infectious arthritis of the radiocarpal joint.

N. B. The radiolucencies dorsal to the radiocarpal joint present on the lateromedial view are a normal anatomical feature resulting from fat, within the joint capsule and the extensor carpi radialis tendon sheath.

Infectious arthritis

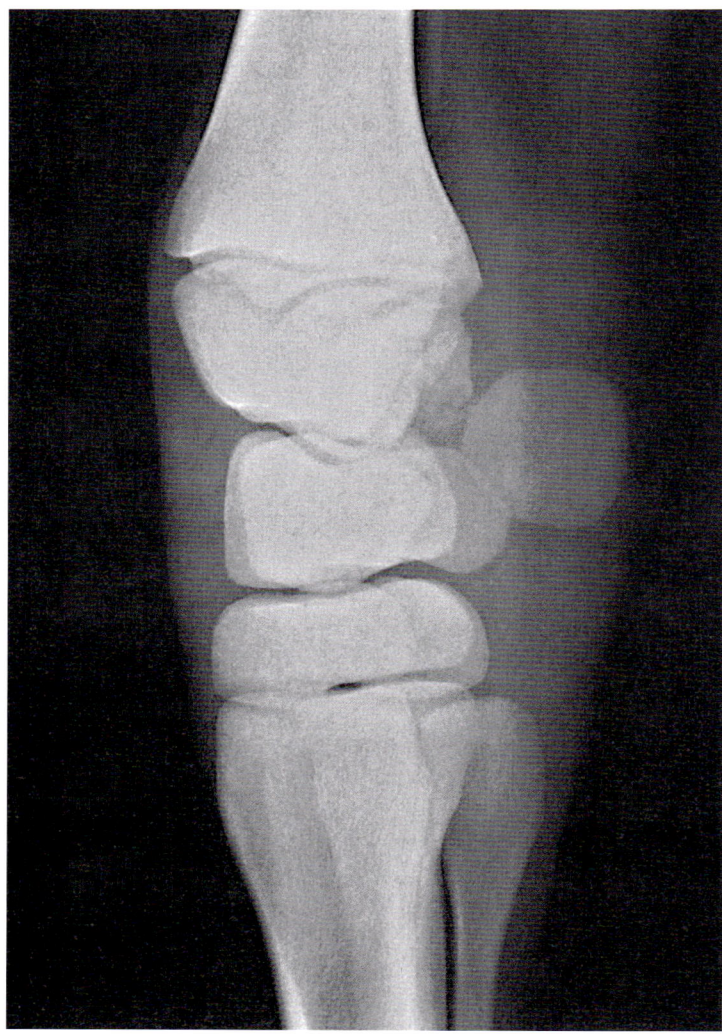

303

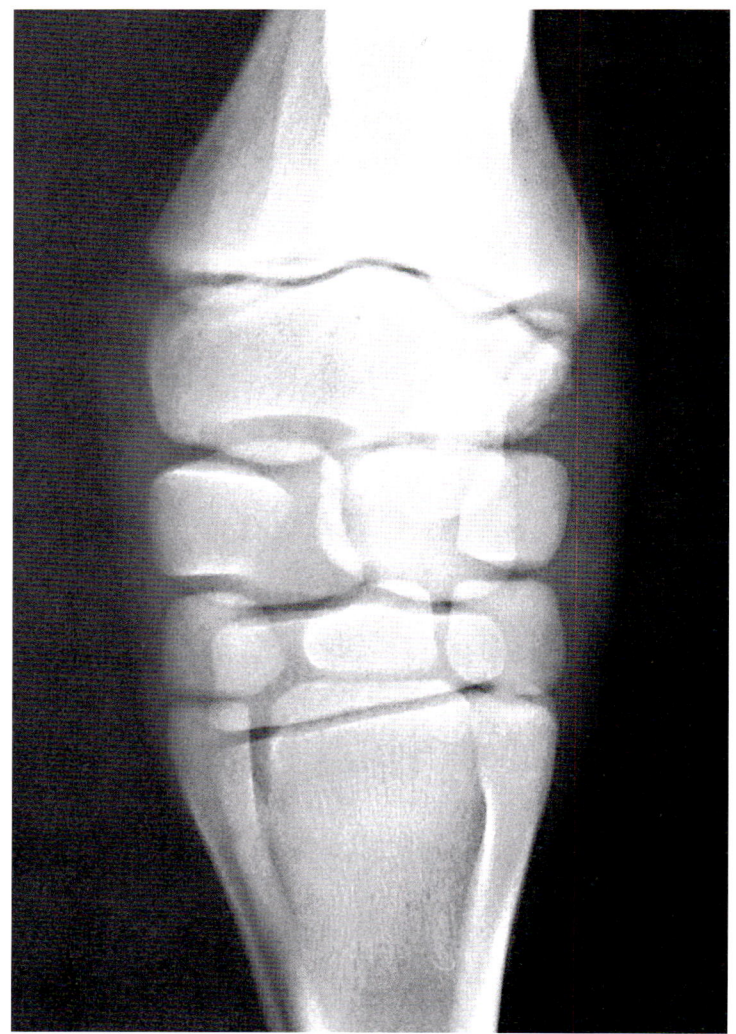

304

303/304 Left carpus, lateromedial (Fig. 303) and dorsopalmar (Fig. 304) view: close-ups.

Foal, 3 ½ weeks.

The irregular, mottled, radiolucent appearance of the lateral styloid process represents either type E osteomyelitis or the normal irregular subchondral ossification pattern of this ossification centre in a young foal. Clinical and laboratory data indicated an infectious bone lesion with associated infectious arthritis, despite the absence of soft tissue swelling. Histological examination confirmed the diagnosis.

N. B. The lateral styloid process is a predilection site for this type of lesion.

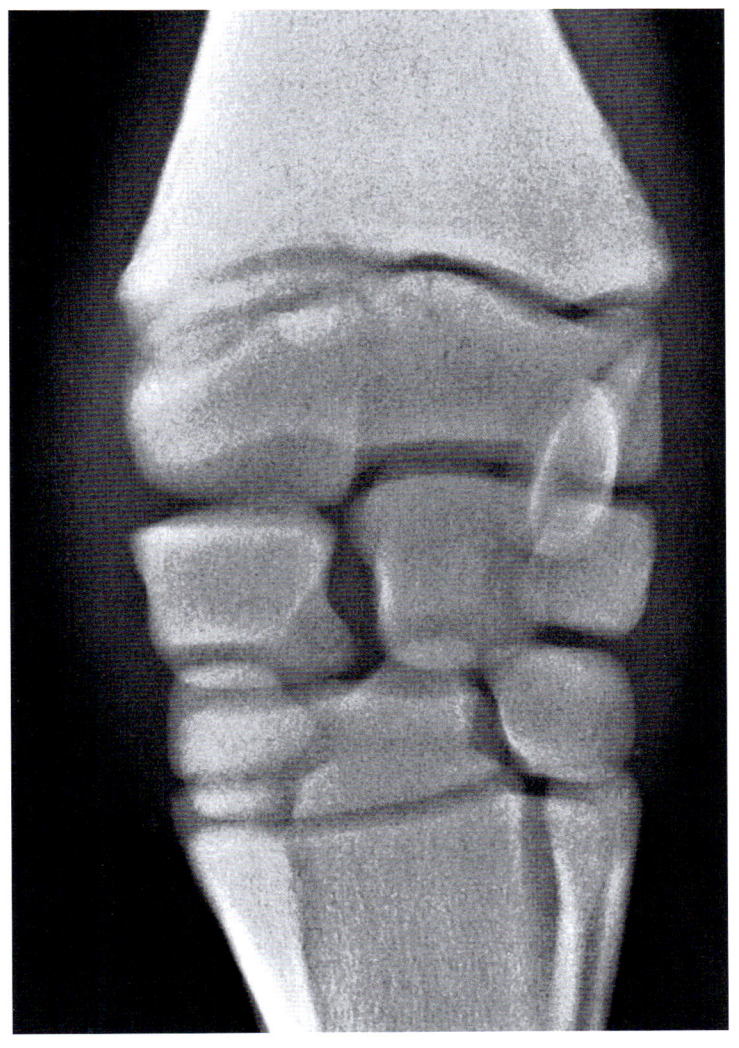

305

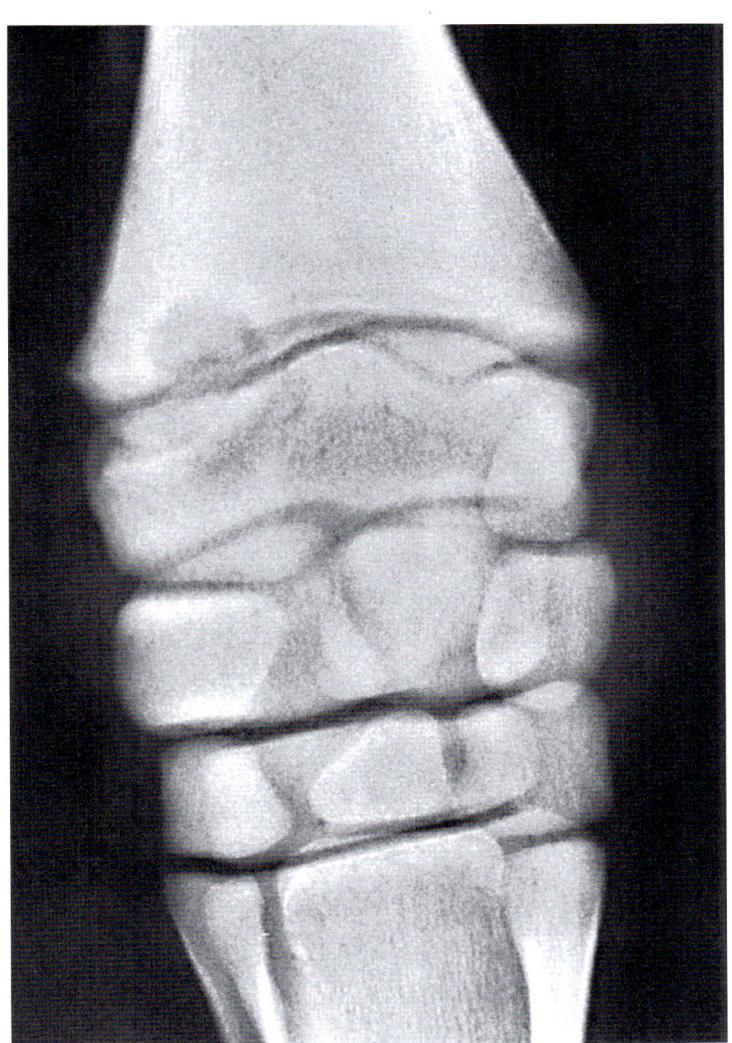

306

305/306 Left carpus, serial dorsopalmar views: close-ups.

Foal, 12 days.

The initial examination (Fig. 305) 1 day after the onset of lameness shows minimal irregularity and blurring of the medial portion of the distal radial growth plate.

A second examination 10 days later (Fig. 306) reveals a well defined cystic radiolucent lesion surrounded by a sclerotic zone in the corresponding area of the metaphysis, characteristic of type P haematogenous osteomyelitis in young foals. The inflammation is restricted to the bone, illustrated by the absence of soft tissue swelling.

Bone cyst

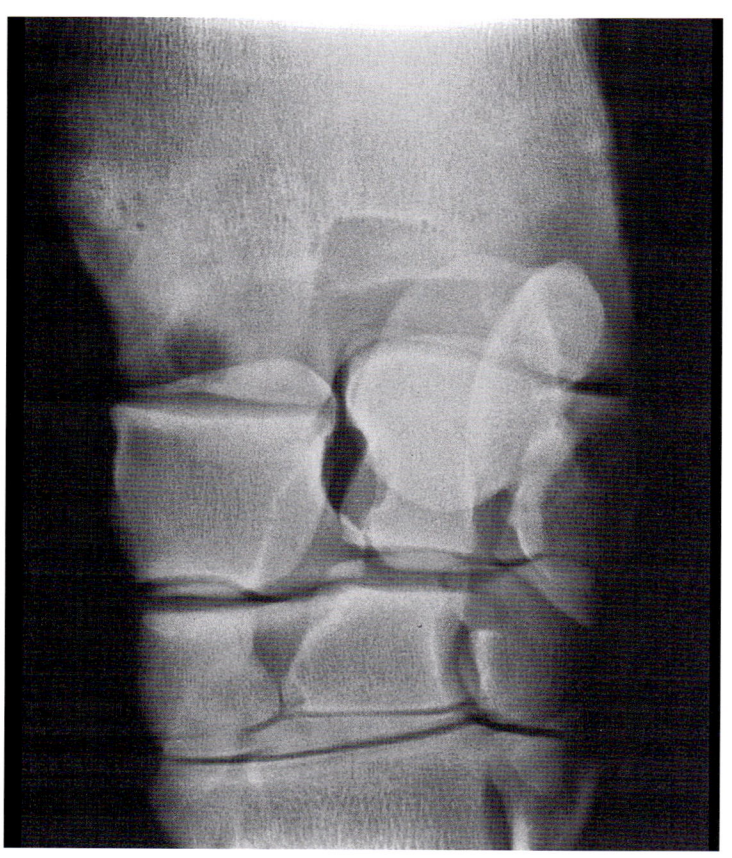

307

307 Left carpus, dorsopalmar view: close-up.

Warmblood, 2 years.

The rounded area of radiolucency in the distomedial aspect of the radius adjacent to the articular surface represents a subchondral bone cyst.

The indistinct, vertical, linear disruption of the underlying subchondral bone suggests communication between the cyst and the radiocarpal joint.

Definitive proof of communication is obtainable by arthrography, i.e. injection of positive contrast material into the joint.

Contrast material injection into a bone cyst is unsuitable, because a valvular mechanism may exist allowing the flow of fluid to proceed only from the articulation to the cyst.

Bone cysts may also be encountered in the radial, ulnar, second, fourth and/or accessory carpal bone.

Generally, cystic bone lesions are of questionable clinical significance.

Lameness is most probable if the cystic lesion has a central weight bearing location, communicates with the joint and is found in a young horse.

Bone sequestration

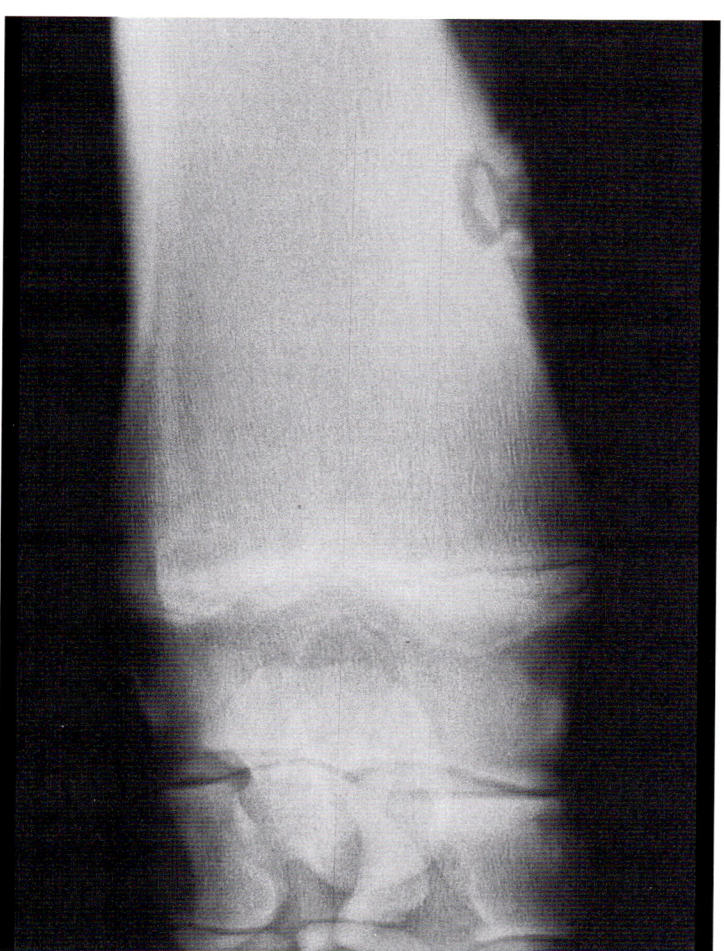

308

308 Right radius, craniocaudal view: close-up.

Warmblood, 2 years.

A well defined dense bone fragment originating from the distomedial radial diaphysis, surrounded by a radiolucent pocket and covered by an interrupted wall of periosteal new bone. This appearance is characteristic of a mature completely separated cortical sequestrum communicating with a fistulous tract.

N.B. In cases of sequestration of the distomedial radius radiographically undetectable fissures may be present, thus increasing the risk for radial fracture during postsurgical recovery.

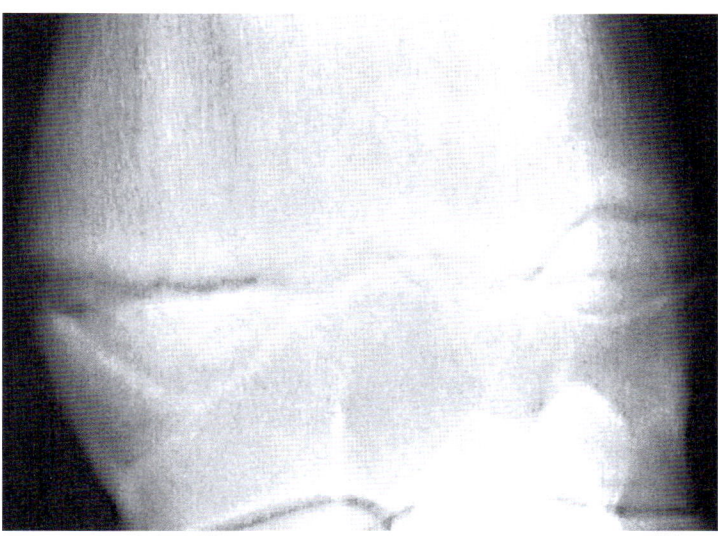

309 Left carpus, dorsopalmar view: close-up.

Foal, 1 year.

Minimal widening and roughness on the medial side of the distal radial growth plate, representing early primary changes of "epiphysitis".

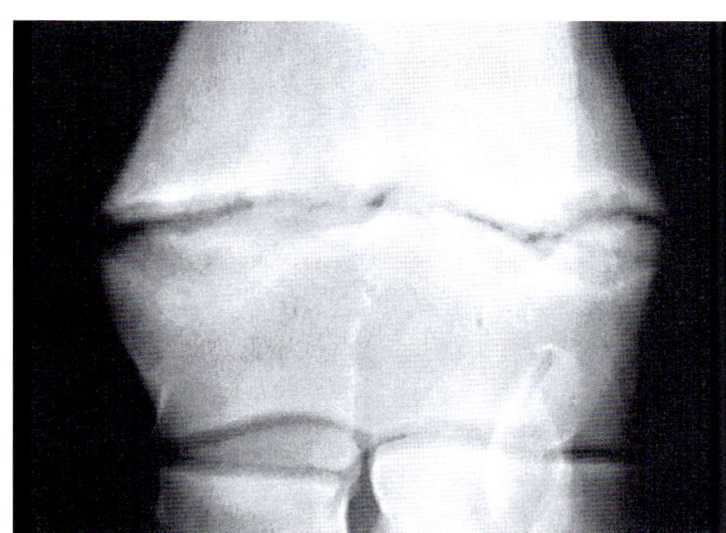

310 Left carpus, dorsopalmar view: close-up.

Foal, 5 months.

Irregular widening of the entire distal radial growth plate, representing more extensive primary changes of "epiphysitis".

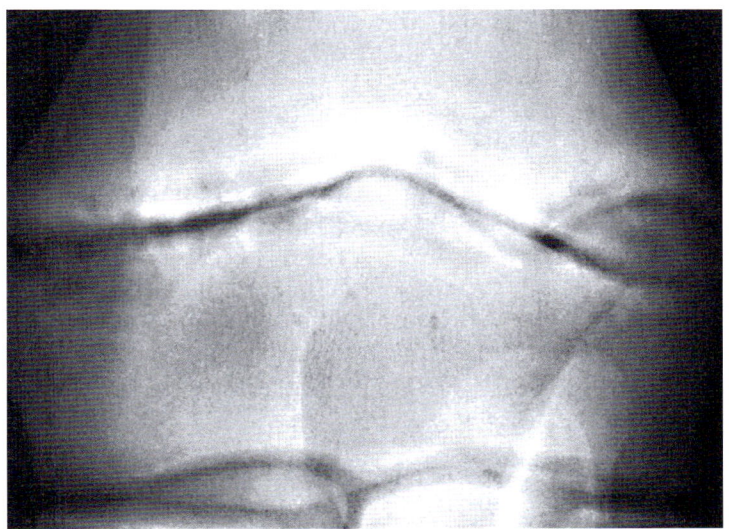

311 Left carpus, dorsopalmar view: close-up.

Foal, 3 months.

Multiple conical radiolucent defects projecting into the medial and central portion of the distal radial metaphysis, representing retained metaphyseal growth plate cartilage, nicely illustrating the similar or identical nature of "epiphysitis" and osteochondrosis (growth plate form).

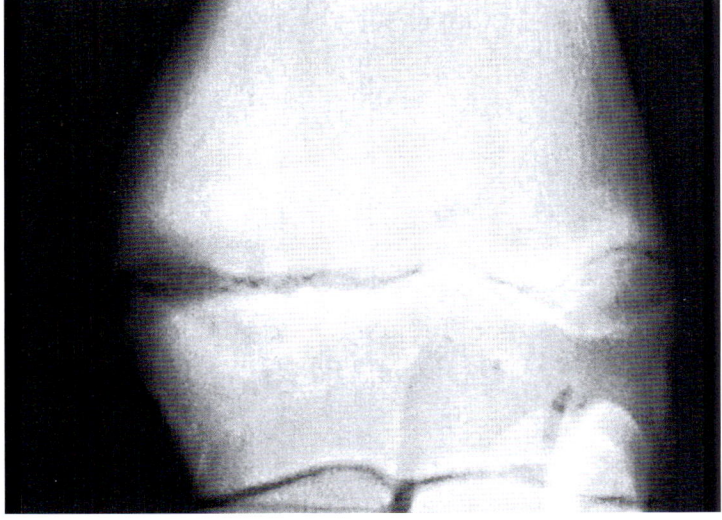

312 Left carpus, dorsopalmar view: close-up.

Foal, 1 year.

Minimal widening, roughness and tipping on the medial side of the distal radial growth plate. The metaphyseal and epiphyseal flaring represent some of the secondary changes of "epiphysitis".

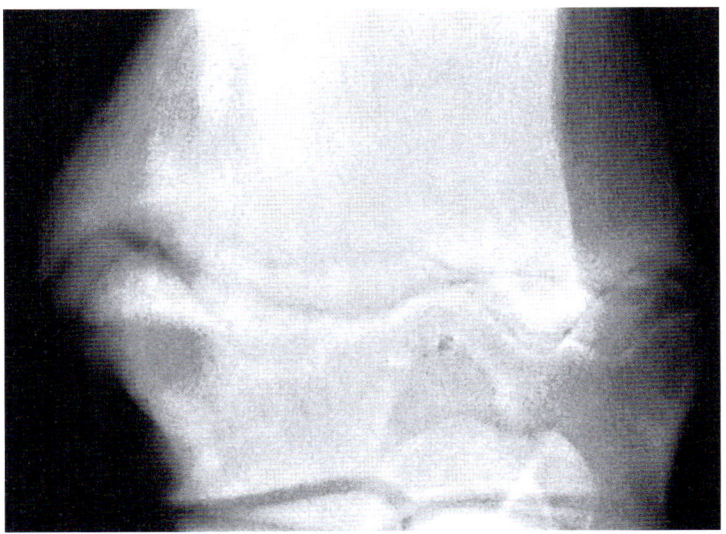

313

313 Left carpus, dorsopalmar view: close-up.

Foal, 1 year.

Widening and marked tipping on the medial side of the distal radial growth plate. The broadened sclerotic metaphysis tends to "flow" over the epiphysis and represents more advanced secondary changes of "epiphysitis".

The Carpus

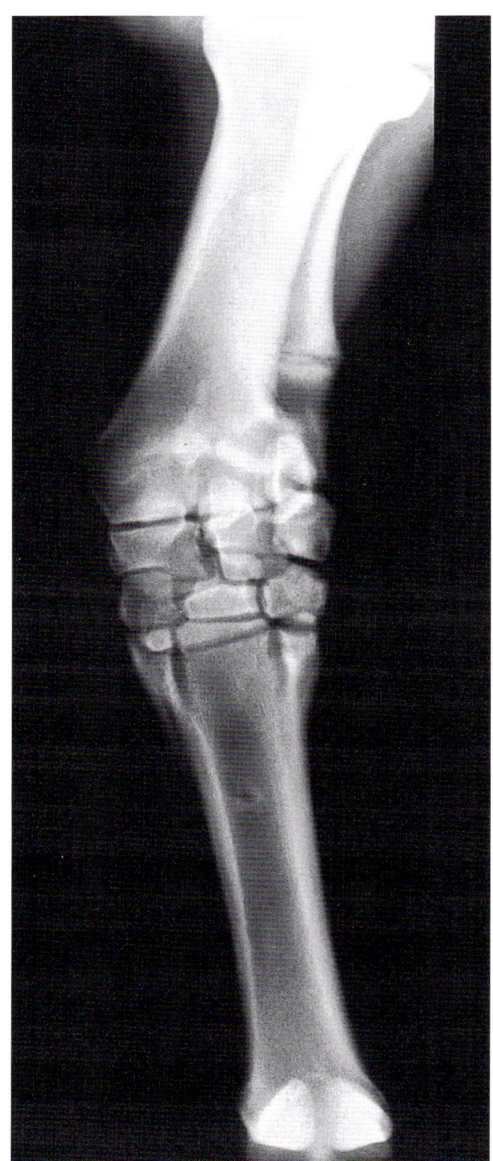

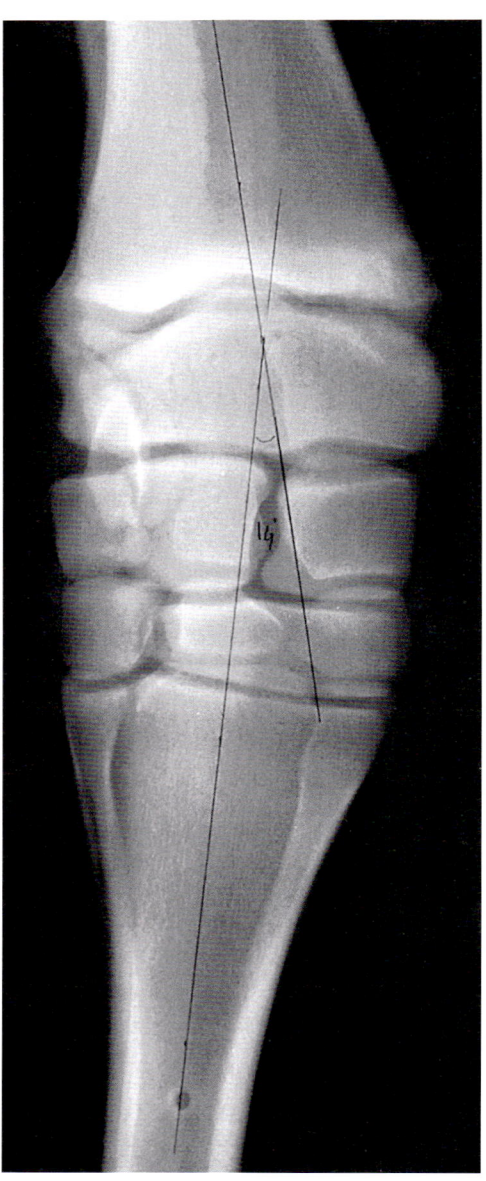

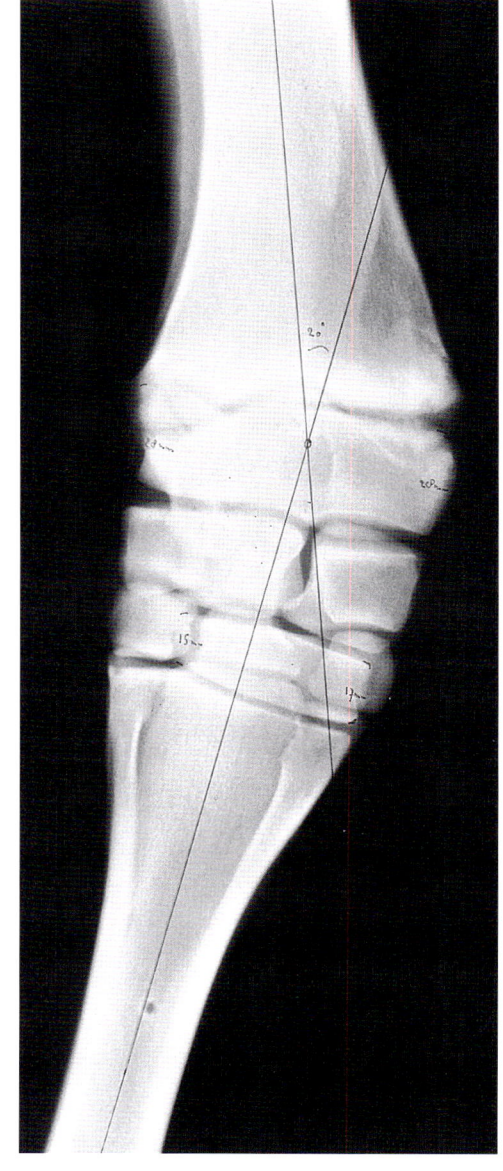

314 Left carpus, dorsopalmar view.

Shetland pony, 7 months.

Valgus deformity associated with a complete ulna. The intact ulna has a distinct distal physis and epiphysis. Due to growth retardation the distal ulnar epiphysis contributes to the radiocarpal joint, but does not extend as far distally as the radial epiphysis thus causing the angulation of the joint.

The presence of a complete ulna and/or fibula is a form of atavism frequently encountered in Shetland ponies. Valgus deformity is commonly associated with this anomaly.

315 Right carpus, dorsopalmar view: close-up.

Foal, 3 ½ weeks.

Minimal widening on the medial side of the distal radial growth plate, mottled radiolucent appearance of the corresponding portion of the metaphysis and a 14° valgus deformity.

The pivot point of mid-sagittal longitudinal lines through the centre of the proximal and distal long bone is located near the distal radial growth plate, indicating primary imbalance in growth at the level of the metaphysis.

316 Right carpus, dorsopalmar view.

Foal, 1 month.

Valgus deformity 20°. The medial width of the radial epiphysis is greater than the lateral width and the pivot point is situated in the proximal aspect of the radial epiphysis, indicating that the angular deformity results from lateral growth retardation of the radial epiphysis.

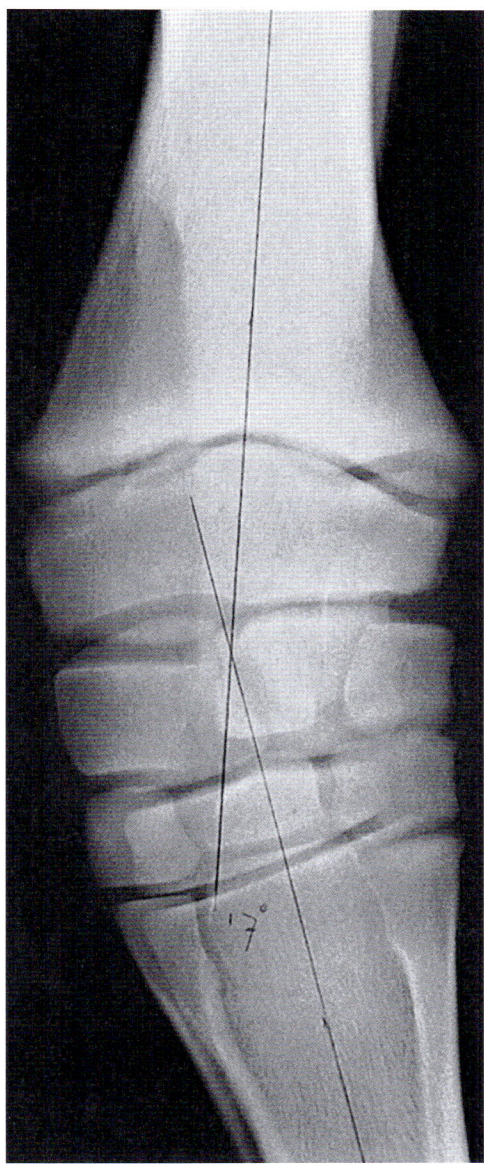

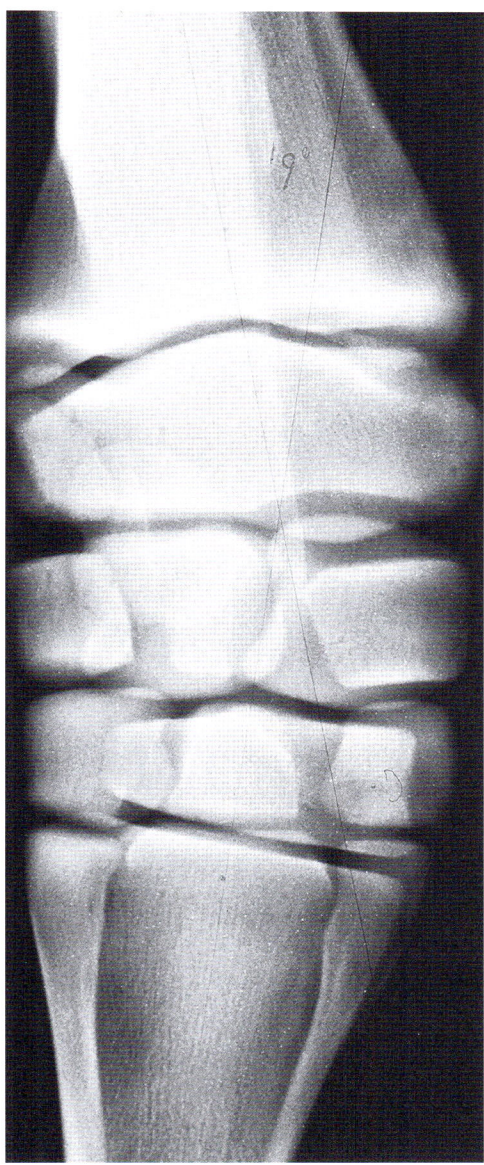

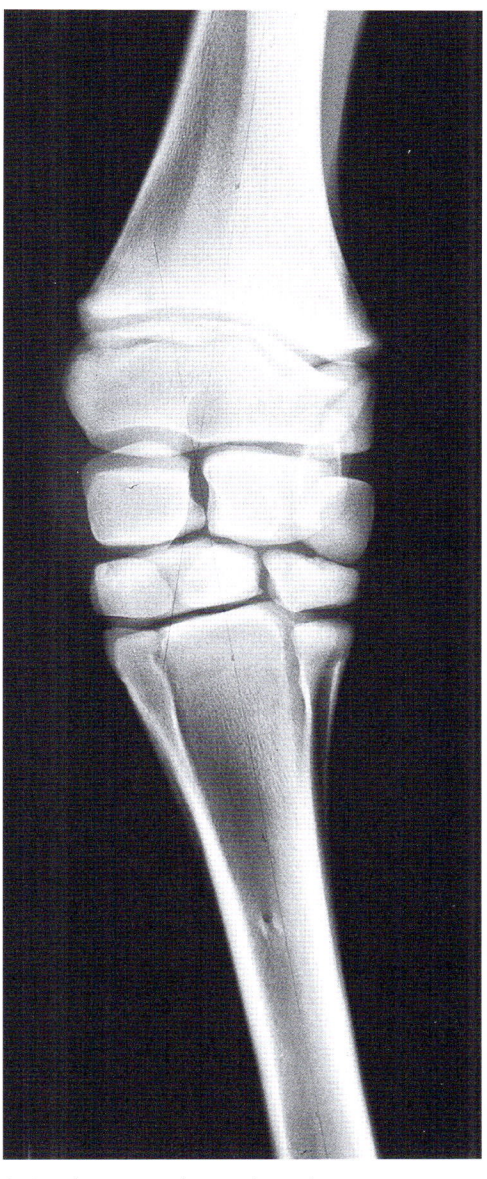

317 Left carpus, dorsopalmar view: close-up.

Foal, 4 weeks.

Valgus deformity 17°. The pivot point rest at the proximal row of carpal bones. Osseous abnormalities are absent indicating that the valgus deformity results from joint instability associated with ligament laxity.

318 Right carpus, dorsopalmar view: close-up.

Foal, 2 weeks.

Valgus deformity 19°. The pivot point is resting at the level of the radiocarpal joint. The latersal width of the third carpal bone is approximately 75% of the medial width thus causing a wedge shaped instead of a rectangular third carpal outline. This angular deformity results from hypoplasia, i.e. incomplete ossification of the third carpal bone.

In normal foals the lateral width of the third carpal bone should be 80 – 90% of the medial width.

319 Left carpus, dorsopalmar view.

Foal, 7 weeks.

Valgus deformity 20°. The pivot point is resting at the level of the radiocarpal joint. The lateral aspect of the fourth carpal bone is reduced in height, thus causing a wedge shaped appearance of this bone.

The proximal head of the lateral splint bone has a uniform radiodensity and a smooth contour but does not extend as far proximally as the cannon bone, thus creating a "stair-step" appearance of the carpometacarpal joint.

These findings indicate angular limb deformity due to hypoplasia and distal displacement of the fourth carpal bone, combined with distal displacement of the fourth metacarpal bone.

If the shortened fourth metacarpal bone has an irregular radiodensity and contour the splint bone changes are categorized as hypoplasia

Angular limb deformities

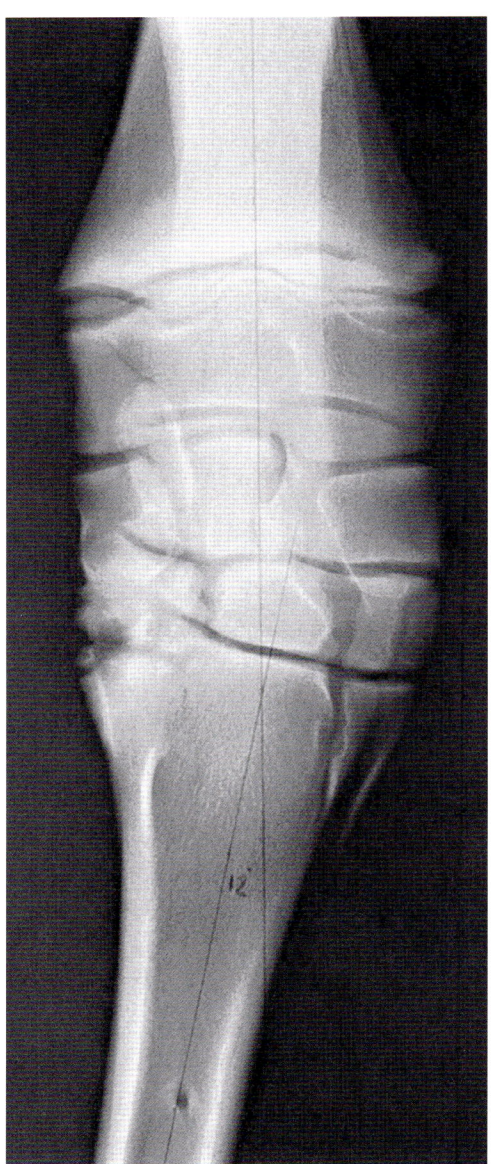

320

320 Right carpus, dorsopalmar view: close-up.

Foal, 8 weeks.

Valgus deformity 12°. The lateral portion of the third carpal bone is compressed dorsoventrally. The lateral portion of the fourth carpal bone has a rough contour and an abnormal radiolucent pattern.

The pivot point is at the proximal end of the cannon bone, indicating that the angular limb deformity is caused by ossification defects of these carpal bones.

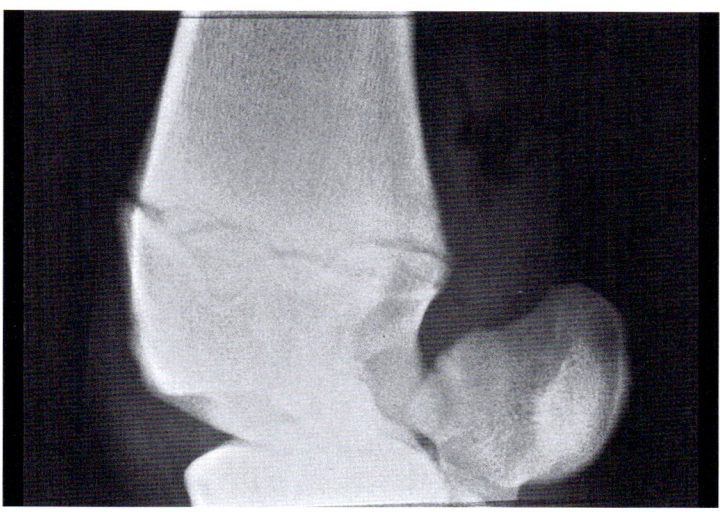

321

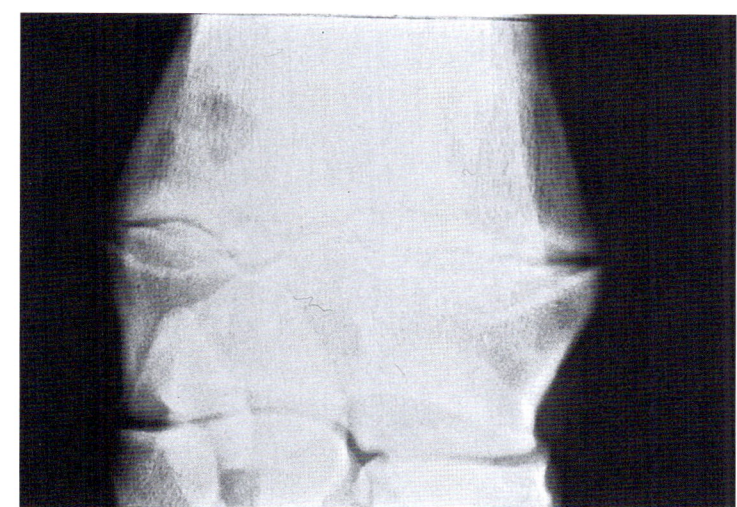

322

321/322 Right carpus, lateromedial and dorsopalmar view: close-ups.

Standardbred, 1½ years.

The lateromedial view (Fig. 321) demonstrates soft tissue swelling proximal to the accessory carpal bone containing both small and large radiolucent areas.

On the dorsopalmar view (Fig. 322) these radiolucencies are superimposed upon the distolateral aspect of the radial metaphysis.

These findings are characteristic of gas accumulation within the caudoproximo-lateral pouch of the radiocarpal joint cavity, resulting from a recent penetrating wound in this horse.

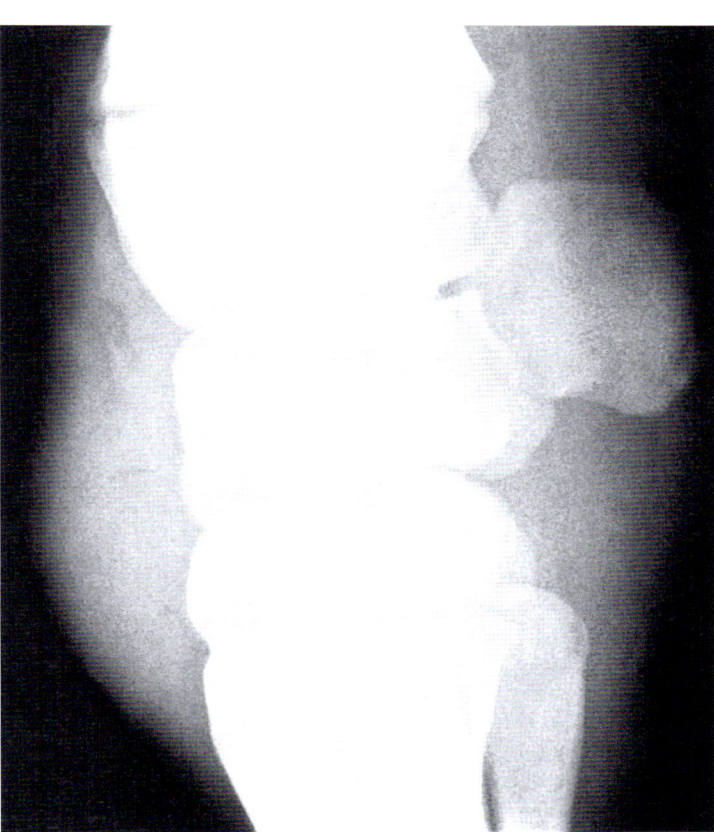

323

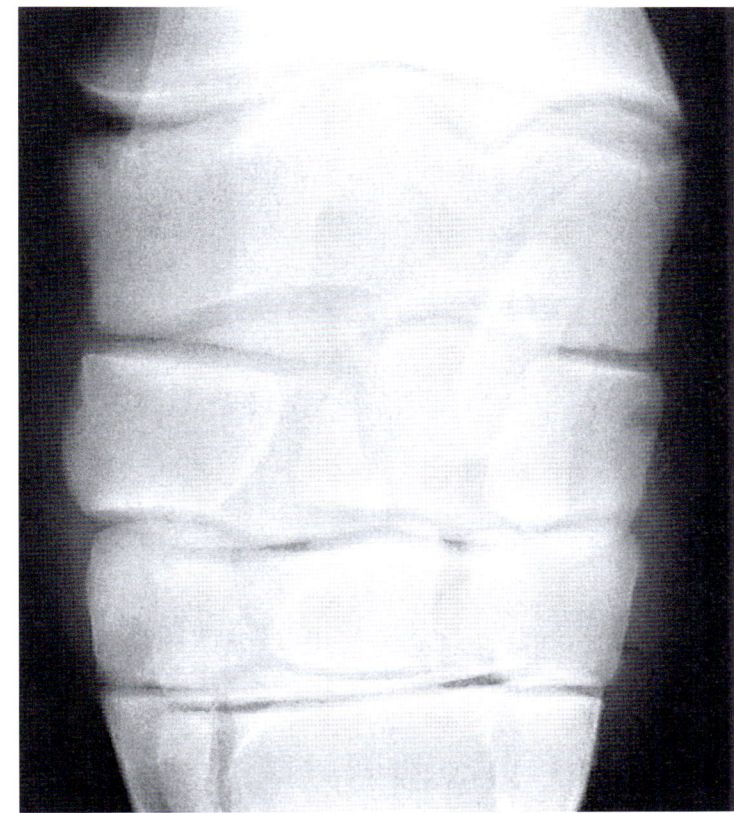

324

323/324 Left carpus, lateromedial and dorsopalmar view: close-ups.

Foal, 2 months.

Soft tissue swelling dorsal to the carpus containing obscure small radiolucent areas, consistent with abscess formation. The soft tissue radiolucencies are more clearly visualized on the dorsopalmar view (Fig. 324) despite the superimposition of the ulnar carpal and fourth carpal bones.

N. B. The linear radiolucencies dorsal to the radiocarpal joint present on the lateromedial view (Fig. 323) are a normal anatomical feature resulting from fat within the joint capsule and the extensor carpi radialis tendon sheath.

Hygroma

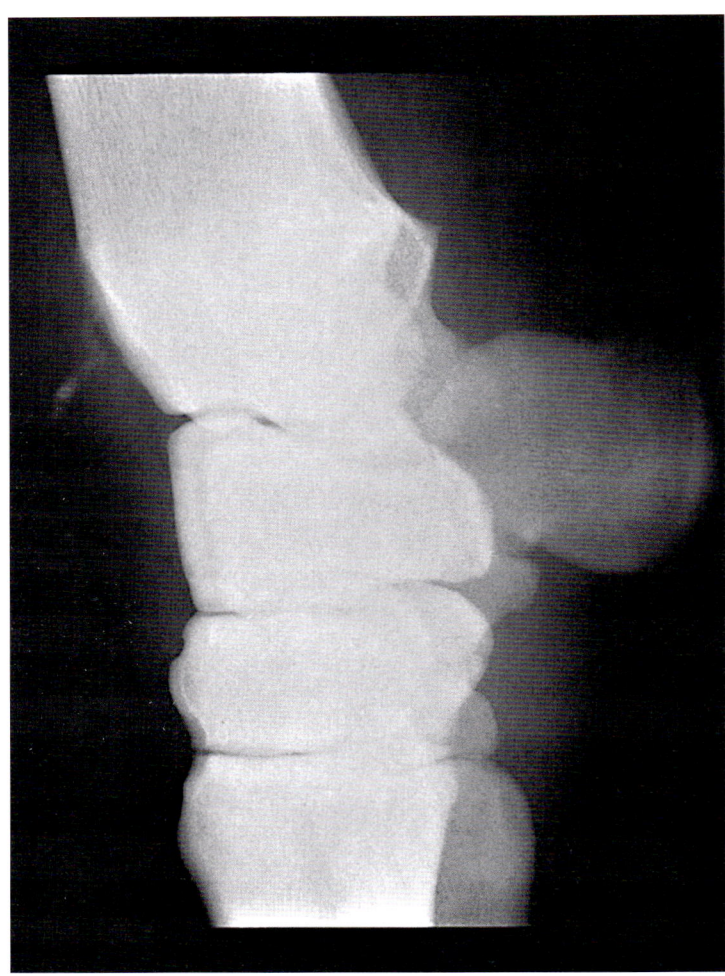

325

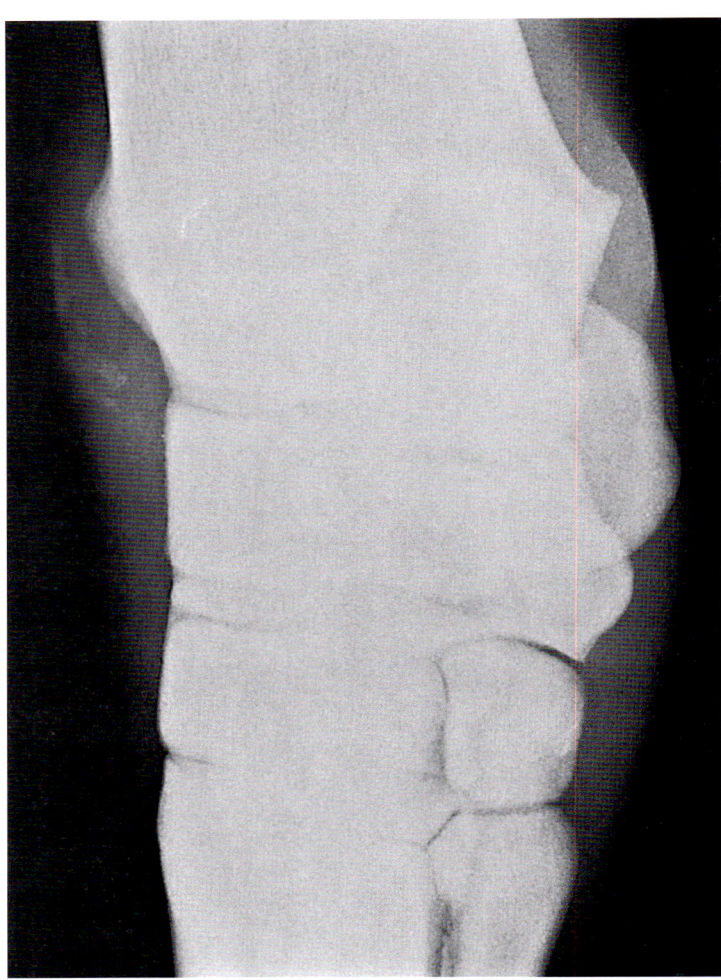

326

325/326 Right carpus, lateromedial and dorsomedial-palmarolateral oblique view.

Warmblood, 8 years.

A clearly defined linear soft tissue opacity apparently connected to the dorsal surface of the distal radius on the lateromedial view (Fig. 325), but isolated on the dorsomedial-palmarolateral oblique view (Fig. 326). The opacity was due to focal calcification of an acquired precarpal bursa.

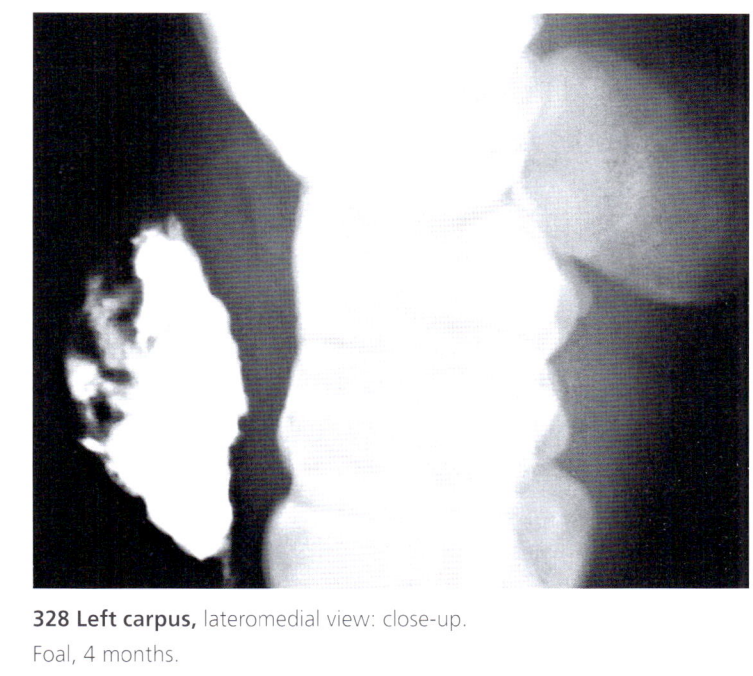

328 Left carpus, lateromedial view: close-up.

Foal, 4 months.

An acquired precarpal bursa dorsal to the carpal bones and the proximal end of the cannon bone, visualized by injection of 10 ml positive contrast material.

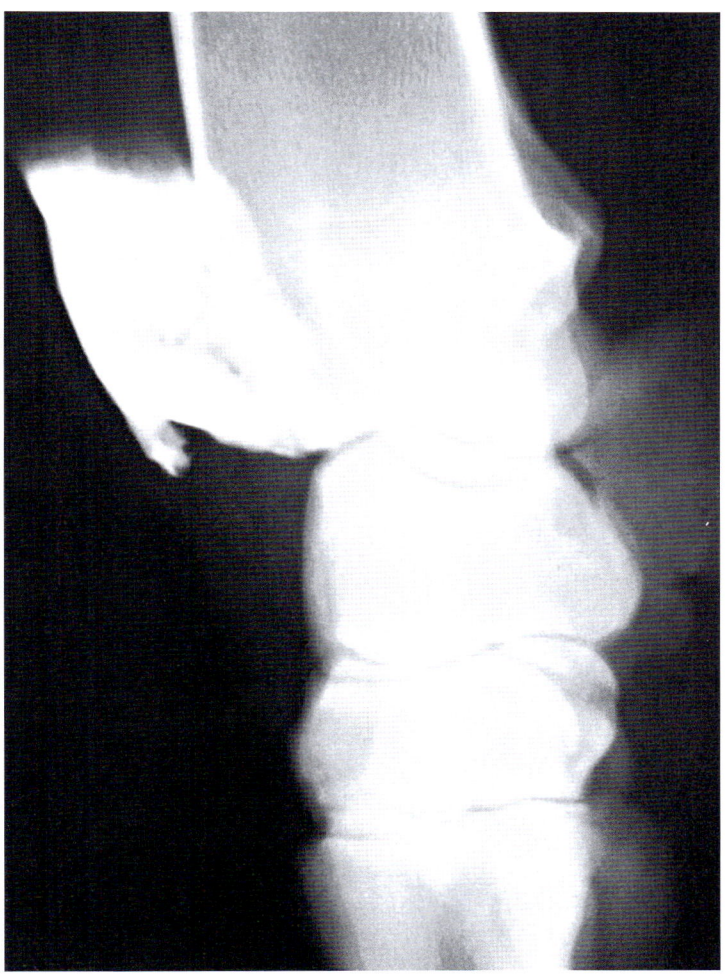

327 Left carpus, lateromedial view.

Warmblood, 5 years.

An acquired precarpal bursa dorsal to the distal end of the radius, visualized by injection of 20 ml positive contrast material.

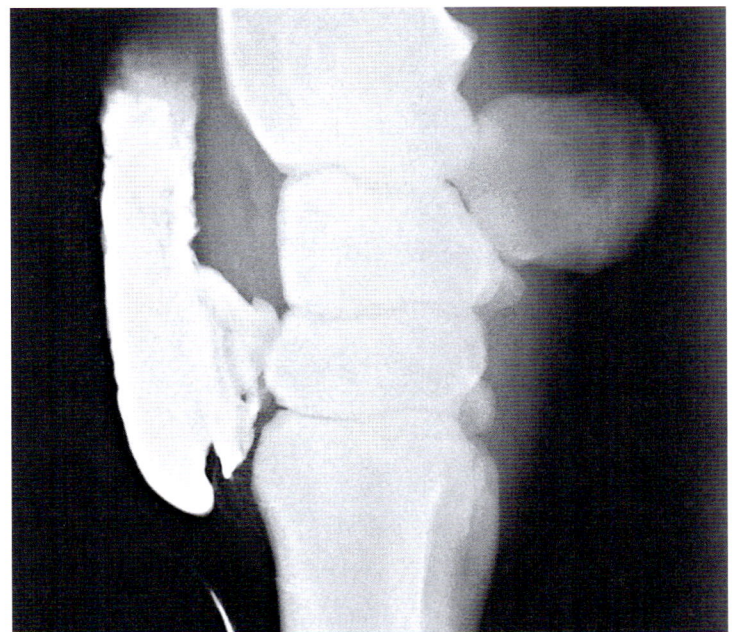

329

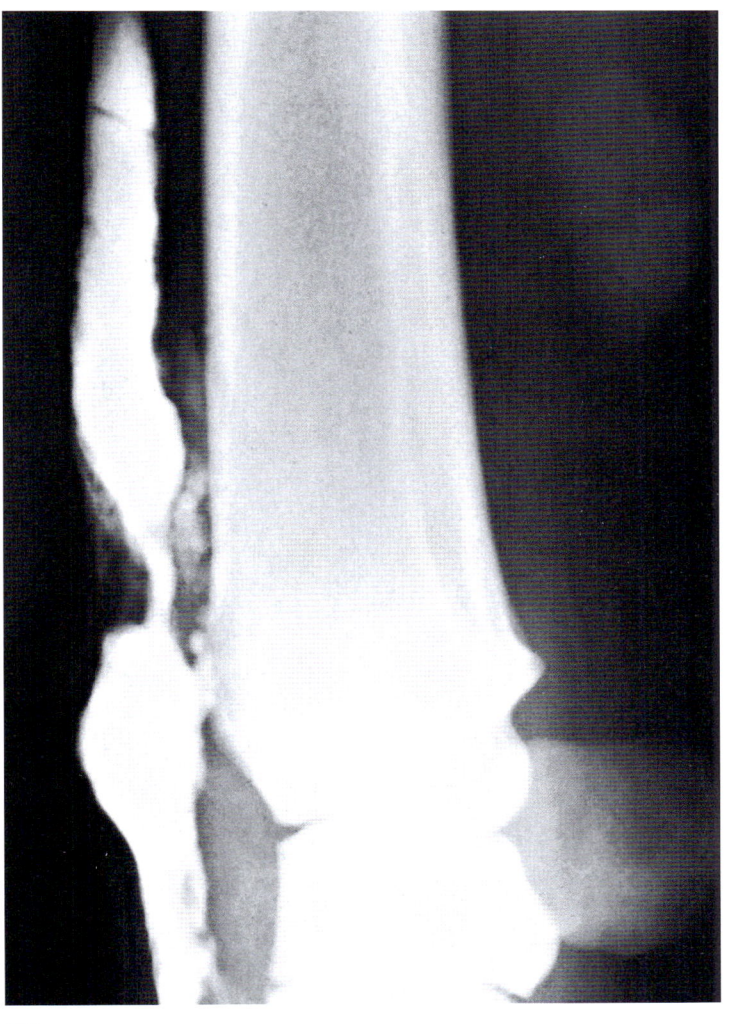

330

329/330 Left carpus, lateromedial views.

Warmblood, 8 years.

A synovial swelling over the dorsal surface of the carpus visualized by injection of 40 ml positive contrast material (Fig. 329). More distally some of the contrast material has leaked through the puncture hole on to the skin. A second radiograph during pressure with an elastic bandage (Fig. 330) reveals involvement of the tendon sheath of the extensor carpi radialis (the constriction of the tendon sheath dorsal to the distal end of the radius results from the overlying tendon of the extensor carpi obliquus).

N. B. Radiographic contrast studies of hygroma are valuable to define the precise location of the synovial swelling, to evaluate its shape and extension and to differentiate acquired bursa, tendon sheath involvement and synovial herniation of the radiocarpal or intercarpal joint capsule.

Osteochondroma

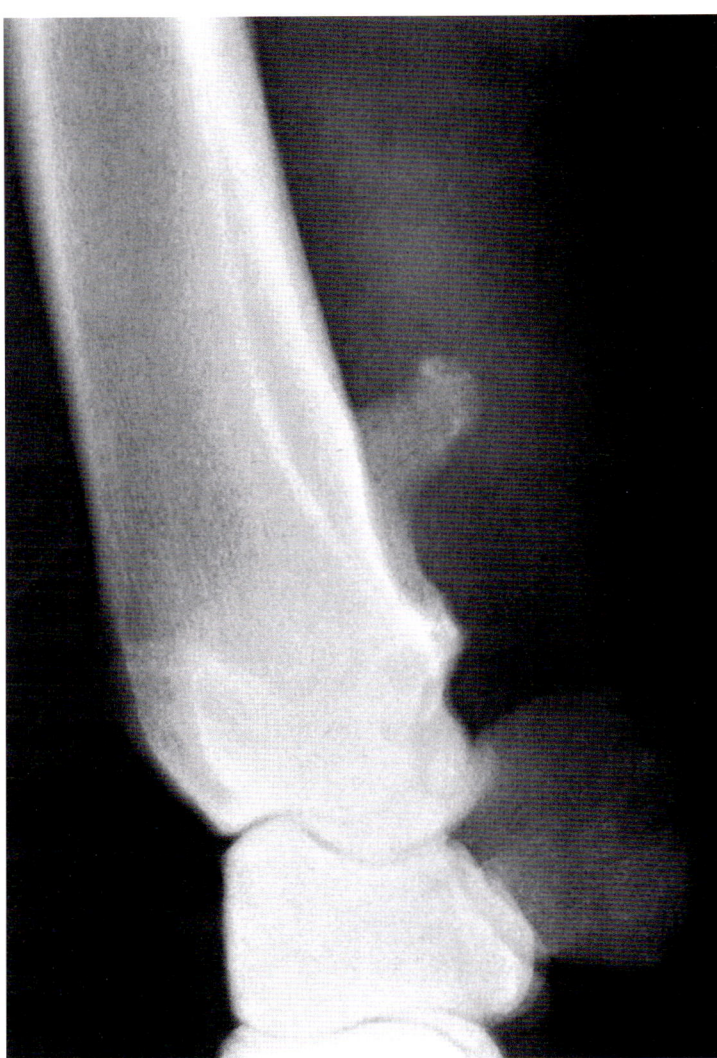

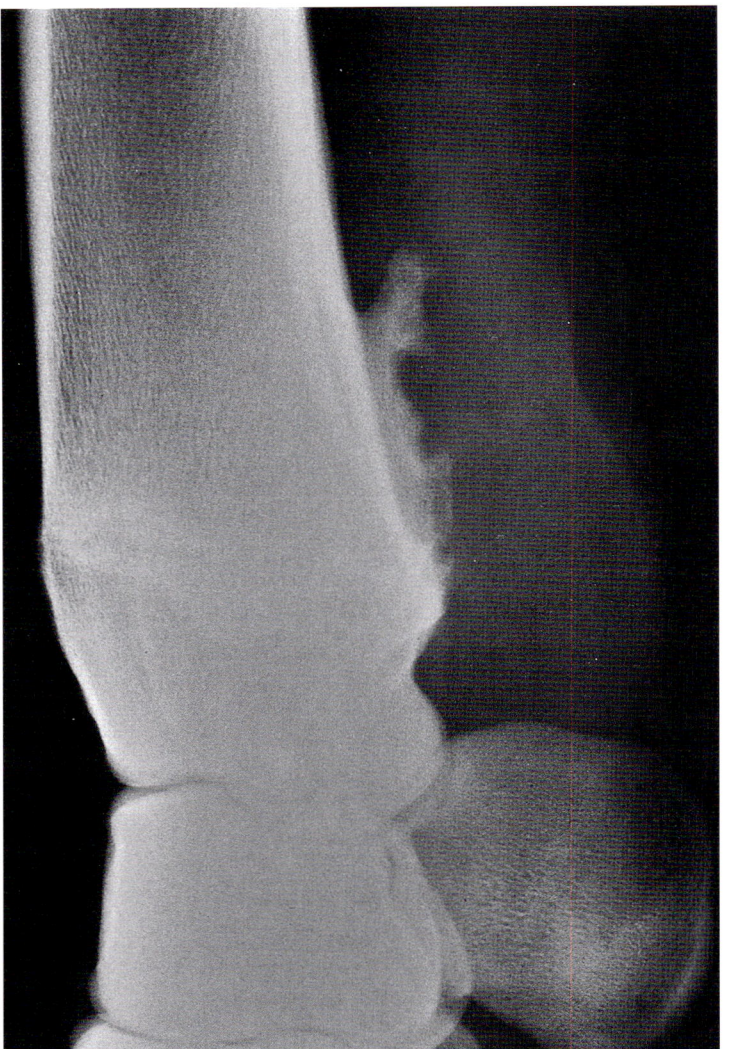

331 Right carpus, lateromedial view.

Standardbred, 4 years.

A large cauliflower-shaped bony spur originating from the palmar metaphyseal region of the radius.

The cortex of the exostosis blends with the cortex of the radius. These radiographic findings are characteristic of an osteochondroma.

332 Right carpus, lateromedial view.

Warmblood, 2 years.

The large irregular exostosis at the caudodistal metaphyseal region of the radius represents an osteochondroma. The overlying soft tissue swelling results from associated distension of the carpal flexor tendon sheath.

Comparison with Fig. 331 demonstrates the variable size and shape of this benign neoplasm.

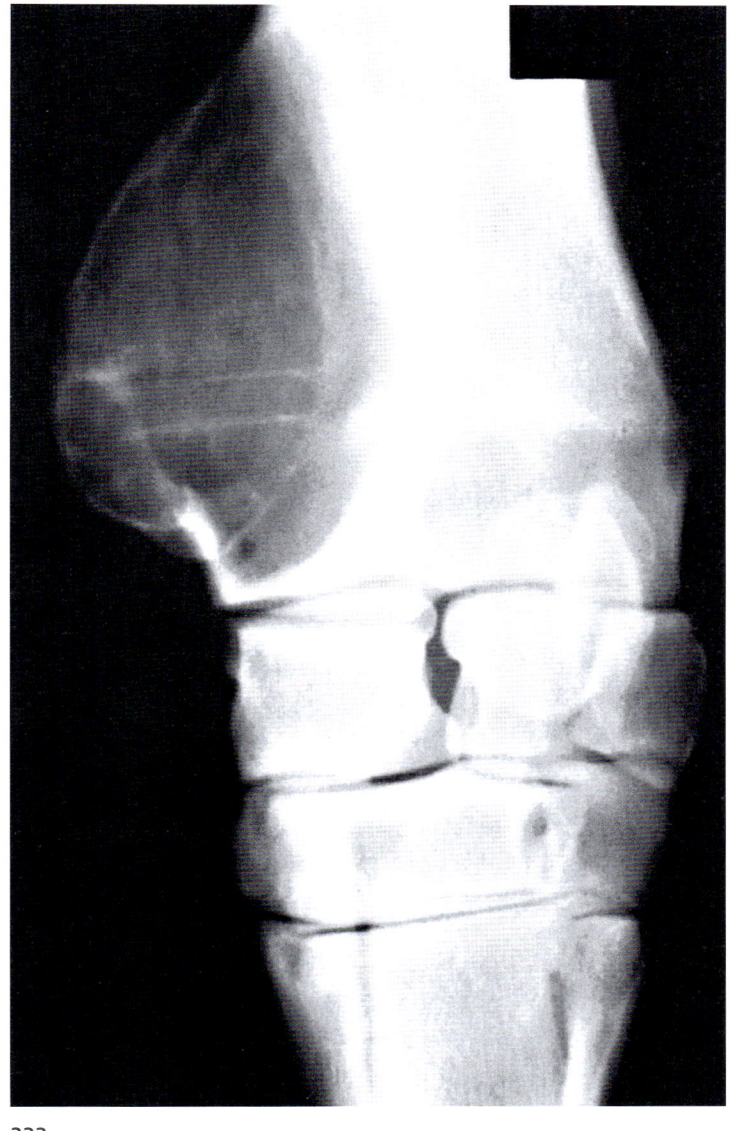

333

333 Left carpus, dorsopalmar view: close-up.

Pony 4 ½ years.

A large well defined radiolucent lesion in the medial distal end of the radius, extending from the metaphysis into the epiphysis, the subchondral bone plate appears to be intact. The lesion, bordered by a thin uninterrupted layer of bone, extends far outside the original cortex ("ballooning out"). The axial aspect of the lesion is bordered by a sclerotic zone. Thin bone septa are present within the radiolucent mass. The radiological features are characteristic of a benign expansive bone tumour and histological examination revealed osteoblastoma.

Synovial sarcoma

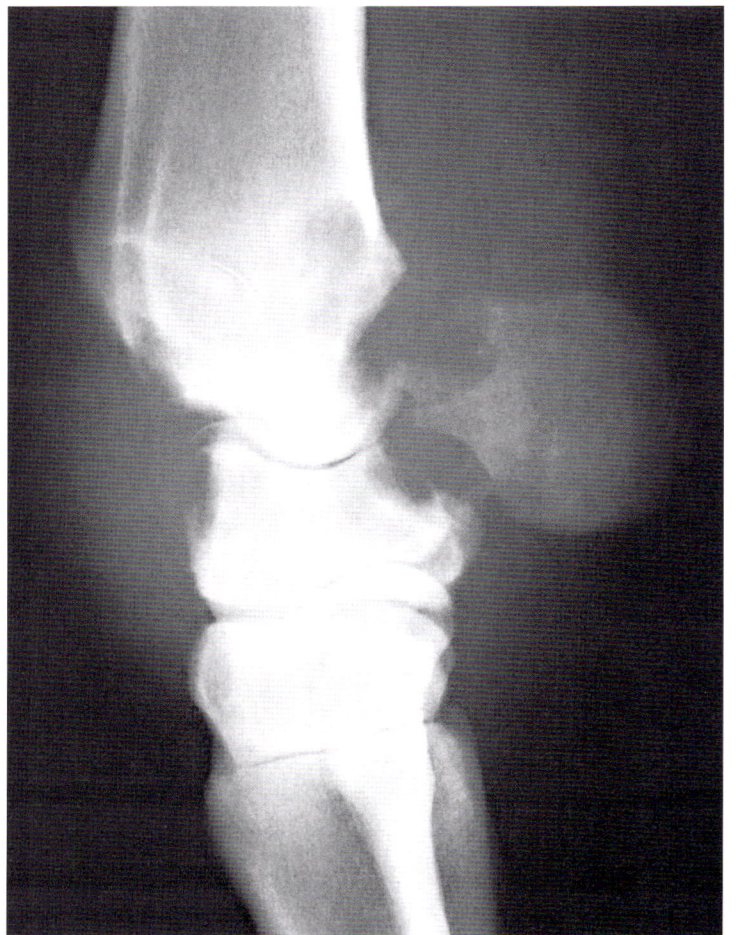

334

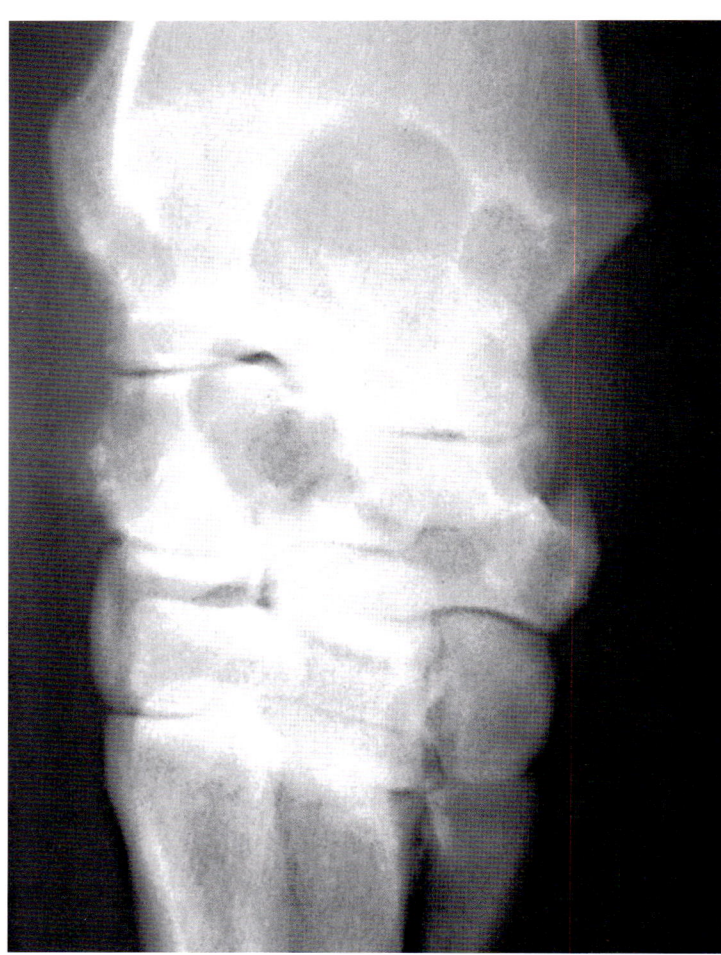

335

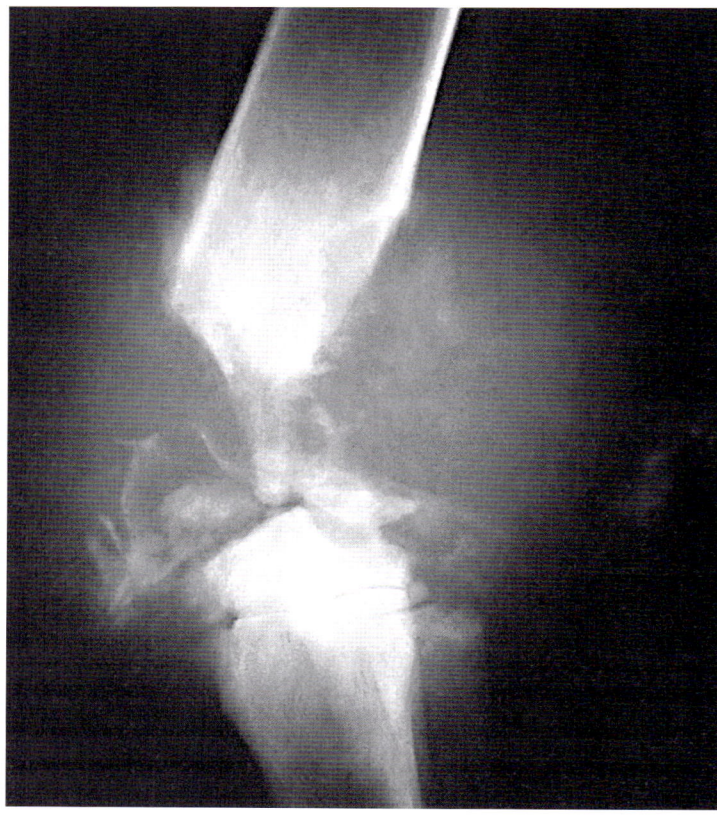

336

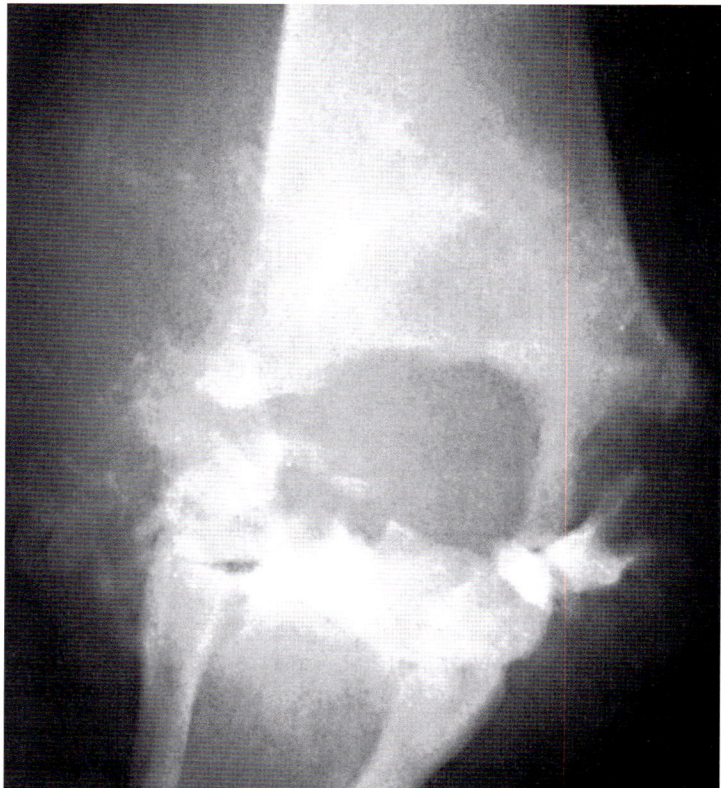

337

334/335/336/337 Left carpus, serial lateromedial and dorsopalmar views.

Standardbred, 16 years.

The initial lateromedial (Fig. 334) and (oblique) dorsopalmar (Fig. 335) view shows soft tissue swelling dorsal and palmar to the radiocarpal joint, multiple "thumb printing" erosive bone lesions involving the distal radius and the proximal row of carpal bones and minimal periosteal reaction on the palmar aspect of the radius and the medial aspect of the radial carpal bone. The radiological features suggest a malignant articular and periarticular soft tissue mass involving the bones adjacent to the joint space. Seven months later (Fig. 336, 337) massive bone destruction resulting in angular deformity is obvious. The periosteal response to the tumour is minimal. Remnants of bone and scattered irregular calcification are present within the soft tissue mass. Histological examination revealed a synovial sarcoma.

The Elbow

Fracture

Fracture / Luxation

Infectious arthritis

Osteomyelitis

Bone cyst

Osteochondrosis

Fracture

Humerus

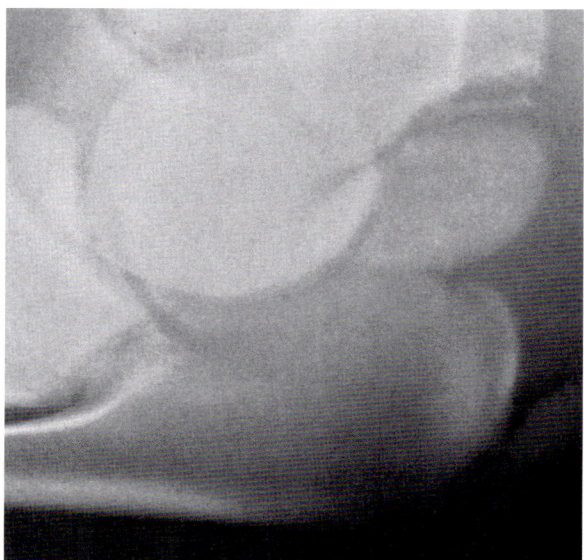

338

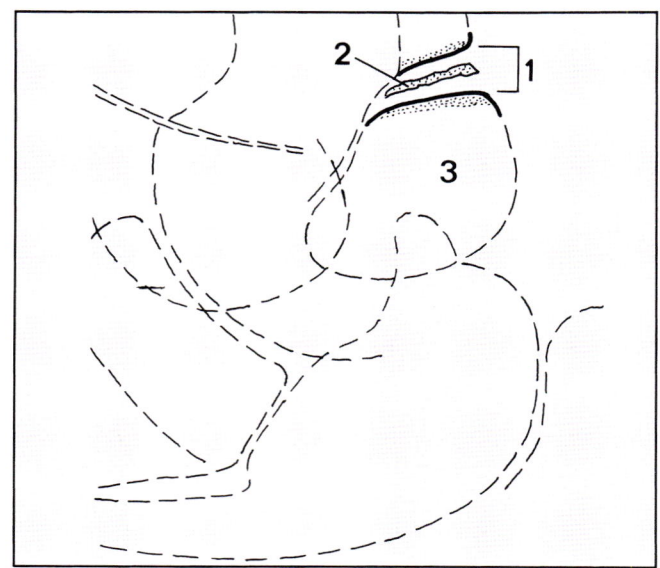

338 a

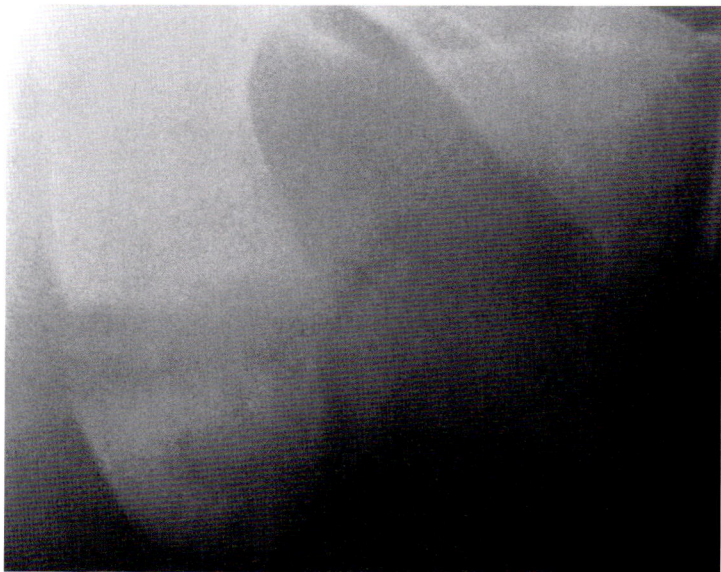
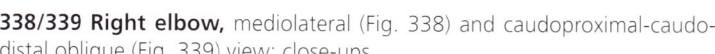

339

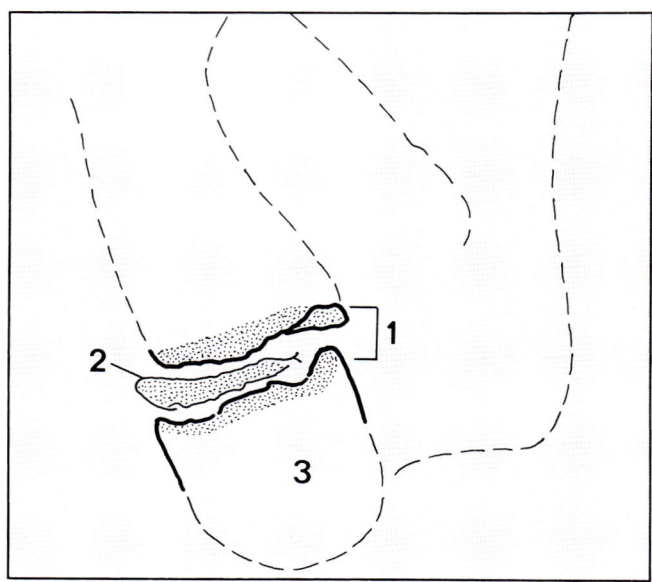

339 a

338/339 Right elbow, mediolateral (Fig. 338) and caudoproximal-caudo-distal oblique (Fig. 339) view: close-ups.

Foal, 3 months.

Both views show widening of the proximal part of the medial epicondylar growth plate **(1)** and a thin, ill bordered layer of bone running parallel with the corresponding portion of the growth plate **(2)**. The radiographic findings result from a recent physeal fracture with minimal distraction and medial shifting of the epicondylar ossification centre **(3)**.

338 a/339 a Schematic drawings

Ulna

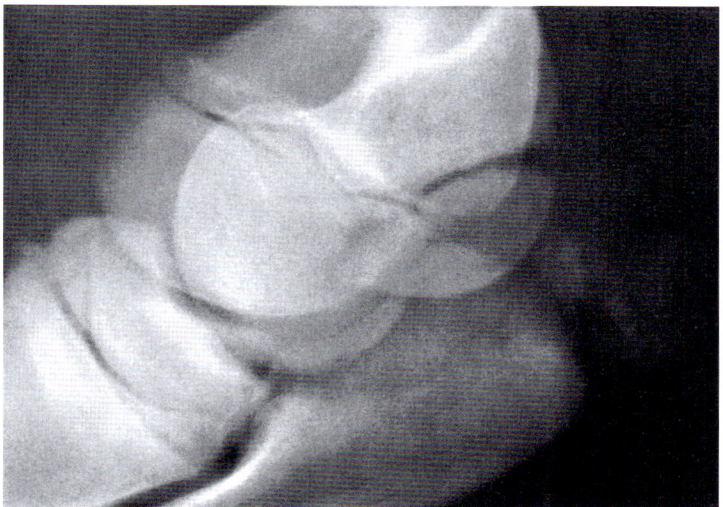

340 Right elbow, mediolateral view: close-up.

Foal, 6 weeks.

Rotation of the ossification centre of the tuber olecrani **(1)** resulting from a recent apophyseal fracture. Thin ill defined additional bone fragments **(2)** are visible superimposing the fracture zone. The site of origin of these fragments is not visible.

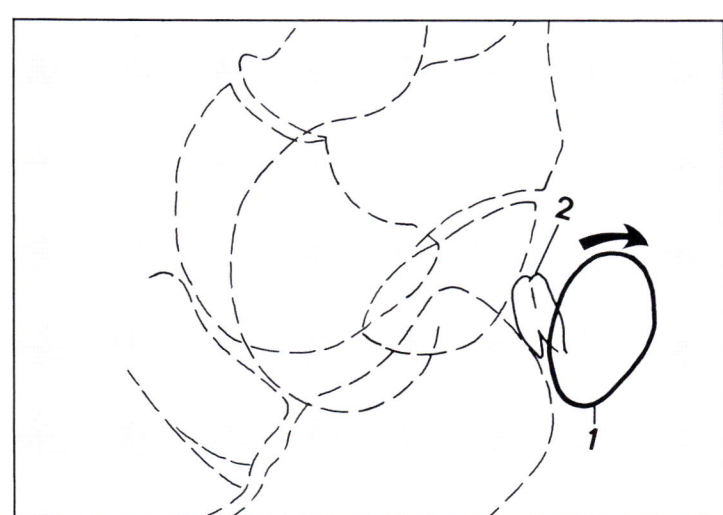

340 a Schematic drawing

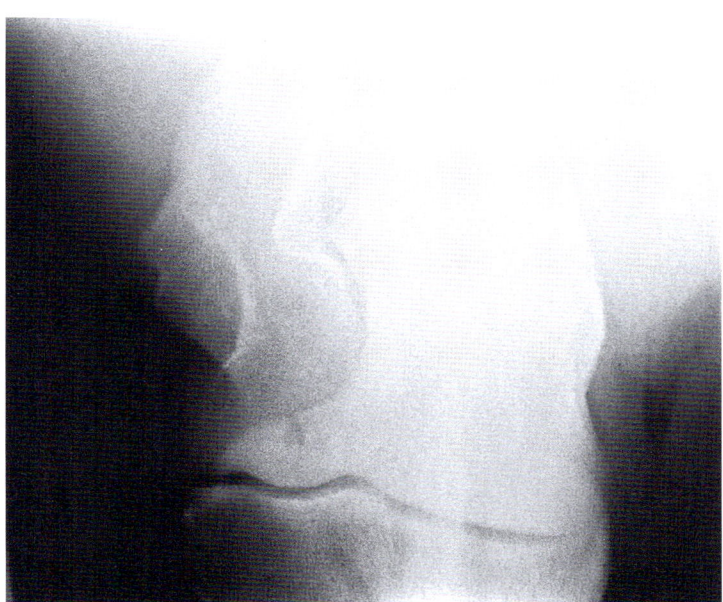

341

341 Right elbow, craniocaudal view: close-up.

Arabian, 9 years.

The linear radiolucent defect extending proximodistally from the distolateral border of the ulnar trochlear notch suggests a (complete or incomplete) fracture of the lateral coronoid process.

The seldom occuring fracture was confirmed by arthroscopic examination.

Fracture

Ulna

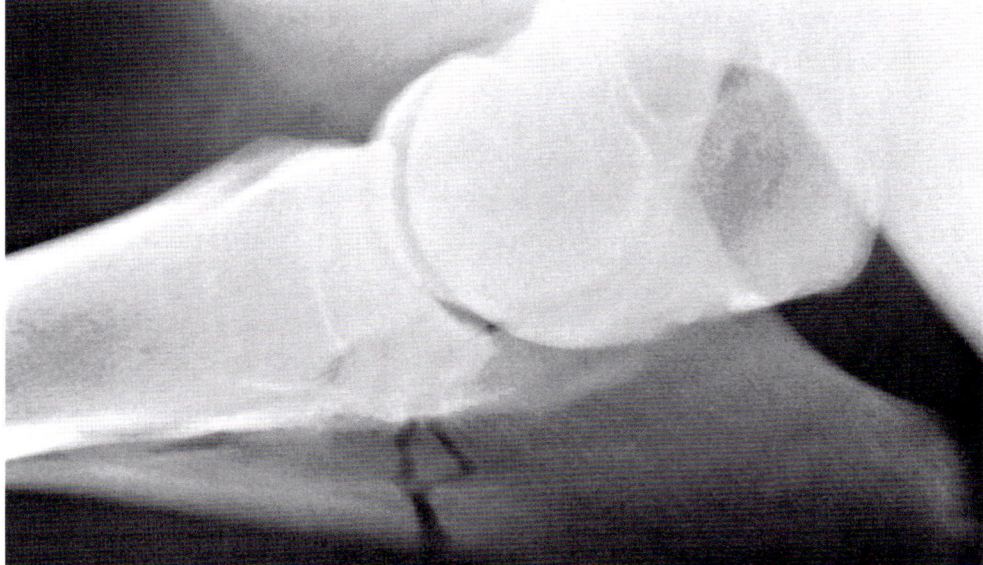

342

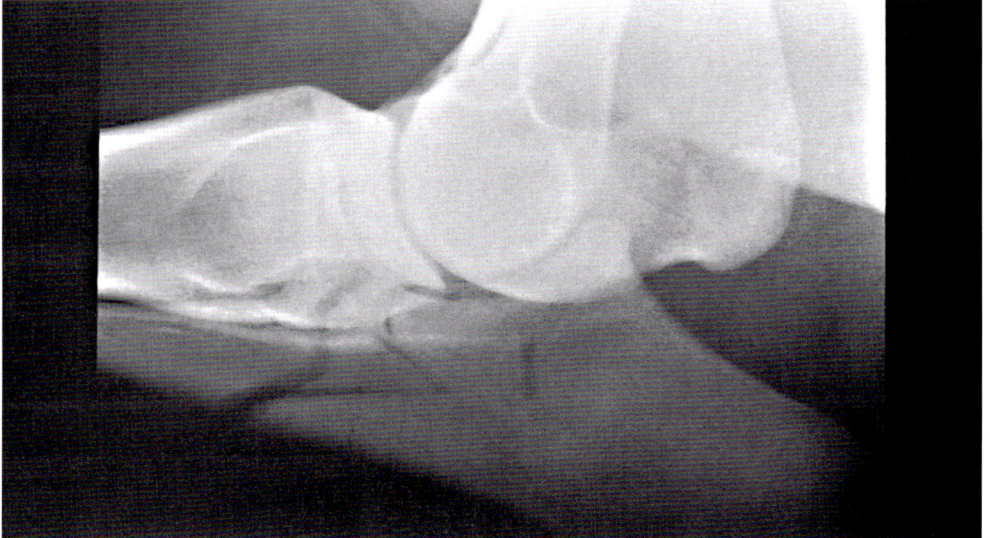

343

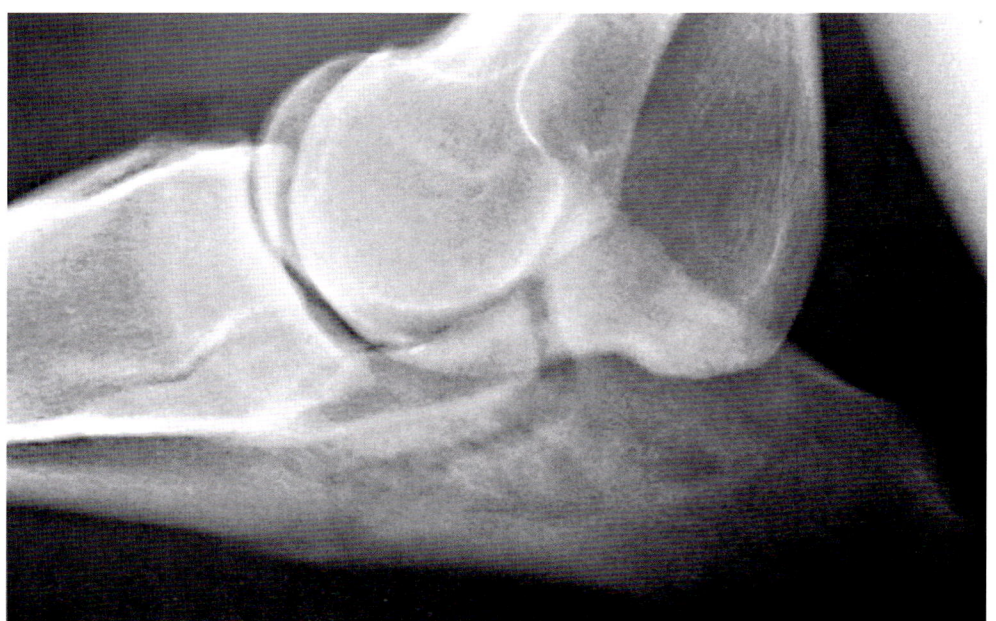

344

342 Left elbow, mediolateral view.

Pony, 8 years.

A sharply bordered radiolucent zone through the proximal ulna, indicating a recent transverse intra-articular fracture.

Disruption of the caudal cortex is obvious but, due to minimal displacement and compression of the cranial cortex, it is more difficult to discern the interruption of the articular surface.

343 Left elbow, mediolateral view.

Warmblood, 8 years.

Multiple, sharply bordered, radiolucent lines in the proximal ulna, some interrupting the articular surface as well as the caudal cortex, indicating a recent comminuted intra-articular fracture.

344 Right elbow, mediolateral view.

Warmblood, 4 years.

Several radiolucent lines through the proximal ulna are clearly defined proximally, interrupting the articular surface distal to the anconeal process and are blurred distally by callus formation overlying and bridging the fracture site. These changes are consistent with a comminuted fracture of some duration.

Radius

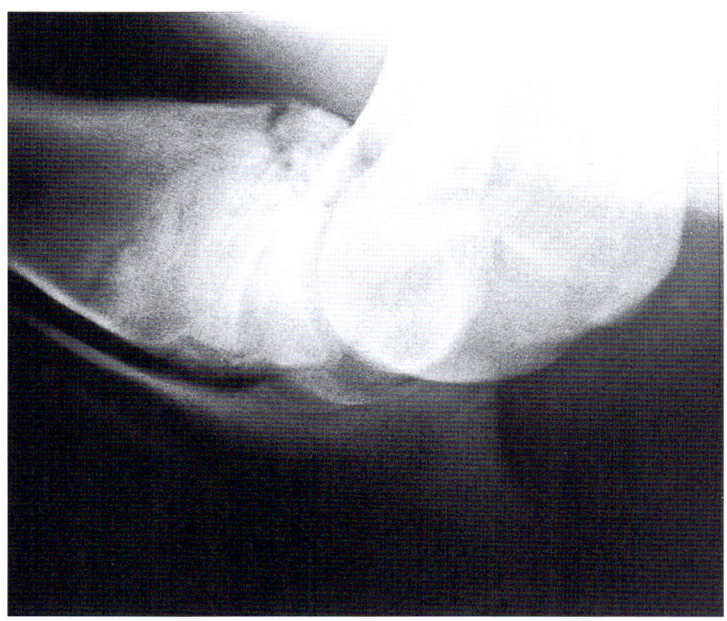

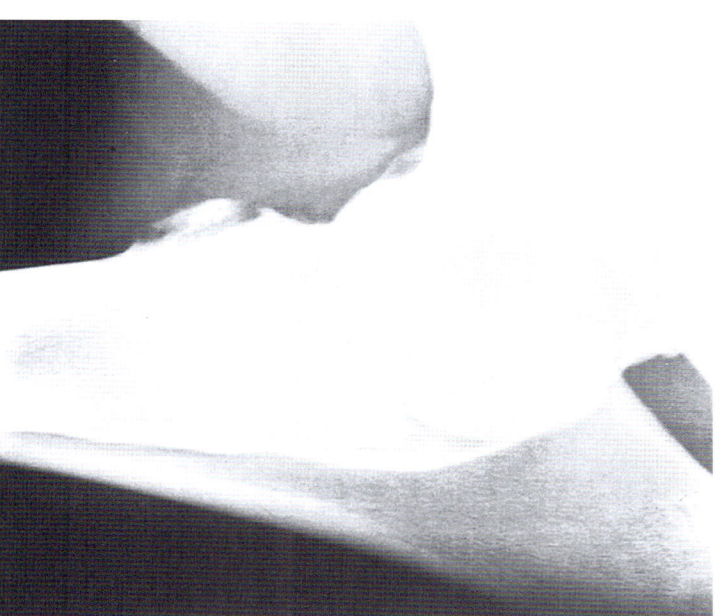

345 Left elbow, mediolateral view: close-up.

Pony, 1 year.

A large bone fragment is separated from the cranial aspect of the radial head, the radiolucent fracture line interrupting the articular surface.

An unusual intra-articular fracture resulting from hyperflexion of the elbow joint.

346 Left elbow, mediolateral view: close-up.

Warmblood, 4 years.

A small extra-articular bone fragment and a corresponding defect of the cranial contour of the radial tuberosity, representing an avulsion fracture caused by overstretching of the biceps brachii tendon insertion.

Radius/ulna

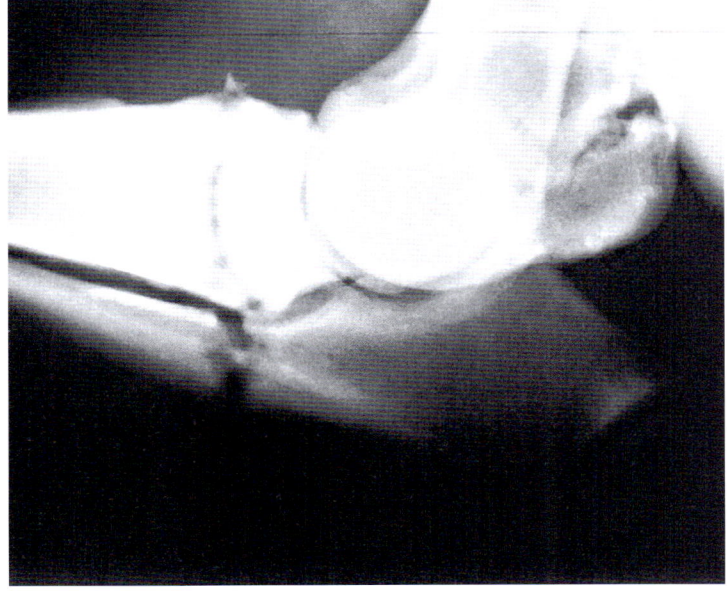

347

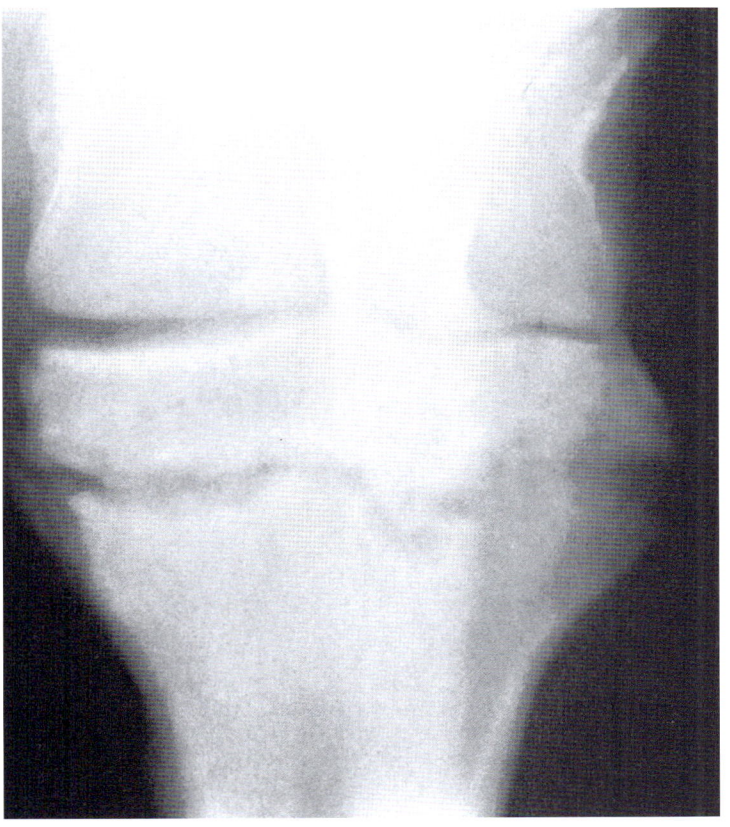

348

347/348 Left elbow, mediolateral and craniocaudal view: close-ups.

Foal, 10 months.

Both views show widening and irregularity of the proximal radial growth plate. The lateral view (Fig. 347) reveals an additional radiolucent zone through the corresponding portion of the ulna and a small isolated bone fragment cranial to the radial physis.

The radiographic changes indicate a Salter-Harris type 1 physeal fracture, with associated fracture of the ulna. The faint, ill bordered layer of periosteal new bone on the caudal surface of the ulna, adjacent to the fracture and around the radial metaphysis, indicates that the fracture occurred several weeks prior to the examination.

Fracture

Radius/ulna

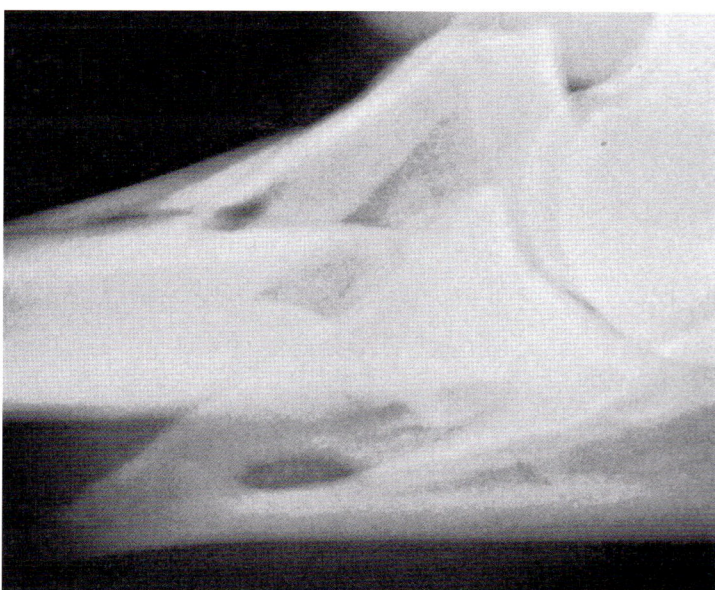

349

349 Right elbow, lateromedial view: close-up.

Warmblood, 6 years.

Fragmentation of the proximal end of the radius with multiple, sharply delineated, displaced and overriding bone fragments, indicating a recent comminuted intra-articular fracture.

The configuration of the fracture suggests an impaction type of injury.

Fracture/Luxation

Radius/ulna

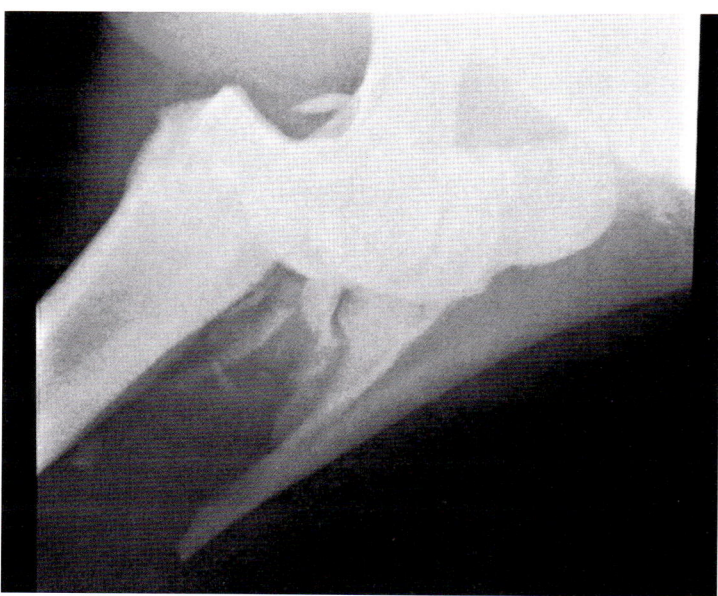

350

350 Left elbow, lateromedial view.

Warmblood, 3 years.

Cranioproximal displacement of the radius and multiple sharply bordered bone fragments between the distracted radius and proximal ulna, indicating a recent Monteggia type fracture, i. e. luxation of the elbow joint with associated fracture of the ulna.

An additional, small fracture fragment is visible cranial to the distal end of the humerus.

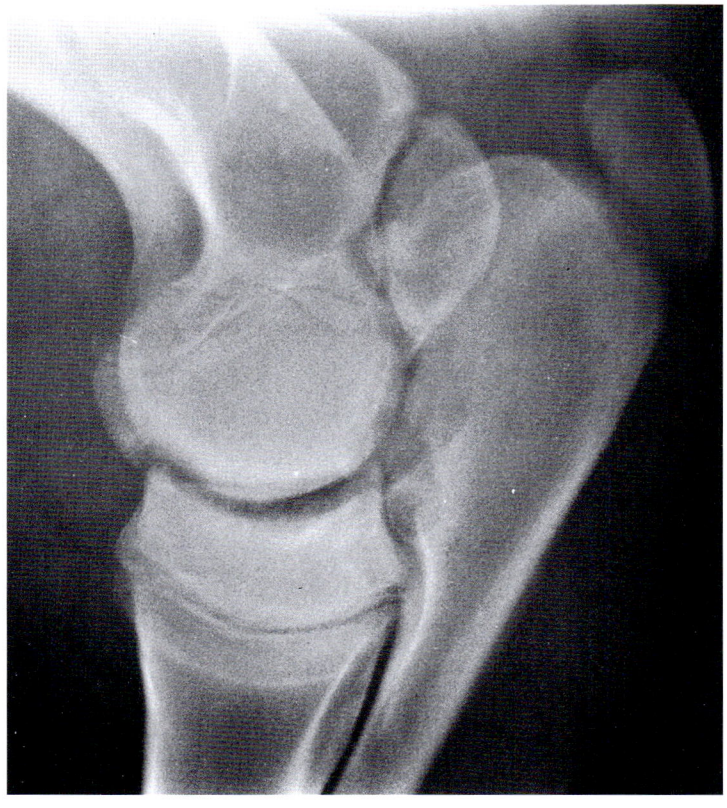

351

351 Right elbow, mediolateral view: close-up.

Foal, 1 month.

The elbow joint appears widened due to irregular loss of subchondral bone along the humeral and radial articular surface.

These changes are consistent with infectious arthritis of some duration. In this foal there was a penetrating wound sustained 3 weeks prior to the examination.

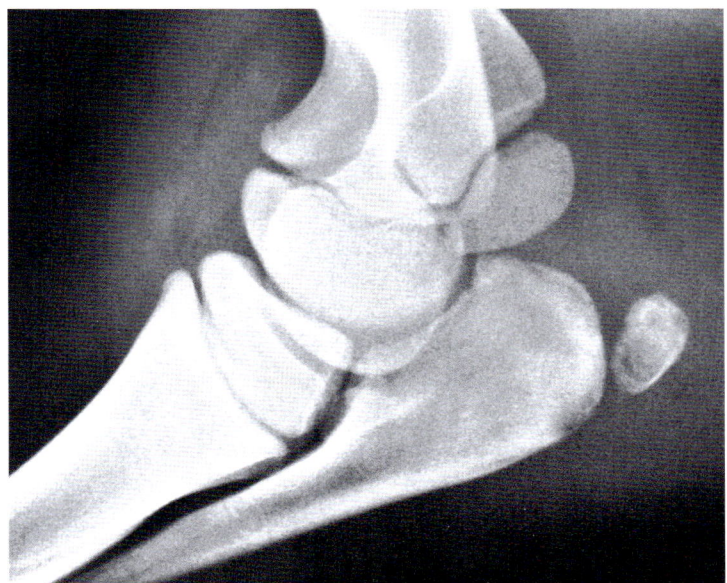

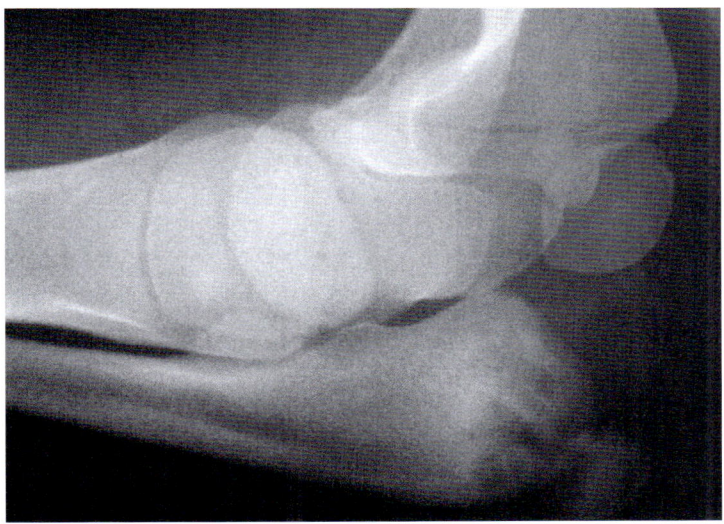

352 Right elbow, mediolateral view.

Foal, 3 weeks.

Extensive soft tissue swelling over the olecranon process and an irregular radiolucent pattern in the apophyseal and metaphyseal bone adjacent to the growth plate of the ulna, characteristic of a recent type P haematogenous osteomyelitis in a young foal.

353 Right elbow, mediolateral view: close-up.

Foal 4 weeks.

Multiple conflueting radiolucent lesions bordered by a sclerotic rim in the apophyseal and metaphyseal bone adjacent to the growth plate of the proximal ulna, indicating a more advanced case of type P osteomyelitis in a young foal.

Osteomyelitis

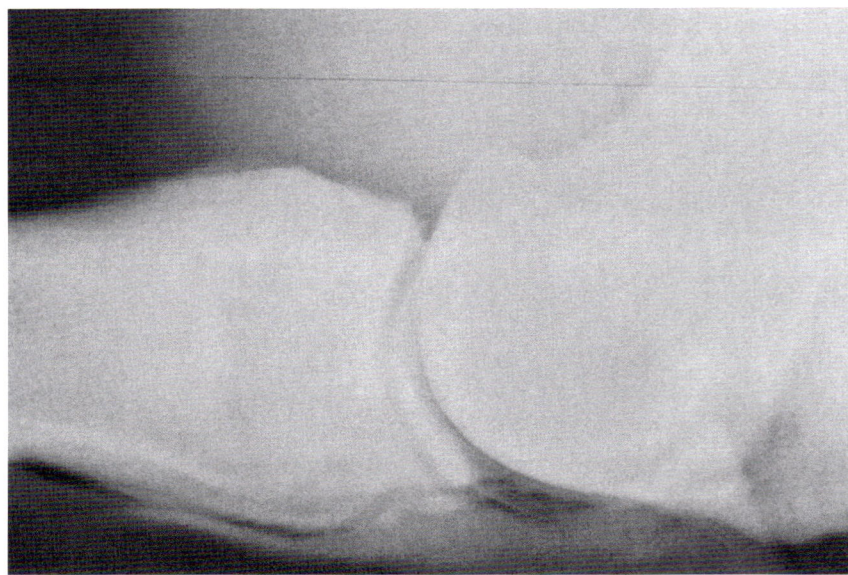

354

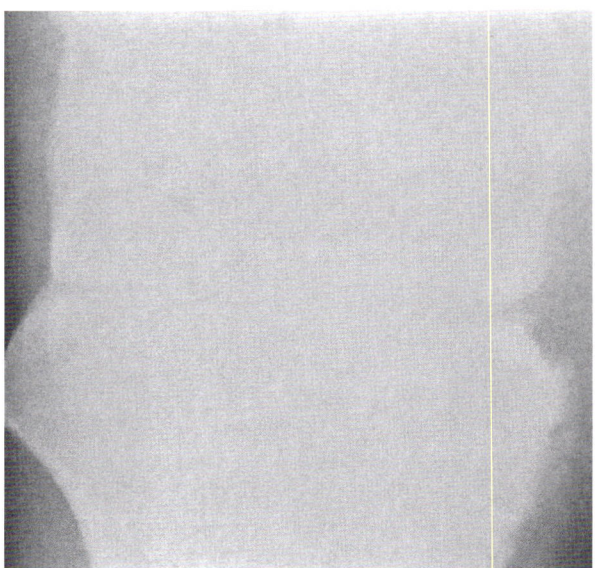

355

354/355 Right elbow, mediolateral and craniocaudal view: close-ups.

Warmblood, 4 ½ years.

The mediolateral view (Fig. 354) shows a very obscure radiolucency in the subchondral bone of the proximal radius and a thin layer of periosteal new bone on the cranial radial surface.

On the craniocaudal view (Fig. 355) irregular radiating periosteal new bone formation on the medial aspect of the proximal radius is obvious.

Failure to identify the associated radiolucency of the proximal radius results from relative underexposure. The brush pattern of the periosteal new bone, perpendicular to the outer cortical surface, suggests either an infectious or malignant disease.

Bone biopsy revealed the presence of an infectious lesion.

Bone cyst

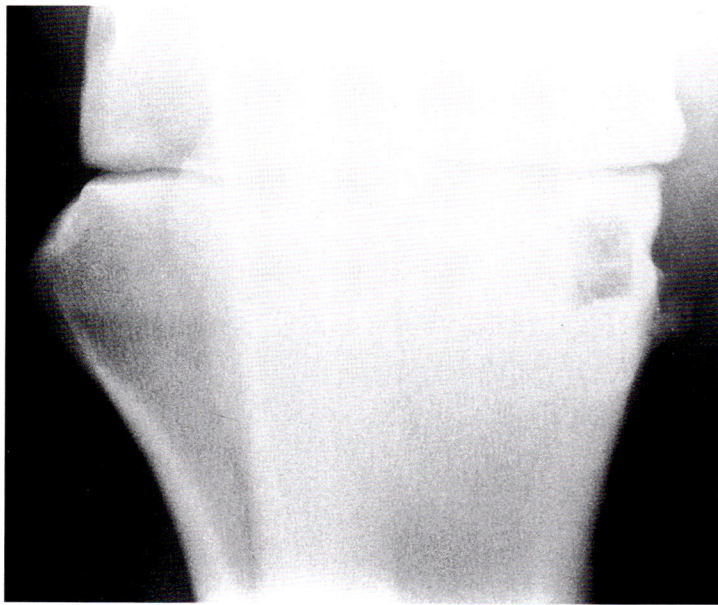

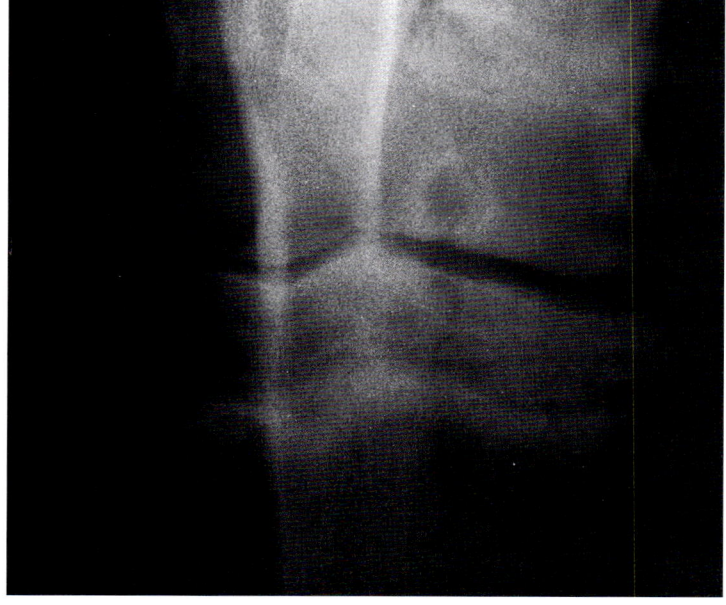

356 Right elbow, craniocaudal view: close-up.

Warmblood, 10 years.

The well defined rounded area of radiolucency in the medial aspect of the proximal radius and the associated periosteal new bone at the site of insertion of the medial collateral joint ligament represent the most common manifestation of a subchondral bone cyst in the elbow region.

Communication between the cyst and the elbow joint is not apparent.

Differential diagnosis includes an infectious lesion (Fig. 354/355)

357 Right elbow, craniocaudal view: close-up.

Pony, 1 year.

The rounded area of radiolucency surrounded by a sclerotic rim in the axial aspect of the distal humeral epiphysis adjacent to the articular surface is consistent with a bone cyst of some duration. The indistinct disruption of the underlying subcondral bone indicates probable communication between the cyst and the elbow joint.

Contrary to a cyst-like lesion in the proximal radius, bone cysts within the distal humerus close to the elbow joint are a rare phenomenon.

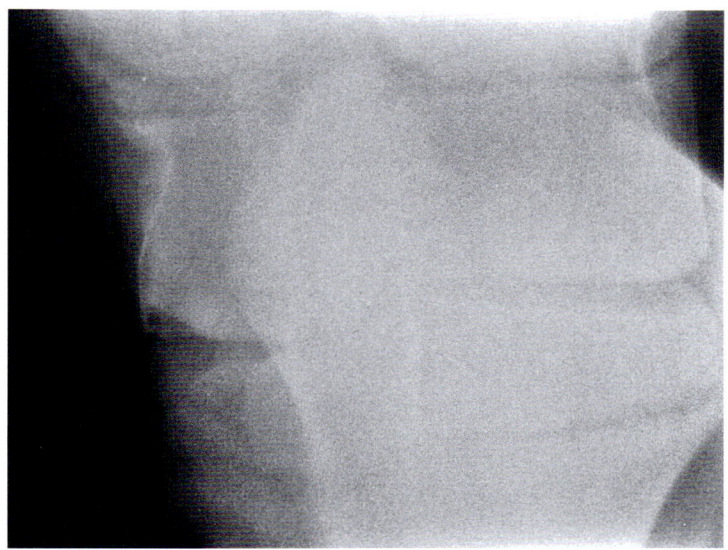

358

358 Right elbow, craniocaudal view: close-up.

Foal, 9 weeks.

The small well defined area of subchondral radiolucency in the lateral aspect of the distal humeral epiphysis is a manifestation of osteochondrosis.

Histological examination confirmed the diagnosis.

In the horse osteochondrosis of the elbow is a rare condition, and only documented previously in the medial aspect of the distal humerus and proximal radius.

The Shoulder

Fracture

Fracture/Luxation

Luxation

Subluxation

Infectious arthritis

Osteomyelitis

Osteochondrosis

Osteoarthrosis

Bone sequestration

Osteosarcoma

Ossification of the biceps brachii tendon

Bicipital bursitis

Shoulder dysplasia

Fracture

Scapula

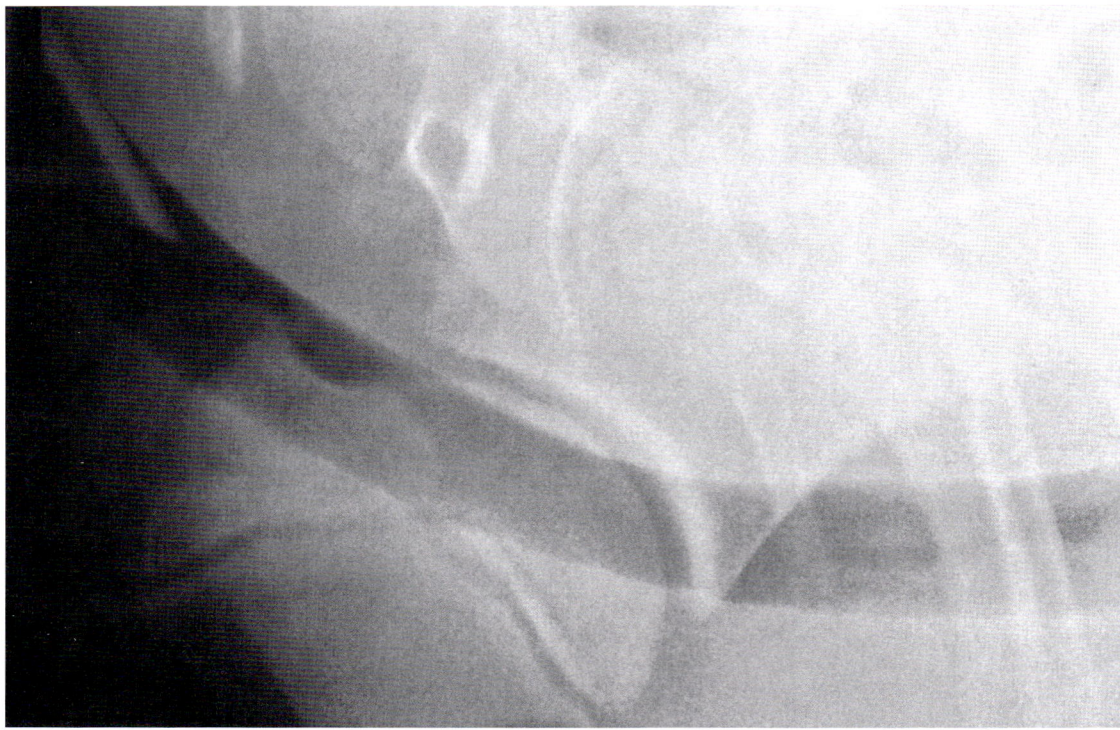

359

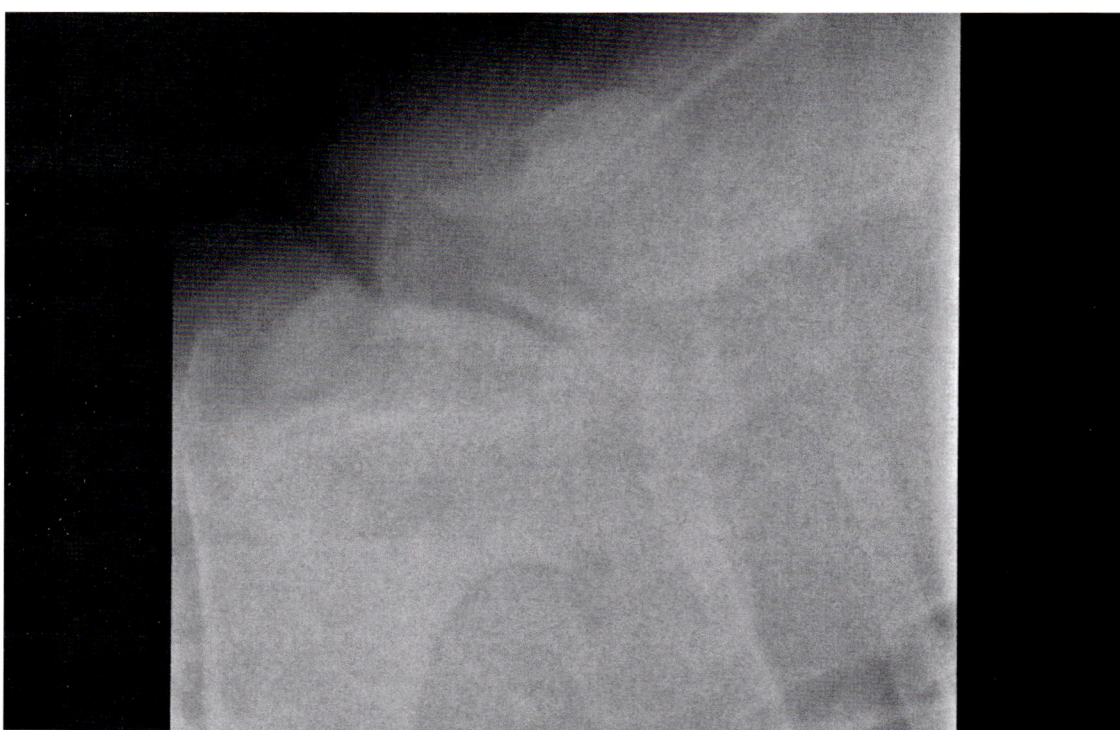

360

Scapula

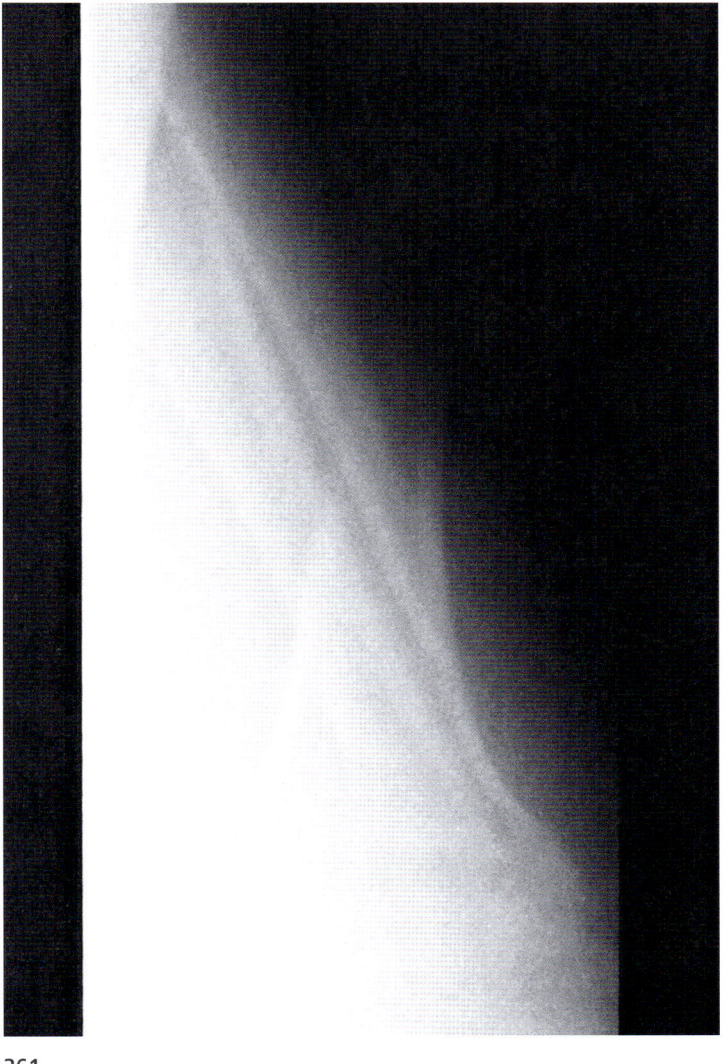

361

359/360/361 Right shoulder, mediolateral and caudocranial views: close-ups.

Foal, 3 months.

The mediolateral view with the anaesthesized horse in lateral recumbency (Fig. 359) shows no abnormality despite the presence of a severe acute shoulder lameness.

An additional mediolateral projection (Fig. 360), with the head and neck fully flexed and the shoulder pushed dorsally, avoids superimposition of the distal end of the scapula over the vertebral column and demonstrates two large overriding bone fragments resulting from a transverse scapular fracture proximal to the supraglenoid tuberosity.

A caudocranial view (Fig. 361) with the horse in dorsal recumbency shows overriding of fracture fragments as well as angular displacement.

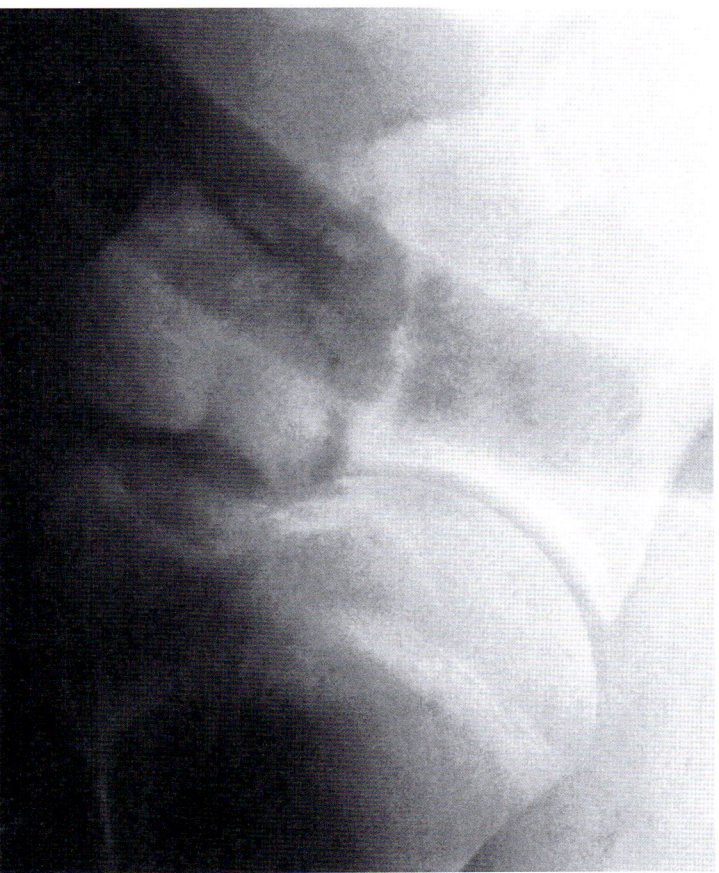
362

362 Right shoulder, mediolateral view: close-up.

Warmblood, 2 years.

The large well defined isolated bone fragment and the corresponding defect in the cranial border of the scapula indicate an intra-articular avulsion fracture of the supraglenoid tuberosity. Small additional fracture fragments are visible superimposing the wide V-shaped fracture zone.

Fracture

Scapula

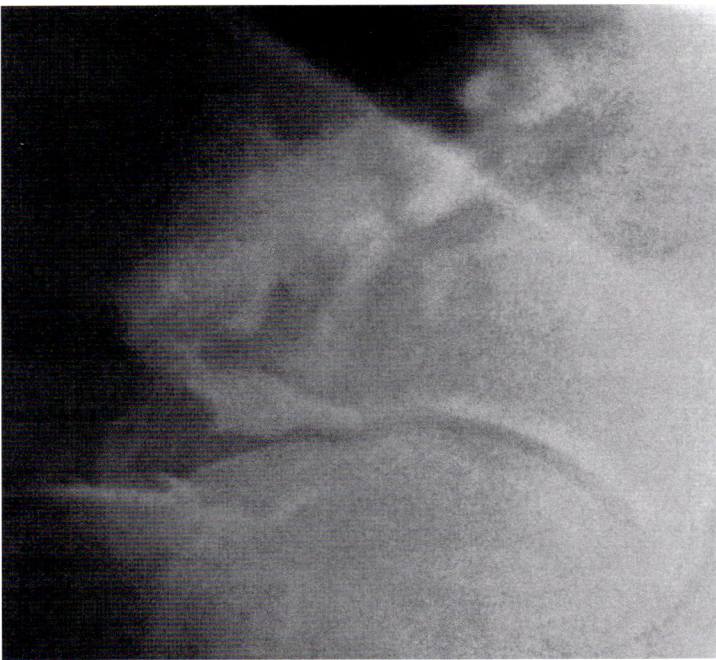

363 Left shoulder, mediolateral view: close-up.

Foal, 11 months.

Severe deformation of the supraglenoid tuberosity and ill defined mixed radiolucent and sclerotic zones within the tuberosity due to an avulsion fracture sustained ½ year previously, resulting in exuberant irregular callus formation. The absence of disruption in the distal border of the scapula suggests an incomplete avulsion.

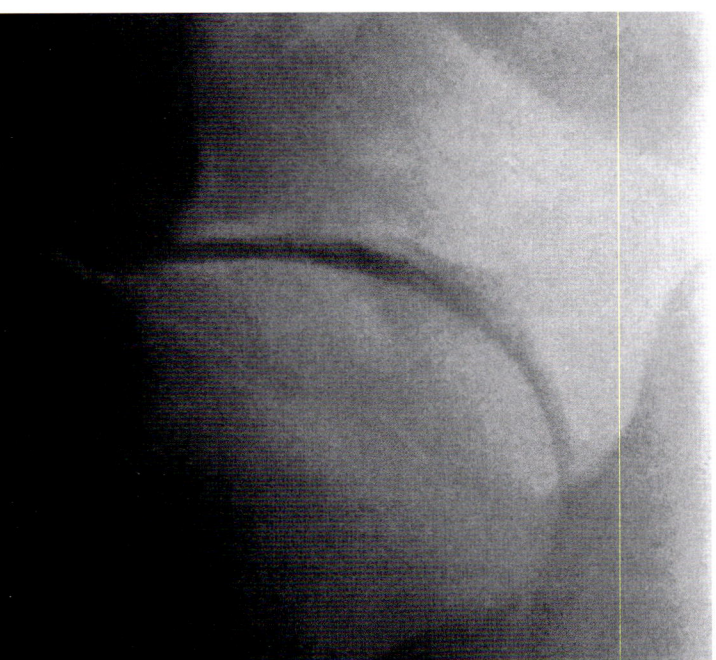

364 Right shoulder, mediolateral view: close-up.

Warmblood, 1 ½ years.

Two small, ill defined bone fragments, the result of a recent chip fracture, are separated from the distal margin of the scapula and disrupt the normally smooth border of the central aspect of the glenoid cavity.

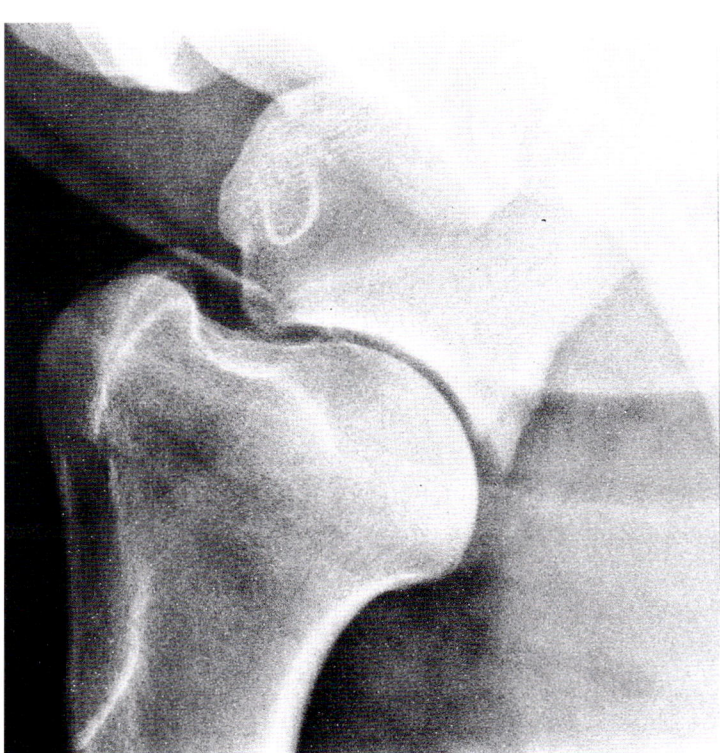

365 Right shoulder, mediolateral view.

Pony, 6 years.

The vertical radiolucent line through the caudodistal aspect of the scapula and the corresponding step-defect disrupting the normally smooth contour of the caudal aspect of the glenoid cavity indicate a fracture of the infraglenoid tuberosity. The ill defined radiolucency of the fracture line suggests a fracture of some duration.

Humerus

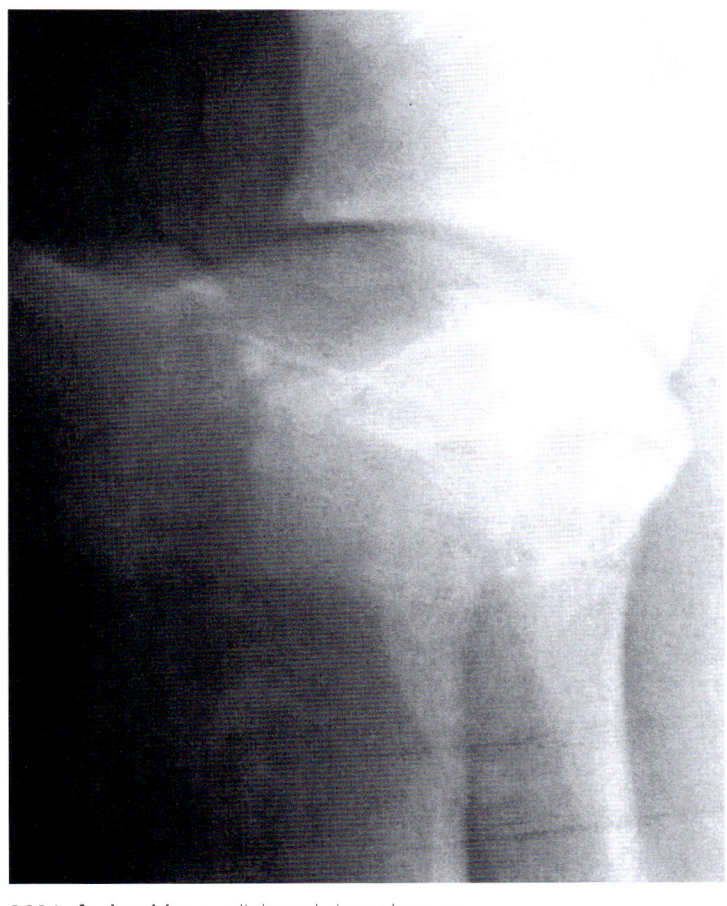

366 Left shoulder, mediolateral view: close-up.

Foal, 11 months.

The humeral head is separated into two overriding, sharply delineated fragments indicating the presence of a recent Salter-Harris type 4 physeal fracture.

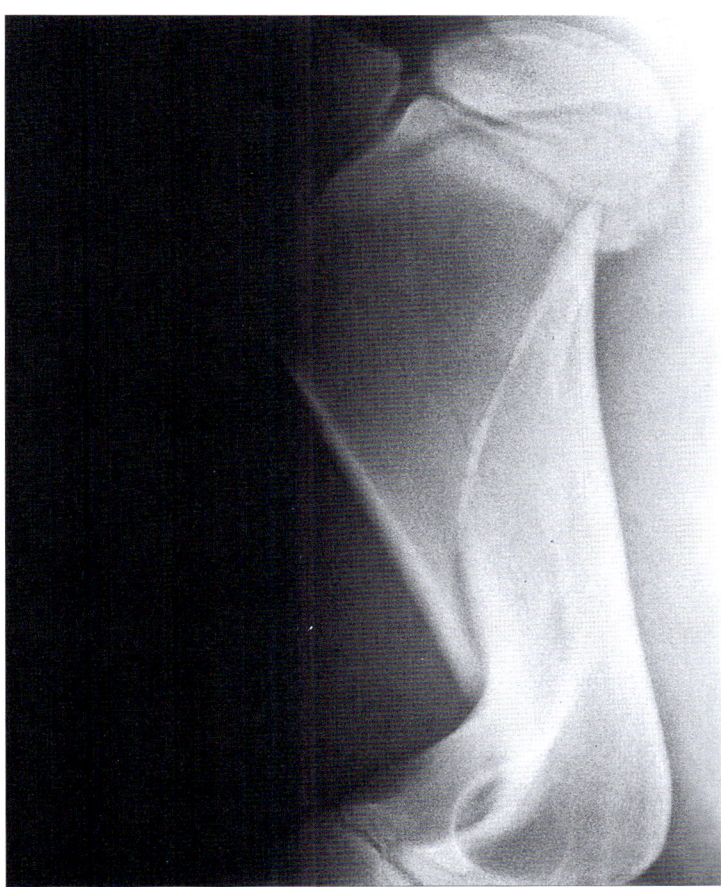

367 Left humerus, mediolateral view.

Foal, 5 weeks.

The oblique radiopaque line extending from the caudoproximal aspect of the humerus just below the humeral head to the craniodistal aspect of the humeral diaphysis represents the most common type of a midshaft humeral fracture. The radiopacity of the fracture line results from overriding of the fracture fragments due to muscle contraction, the craniodistal overriding being most prominent. Radial nerve paralysis often occurs secondary to these fractures because of its location in the musculospiral groove of the humerus.

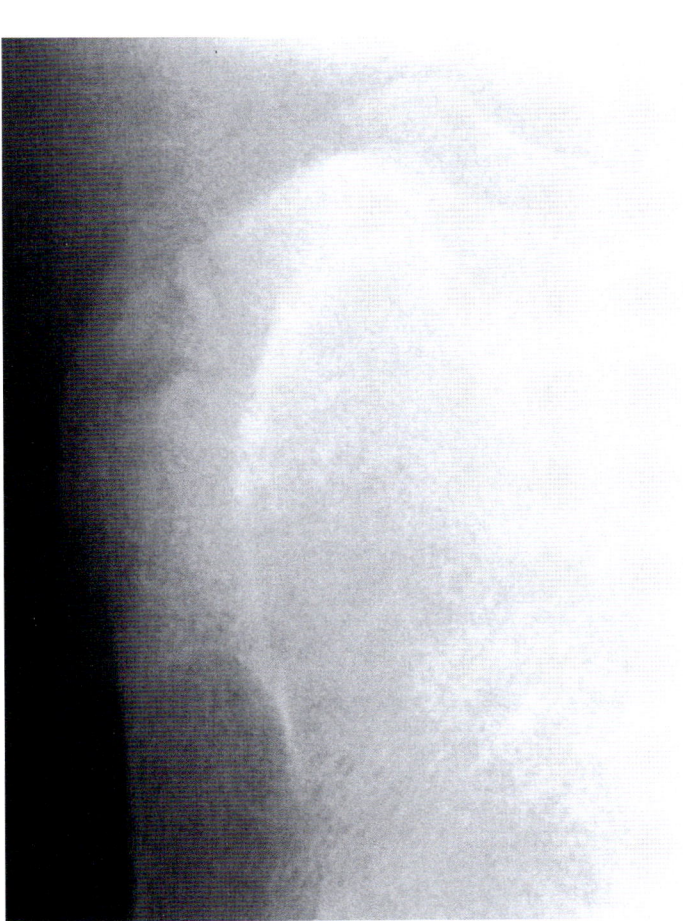

368

368 Right shoulder, mediolateral view: close-up of the humeral tuberosities.

Warmblood, 9 years.

Partial fragmentation of the cranial surface of the lateral tuberosity of the humerus, caused by a kick by another horse 2 weeks prior to the examination.

Fracture

Humerus

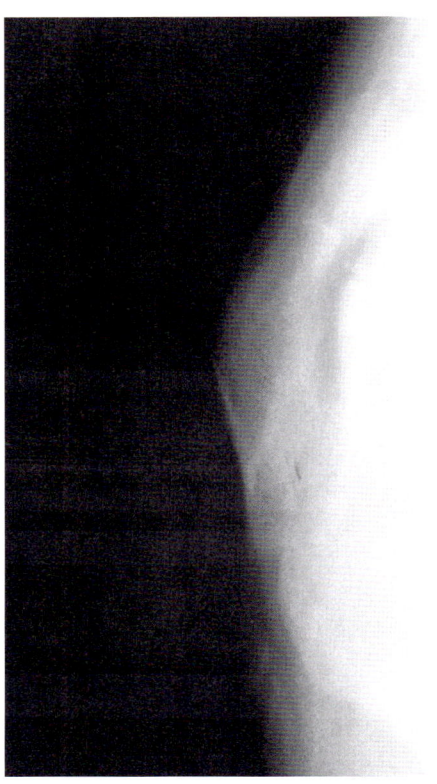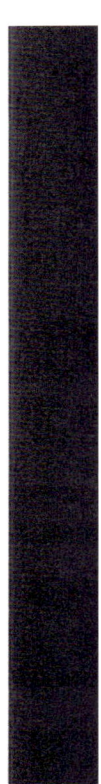

369

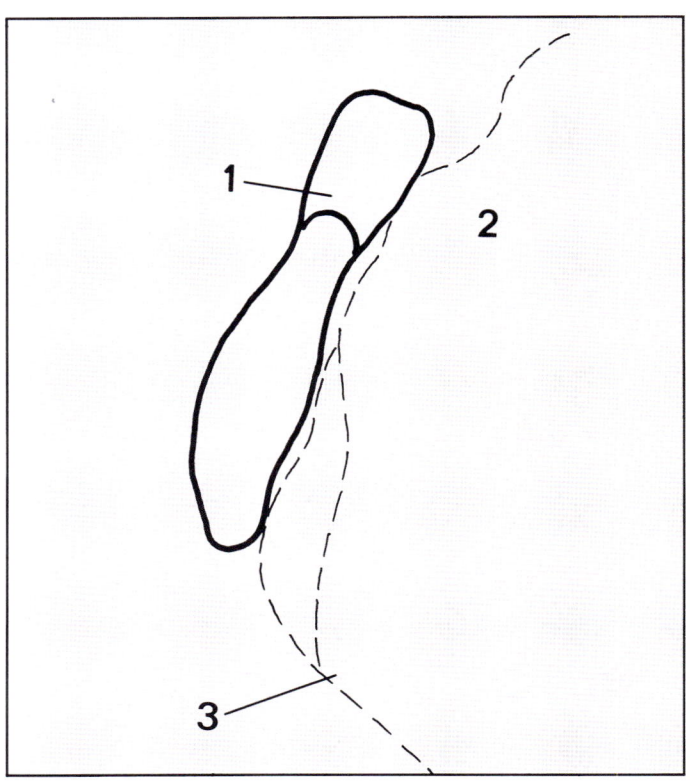

369 a

369 Right shoulder, caudolateral-craniomedial oblique "skyline" view: close-up.

Warmblood, 5 years.

A wide ill bordered radiolucent zone running between the caudal portion of the lateral tuberosity **(1)** and the humeral head **(2)** and extending distally to the deltoid tuberosity **(3)**. This was the result of a recent intra-articular fracture of the lateral tuberosity. The fracture plane is not strictly parallel with the central beam and the fracture zone is therefore indistinct and not clearly demonstrable distally.

The reason for this special skyline projection was the absence of radiographic abnormalities on the mediolateral view despite a severe and acute shoulder lameness.

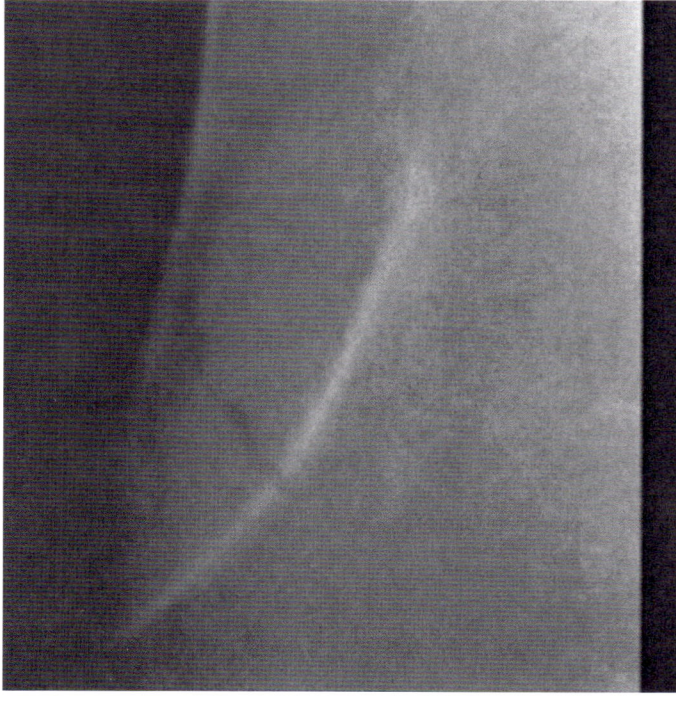

370

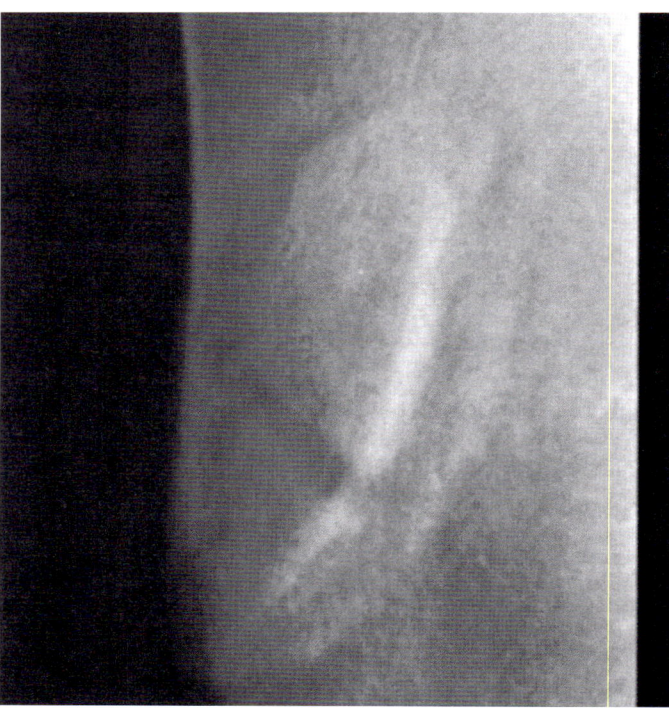

371

370/371 Left shoulder, serial mediolateral views: close-ups of the deltoid tuberosity.

Standardbred, 5 years.

The initial examination (Fig. 370), 1 day after the onset of lameness, reveals distinct, distally diverging, radiolucent zones in the deltoid tuberosity, which do not interrupt the continuity of the cranial surface of the humerus. These indicate the presence of an incomplete fracture. The second examination (Fig. 371) 2 weeks later, demonstrates widening of the fracture zone, due to bone resorption and a faint thin layer of periosteal new bone on the cranial aspect of the humerus.

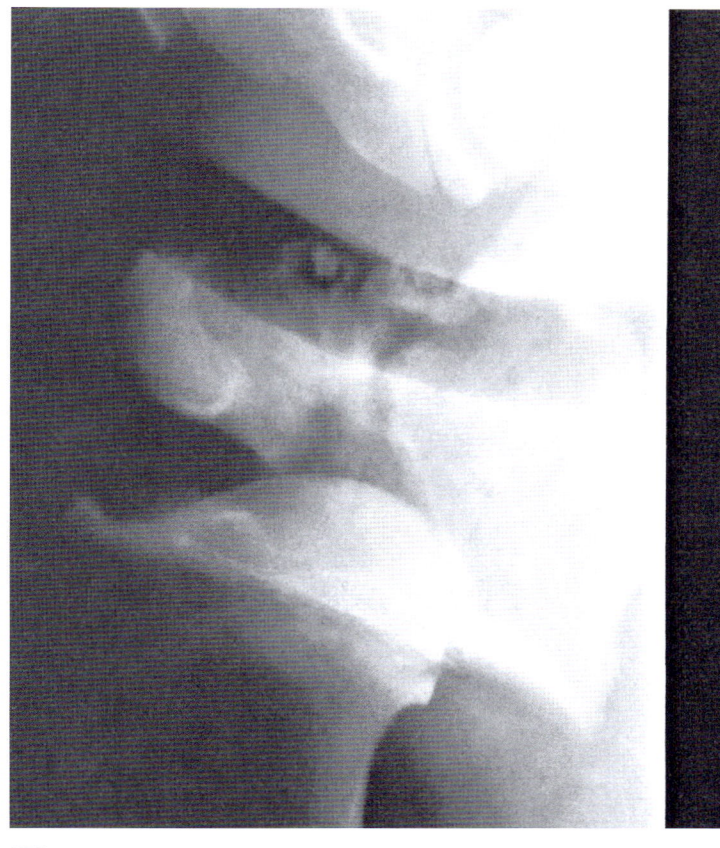

372

372 Right shoulder, mediolateral view.

Pony, 1 ½ year.

Complete luxation of the shoulder joint with cranioproximal displacement of the humerus and overriding of the distal end of the scapula.

The bone fragments proximal to the humerus indicate that dislocation occurred together with associated fracture of the supraglenoid tuberosity and the cranial aspect of the glenoid cavity.

Luxation

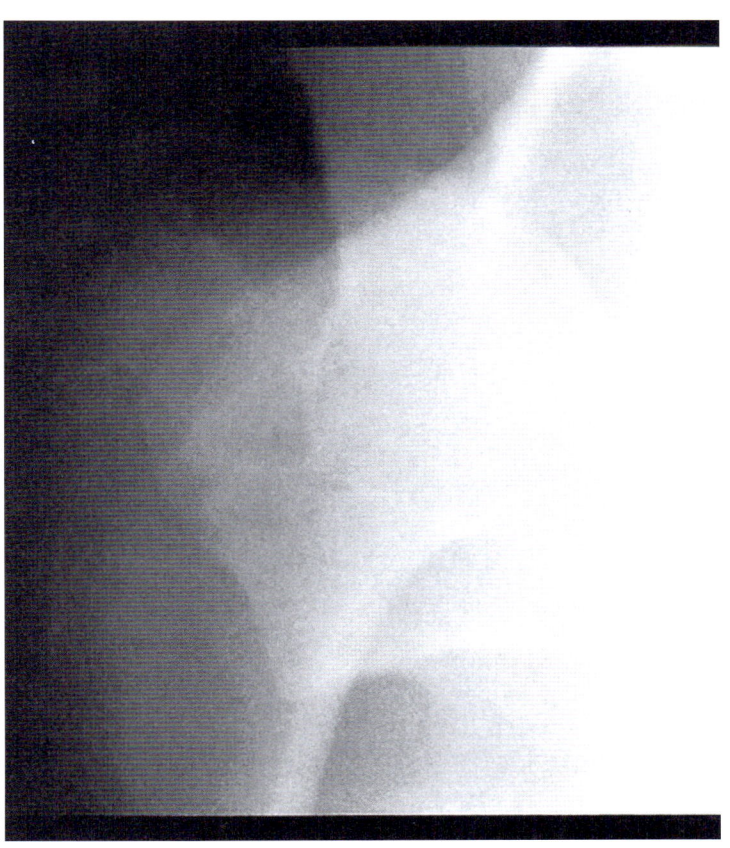

373

373 Left shoulder, mediolateral view: close-up.

Warmblood, 15 years.

Complete luxation of the shoulder joint without associated fracture.

Subluxation

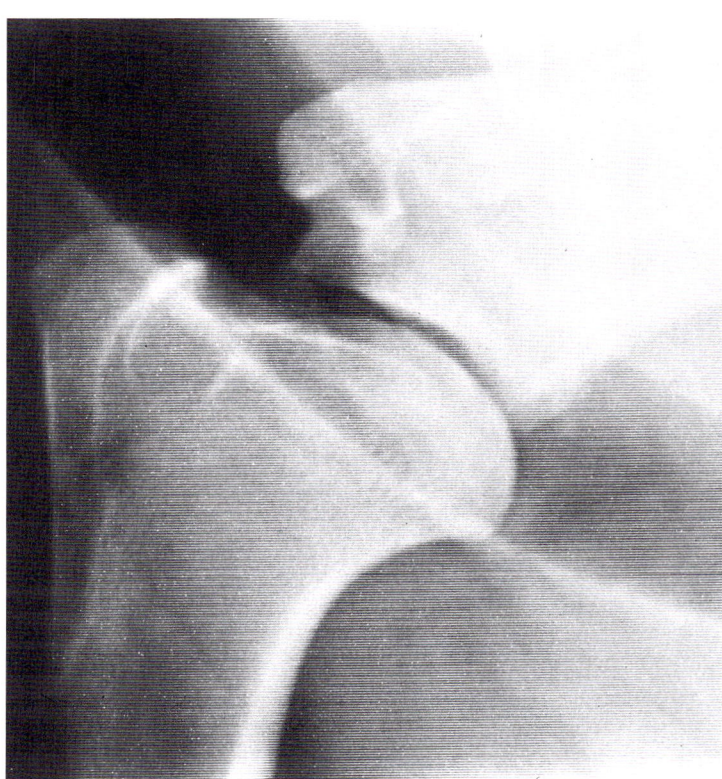

374

374 Left shoulder, mediolateral view.

Pony, 2 years.

The loss of congruity between the outlines of the glenoid cavity of the scapula and the humeral head and the caudal displacement of the humerus indicate subluxation of the shoulder joint.

Blunting of the normally pointed contour of the caudal border of the glenoid cavity and the adjacent soft tissue opacity indicate associated mild fragmentation of the infraglenoid tuberosity.

Infectious arthritis

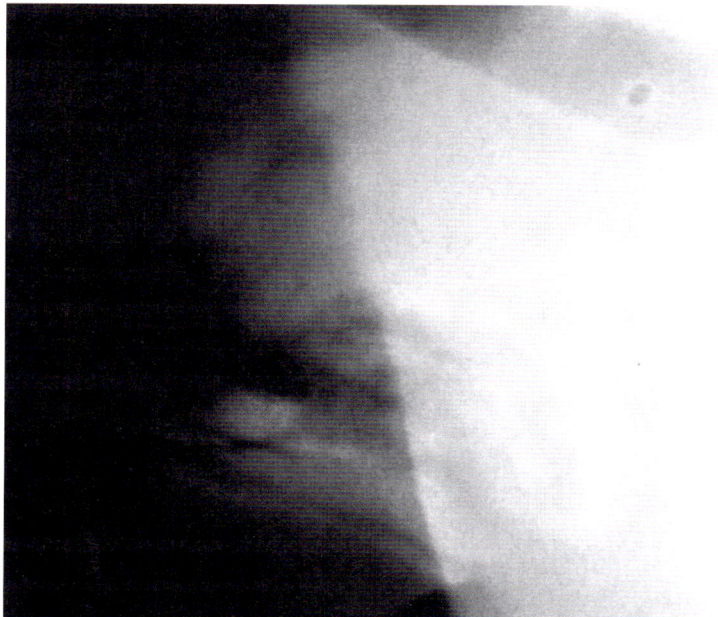

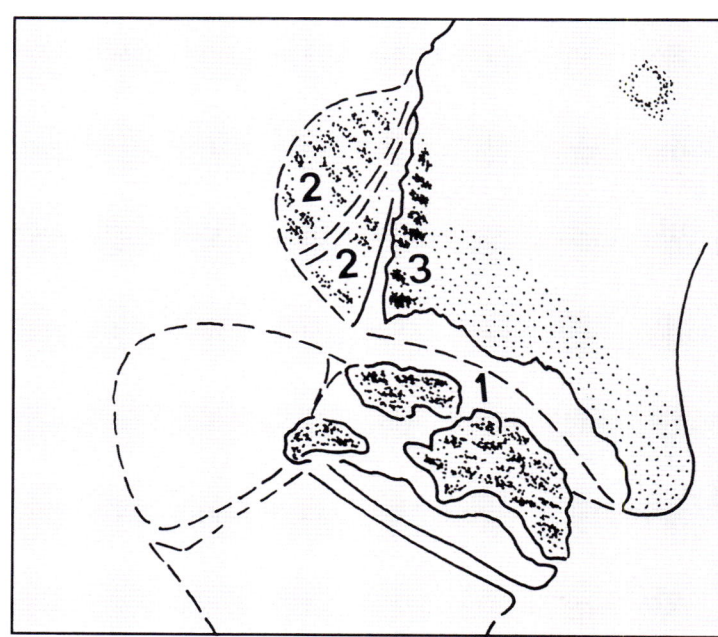

375 Right shoulder, mediolateral view: close-up.

Foal, 2 months.

Severe destruction of subchondral bone on both sides of the unequally widened joint space **(1)** indicating infectious arthritis.

Joint infection resulted from extension of peri-articular abscess formation.

N. B. The irregular mottled appearance of the supraglenoid tuberosity of the scapula **(2)** and the cranial aspect of the glenoid cavity **(3)** represents the normal irregular subchondral ossification pattern of these ossification centres in the young foal.

375 a Schematic drawing

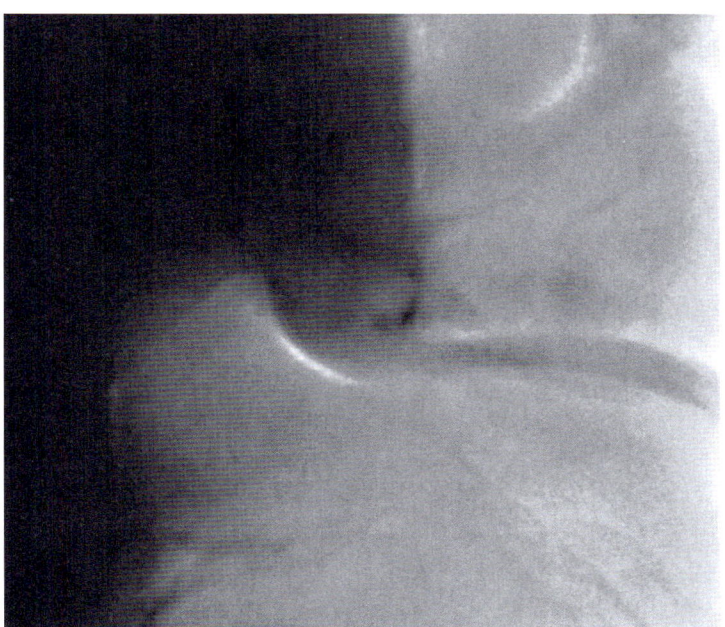

376

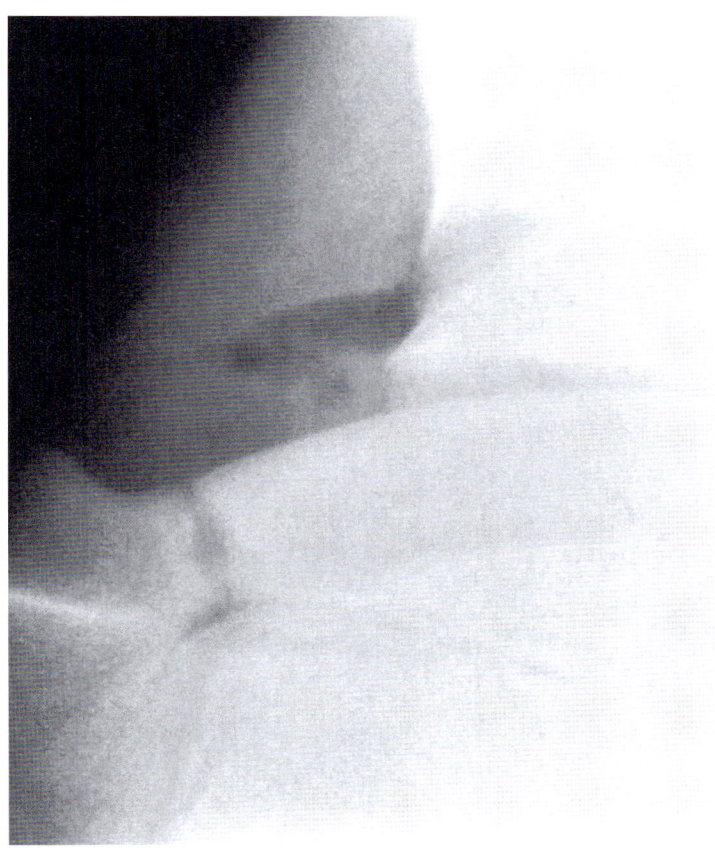

377

376/377 Right shoulder, mediolateral and caudolateral-craniomedial oblique view.

Foal, 6 months.

The mediolateral view (Fig. 376) shows radiolucent areas suggestive of destructive bone lesions in the lateral tuberosity of the humerus and the cranial part of the glenoid cavity of the scapula. On a caudolateral-craniomedial oblique projection (Fig. 377) the radiolucent areas shift cranially and are situated within the joint cavity. Differential diagnosis includes intra-articular air or gas accumulation resulting from infectious arthritis, penetrating wound or intra-articular injection. In this foal a local anaesthetic block of the shoulder joint had resulted in artefactual intra-articular air accumulation.

Osteomyelitis

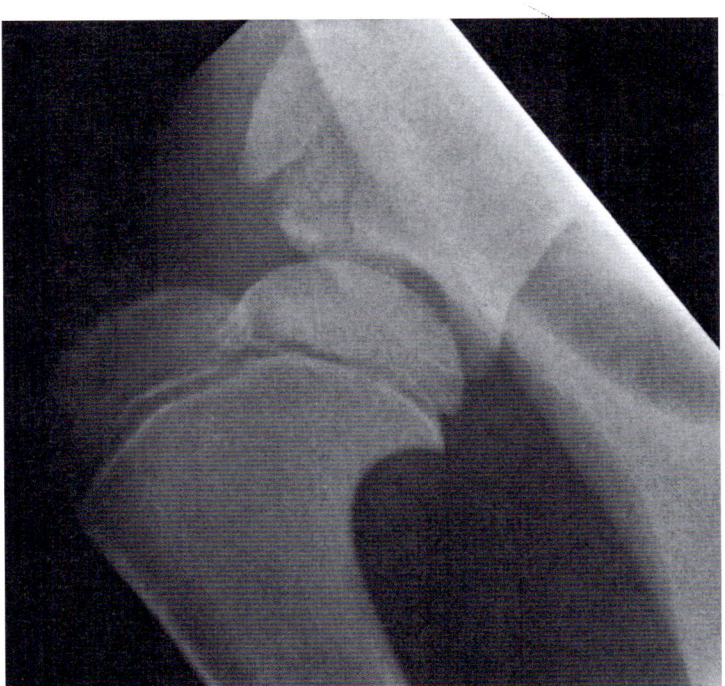

378

378 Right shoulder, mediolateral view.

Foal, 2 weeks.

A clearly defined, cystic, radiolucent defect in the central area of the glenoid cavity. Soft tissue swelling is not apparent.

Differential diagnosis includes an infectious, cyst-like, or osteochondral lesion. Clinical and laboratory data indicated the presence of an infectious lesion, despite the absence of soft tissue swelling.

Histological examination confirmed the diagnosis.

Osteomyelitis

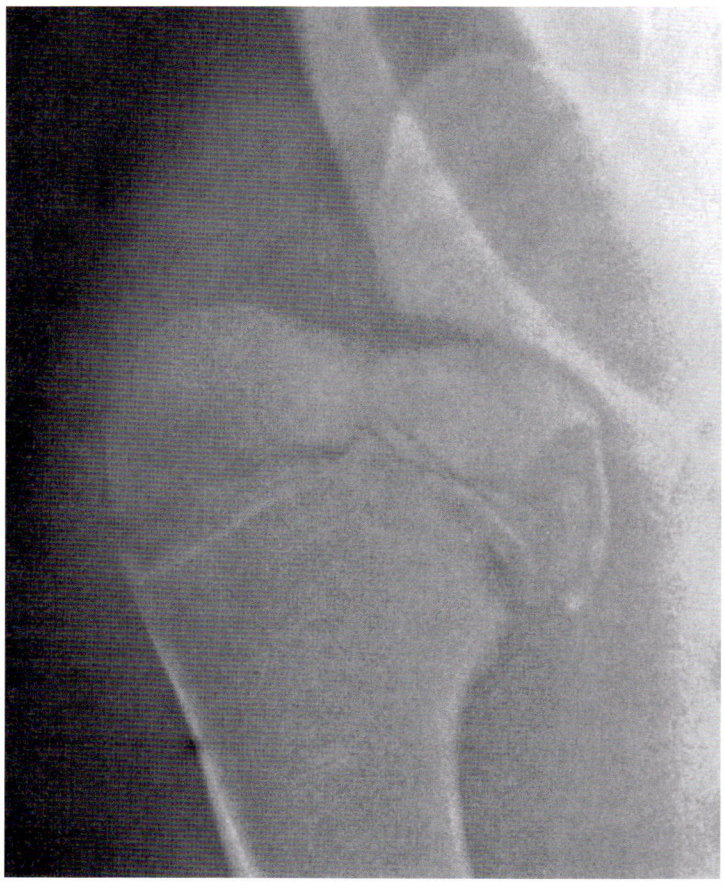

379

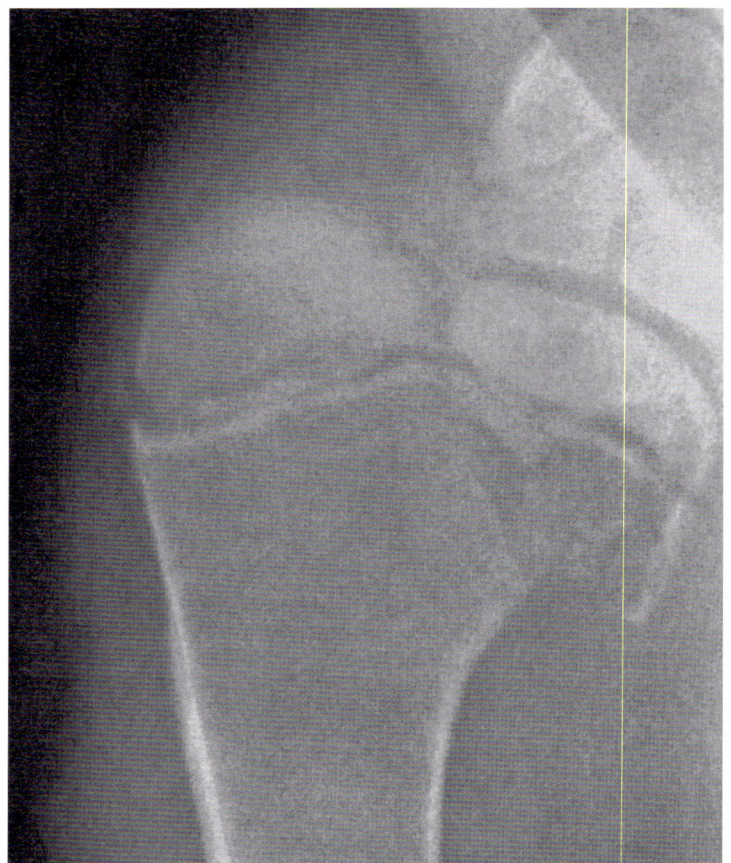

380

379/380 Right shoulder, serial mediolateral views: close-ups.

Foal, 6 weeks.

The initial examination (Fig. 379), 12 days after the onset of lameness, reveals peri-articular soft tissue swelling and a large radiolucent bone lesion involving the epi- and metaphyseal bone of the caudal aspect of the humeral head, characteristic of type P haematogenous osteomyelitis in a young foal. The radiopaque centre of the lesion, the linear radiopacity and flattening of the subchondral bone indicates sequestrum formation, collapse of the humeral head and direct communication of the focus of osteomyelitis with the joint cavity.

A second examination 1 week later (Fig. 380), demonstrates more advanced lysis and disintegration of the sequestra.

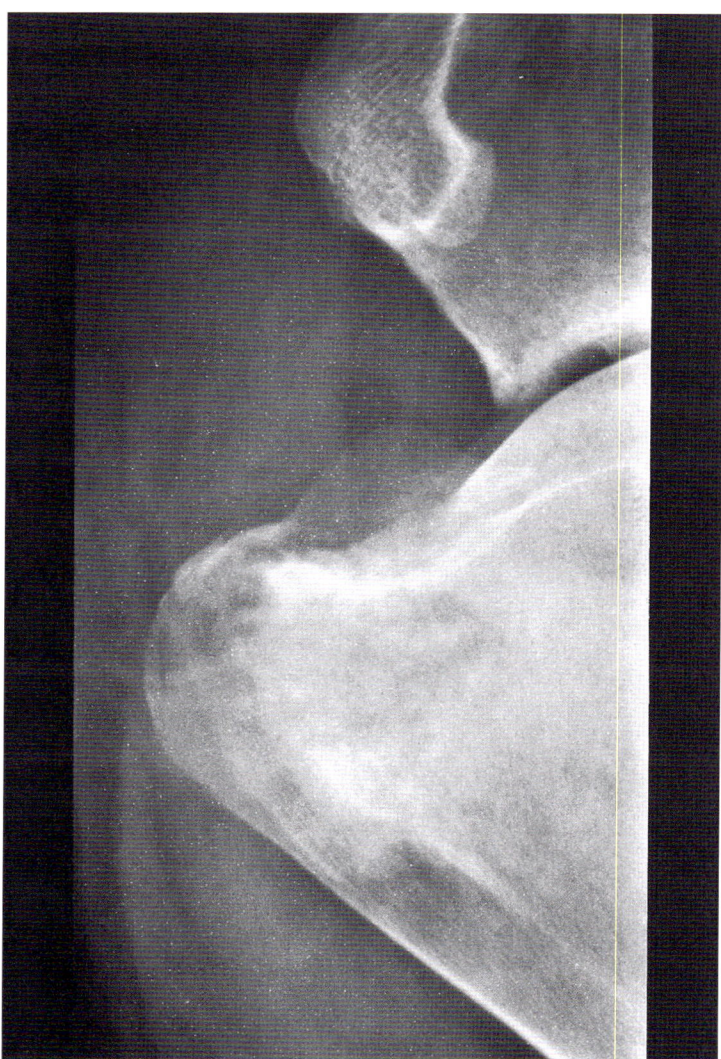

381 Shoulder joint specimen, mediolateral appearance.

Warmblood, 5 years.

The patchy radiopacity of the bone texture in the region of the lateral, intermediate and medial humeral tuberosity results from osteomyelitis and sequestrum formation; in this horse introduced by infection of the overlying bicipital bursa.

381

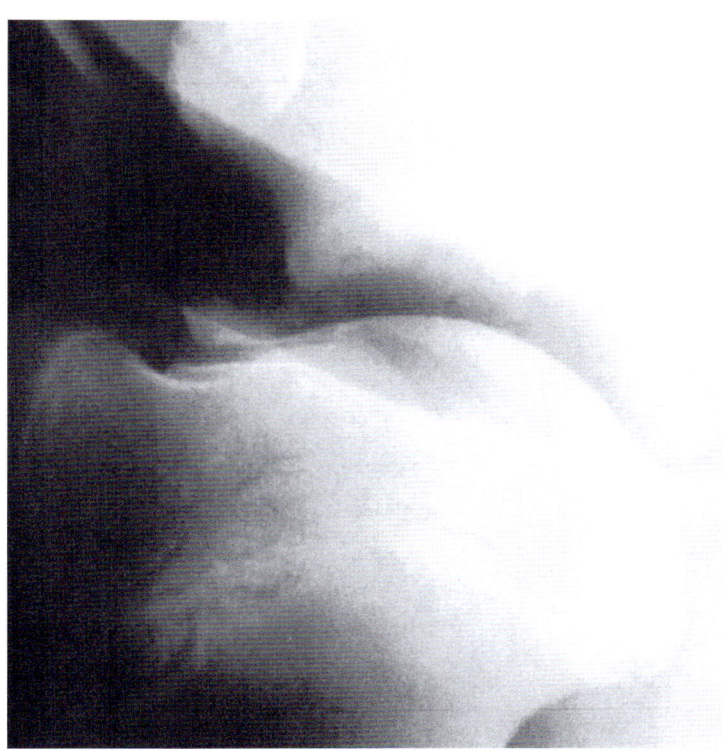

382 Right shoulder, mediolateral view: close-up.

Foal, 8 months.

The patchy radiolucent areas within the glenoid cavity are a manifestation of osteochondrosis.

N. B. In most cases the major radiographic changes of osteochondrosis are centred on the caudal aspect of the humeral head, radiographic changes of only the glenoid cavity are infrequent.

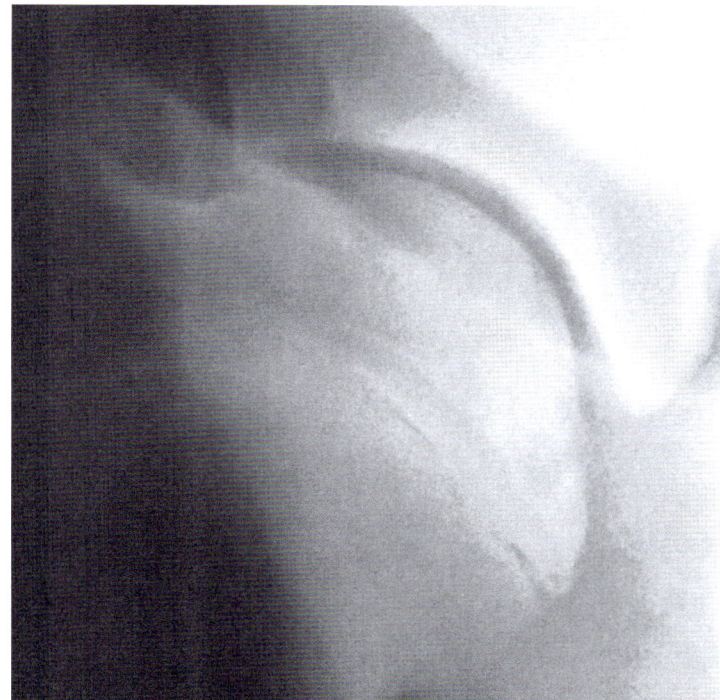

383 Left shoulder, mediolateral view: close-up.

Warmblood, 1 ½ years.

Marked flattening of the caudal aspect of the arcuate margin of the humeral head and sclerosis of the subchondral bone surrounding an obscure radiolucent defect extending in the humeral head, indicating osteochondrosis.

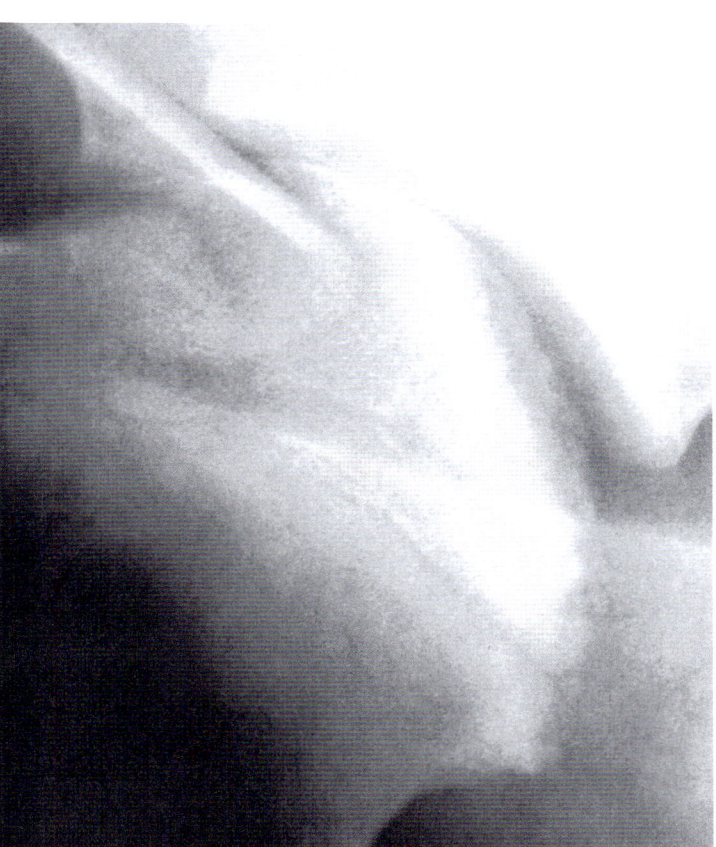

384

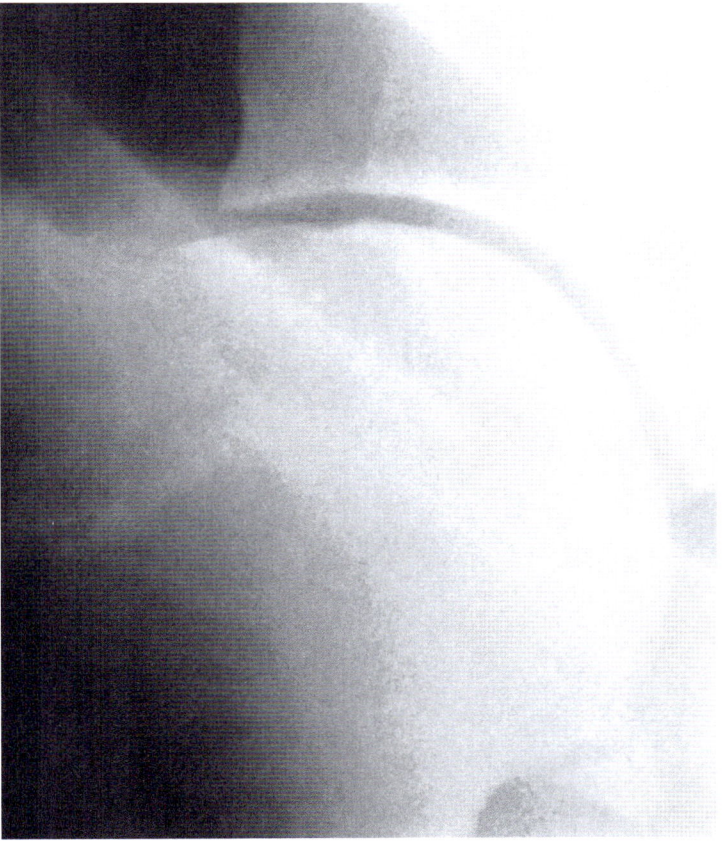

385

384/385 Right shoulder, serial mediolateral views: close-ups.

Foal, 6 months.

The initial examination (Fig. 384) at the age of 6 months, shows flattening and extensive irregularity of the caudal aspect of the humeral head with a patchy radiolucency in the subchondral bone, associated with osteochondrosis. The second examination 2 years later (Fig. 385), reveals a large bony fragment in the caudal pouch of the joint capsule, probably resulting from a calcified cartilage flap which has separated and is "free" in the joint cavity. The defect in the humeral head has repaired to a great extent.

N. B. The presence of a free fragment is not a common finding in osteochondrosis of the equine shoulder joint.

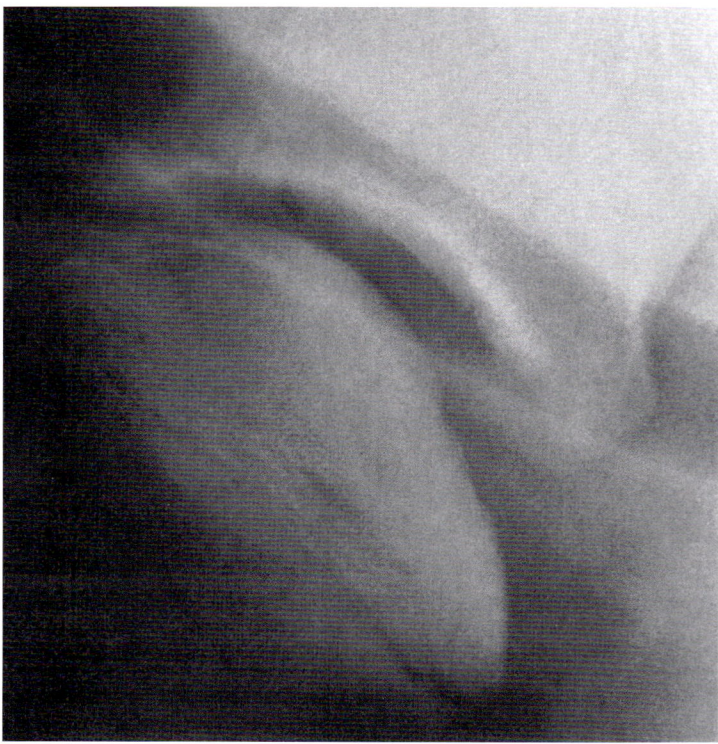

386

386 Left shoulder, mediolateral view: close-up.

Foal, 9 months.

Flattening of the caudal portion of the humeral head, with cystic radiolucent areas surrounded by a sclerotic rim in the subchondral bone and radiolucent irregularity of the margin of the glenoid cavity. These findings are characteristic of osteochondrosis affecting the humeral head and glenoid cavity.

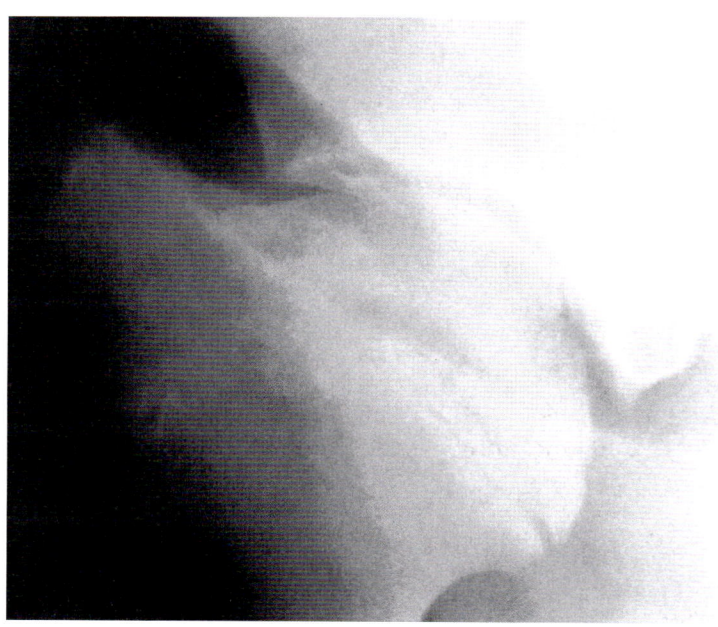

387 Left shoulder, mediolateral view: close-up.

Foal, 1 year.

Flattening and irregularity of the caudal aspect of the articular margin of the humeral head indicates osteochondrosis. The linear radiopacity **(1)** opposite the "dished-out" area in the contour of the humeral head represents a calcified cartilage flap.

Spur formation **(2)** at the caudal aspect of the glenoid cavity indicates associated secondary osteoarthrosis, resulting from instability due to incongruency of the articular surfaces.

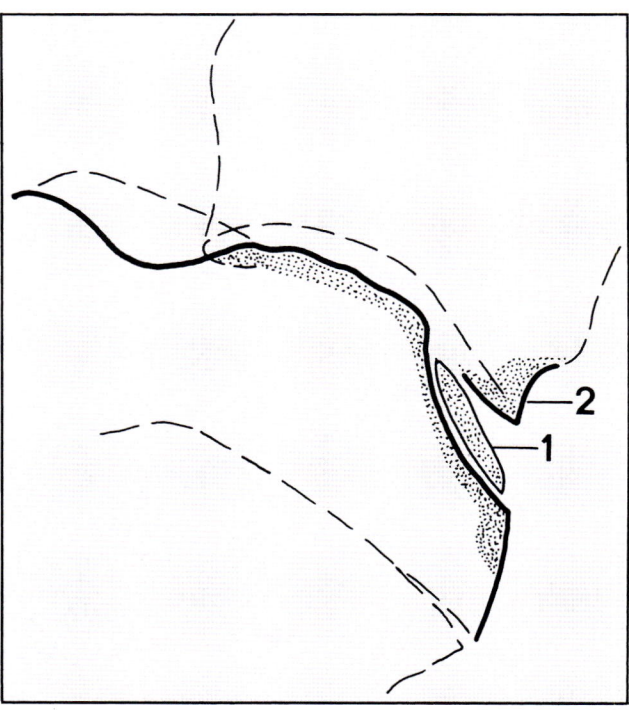

387 a Schematic drawing

Osteoarthrosis

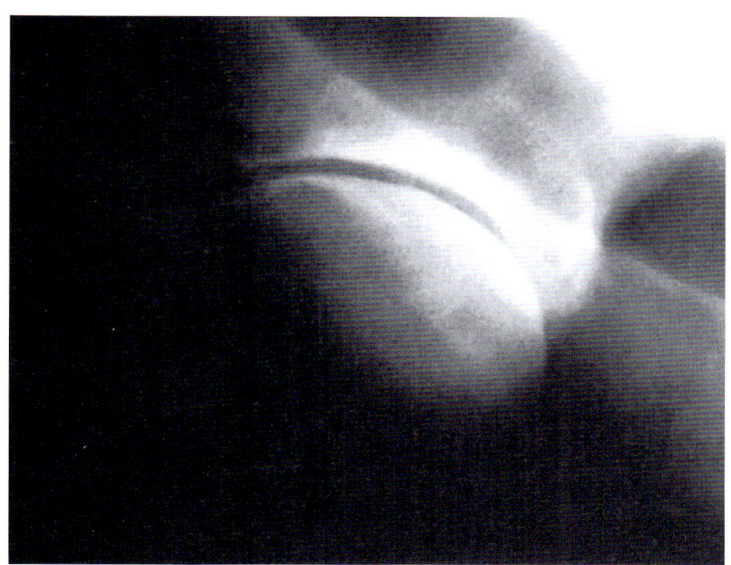

388 Right shoulder, mediolateral view.

Pony, 3 years.

Prominent narrowing of the caudal part of the joint space and irregular new bone formation on the caudal aspect of the glenoid cavity indicate osteoarthrosis, which may have resulted from the horse having slipped 2 months prior to the examination.

Bone sequestration

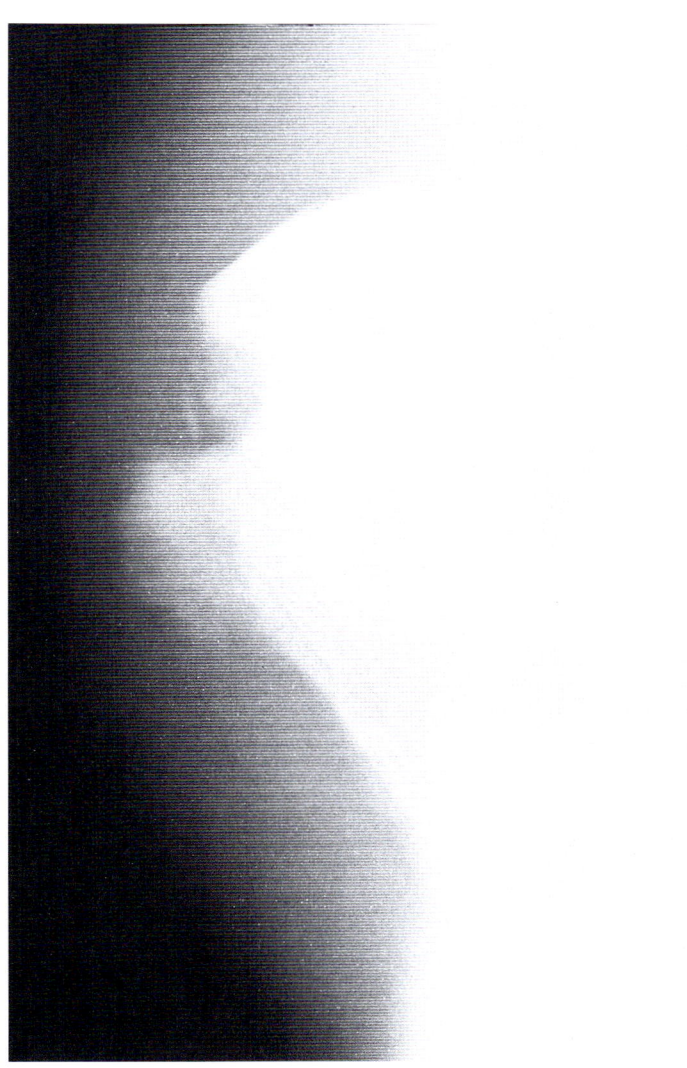

389 Right shoulder, craniomedial-caudolateral oblique view: close-up of the lateral humeral tuberosity.

Warmblood, 1 year.

The deep, clearly defined defect in the cranial contour of the lateral humeral tuberosity, completely separating thin fragments from the underlying bone and the dense ill bordered periosteal new bone distal to this defect indicate mature sequestration; in this horse resulting from a penetrating wound sustained 4 weeks previously.

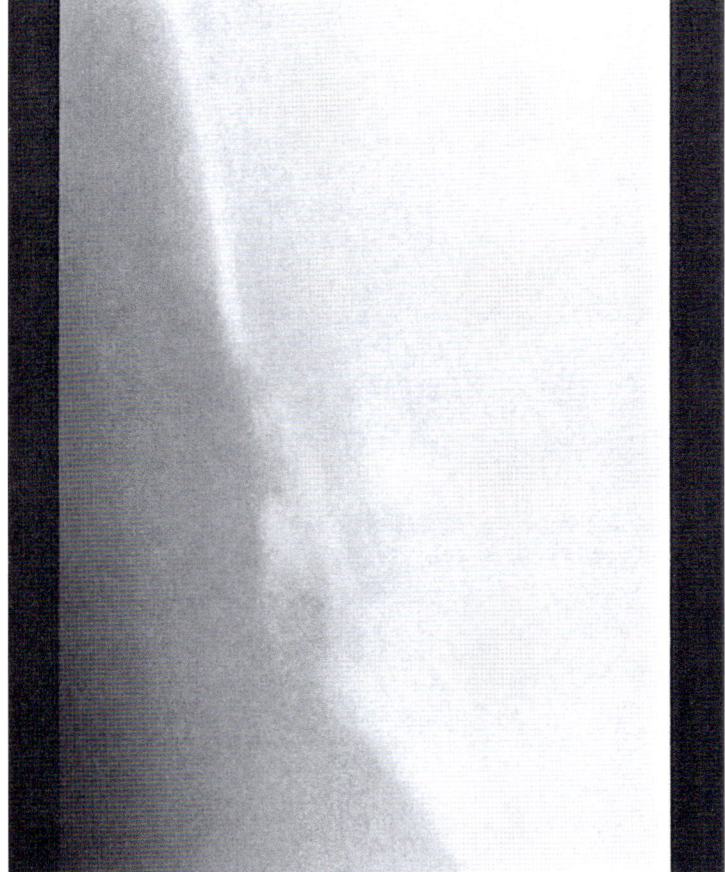

390 Left shoulder, mediolateral view: close-up of the deltoid tuberosity.

Warmblood, 7 years.

The superficial, ill defined, radiolucent defect in the deltoid tuberosity, separating ill bordered fragments from the underlying bone and the layer of periosteal new bone proximal to the destructive bone lesion indicates sequestrum formation.

The sequestrum, associated with a puncture wound sustained 2 weeks prior to the examination, is immature, as indicated by the incomplete separation of the abnormal from the normal bone.

The faint ill bordered periosteal new bone indicates a recently developed, active periosteal reaction.

Osteosarcoma

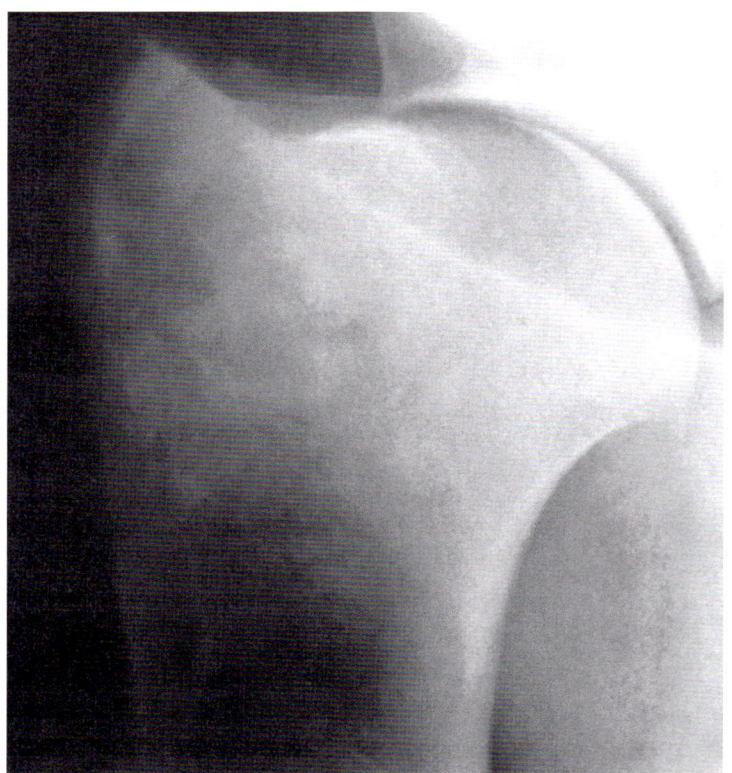

391

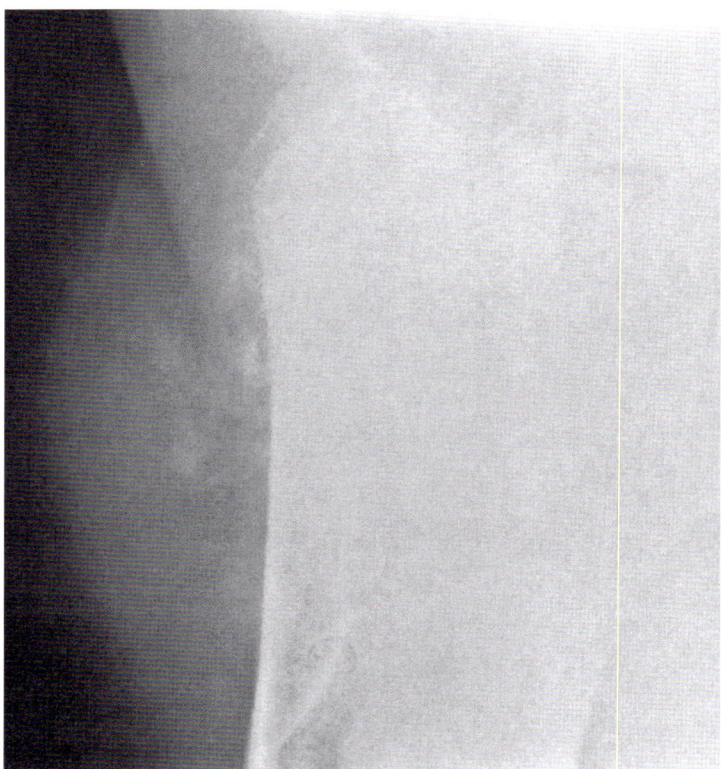

392

391/392 Left shoulder, mediolateral views.

Warmblood, 8 years.

The more penetrating exposure (Fig. 391) shows a patchy, radiopaque trabecular pattern of the cranioproximal portion of the humerus.

An additional radiograph (Fig. 392), deliberately underexposed to highlight the soft tissues, reveals soft tissue swelling cranial to the proximal humerus, linear soft tissue opacities opposite the humeral tuberosities and amorphous scattered and "sunbursting" periosteal new bone at the cranial aspect of the proximal humerus, suggestive of a malignant lesion. Histological examination revealed an osteosarcoma.

N. B. In horses osteosarcoma is rare and usually occurs on the bones of the skull.

Ossification of the biceps brachii tendon

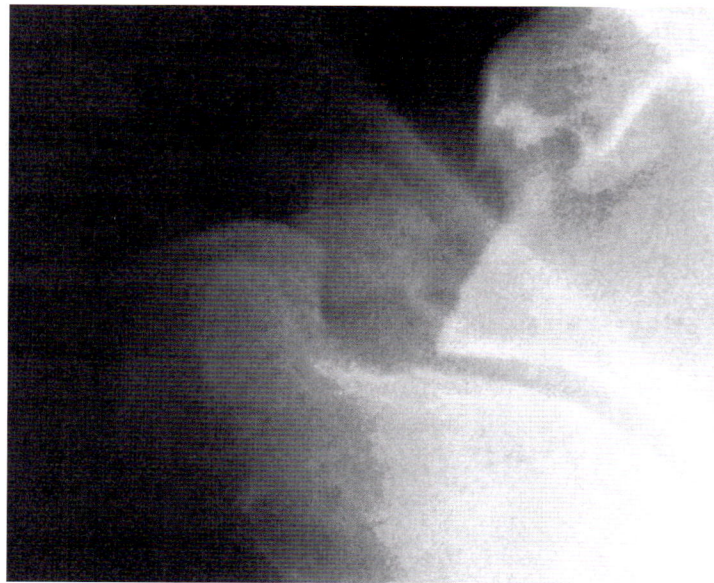

393 Right shoulder, mediolateral view: close-up.

Warmblood, 3 years.

The large, well defined, isolated, radiopaque area **(1)** superimposed on the lateral tuberosity of the humerus does not result from a fracture because of the absence of a corresponding fracture "bed" in the adjacent bone. The radiopaque area represents a calcified mass in the region of the tendon of the biceps brachii muscle.

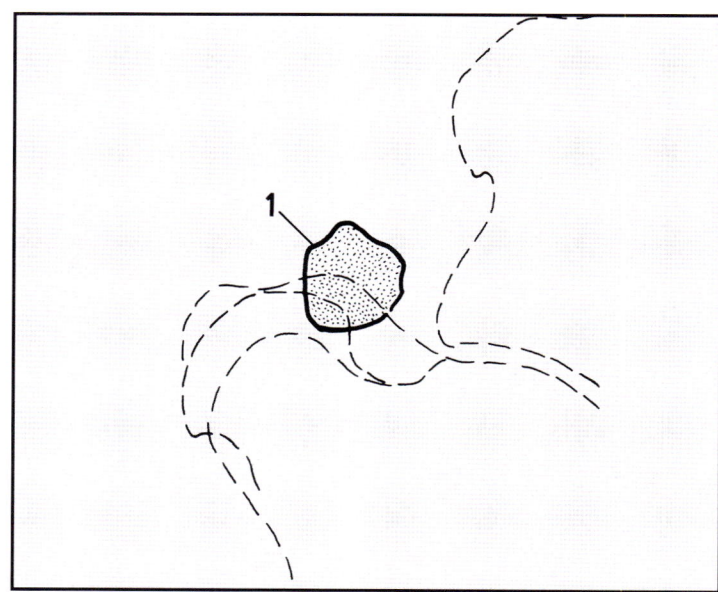

393 a Schematic drawing

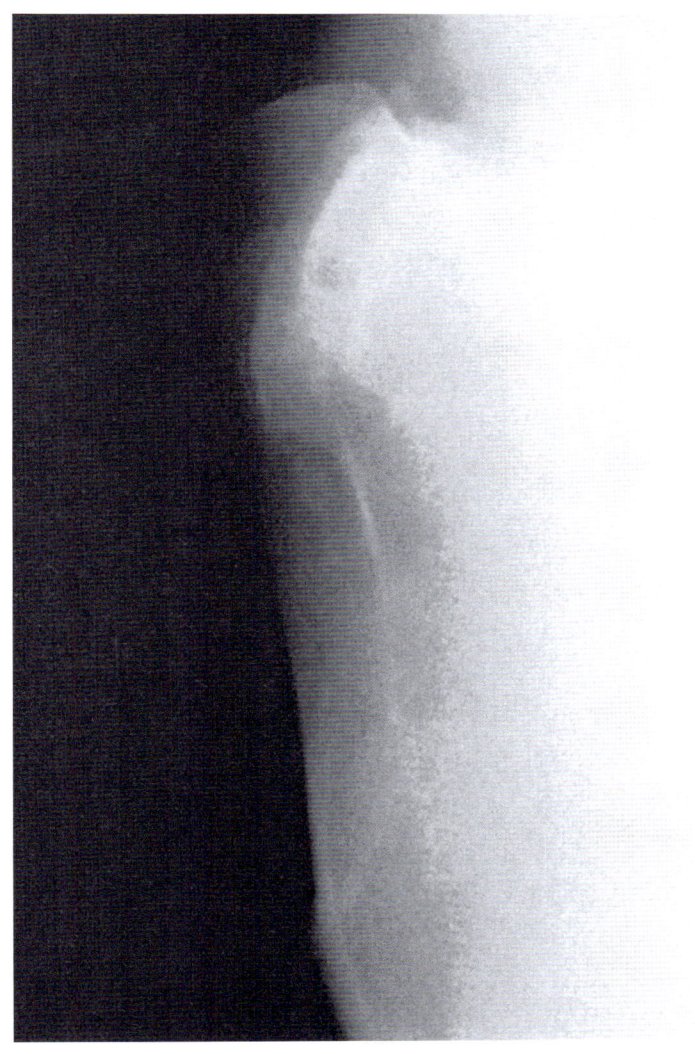

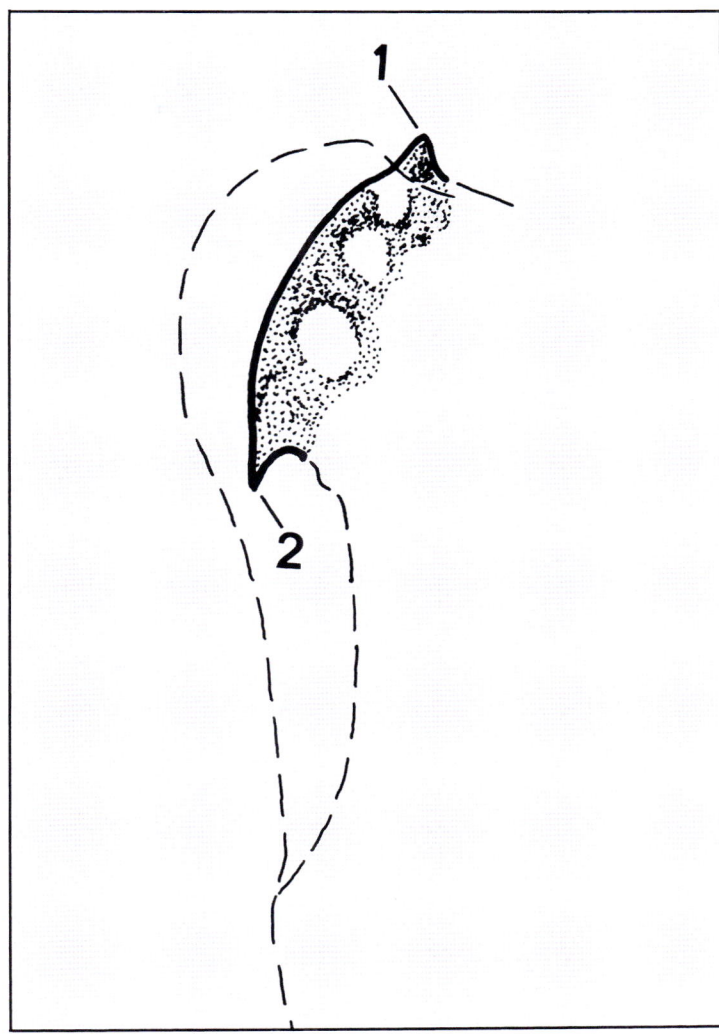

394 Right shoulder, mediolateral view: close-up of the humeral tuberosities.
Warmblood, 4 years.

Minimal, irregular radiolucency of the subchondral bone of the intermediate tuberosity and obvious spurring of the proximal **(1)** and distal **(2)** end of the tuberosity associated with bicipital bursitis.

Lameness disappeared after a local anaesthetic block of the bicipital bursa.

394 a Schematic drawing

Shoulder dysplasia

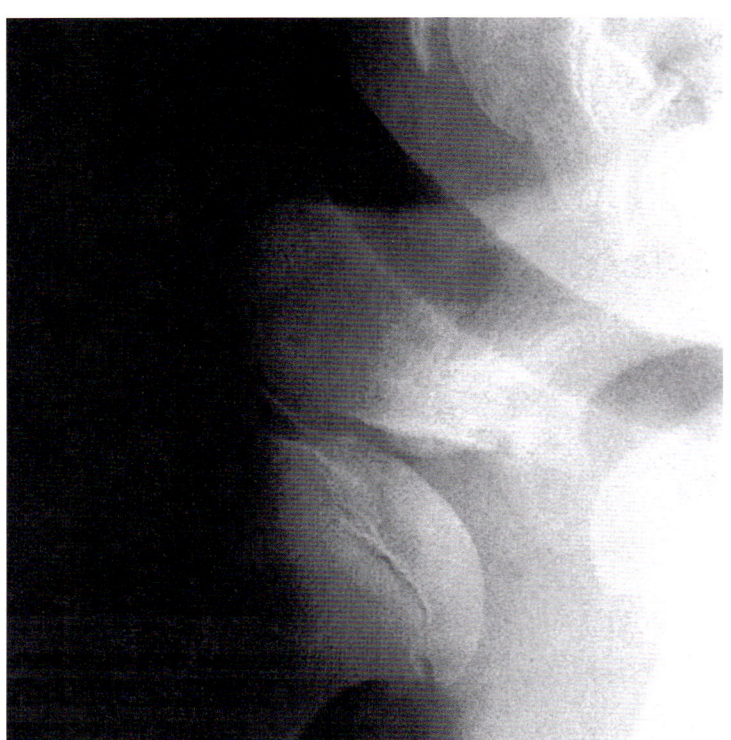

395

395 Right shoulder, mediolateral view: close-up.

Pony foal, 6 months.

Marked flattening and deformity of the glenoid cavity resulting from dysplasia. Superimposition of the cranial part of the lateral tuberosity of the humerus by the craniodistal aspect of the scapula indicates minimal subluxation.

Similar radiographic changes were present in the contralateral shoulder.

N. B. In horses shoulder dysplasia is a rare and poorly described disease.

The Hock Joint

Fracture

Fracture/Luxation

Ligamentous injury

Osteoarthrosis

Tarsal bone collapse

Infectious arthritis

Osteomyelitis

Bone sequestration

Osteochondrosis

Villonodular synovitis

Bone cyst

Thoroughpin

False thoroughpin

Superficial digital flexor tendon luxation

Puncture wound

Interosseous strain

Fracture

Tibia

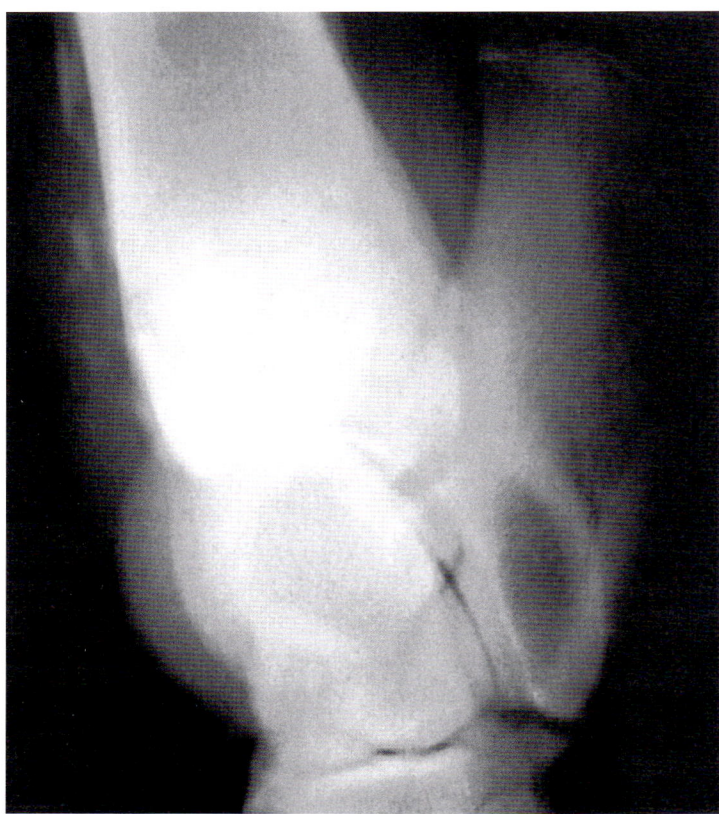

396

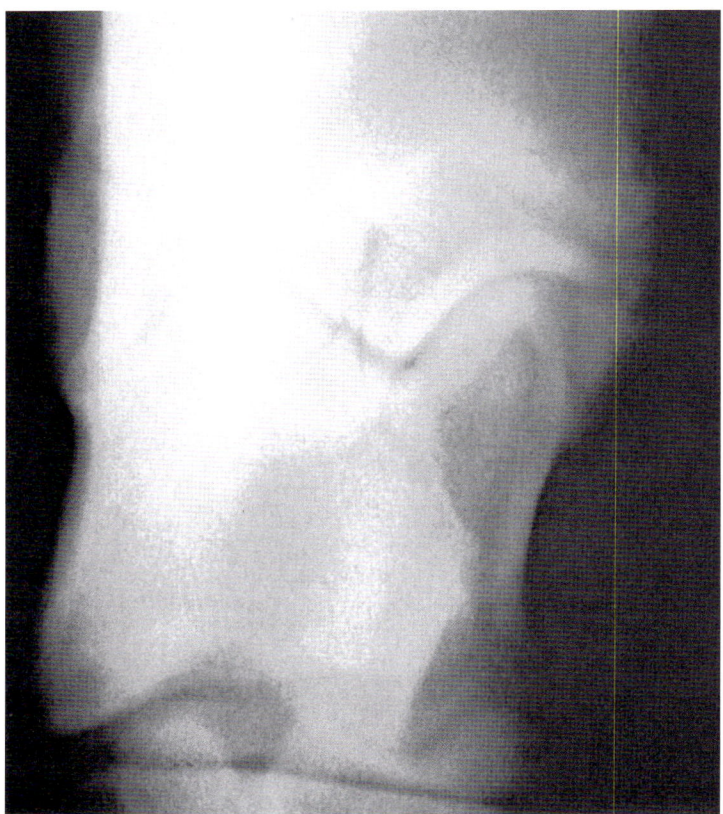

397

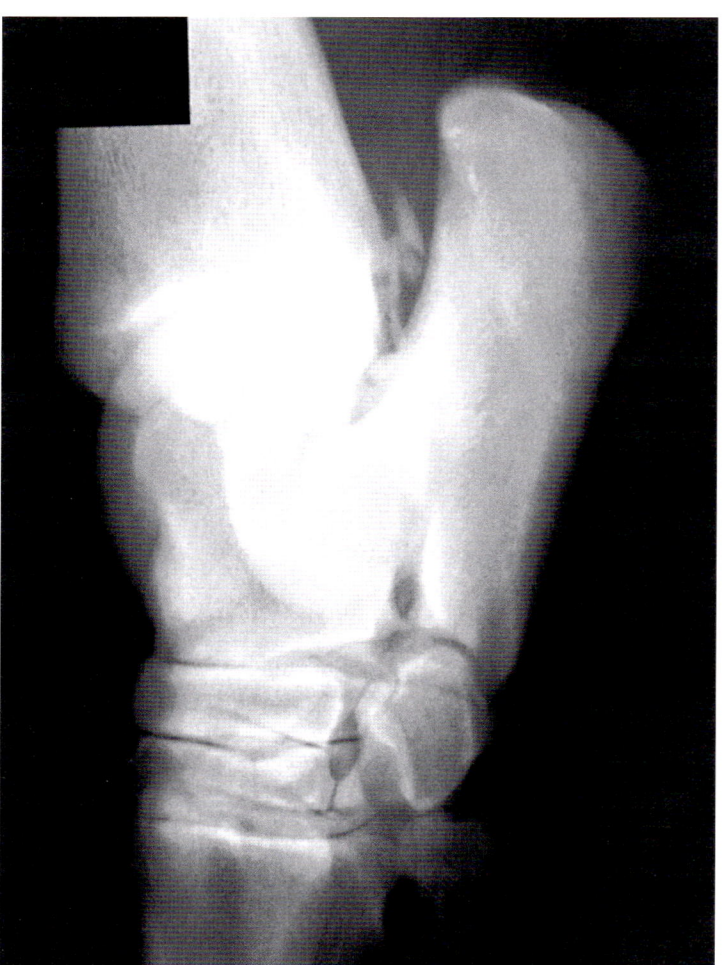

396/397 Right hock joint, lateromedial and dorsoplantar view: close-ups. Warmblood, 14 months.

The lateromedial view (Fig. 396) revals indistinct soft tissue swelling cranial and caudal to the distal end of the tibia, a zone of periosteal new bone along the cranial and caudal tibial border, and soft tissue calcification adjacent to the dorsal aspect of the tibia.

The tibial physis, normally not "closed" at this age, is not visible. On the dorsalplantar view (Fig. 397) the tibial physis is narrowed and obscured. A vertical radiolucent line through the midportion of the distal tibial epiphysis extends from the physis to the tibial intermediate ridge and is superimposed on the tibiotarsal joint space.

These findings indicate a compression type physeal injury (Salter-Harris type 3 physeal fracture). The accompanying periosteal reaction and soft tissue calcification suggest a fracture of some duration.

398 Right hock joint, dorsolateral-plantaromedial oblique view. Warmblood, 3 years.

Multiple, small, sharply bordered, slightly displaced fracture fragments, originating from the caudolateral aspect of the distal tibia, are visible.

Tibia

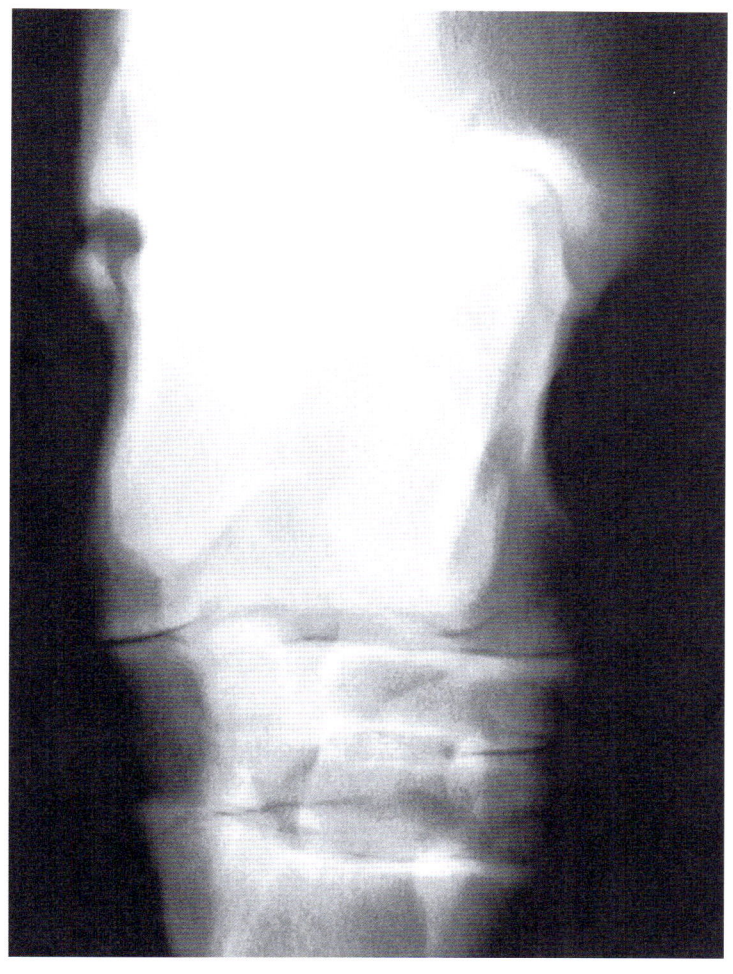

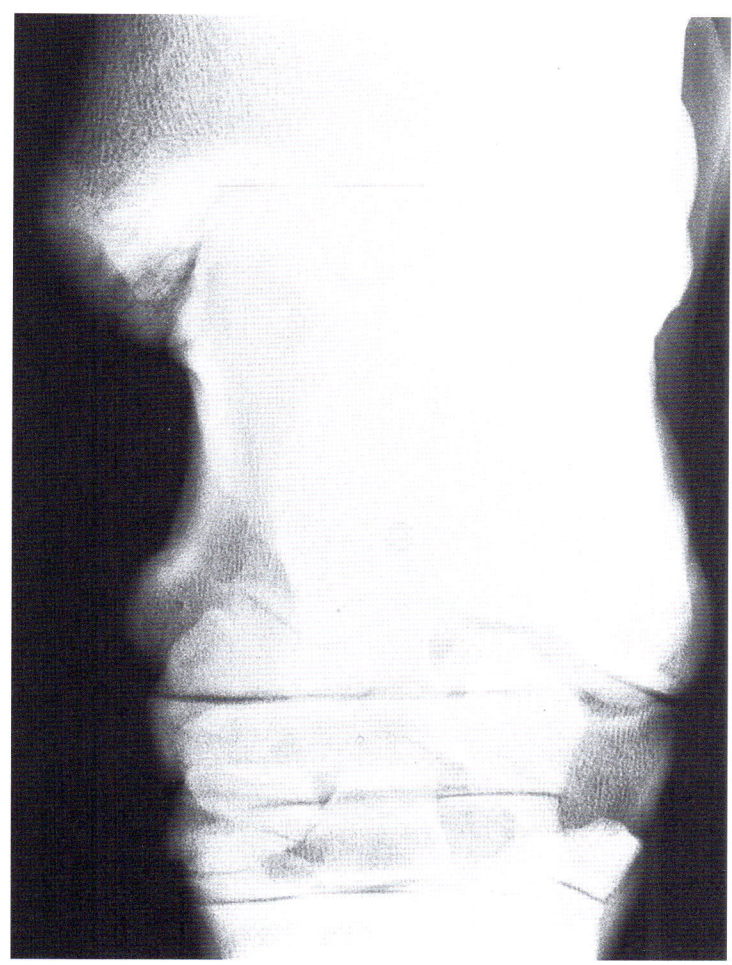

399 Right hock joint, dorsoplantar view: close-up.

Warmblood, 9 years.

The well defined, irregular, slightly displaced bone fragment and correspond-ing defect of the distolateral aspect of the tibia indicates a recent fracture of the lateral malleolus.

Differential diagnosis includes ligamentous calcification (Fig. 432) and osteochondrosis (Fig. 501).

400 Left hock joint, dorsoplantar view.

Warmblood, 3 years.

Multiple horizontal radiolucent lines through the medial malleolus involving the articular surface, indicating recent incomplete fracture.

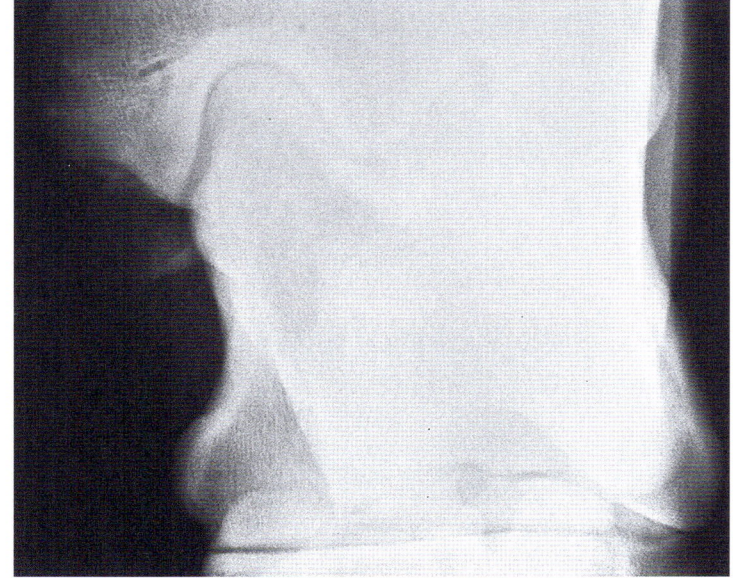

401 Left hock joint, dorsoplantar view: close-up.

Warmblood, 16 months.

Small fragments within a corresponding defect of the distal aspect of the medial malleolus, as well as a large irregular displaced bone fragment ad-jacent to the proximal tuberosity of the tibial tarsal bone. These findings are consistent with recent avulsion fracture caused by overstretching of the medial collateral ligaments of the tibiotarsal joint. The differential diagnosis includes osteochondrosis. However, an osteochondrosis fragment of the medial malleolus is more rounded in shape, usually not displaced and in-volves the inner, i.e. articular aspect of the malleolus (Fig. 499/500).

Fibular tarsal bone

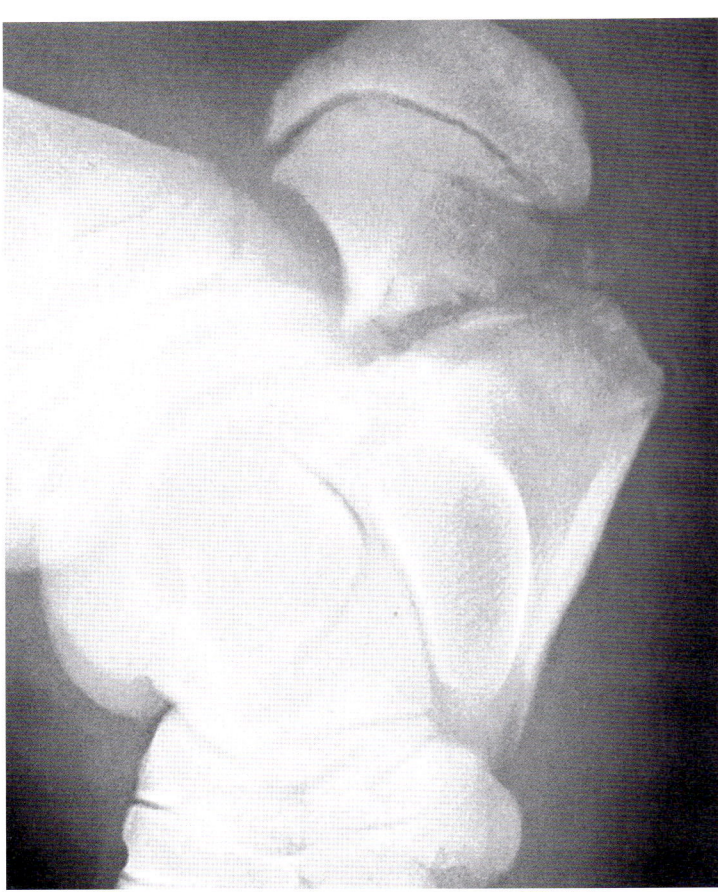

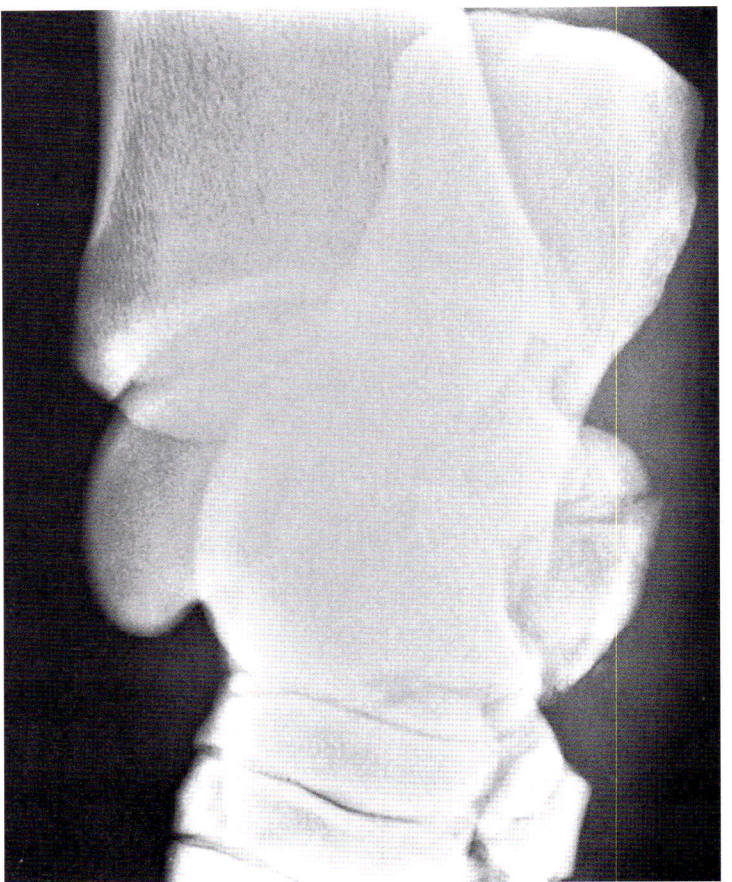

402 Right hock joint, lateromedial view: close-up.

Foal, 2 months.

Dorsal displacement of the proximal portion of the fibular tarsal bone, due to a recent oblique fracture. The fracture zone is ill defined because of obliquity of the fracture plane to the lateromedial directed central beam and minimal overriding of the fracture fragments. Small additional bone fragments superimposed on the fracture zone are visible.

403 Left hock joint, dorsomedial-plantarolateral oblique view.

Warmblood, 5 years.

The proximomedial border of the sustentaculum tali is interrupted by a well defined radiolucent line, resulting from a recent horizontal fracture, associated with a draining wound on the plantaromedial aspect of the hock.

Minimal displacement produces a "step" defect in the medial border of the sustentaculum tali.

Fibular tarsal bone

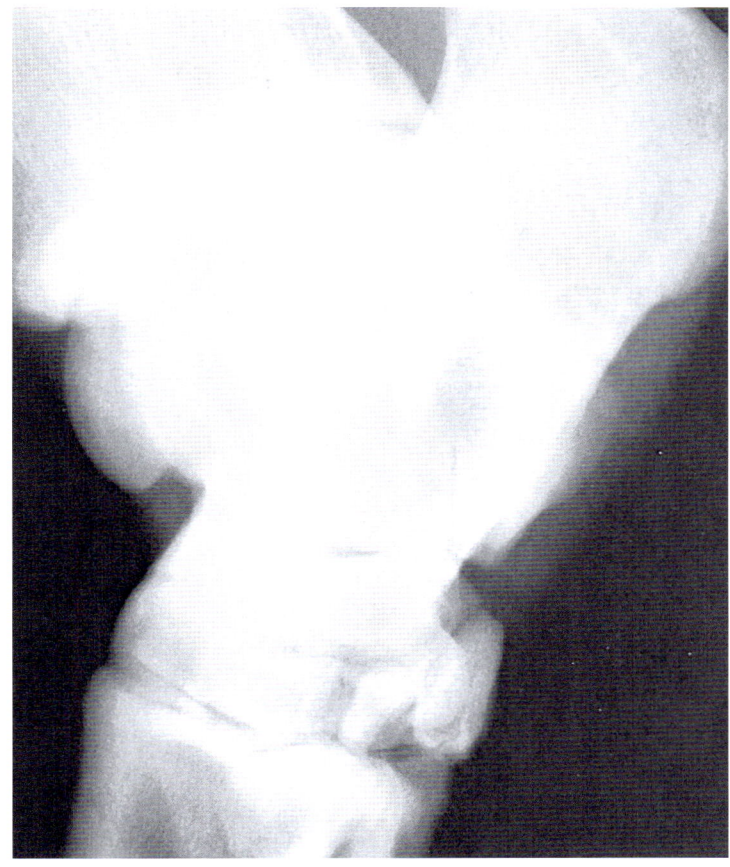

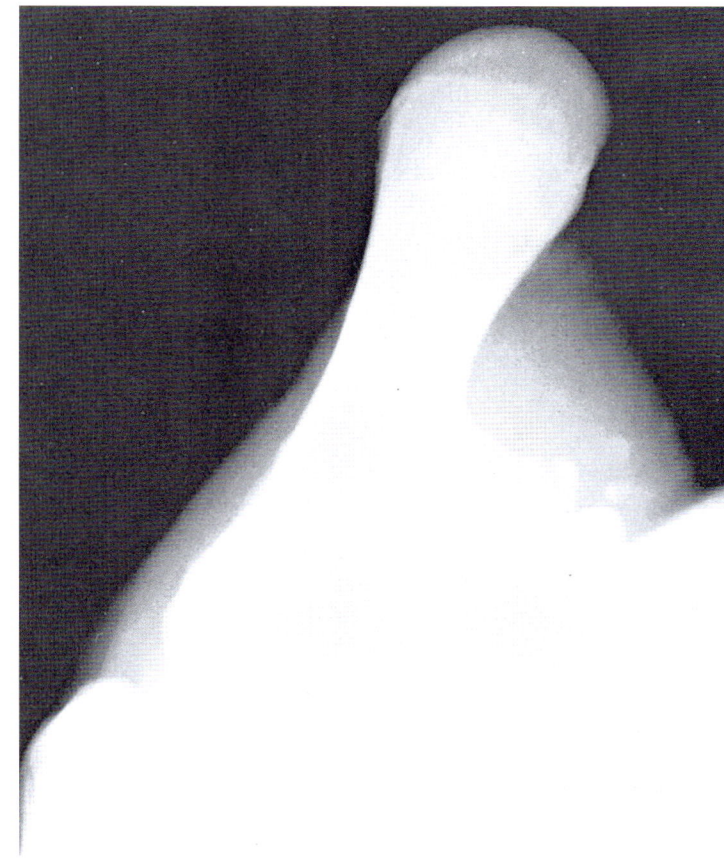

404

405

404/405 Right hock joint, dorsomedial-plantarolateral oblique and dorsoplantar (flexed) "skyline" view.

Warmblood, 7 years.

The dorsomedial-plantarolateral oblique view (Fig. 404) shows very obscure, small bone fragments close to the proximal aspect of sustentaculum tali and irregularity of the corresponding portion of the normally smooth sustentaculum border.

The additional "skyline" view (Fig. 405) clearly demonstrates two small chip fragments and a fracture line through the medial border of the sustentaculum tali. The soft tissue swelling plantar to the sustentaculum results from distension of the tarsal sheath.

Fracture

Tibial tarsal bone

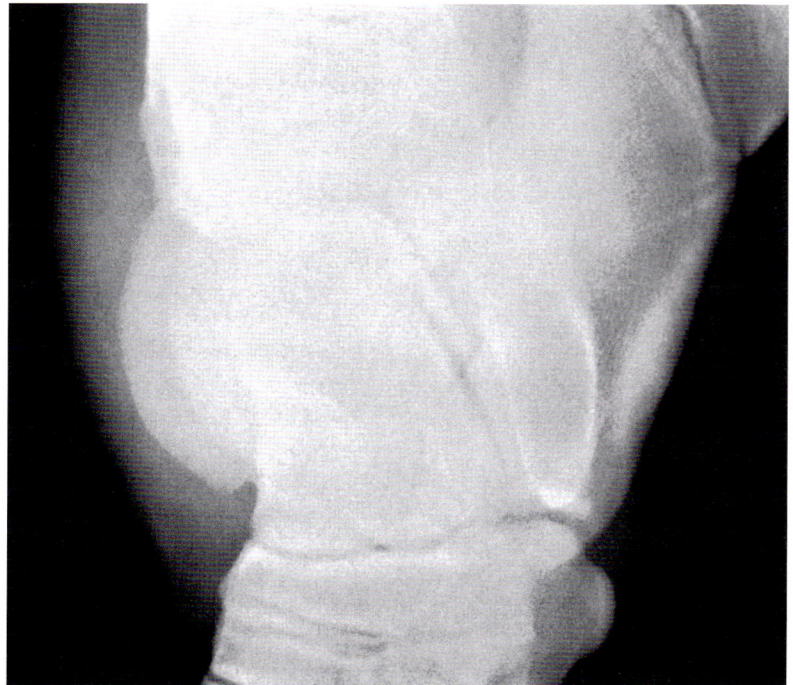

406

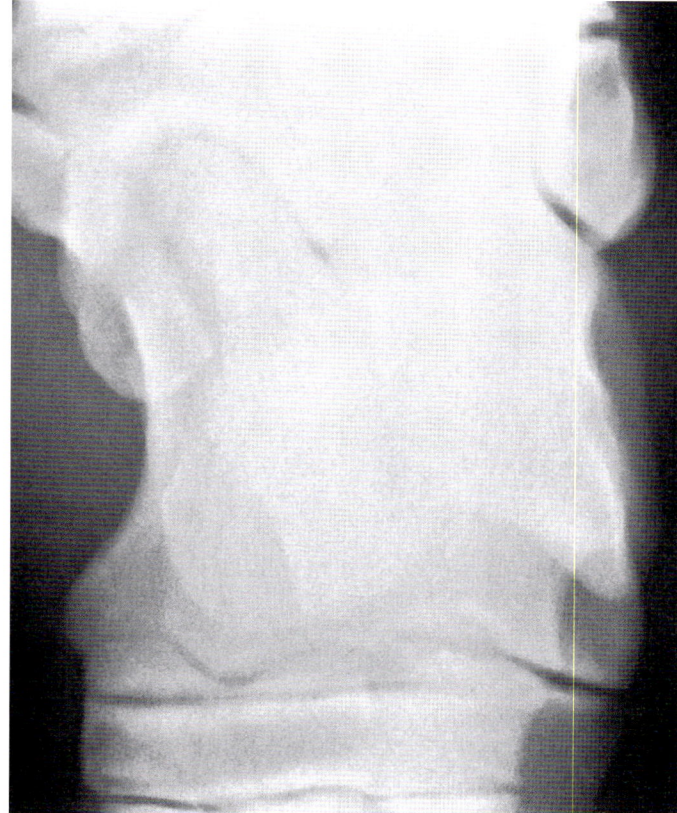

407

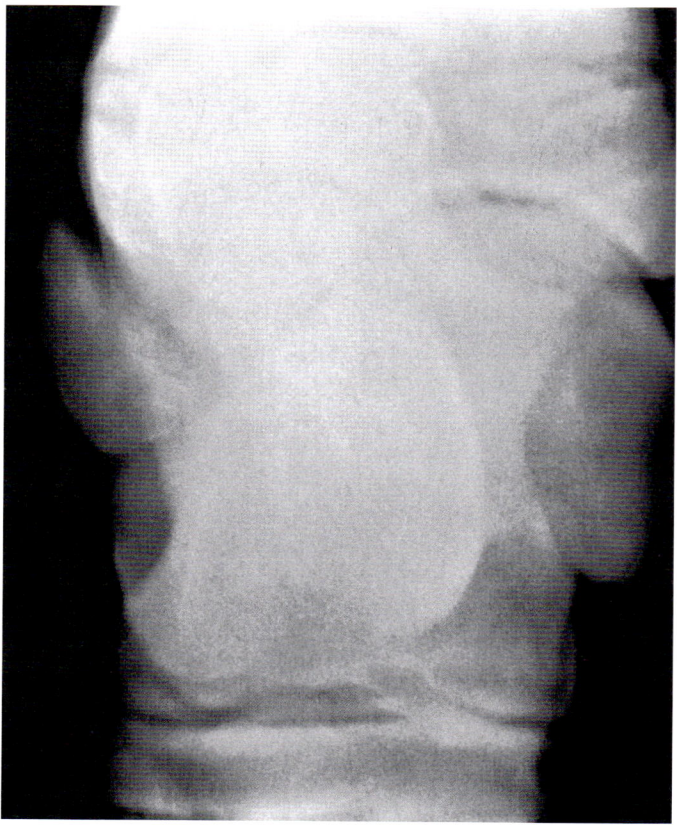

408

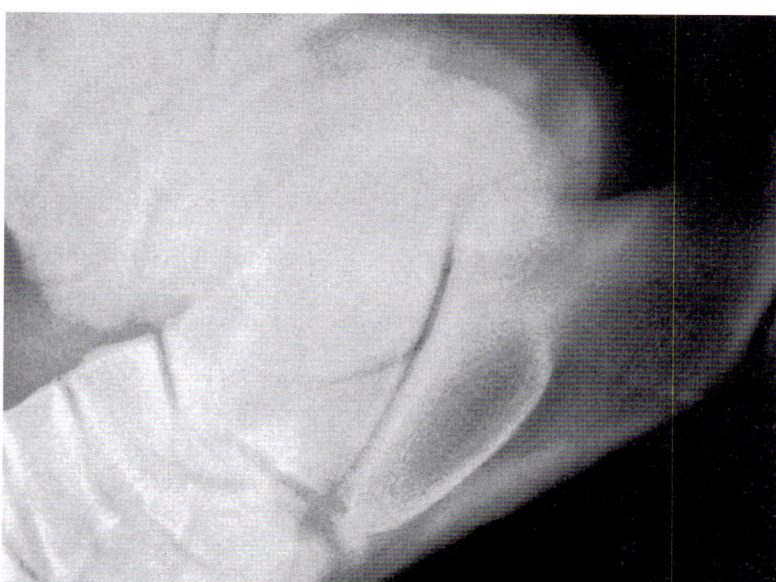

409

406/407/408/409 Left hock joint, lateromedial, dorsoplantar, dorsomedial-plantarolateral oblique and plantarolateral-dorsomedial oblique (flexed) view: close-ups.

Foal, 4 months.

The slightly underexposed lateromedial view (Fig. 406) reveals only soft tissue swelling dorsal and plantaroproximal to the tibial tarsal bone superimposed on the fibular tarsal bone, characteristic of effusion of the tibiotarsal joint. The dorsoplantar view (Fig. 407) presents a large well defined semicircular bone fragment partly superimposed on the medial malleolus and tibial tarsal bone.

A dorsomedial-plantarolateral projection (Fig. 408) results in less superimposition of the fragment, indicating that the fracture fragment originates from the plantaromedial aspect of the tibial tarsal bone. The plantarolateral-dorsomedical oblique (flexed) view (Fig. 409) demonstrates more precisely that the fragment originates from the plantaroproximal aspect of the medial trochlear ridge of the tibial tarsal bone.

Displacement of the bone fragments results in a "step" defect in the proximal border of the medial trochlear ridge.

Tibial tarsal bone

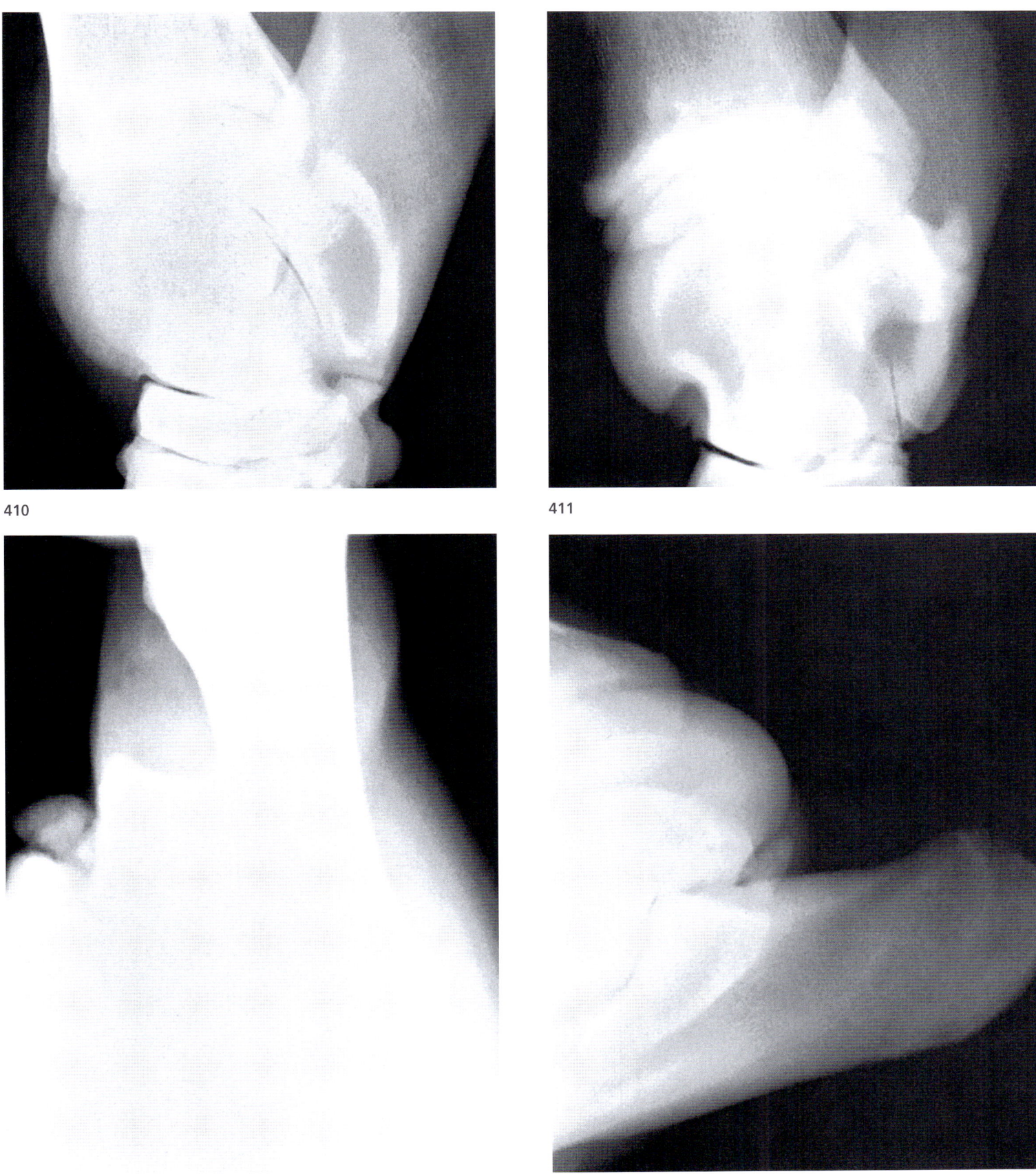

410

411

412

413

410/411/412/413 Left hock joint, lateromedial, dorsomedial-plantarolateral oblique, dorsoplantar (flexed) "skyline" and proximolateral-distomedial oblique (flexed) view: close-ups.

Warmblood, 7 years.

The lateromedial view (Fig. 410) presents soft tissue swelling dorsal to the tibial tarsal bone, resulting from effusion of the tibial tarsal joint and an obscure opacity superimposed on the dorsoproximal aspect of the sustentaculum tali.

A more penetrating dorsomedial-plantarolateral oblique view (Fig. 411) results in a clearer visualization of the opacity, which is a small bone fragment medial to the sustentaculum, demonstrated by the "skyline" view (Fig. 412). The fragment originates from the plantaroproximal aspect of the medial trochlear ridge of the tibial tarsal bone, clearly shown in the proximolateral-distomedial oblique (flexed) view (Fig. 413).

Fracture

Tibial tarsal bone

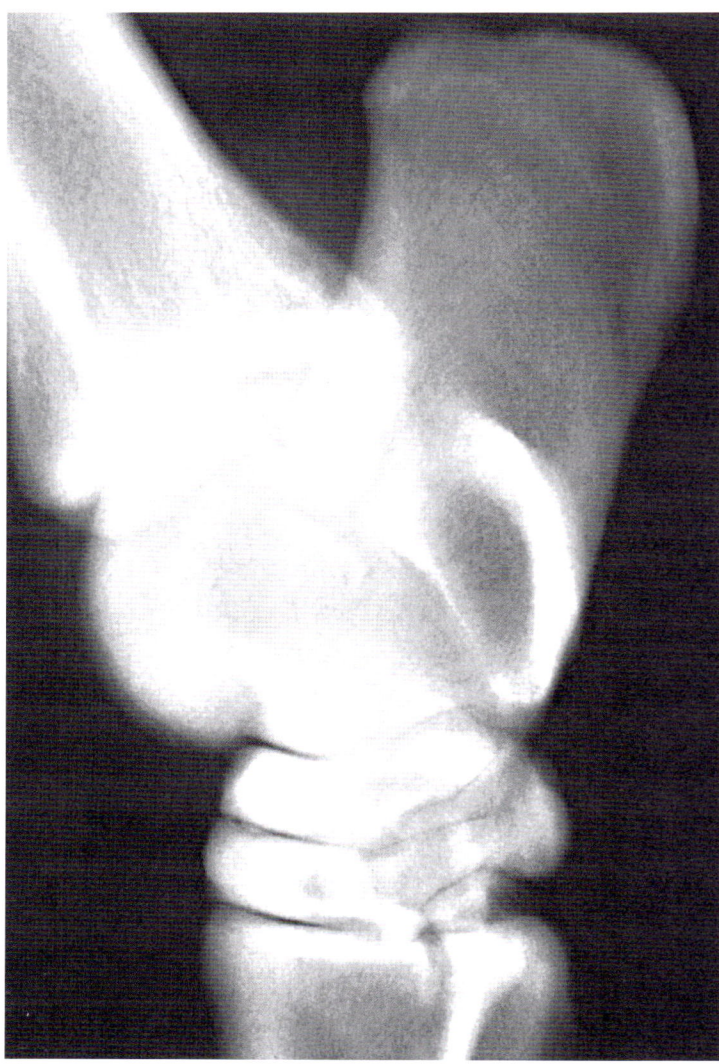

414

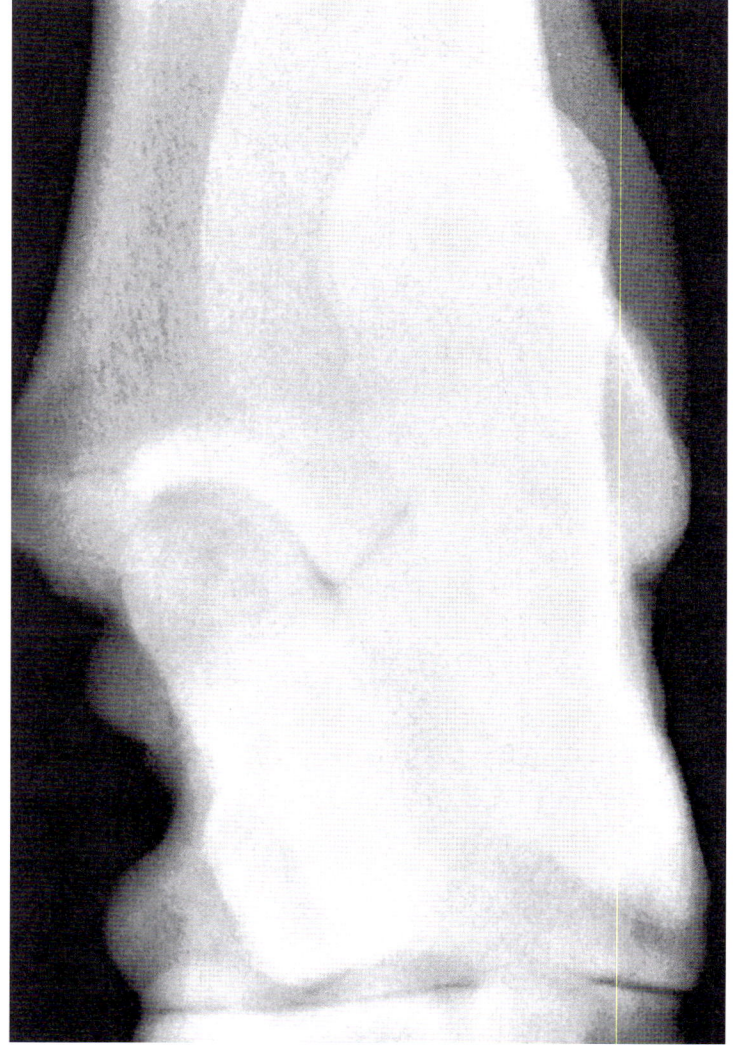

415

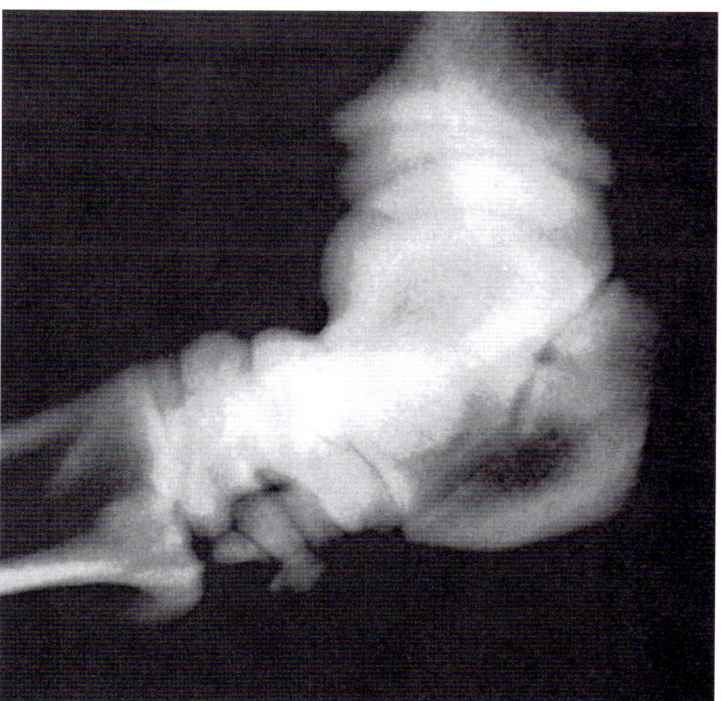

416

414/415/416 Left hock joint, lateromedial, dorsoplantar: close-up and plantarolateral-dorsomedial oblique (flexed) view.

Pony, 5 years.

The lateromedial view (Fig. 414) reveals an obscure oblique radiolucent line through the plantaroproximal aspect of the trochlea of the tibial tarsal bone interrupting the articular surface. The dorsoplantar projection (Fig. 415) presents only an indistinct irregularity of the contour and texture of the proximal aspect of the medial trochlear ridge. On a deliberately overexposed plantarolateral-dorsomedial oblique (flexed) projection (Fig. 416) the radiolucent line is identified as a fracture through the medial trochlear ridge.

Tibial tarsal bone

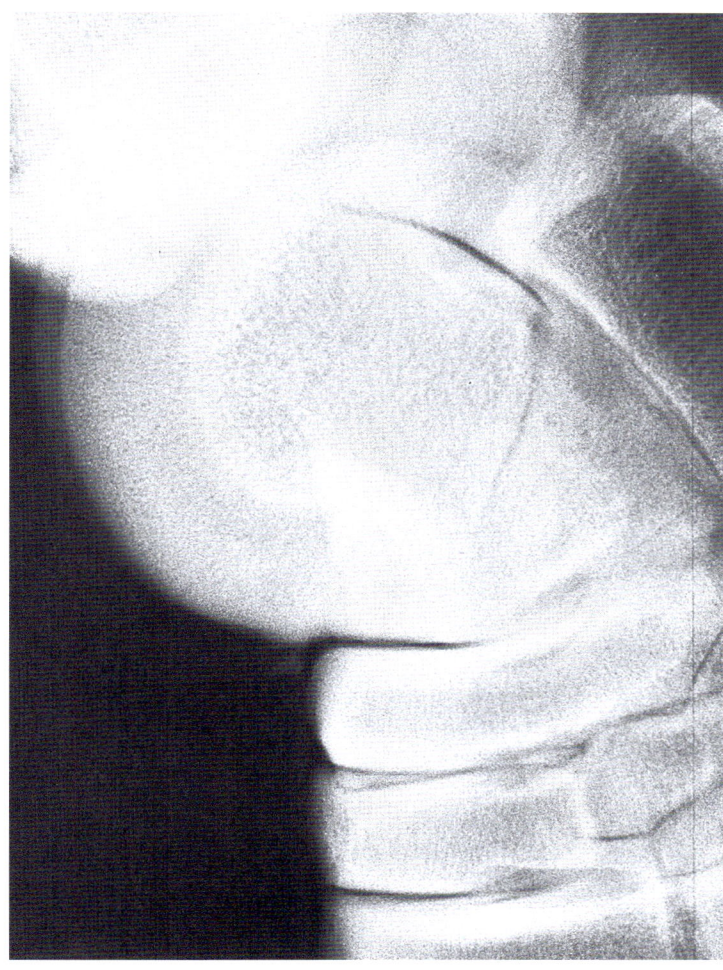

417 Left hock joint, lateromedial view: close-up.

Warmblood, 3 years.

The small distinct radiopacity distal to the trochlear ridges of the tibial tarsal bone represents a "spur fragment" of the distal protuberance of the medial trochlear ridge. One or two of these bony opacities are occasionally seen.

This fracture appearance may be true, or false, i.e. resulting from incomplete ossification. It usually has no clinical significance and should not be confused with osteochondrosis.

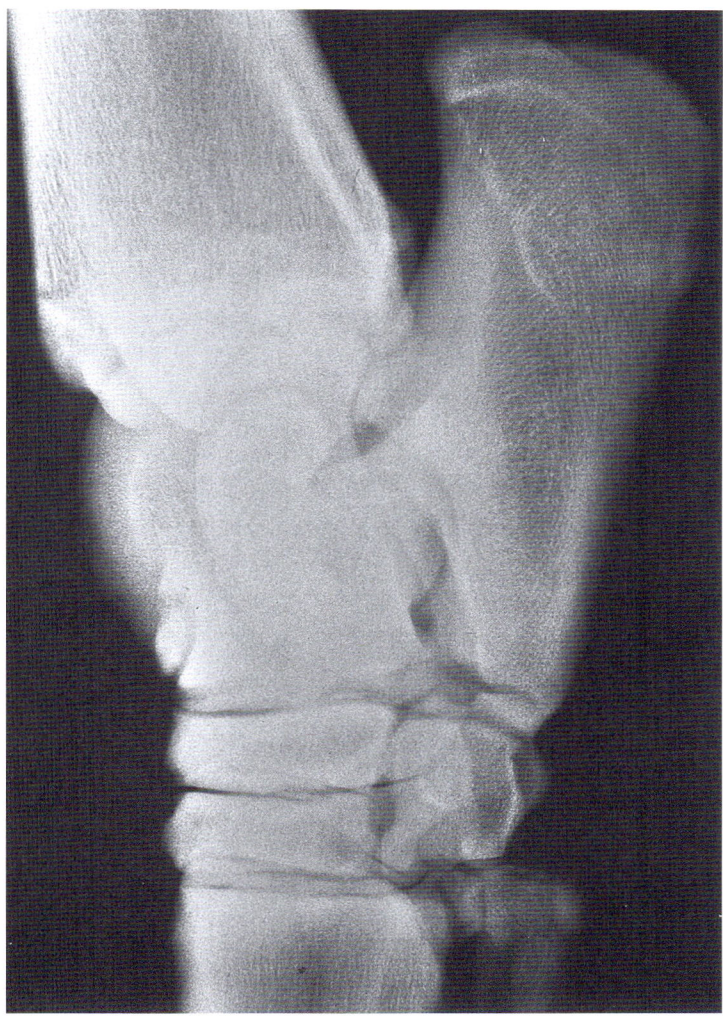

418 Left hock joint, dorsolateral-plantaromedial oblique view.

Warmblood, 3 years.

The well defined oval fragment within a corresponding defect of the disto-medial aspect of the tibial tarsal bone, superimposed on the distal aspect of the medial trochlear ridge, results from avulsion of the origin of the dorsal ligament.

This seldom occuring injury should not be confused with osteochondrosis.

Fracture

Tibial tarsal bone

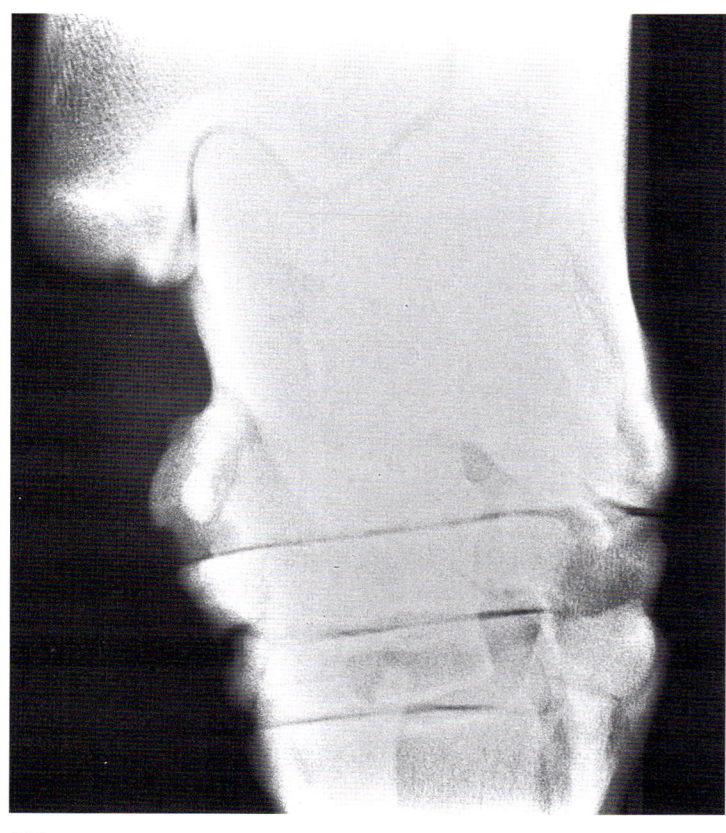

419

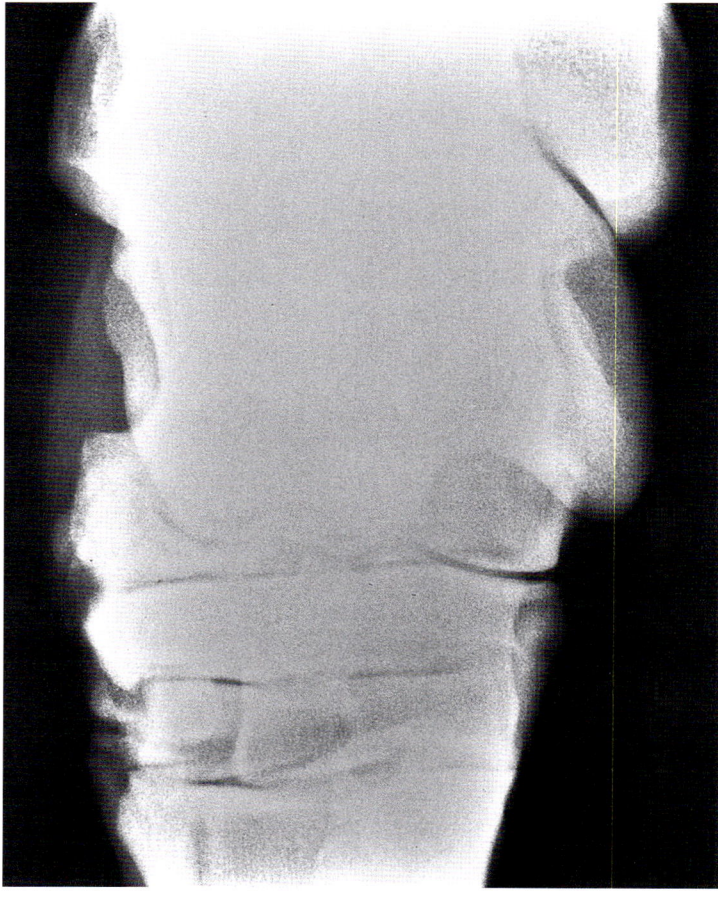

420

419/420 Left hock joint, dorsolateral-plantaromedial oblique and dorsomedial-plantaro-lateral oblique view.

Standardbred, 5 years.

The dorsomedial-plantarolateral oblique view (Fig. 420) reveals an obscure rounded fragment partly superimposed on the distal tuberosity of the tibial tarsal bone.

The dorsolateral-plantaromedial oblique radiograph (Fig. 419) results in more superimposition of the fragment. Nevertheless, the fragment is recognizable on this view as a distinct rounded opacity in the central region of the distal tuberosity.

Apparently this fragment, is avulsed from the plantaromedial aspect of the distal tuberosity and, therefore, associated with sprain of the medial collateral ligaments of the tibiotarsal joint.

Central tarsal bone

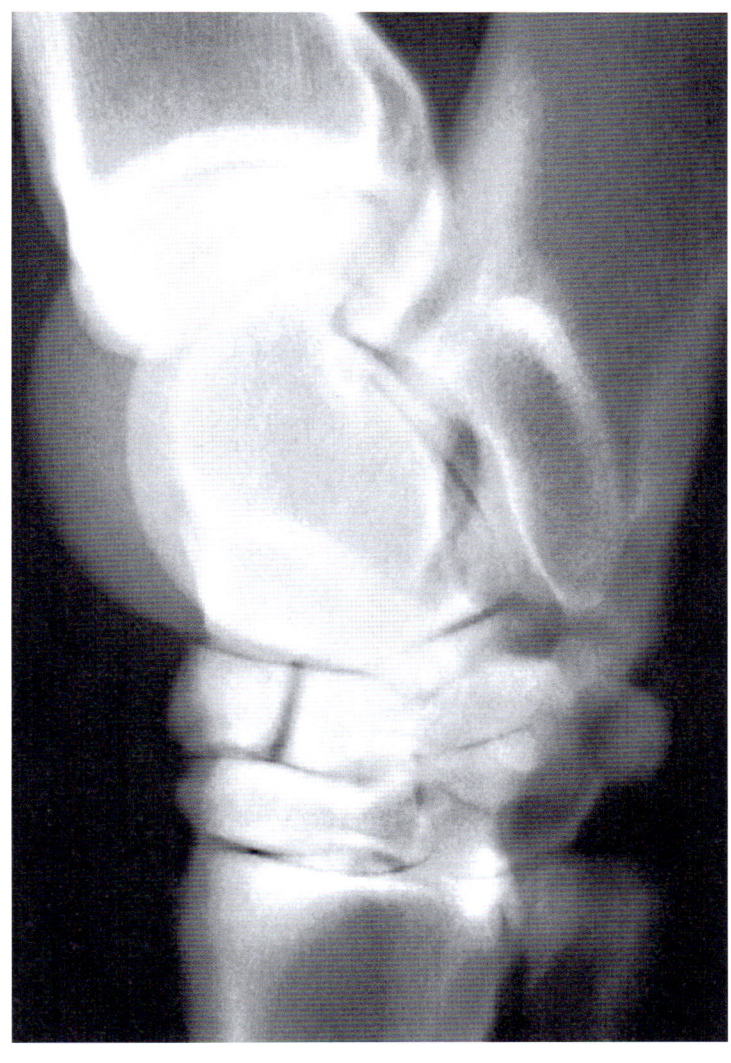

421 Left hock joint, lateromedial view: close-up.

Standardbred, 6 years.

The vertical radiolucent line through the dorsal portion of the central tarsal bone, extending from the proximal intertarsal joint to the distal intertarsal joint, indicates the presence of a recent slab fracture.

Fracture

Splint bone

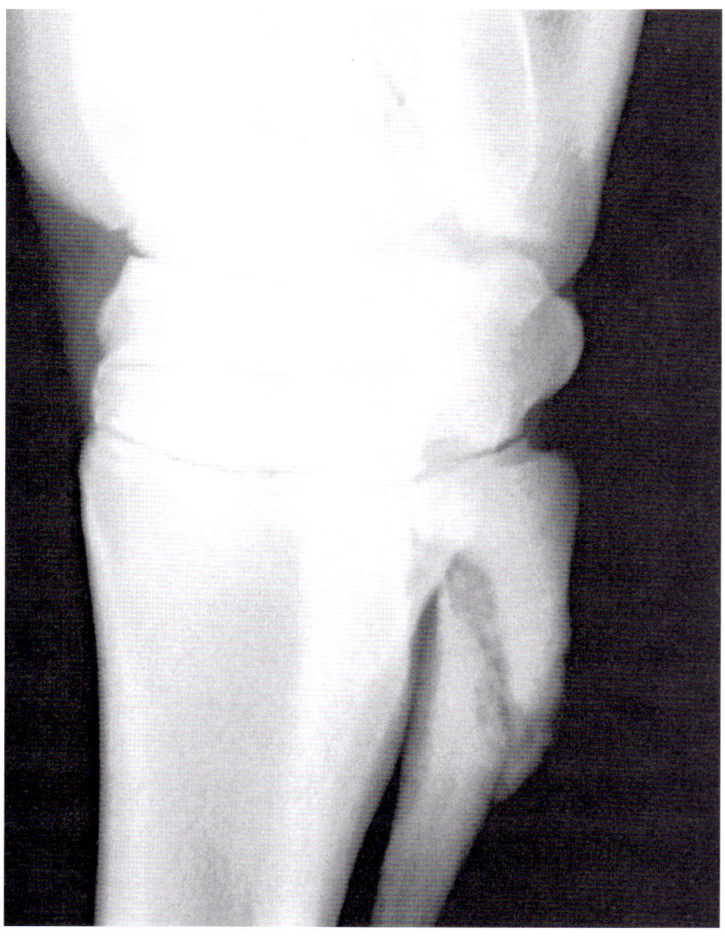

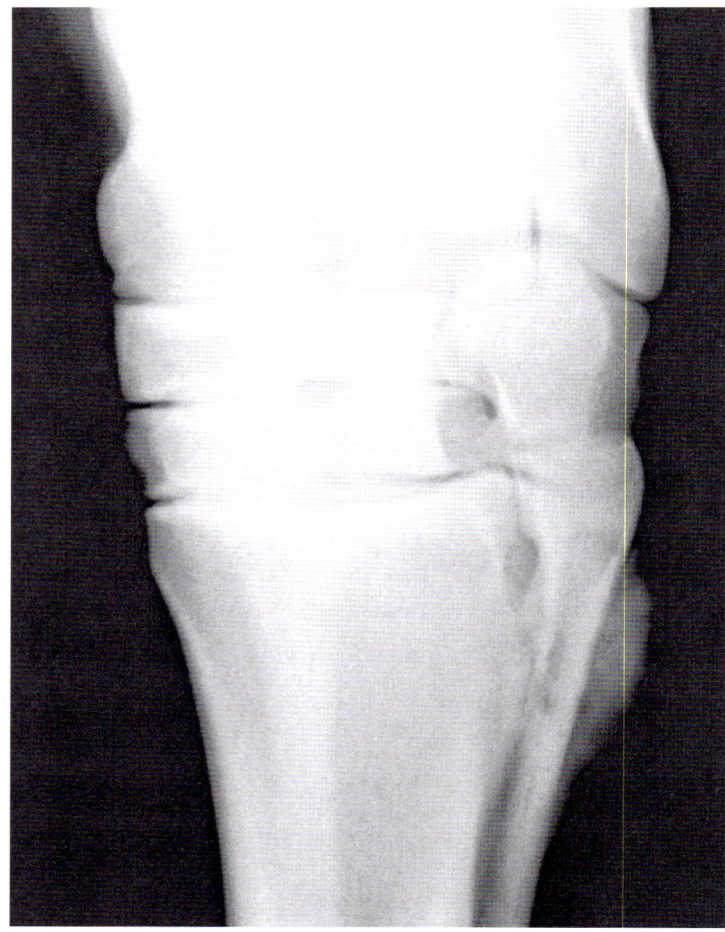

422

423

422/423 Right hock joint, lateromedial and dorsolateral-plantaromedical oblique view: close-ups.

Foal, 5 months.

The lateromedial view (Fig. 422) shows an oblique radiolucent zone through the proximal aspect of the lateral splint bone, due to a simple complete fracture of some duration, indicated by the periosteal callus formation overlying the fracture site. On the dorsolateral-plantaromedial oblique view (Fig. 423) the fracture zone is obscured, but the callus formation is more obvious. The periosteal callus is active and immature, as indicated by its ill bordered faint appearance.

Cannon bone

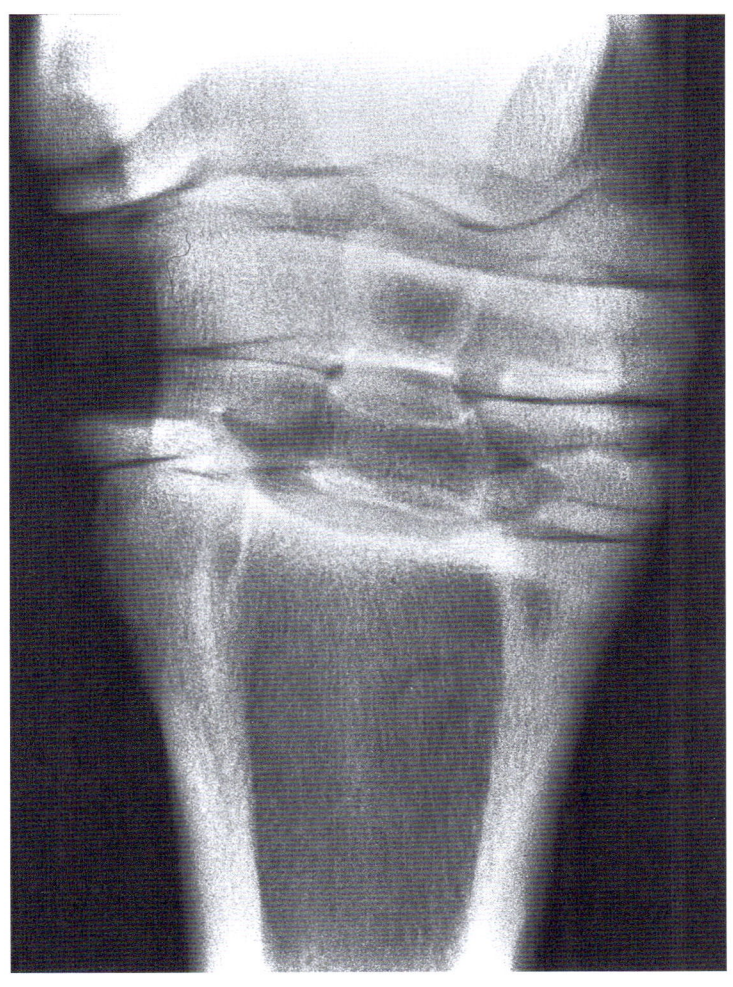

424 Right hock joint, dorsoplantar view: close-up.

Warmblood, 11 years.

The semicircular radiolucent line in the proximomedial aspect of the third metatarsal bone is characteristic of an avulsion fracture of the origin of the suspensory ligament. This may be accompanied by proximal suspensory ligament desmitis.

Therefore, additional ultrasonographic examination is important to demonstrate or rule out associated suspensory ligament injury.

Fracture/Luxation

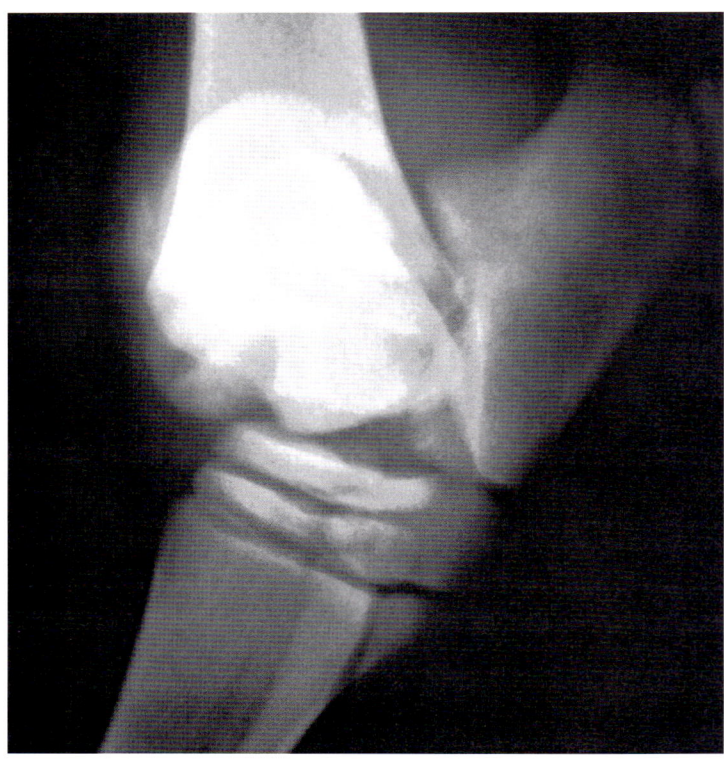
425

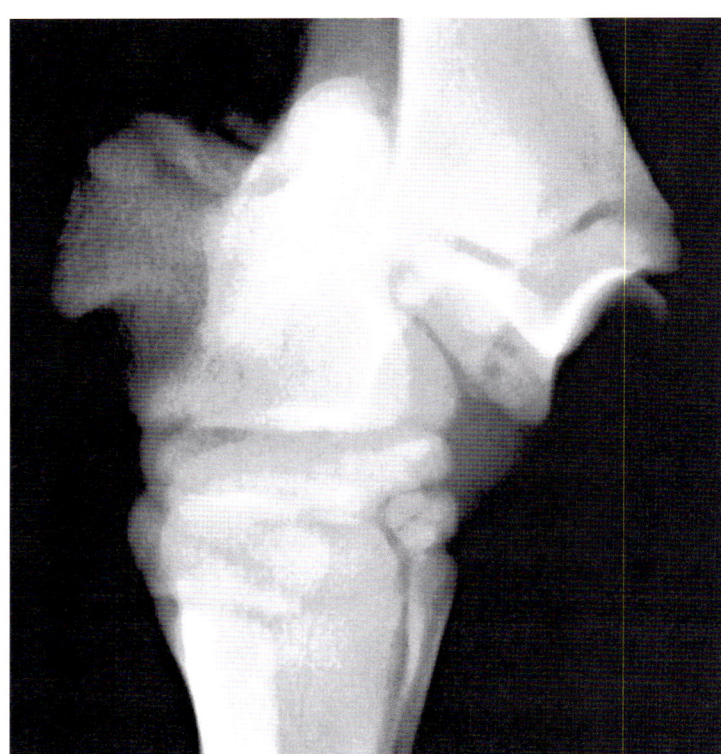
426

425/426 Right hock joint, lateromedial (Fig. 425) and dorsoplantar view (Fig. 426).

Foal, 1 week.

Complete luxation of the tibiotarsal joint and subluxation of the proximal intertarsal joint with rotation and lateral displacement of the tibial tarsal bone and over-riding of the distal end of the tibia. The bone fragments superimposed on the tibial tarsal bone and distal tibia and proximal to the articular surface of the tibial tarsal bone indicate that dislocation was accompanied by fracture.

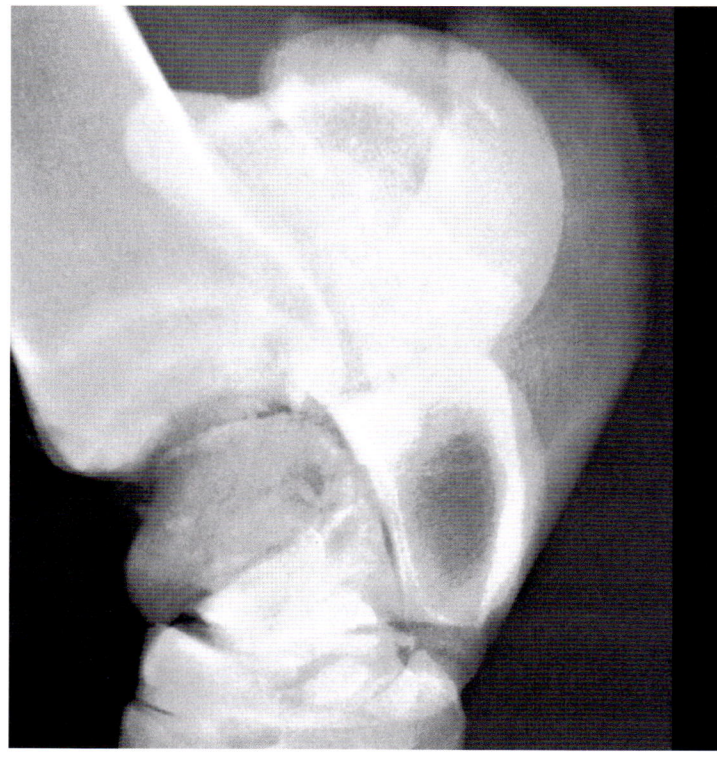
427

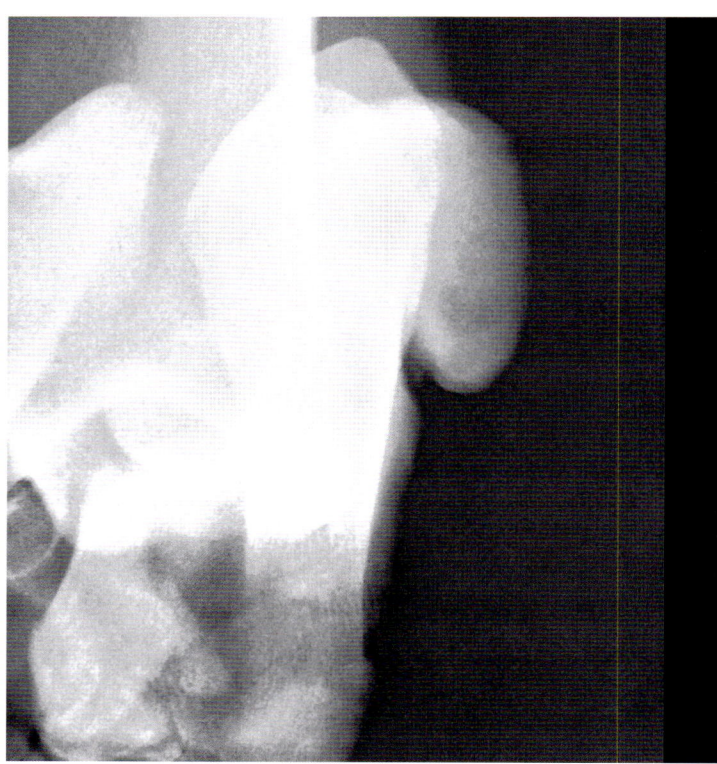
428

427/428 Left hock joint, lateromedial (Fig. 427) and dorsoplantar (Fig. 428) view: close-ups.

Warmblood, 15 years.

Fragmentation, rotation and upward, abaxial luxation of large tibial tarsal bone fragments, and overriding of the distal end of the tibia.

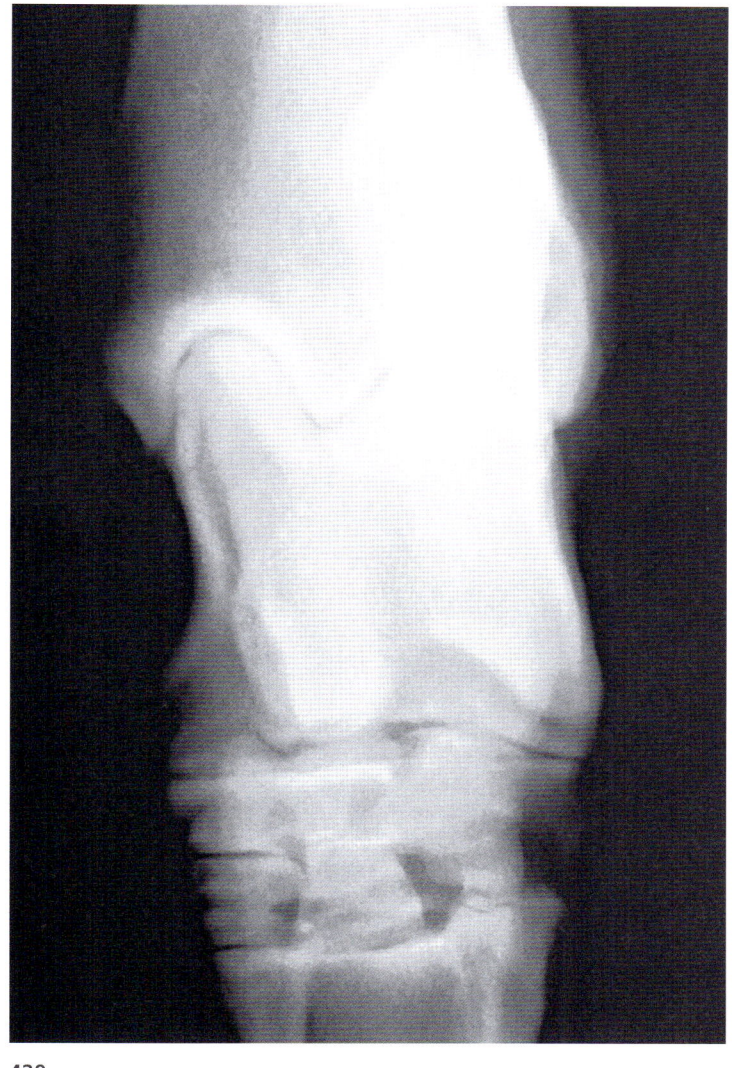 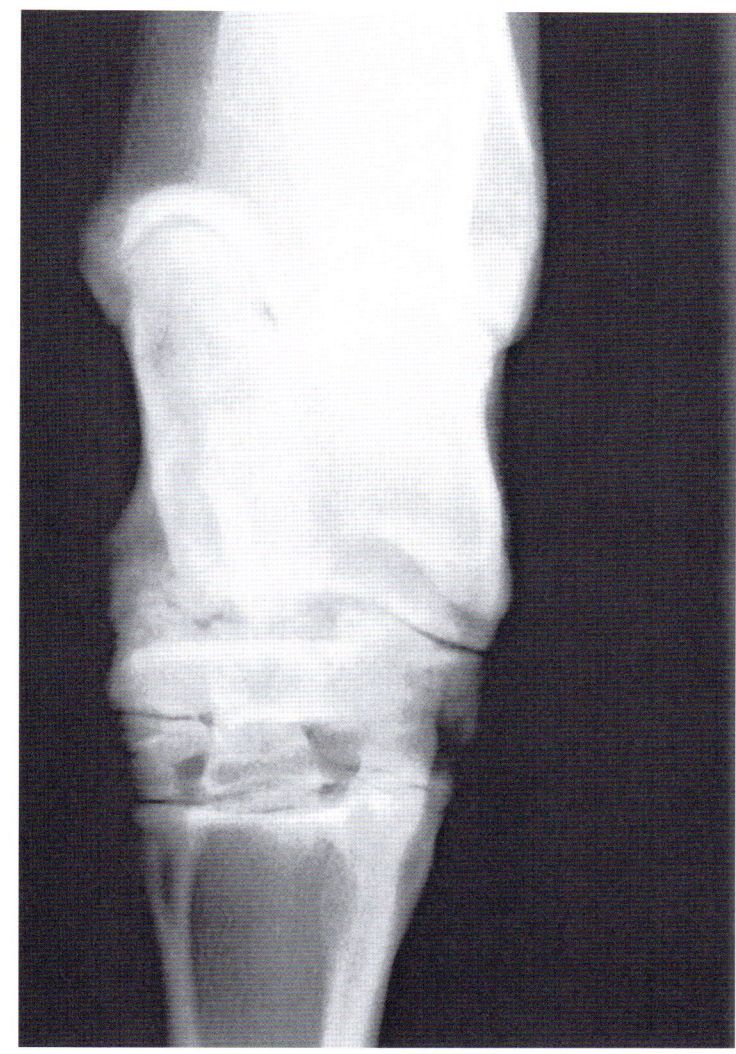

429   430

429/430 Left hock joint, serial dorsoplantar views.

Standardbred, 8 years.

The initial examination (Fig. 429), 1 day after the abrupt onset of severe lameness during training, reveals minimal widening of the medial part of the proximal intertarsal joint space, indicative of ligamentous injury (moderate sprain).

Joint instability resulted in osteoarthrosis, demonstrated 1 year later by the irregularity of the joint margins of the medial and dorsal part of the proximal intertarsal joint (Fig. 430).

Ligamentous injury

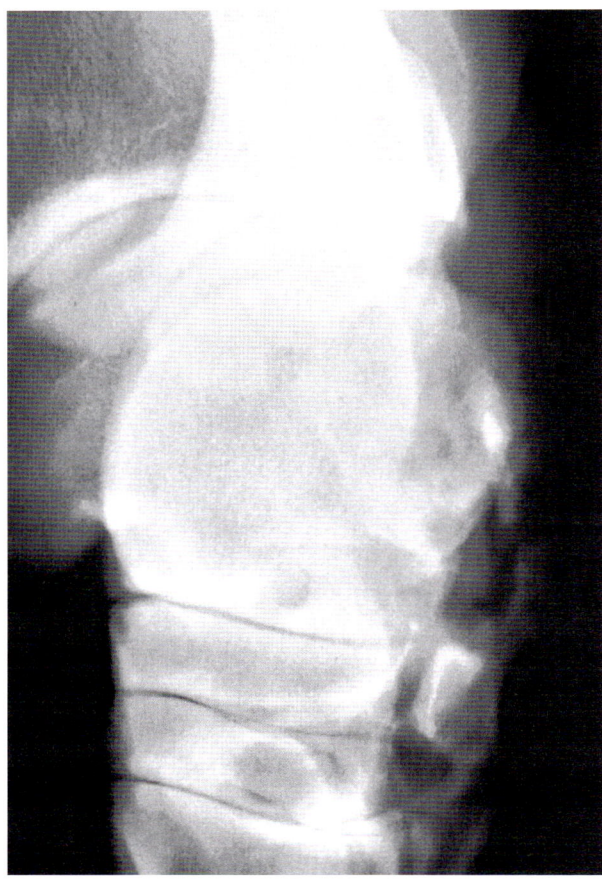

431 Right hock joint, dorsomedial-plantarolateral oblique view: close-ups.
Warmblood, 10 years.

Extensive calcification in the fibro-osseous attachment of the tarsometatarsal ligament into the sustentaculum tali and the second tarsal bone, probably due to severe trauma with haemorrhage in the damaged ligament.

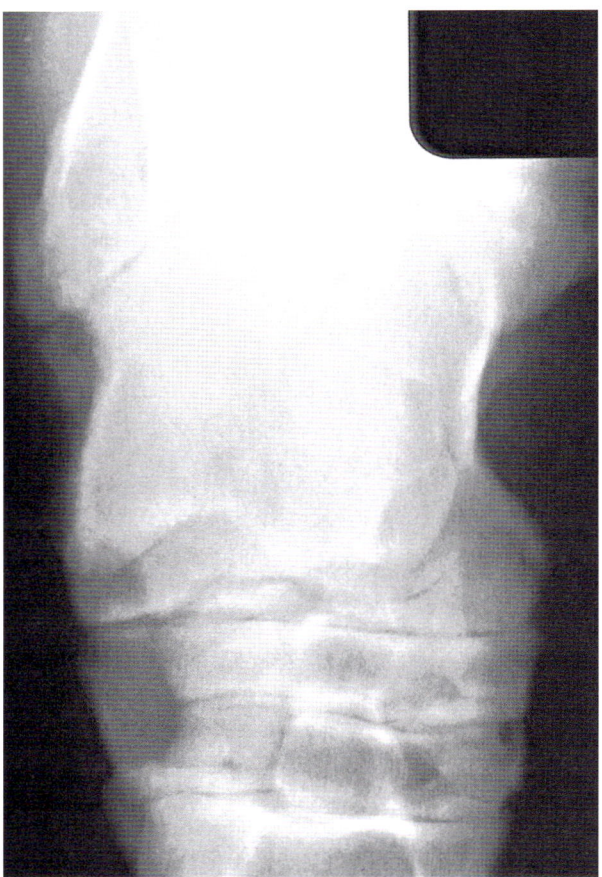

432 Right hock joint, dorsoplantar view: close-up.
Warmblood, 6 years.

Local calcification in the short lateral collateral tarsocrural ligament adjacent to the distolateral aspect of the tibia. Irregularity of the contour and texture of the corresponding portion of the distal tibia indicates that ligamentous injury occurred with periosteal reaction at the ligamentous insertion on the lateral malleolus.

Differential diagnosis includes fracture of the lateral malleolus (Fig. 399) and osteochondrosis (Fig. 501).

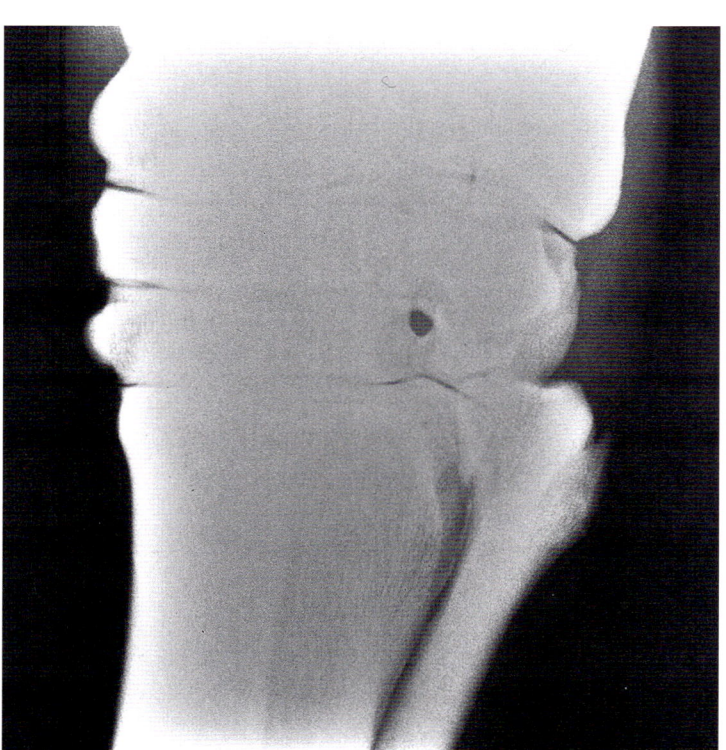

433 Left hock joint, dorsolateral-plantaromedial oblique view: close-up.
Warmblood, 10 years.

Pointed, dense, clearly bordered periosteal new bone formation at the site of attachment of the plantar ligament to the proximal extremity of the fourth metatarsal bone.

"Curby" swellings due to injury of the plantar ligament are not uncommon, but associated enthesophytosis is seldom.

Tibiotarsal joint

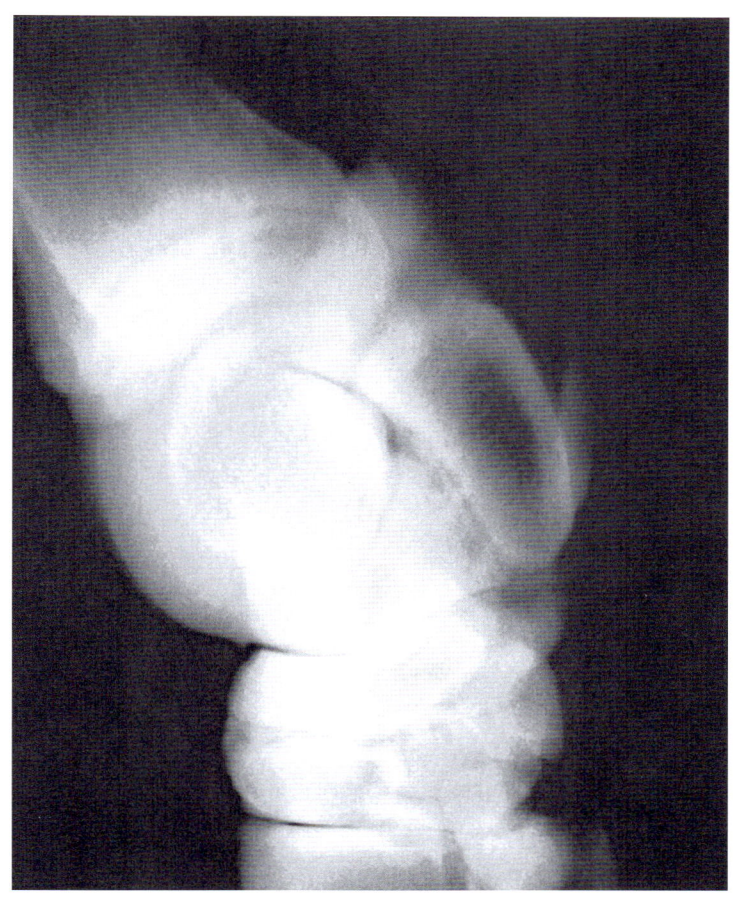

434 Right hock joint, lateromedial view; close-up.

Warmblood, 9 years.

The irregularity of the distal part of the normall smooth bordered articulation between the calcaneus and talus and patchy radiolucency in the corresponding subchondral bone of the talus indicate destructive osteoarthrosis of the talocalcaneal articulation.

This is a seldom occuring disease, probably caused by sudden traumatic injury rather than by chronic use.

Additional finding: ankylosing osteoarthrosis of the distal intertarsal joint, indicated by the smoothy rounded and fused dorsal contour of the central and third tarsal bone, collapse and hazy appearance of the distal intertarsal joint space.

Osteoarthrosis (bone spavin)

Proximal intertarsal joint

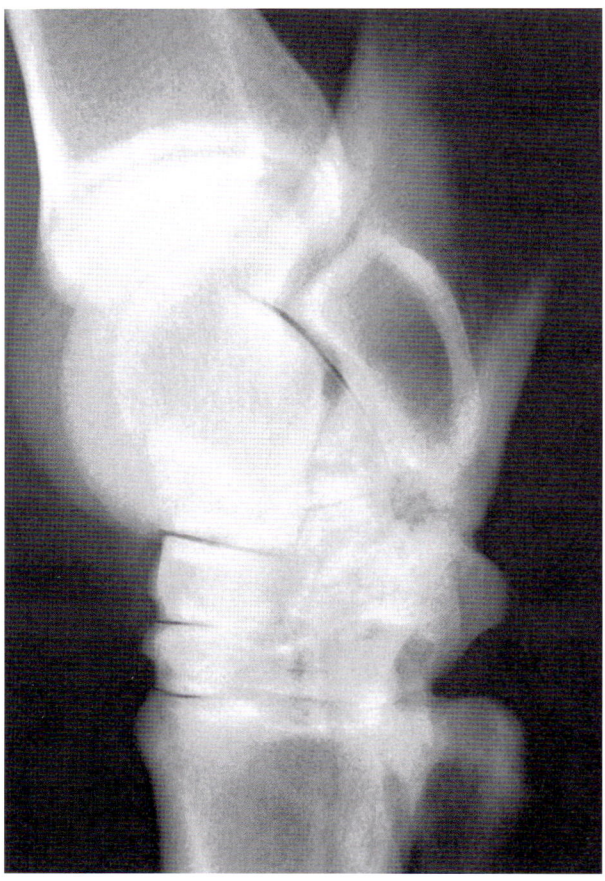

435

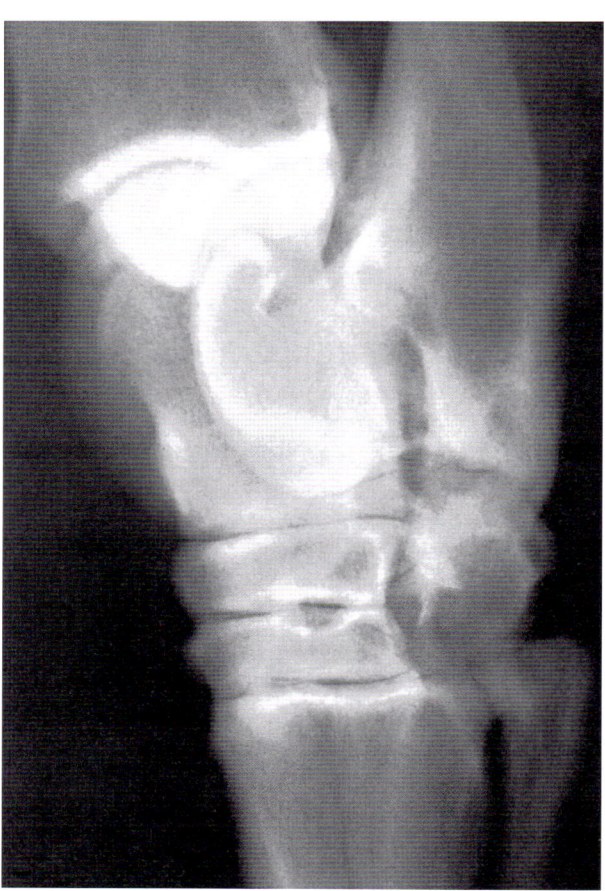

437

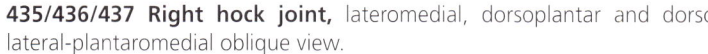

436

435/436/437 Right hock joint, lateromedial, dorsoplantar and dorso-lateral-plantaromedial oblique view.

Warmblood, 9 years.

The irregularity of the distal calcaneal border indicates osteoarthrosis of the plantarolateral aspect of the proximal intertarsal joint, i. e. the articulation between the calcaneus and fourth tarsal bone.

The degenerative changes extend into the sinus tarsi, indicated by the irregularity of the dorsolateral aspect of the calcaneus. This is a seldom occurring disease, probably arising from ligamentous injury.

The radiographic changes are clearly demonstrated by the dorsolateral-plantaromedial oblique view (Fig. 437). On the lateromedial (Fig. 435) and dorsoplantar (Fig. 436) projection the lesions are less obvious and difficult to localize.

Proximal intertarsal joint

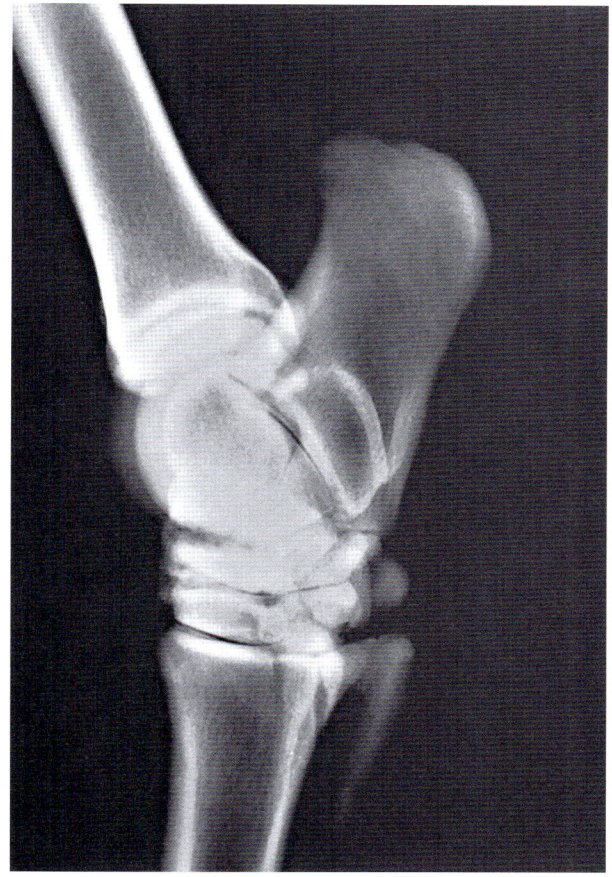

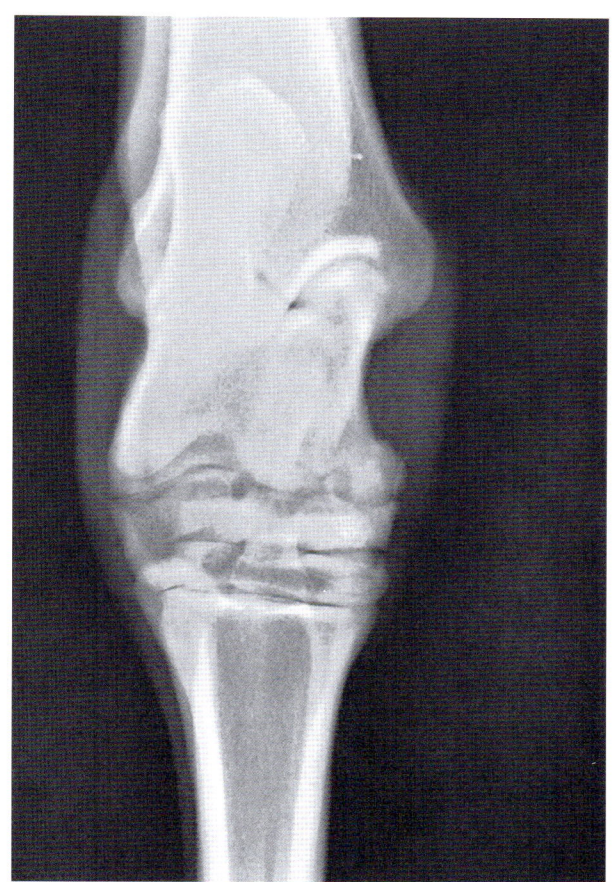

438

439

438/439 Right hock joint, lateromedial (Fig. 438) and dorsoplantar (Fig. 439) view.

Pony, 13 years.

The widened, irregular, ill bordered, proximal intertarsal joint space indicates a severe destructive type of osteoarthrosis. Osteoarthrosis of the proximal intertarsal joint has a poor prognosis.

A predominantly destructive type of osteoarthrosis is more frequently encountered in ponies than in horses and clinical signs are likely to be severe.

Osteoarthrosis (bone spavin)

Distal intertarsal joint

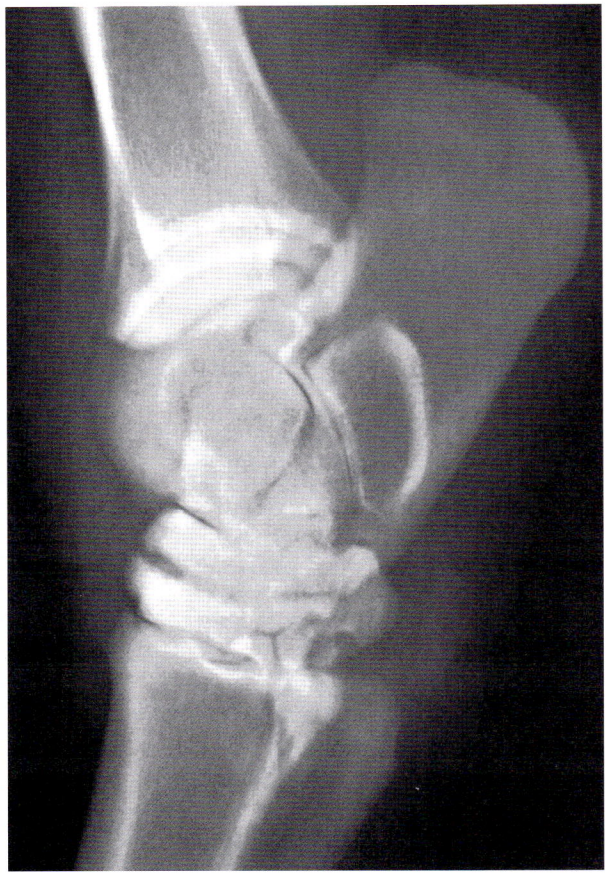

440

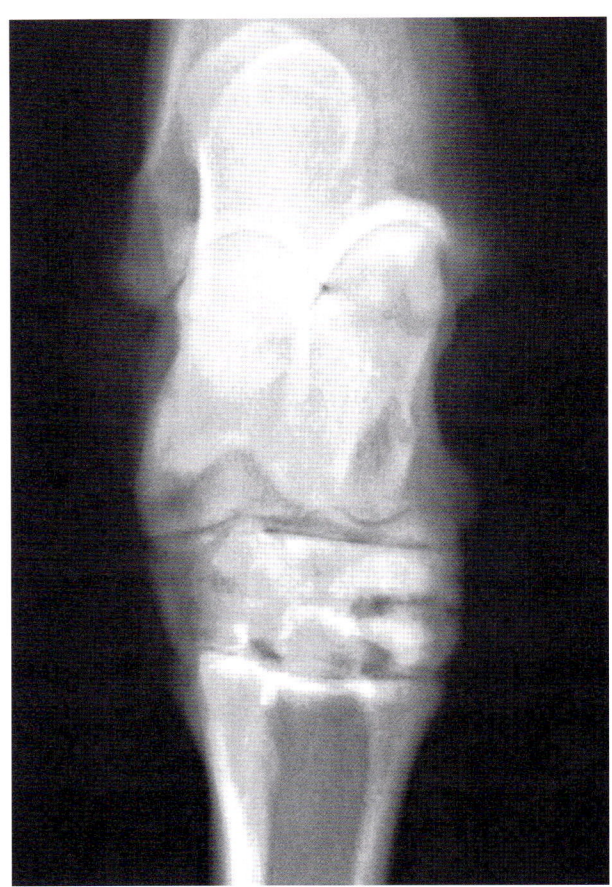

441

440/441 Right hock joint, lateromedial (Fig. 440) and dorsoplantar (Fig. 441) view.

Warmblood, 4 years.

The dorsal and medial part of the distal intertarsal joint are widened, irregular and ill bordered due to subchondral bone destruction.

The remaining portion of the joint space is obliterated by bony proliferation bridging the distal intertarsal joint. Small additional spurs are present on the dorso-proximal aspect of the third tarsal and the third metatarsal bones. Osteoarthrosis characterized by a mixture of destructive and proliferative changes is a significant finding, the more destructive the lesion is, the more likely clinical signs are to be present.

Distal intertarsal joint

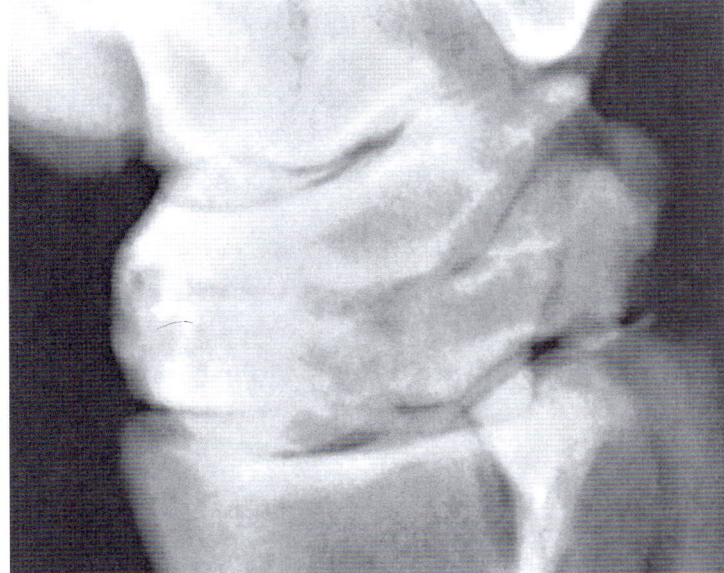 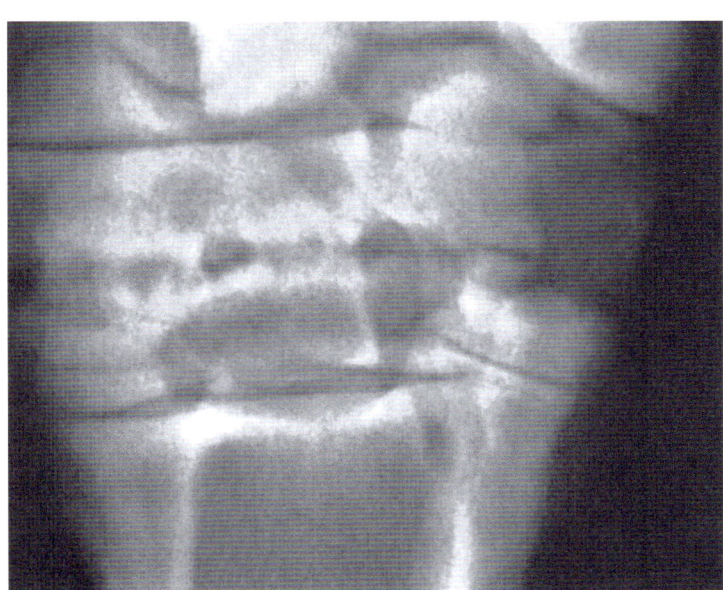

442

443

442/443 Left hock joint, lateromedial and dorsoplantar view: close-ups.

Warmblood, 6 years.

On the lateromedial view (Fig. 442) the distal intertarsal joint space is irregular, narrow and poorly defined. In addition, a small area of radiolucency is visible in the region of the distal intertarsal joint adjacent to the rounded, fused dorsal contour of the central and third tarsal bones.

The dorsoplantar view (Fig. 443) shows multiple cystic and irregular radiolucent areas in the subchondral region of the distal intertarsal joint space and areas of new bone bridging the distal intertarsal joint space, resulting in spur formation on the lateral aspect of the joint.

The radiographic changes indicate an ankylosing osteoarthrosis of the entire distal intertarsal joint.

Partial ankylosis may occur without lameness, but clinical signs are likely to the present due to the associated destructive changes.

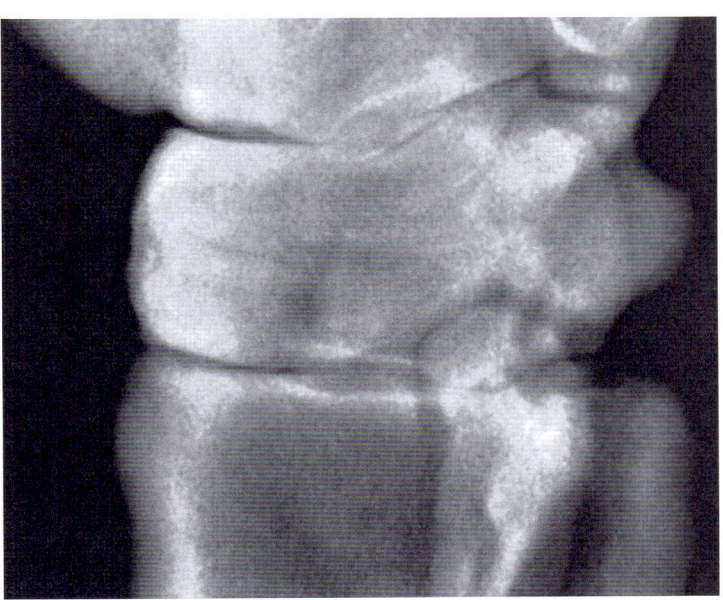 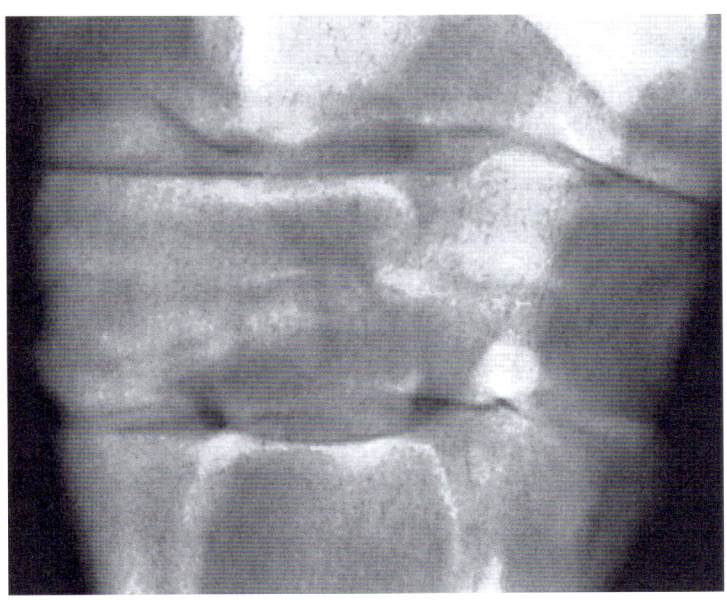

444

445

444/445 Left hock joint, lateromedial (Fg. 444) and dorsoplantar (Fig. 445) view: close-ups.

Warmblood, 8 years.

The rounded, fused dorsal contour of the central and third tarsal bones and diffuse obliteration of the entire intertarsal joint space indicate complete ankylosis without destructive changes. This is regarded as an „end stage" of bone spavin and may be present in sound horses.

Osteoarthrosis (bone spavin)

Distal intertarsal joint

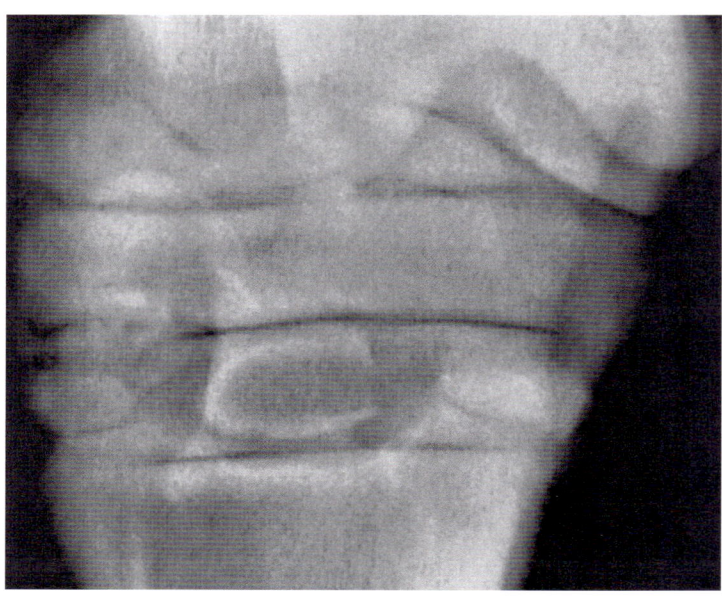

446 Left hock joint, dorsoplantar view: close-up.

Warmblood, 4 years.

The roughened, narrowed and hazy appearance of the medial aspect of the distal intertarsal joint space indicates osteoarthrosis; such changes are of variable clinical significance and may be present in both lame as well as sound horses.

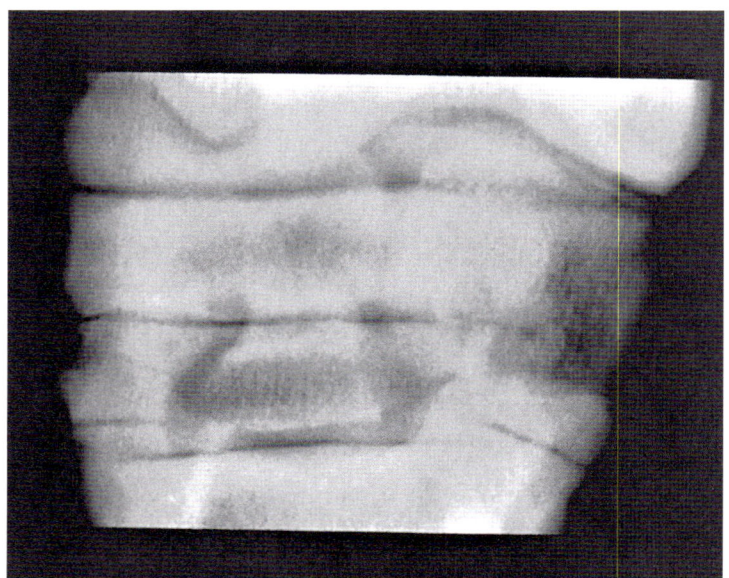

447 Left hock joint, dorsoplantar view: close-up.

Pony, 10 years.

The irregular, hazy appearance of the lateral region of the distal intertarsal joint space and spur formation on the lateral aspect of the joint indicate osteoarthrosis; such changes are of variable clinical significance and may or may not be associated with lameness.

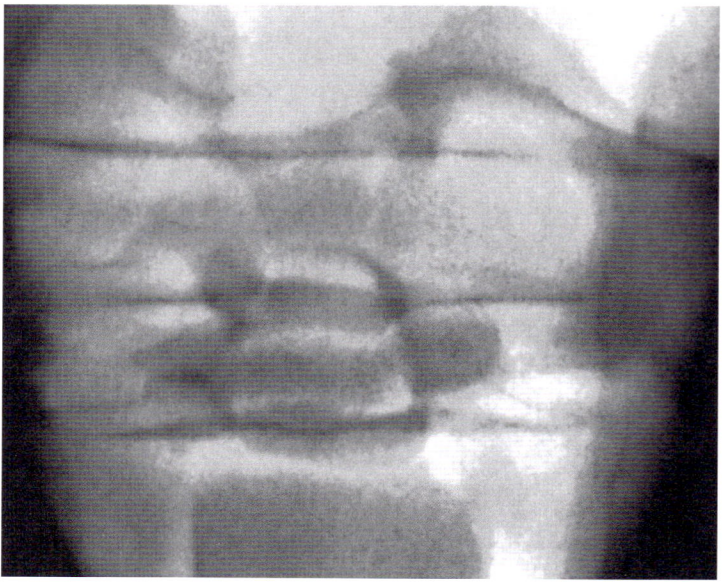

448 Left hock joint, dorsoplantar view: close-up.

Warmblood, 3 years.

Blurring of the medial aspect of the distal intertarsal joint space; such changes are insignificant and may be present in sound horses.

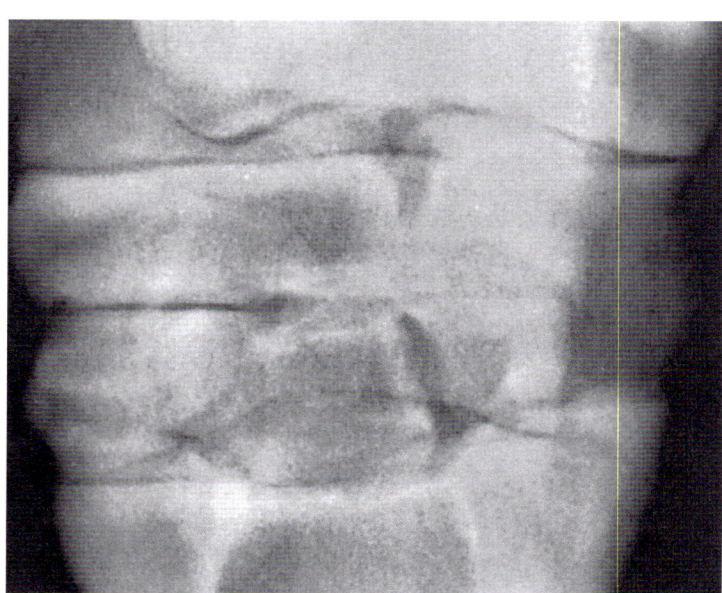

449 Left hock joint, dorsoplantar view: close-up.

Warmblood, 5 years.

A small cystic indentation in the proximal medial border of the distal intertarsal joint; this change is of little or no clinical significance.

Additional finding: The blurring of the lateral aspect of the distal intertarsal joint space is artefactual, caused by centring the dorsoplantar directed beam at a point approximately 2 cm distal to the distal intertarsal joint; this artefact should not be confused with partail ankylosis.

Tarsometatarsal joint

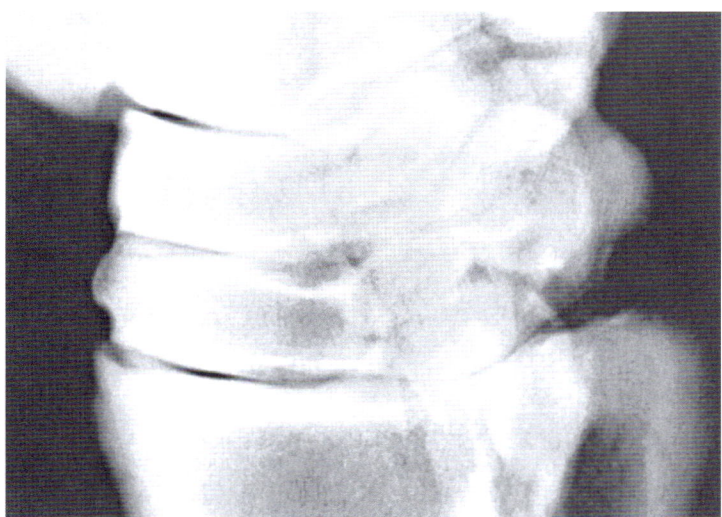

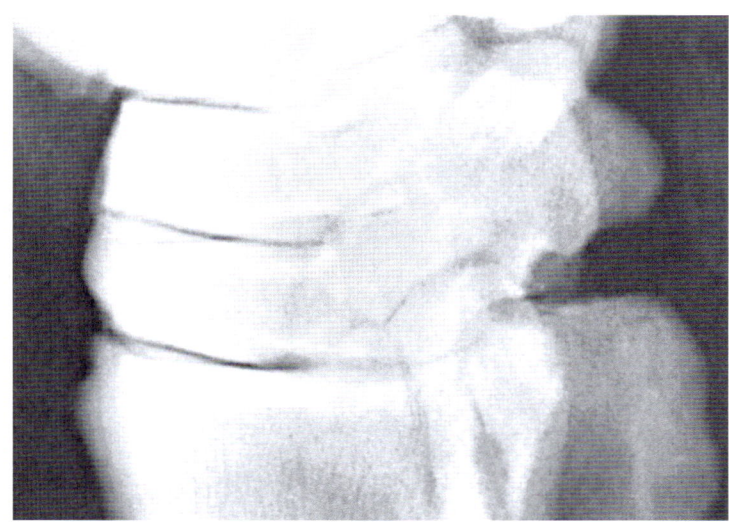

450 Right hock-joint, lateromedial view: close-up.

Warmblood, 5 years.

A large bony spur on the dorsoproximal aspect of the third metatarsal bone; such changes are of variable clinical significance and may be present in both lame and sound horses.

Intra-articular anaesthesia of this tarsometatarsal joint rendered the horse sound.

451 Right hock joint, lateromedial view: close-up.

Warmblood, 4 years.

The small bony spur on the dorsoproximal aspect of the third metatarsal bone is a change of little or no clinical significance.

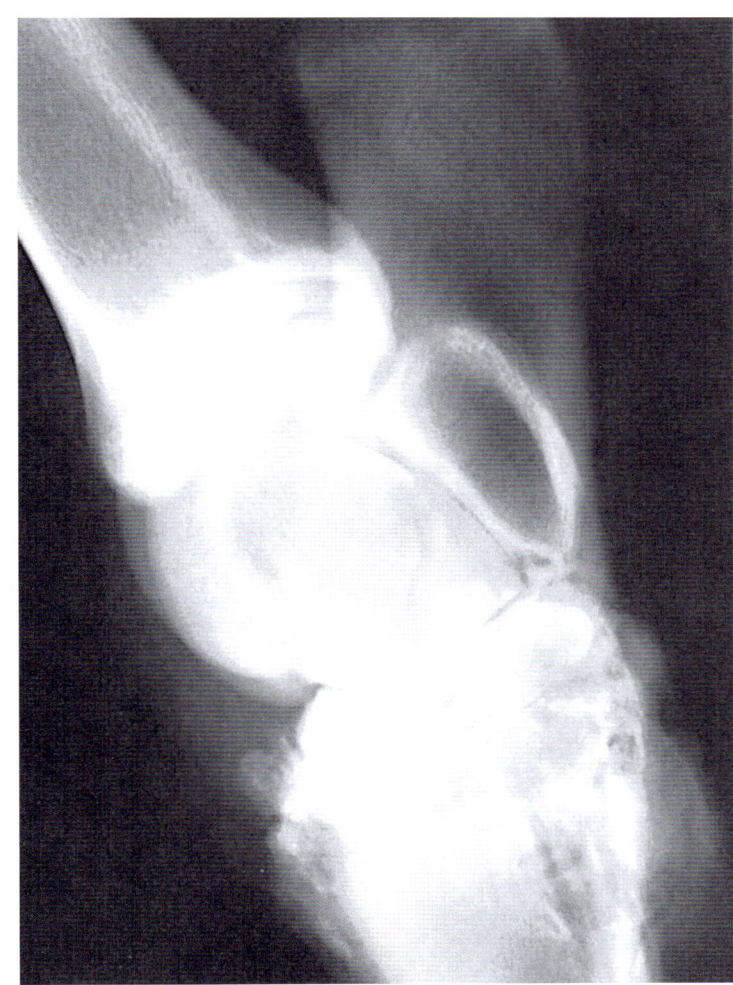

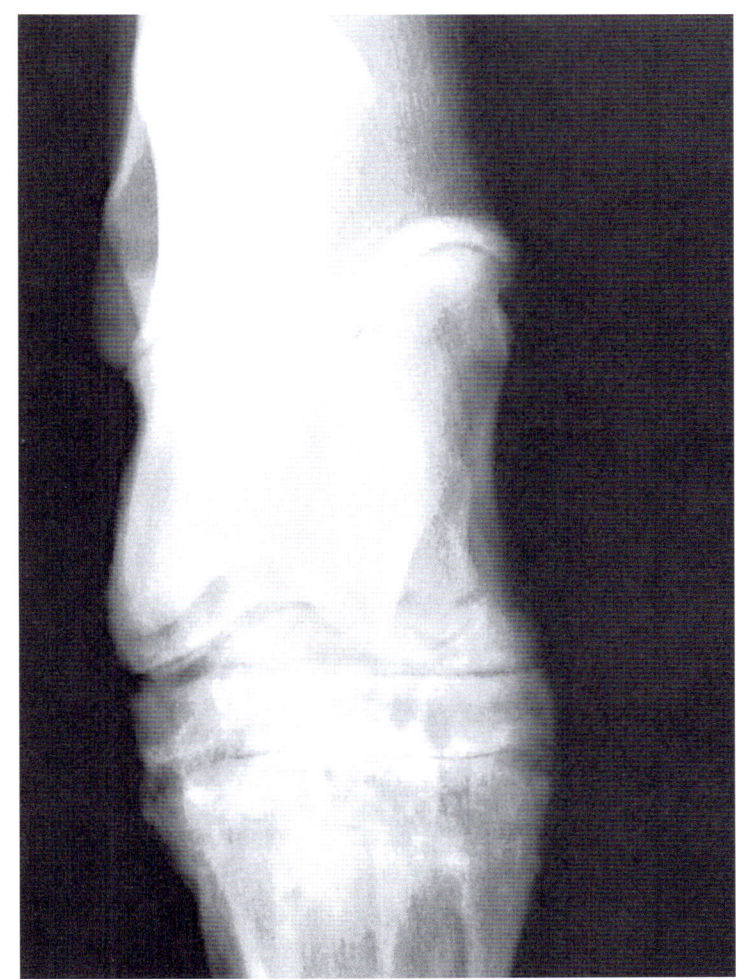

452

453

452/453 Right hock joint, lateromedial (Fig. 452) and dorsoplantar (Fig. 453) view.

Warmblood, 6 years.

Collapse of the distal intertarsal joint space, obliteration of the tarsometatarsal joint, and extensive irregular articular and peri-articular new bone formation bridging both joints and resulting in ankylosis.

The osteoarthrosis resulted from a traumatic injury 1 year previously.

Tarsal bone collapse

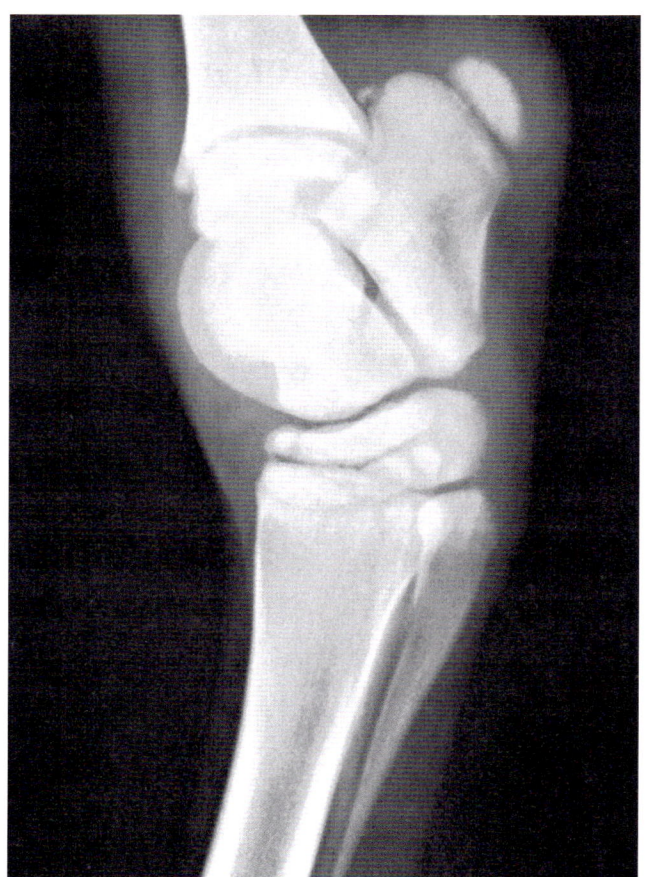

454

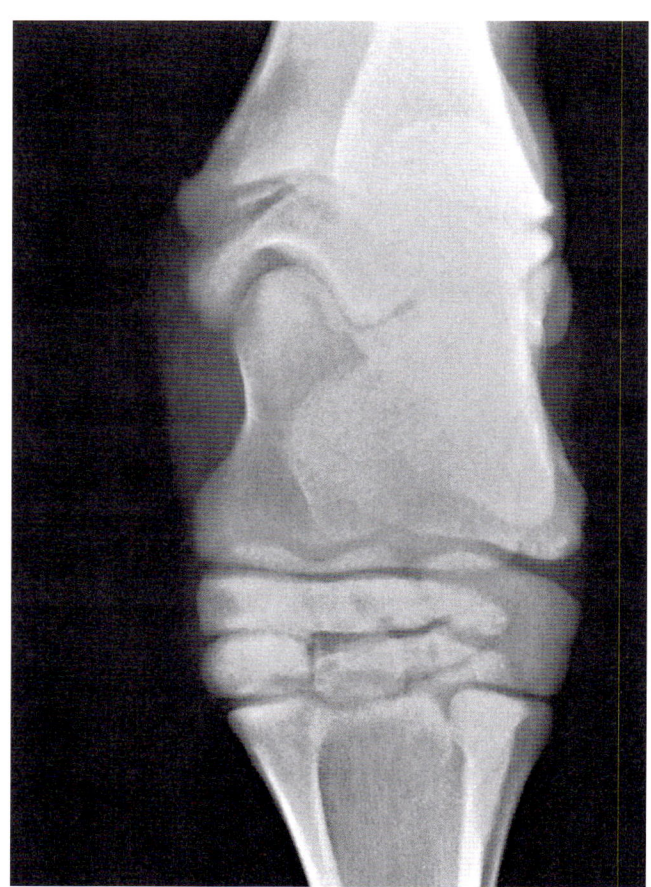

455

454/455/456/457 Left hock joint, serial lateromedial and dorsoplantar views.

Foal, 1 month.

On the initial lateromedial view (Fig. 454) the hock appears sickled and there is soft tissue swelling over the small tarsal bones. The dorsal aspect of the central tarsal bone is more rounded than usual and shows a vertical radiolucent line, suggestive of fragmentation. It is difficult to identify the third tarsal bone and the tarsometatarsal joint space on the lateromedial view, due to wedging of the lateral aspect of the central and third tarsal bones, clearly demonstrated by the initial dorsoplantar projection (Fig. 455). This view also reveals small, ill defined radiolucent areas in the dorsal and lateral aspect of the central and third tarsal bones.

The radiographic changes indicate incomplete ossification of the central and third tarsal bones. Weight-bearing upon the weakened bones resulted in compression, collapse and deformation of the third tarsal bone, demonstrated by the second examination 8 months later (Fig. 456, 457). On the dorsoplantar view the distal intertarsal joint space is narrowed and obliterated, due to superimposition of the deformed, crushed dorsal aspect of the third tarsal bone and ankylosing osteoarthrosis. Collapse and deformation of the central tarsal bone did not occur, despite the fragmentation suggested on the initial lateromedial view.

Additional finding (lateromedial views): the small bone fragment dorsal to the proximal aspect of the body of the fibular tarsal bone, visible on the initial lateromedial view, results from incomplete ossification and is no longer obvious on the second examination.

N. B. Incomplete ossification of the central and third tarsal bones is most common in foals born either prematurely or as one of twins, or may result from hypothyroidism. Tarsal bone collapse has also been associated with osteomyelitis (Fig. 497/480/481/482) and aseptic necrosis of the small tarsal bones.

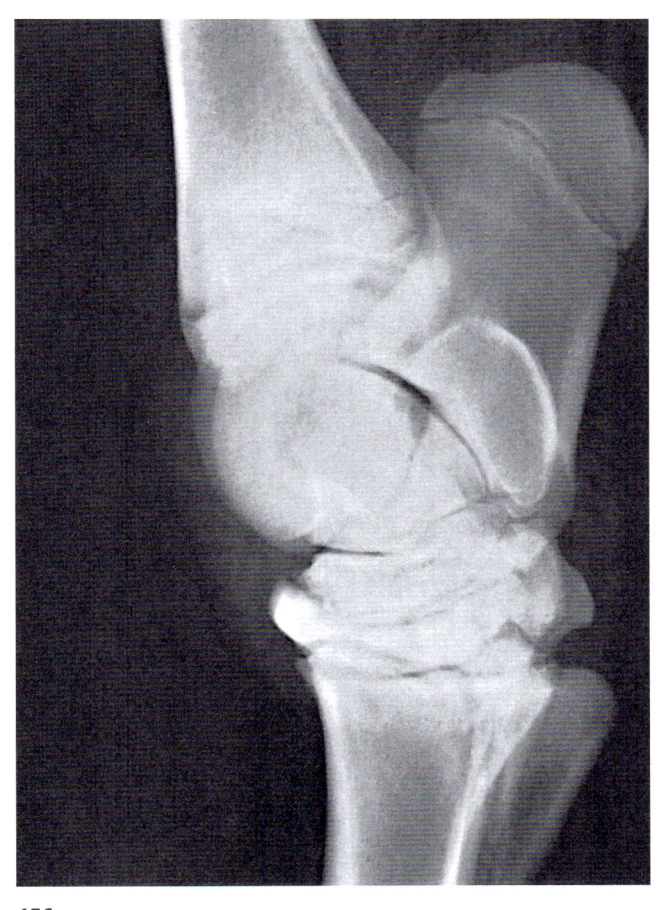

456

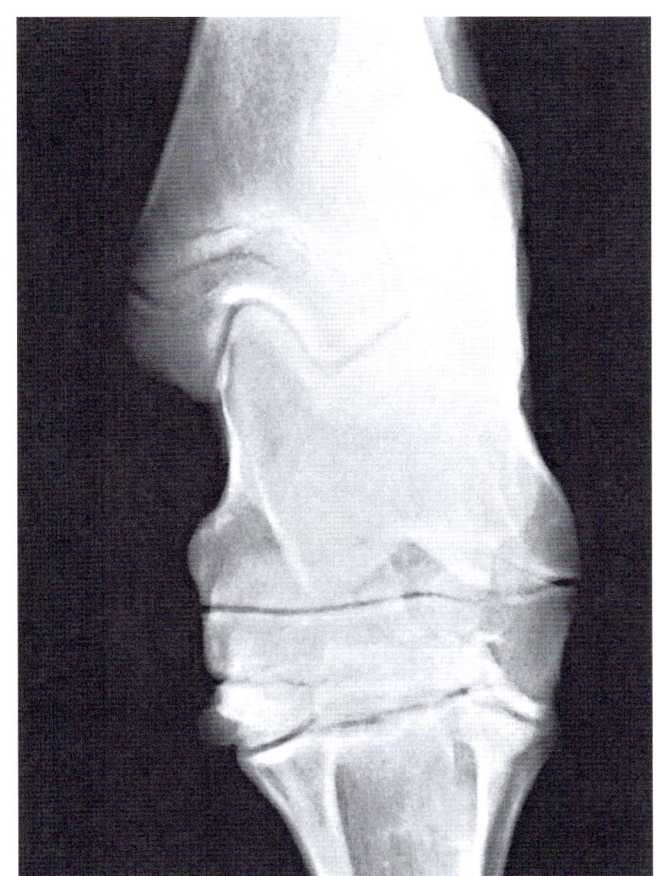

457

Infectious arthritis

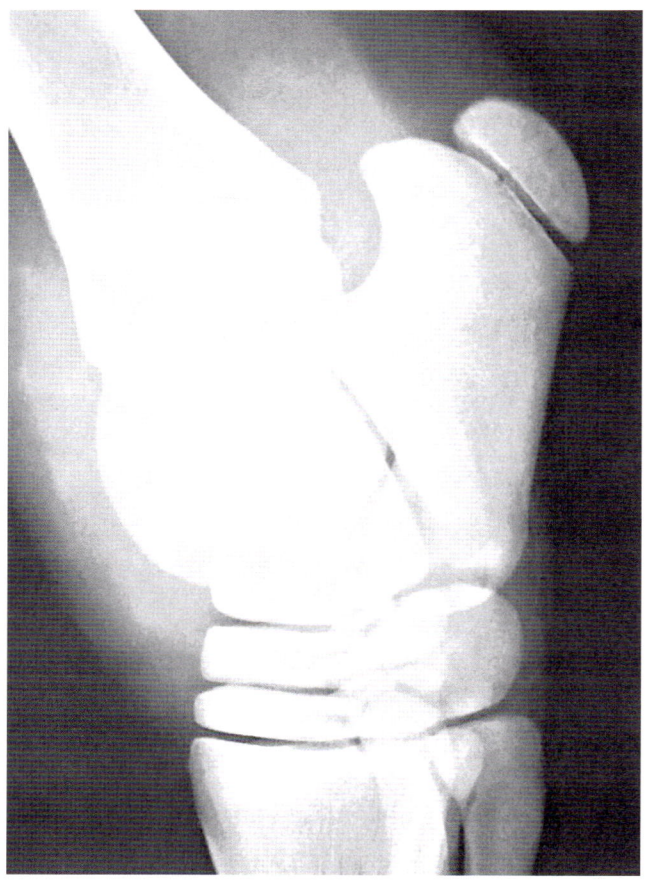

458

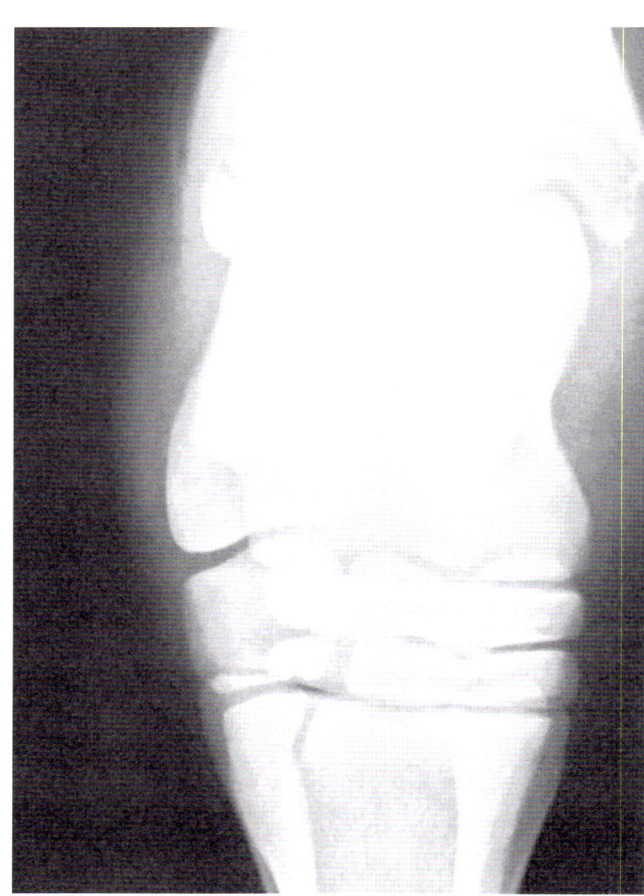

459

458/459 Right hock joint, lateromedial (Fig. 458) and dorsoplantar (Fig. 459) view.

Foal, 2 weeks.

The soft tissue swelling dorsal and medial to the tibial tarsal bone and the subchondral radiolucent area in the medial malleolus are consequences of haemato-geneous osteomyelitis type E in a young foal with concomitant infectious arthritis of the tibiotarsal joint.

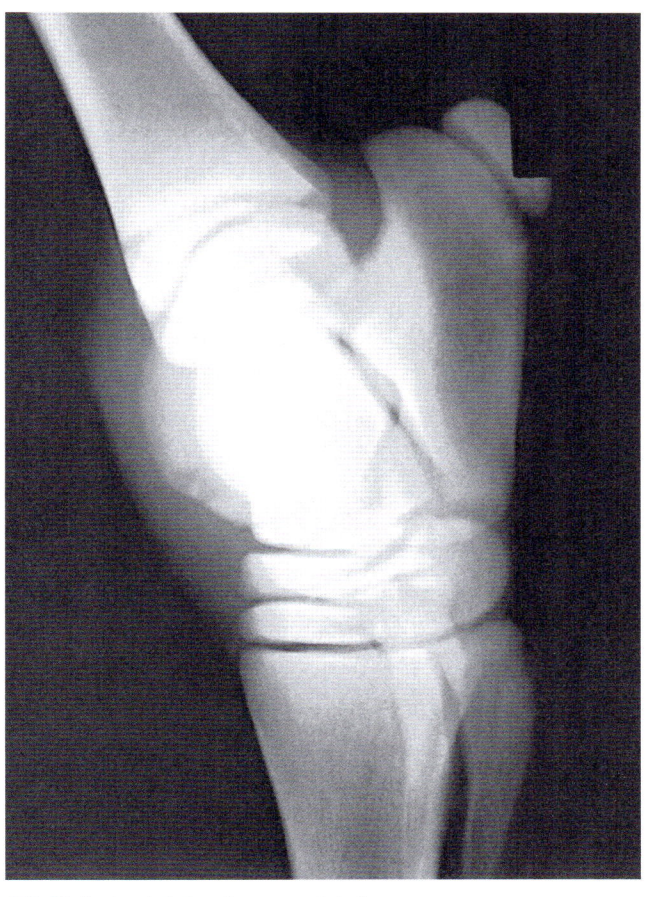

460 Right hock joint, lateromedial view.

Foal, 2 weeks.

The large radiolucent area in the distal aspect of the medial trochlear ridge of the tibial tarsal bone represents either type E osteomyelitis or delayed ossification.

Histological examination revealed an osteomyelitic lesion. The concomitant effusion of the tibiotarsal joint resulted from infectious arthritis, indicated by the clinical and laboratory data.

N. B. Infectious arthritis in a young foal may occur with or without accompanying type E osteomyelitic lesions, so radiographic differentiation between type E osteomyelitis and delayed ossification is impossible if joint effusion is present.

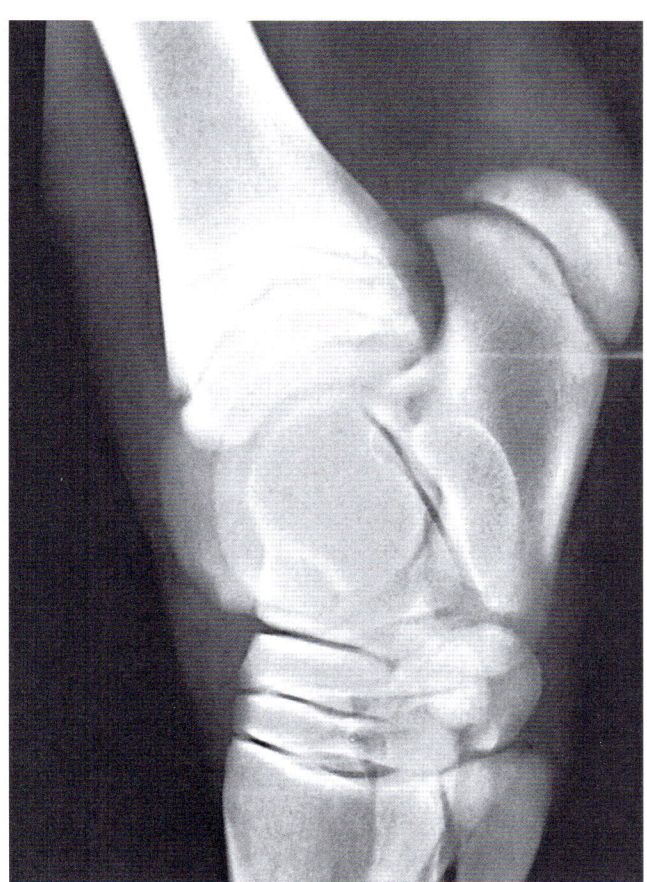

461 Right hock joint, lateromedial view.

Foal, 6 weeks.

A small radiolucent area in the distal aspect of the medial trochlear ridge of the tibial tarsal bone. The differential diagnosis includes type E osteomyelitis and delayed ossification. Type E osteomyelitis is always accompanied by infectious arthritis. The absence of joint effusion indicates the presence of delayed ossification. Histological examination confirmed the diagnosis.

N. B. Delayed ossification of the distal aspect of the medial or lateral trochlear ridge of the tibial tarsal bone is a coincidental finding of little or no clinical significance. Spontaneous healing usually occurs within 1 or 2 months.

Infectious arthritis

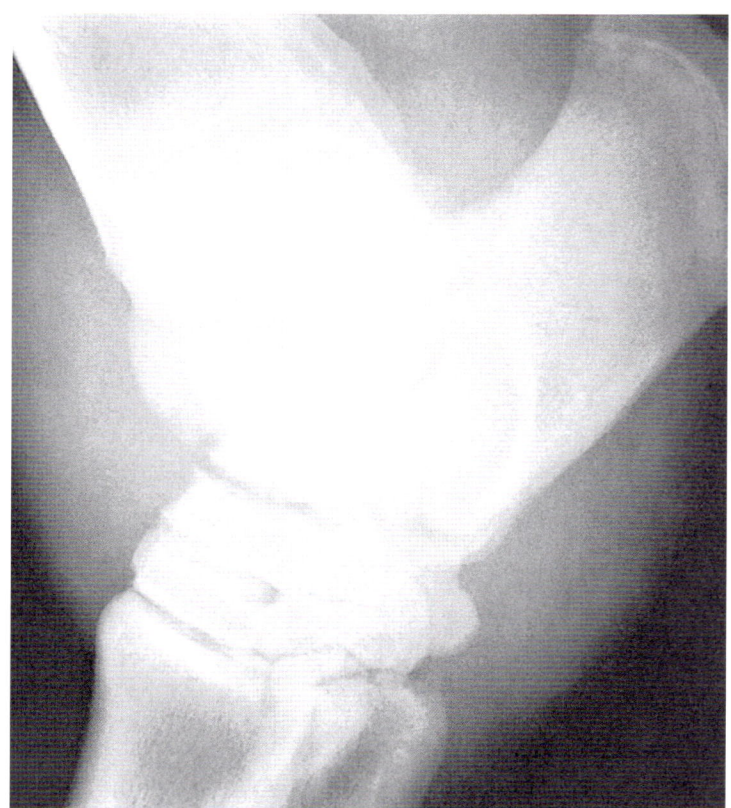

462

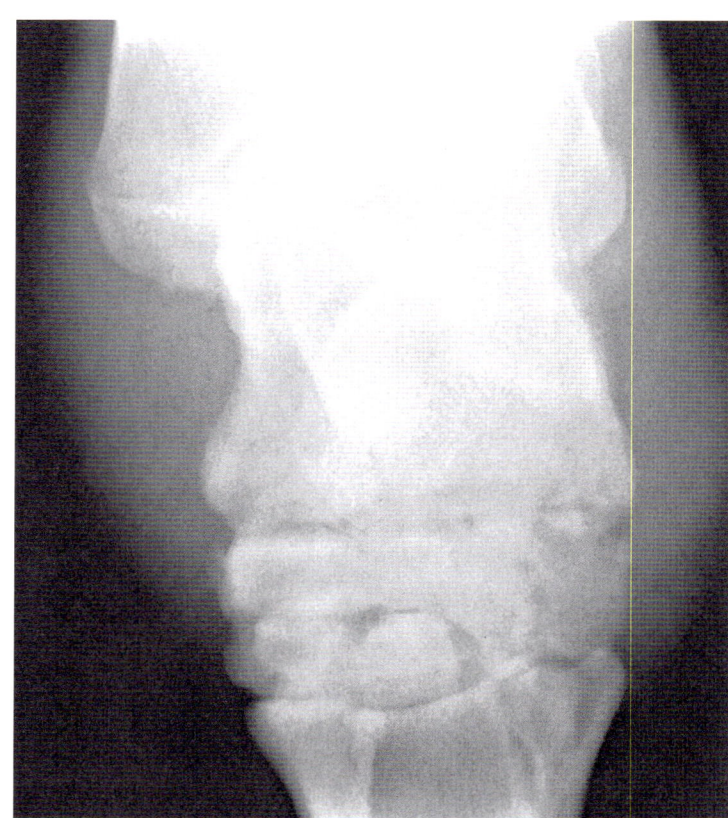

463

462/463 Left hock joint, lateromedial (Fig. 462) and dorsoplantar (Fig. 463) view.

Warmblood, 1½ years.

Extensive soft tissue swelling over the small tarsal bones and widening of the proximal intertarsal joint space, caused by infectious arthritis, resulting from a puncture wound 4 weeks prior to the examination. The irregular radiolucency in the subchondral region of the joint, visible on the dorsoplantar view, indicates subchondral bone destruction, usually noticed within 3 – 6 weeks after the onset of the disease. The concomitant effusion of the tibiotarsal joint is due to the communication between the tibiotarsal and proximal intertarsal joint.

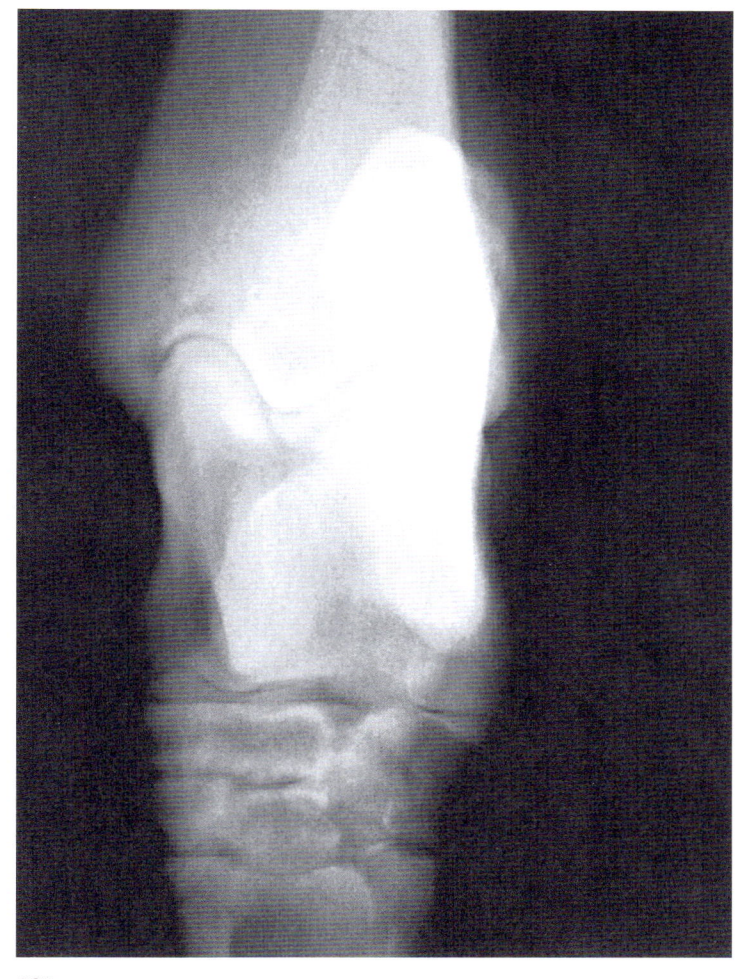

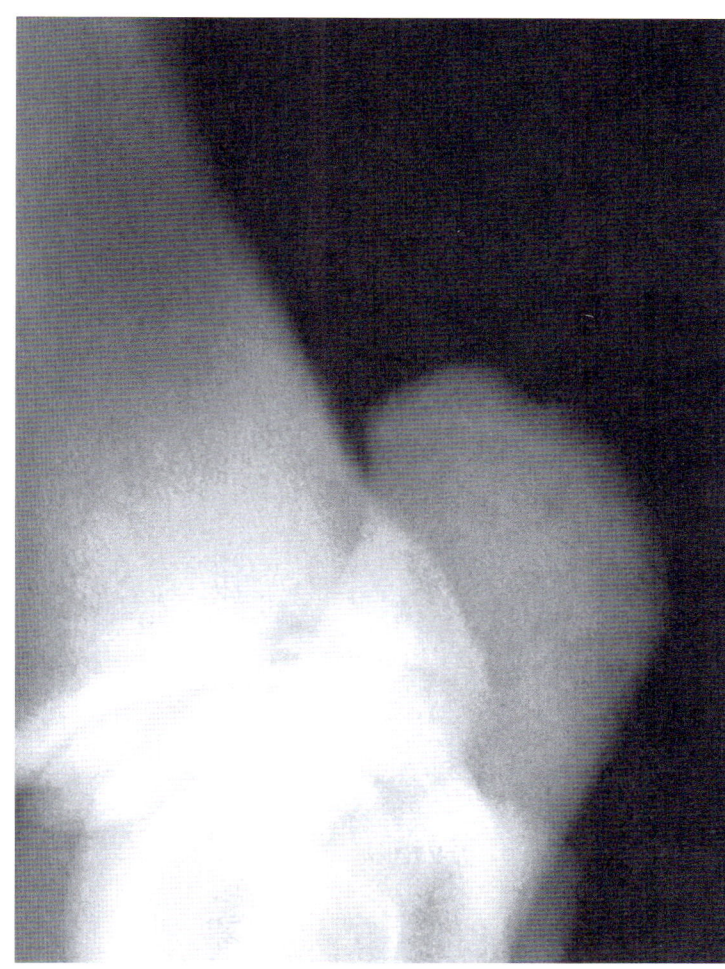

464

465

464/465 Left hock joint, dorsoplantar and dorsomedial-plantarolateral oblique view: close-up.

Pony, 4 years.

The dorsoplantar view (Fig. 464) shows a small subchondral bone fragment surrounded by a radiolucent zone within the distomedial end of the tibia, also clearly demonstrated on the dorsomedial-plantarolateral oblique projection (Fig. 465). The radiographic changes indicate bone sequestration. Clinical and laboratory data revealed infectious arthritis.

N. B. Infectious arthritis is rarely accompanied by focal subchondral bone sequestration, so sequestration in such cases may thus be associated with concomitant trauma.

Infectious arthritis

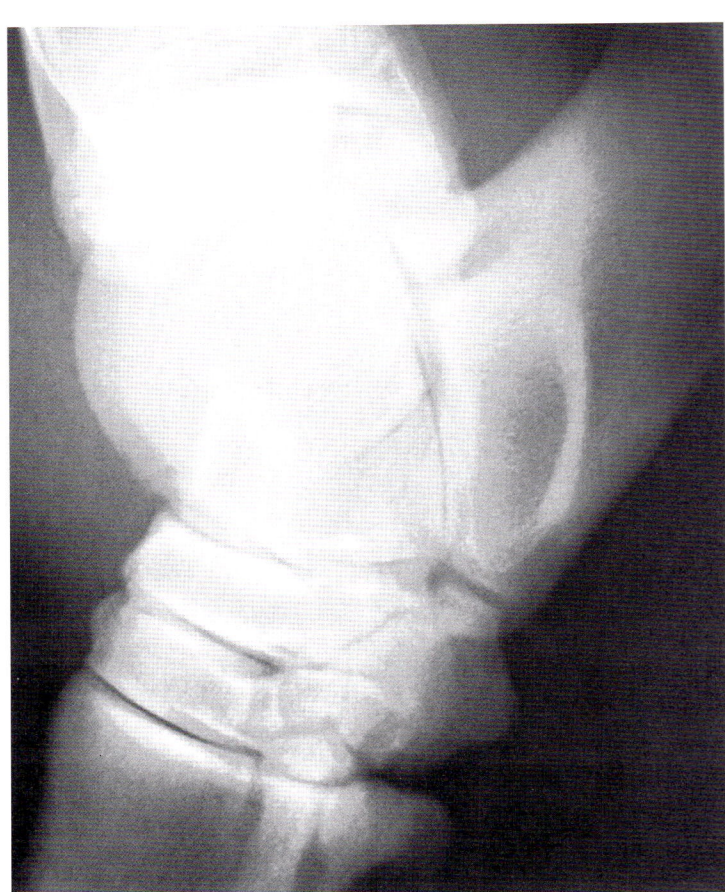

466

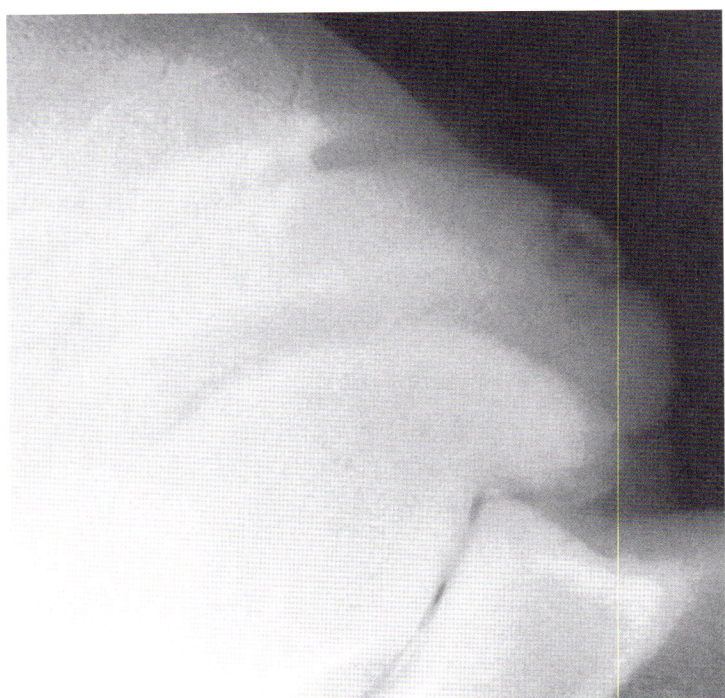

467

466/467 Right hock joint, lateromedial and proximolateral-distomedial oblique (flexed) view: close-ups.

Warmblood, 1½ years.

Effusion of the tibiotarsal joint demonstrated by the lateromedial view (Fig. 466), and an irregular subchondral bone fragment surrounded by a radiolucent zone within the proximal aspect of the medial trochlear ridge of the tibial tarsal bone, more clearly demonstrated by the proximolateral-distomedial oblique (flexed) projection (Fig. 467).

The radiographic changes indicate focal subchondral bone sequestration. Clinical and labaratory data revealed infectious arthritis.

The reason for the special oblique (flexed) projection was the presence of a very obscure bone lesion within the plantaro-proximal aspect of the tibial tarsal bone on the lateromedial view.

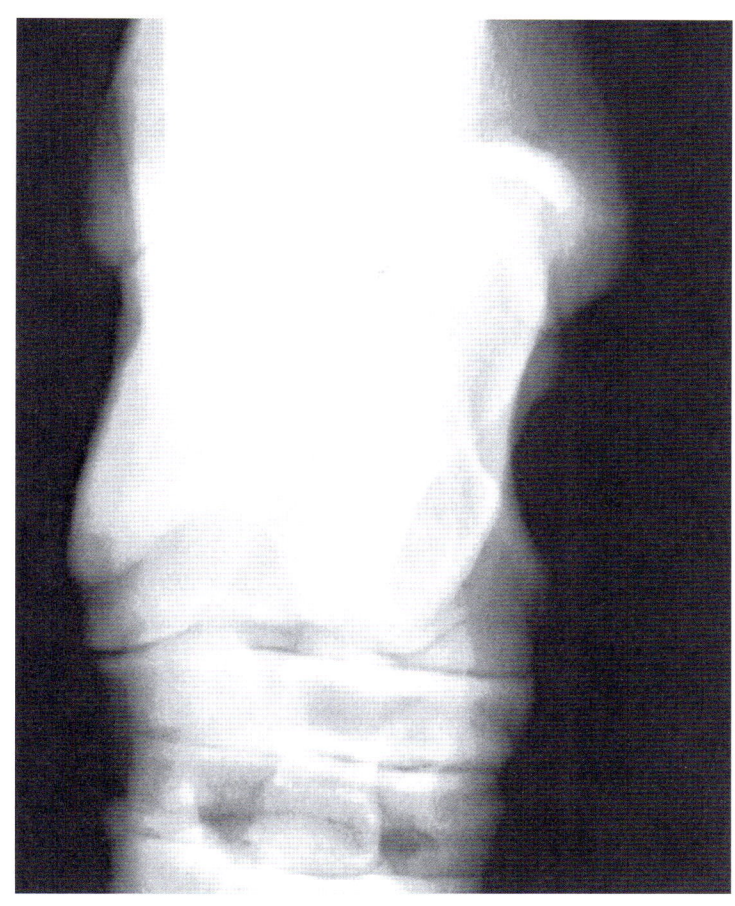

468

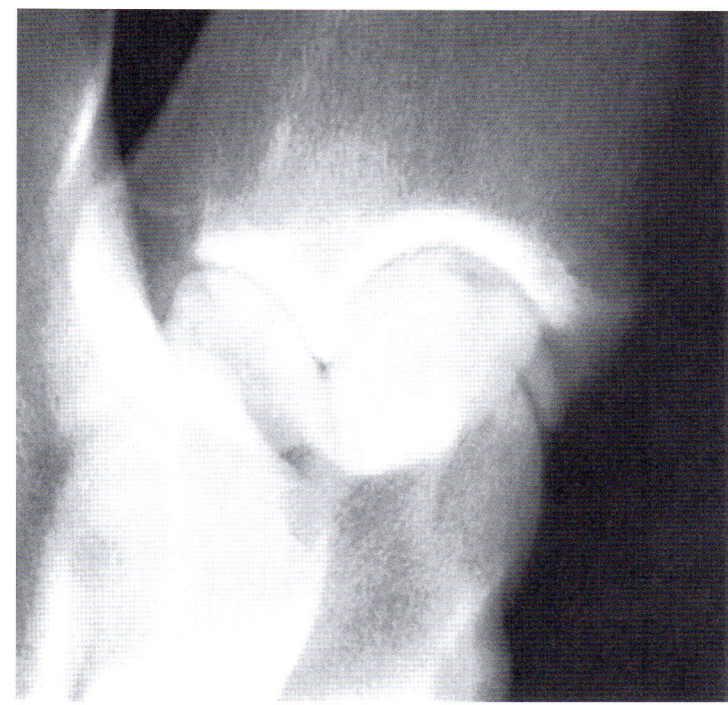

469

468/469 Right hock joint, dorsoplantar and dorsolateral-plantaromedial oblique view: close-up.

Warmblood, 3 years.

The dorsoplantar view (Fig. 468), 3 weeks after the onset of clinical symptoms, shows an ill defined, small subchondral bone sequestrum in the proximal aspect of the medial trochlear ridge of the tibial tarsal bone. The bone fragment is more obvious on the dorsolateral-plantaromedial oblique projection (Fig. 469). Clinical and laboratory data revealed infectious arthritis.

Infectious arthritis

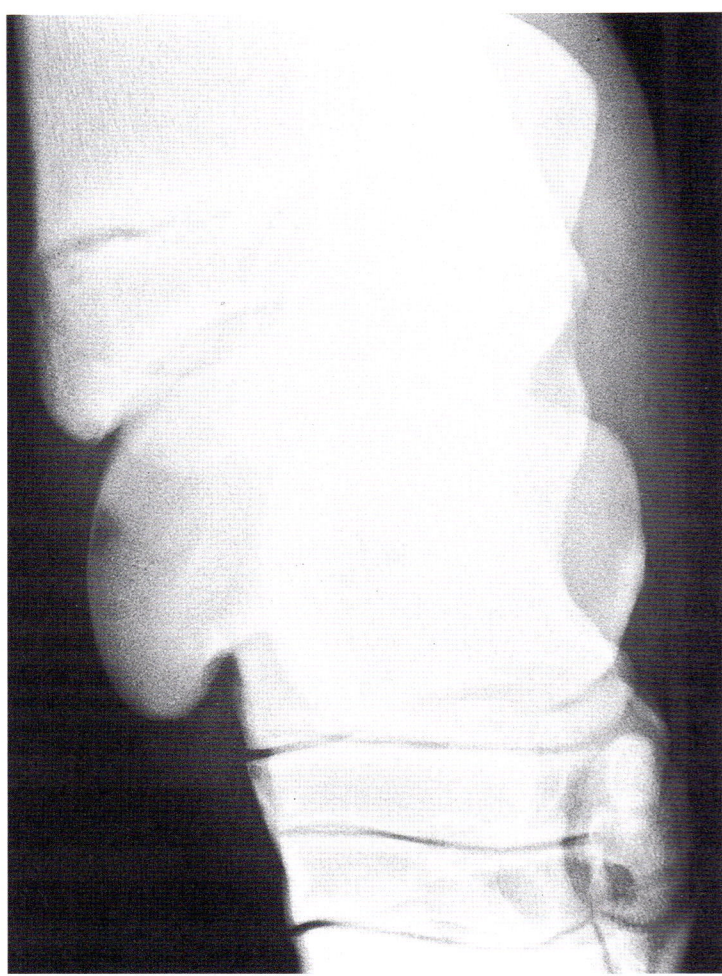

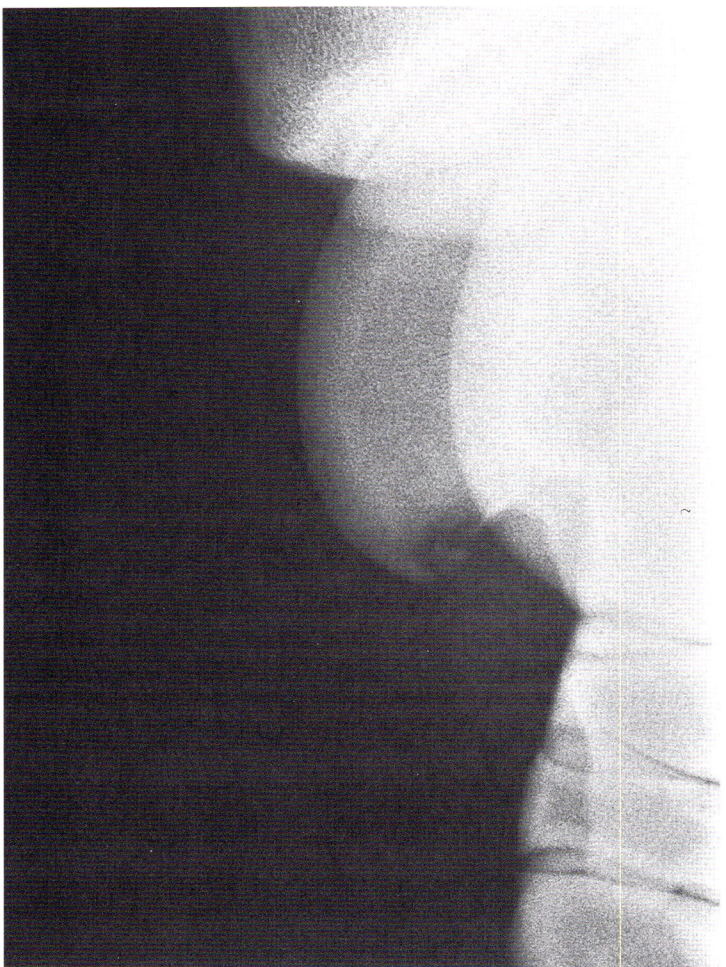

470 Right hock joint, dorsomedial-plantarolateral oblique view. Warmblood, 1 year.

An obvious, small, ill bordered area of subchondral lucency in the mid region of the lateral trochlear ridge of the tibial tarsal bone.

The absence of a corresponding defect of the overlying bony outline is uncommon with osteochondrosis.

Bacterial culture of synovial fluid was negative. However, cytologic synovial fluid analysis demonstrated a neutrophil count of ≥90%, thus implying focal subchondral bony lysis associated with infectious arthritis.

471 Right hock joint, dorsomedial-plantarolateral oblique view: close-up. Warmblood, 3 years.

The small bony fragment at the distal end of the lateral trochlear ridge of the tibial tarsal bone suggest osteochondrosis (Fig. 495). However, the indistinct outline of the corresponding bony defect versus the sharp definition of the fragment are unusual for this condition.

E-coli was isolated from the synovial fluid. Therefore, the bony fragment actually represents focal subchondral sequestration introduced by infectious arthritis. Concomitant trauma was not apparent.

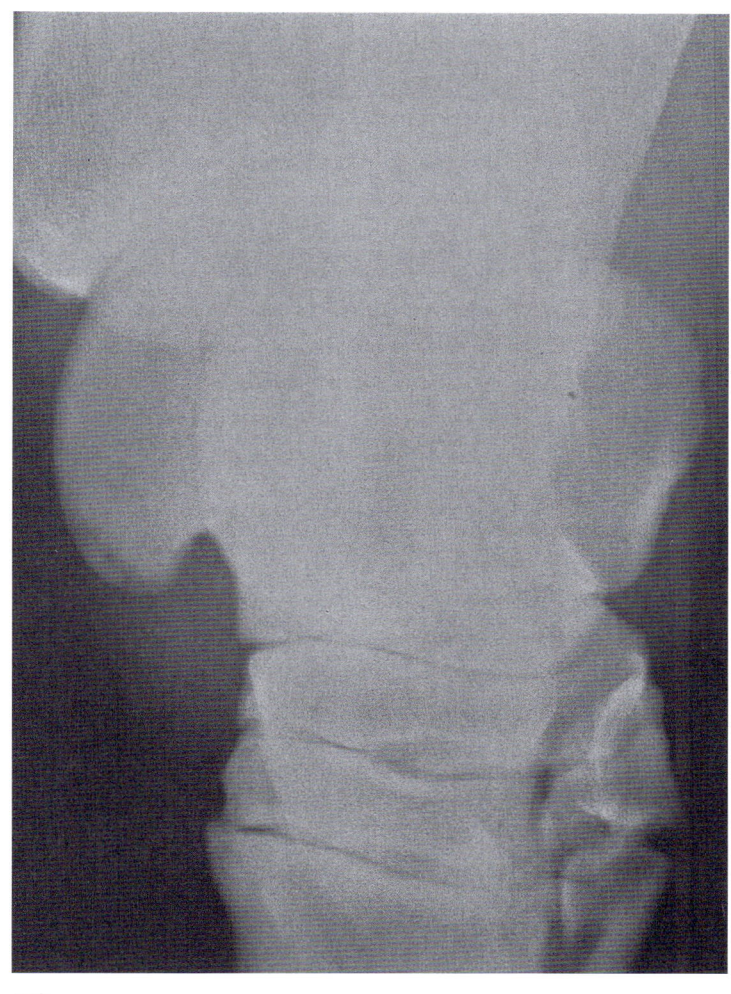

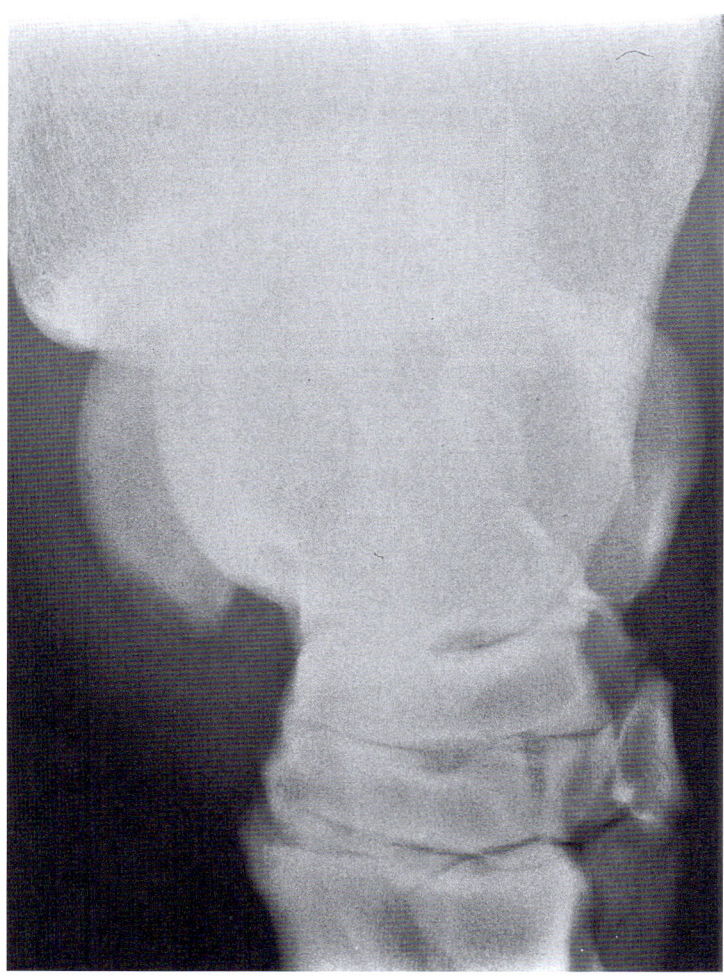

472

473

472/473 Right hock joint, serial dorsomedial-plantarolateral oblique views.

Warmblood, 4 years.

The initial view (Fig. 472), 2 weeks after the onset of acute severe lameness, reveals a bony fragment at the distal end of the lateral trochlear ridge of the tibial tarsal bone, separated from the underlying bone tissue by a narrow ill defined radiolucent zone.

Three weeks later (Fig. 473) the fragment has almost disappeared. Contrary to foals (Fig. 505, 514), in adult horses spontaneous disappearance of an osteochondrosis fragment is improbable. Clinical examination demonstrated a penetrating wound and synovial fluid analysis indicated infectious arthritis. Therefore, the fragment disappearance actually represents spontaneous resolution of a sequestrum, the focal subchondral sequestration possibly introduced by the perforating trauma.

Osteomyelitis

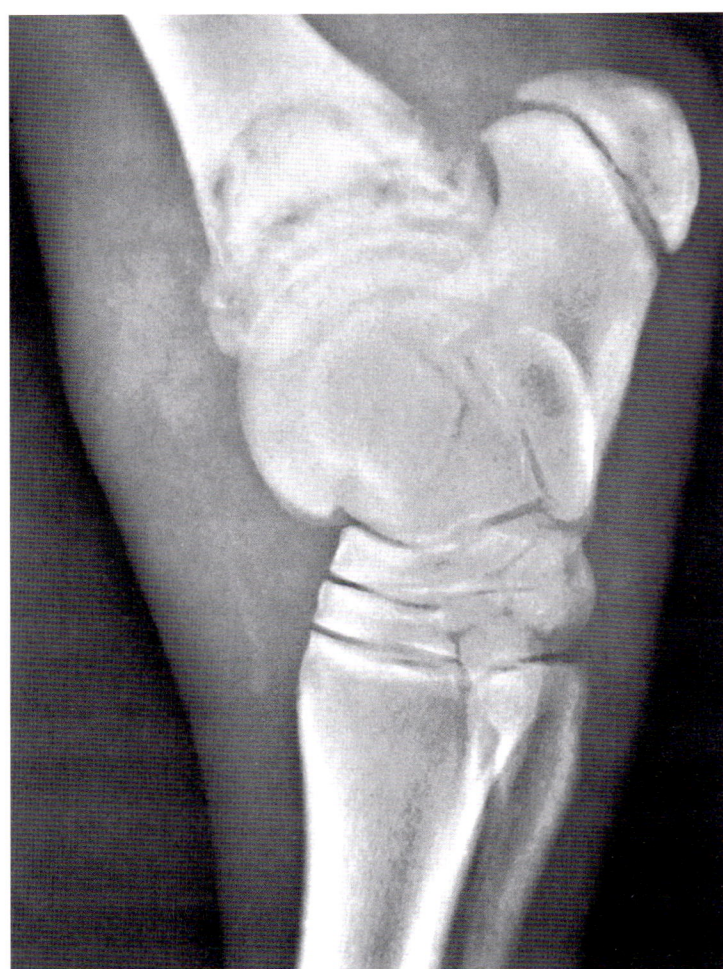

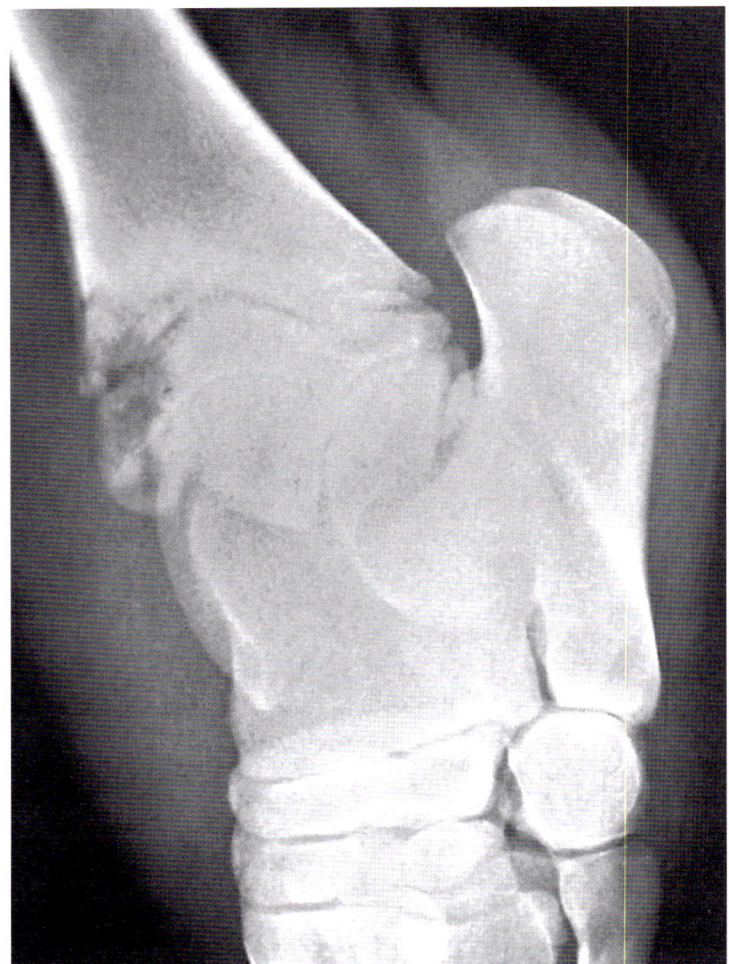

474 Left hock joint, lateromedial view.

Foal, 2 months.

Soft tissue swelling, most prominent dorsal to the distal tibia, and a zone of irregular radiolucency extending along the entire tibial physis, characteristic of haematogeneous osteomyelitis type P in young foals. The lesion shows an irregular radiopaque pattern surrounded by a radiolucent zone, indicative of sequestrum formation.

475 Right hock joint, dorsolateral-plantaromedial oblique view.

Foal, 1 month.

Minimal subperiosteal new bone along the dorsomedial aspect of the metaphysis and a large area of irregular radiolucency in the corresponding portion of the tibial metaphysis and epiphysis, indicating focal osteomyelitis type P. Effusion of the tibiotarsal joint suggests concomitant infectious arthritis.

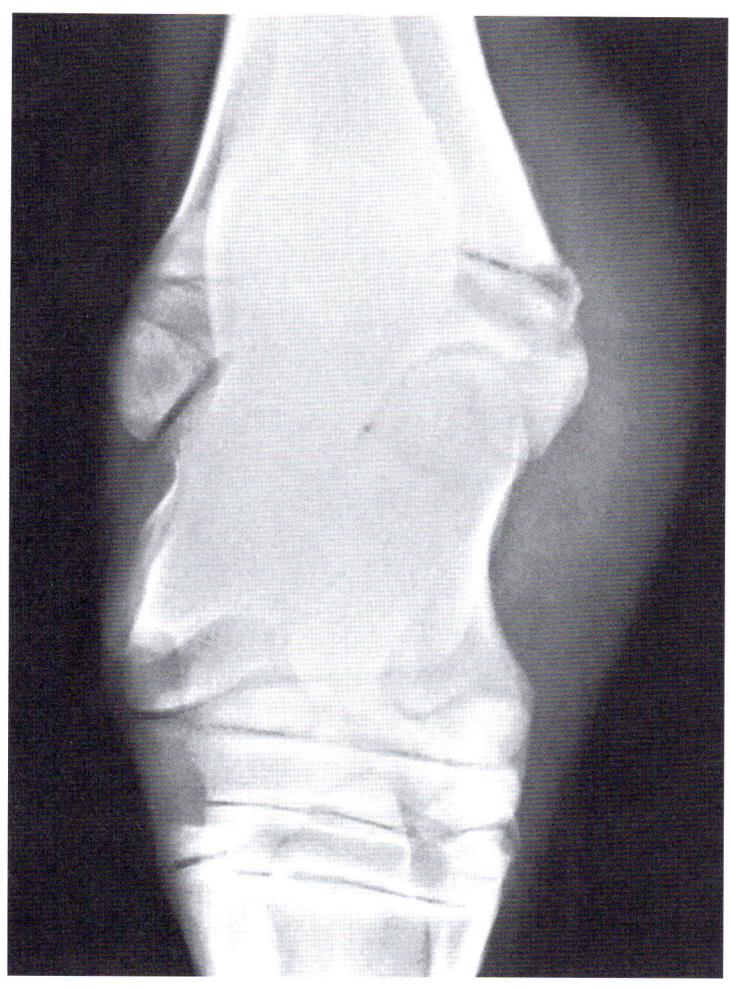

476 Right hock joint, dorsoplantar view.

Foal, 7 weeks.

Extensive soft tissue swelling along the medial aspect of the hock joint and most prominent over the distal tibial physis, minimal subperiosteal new bone along the medial aspect of metaphysis, and an ill bordered radiolucent area within the medial part of the tibial metaphysis in close connection with the physis, indicating focal osteomyelitis type P.

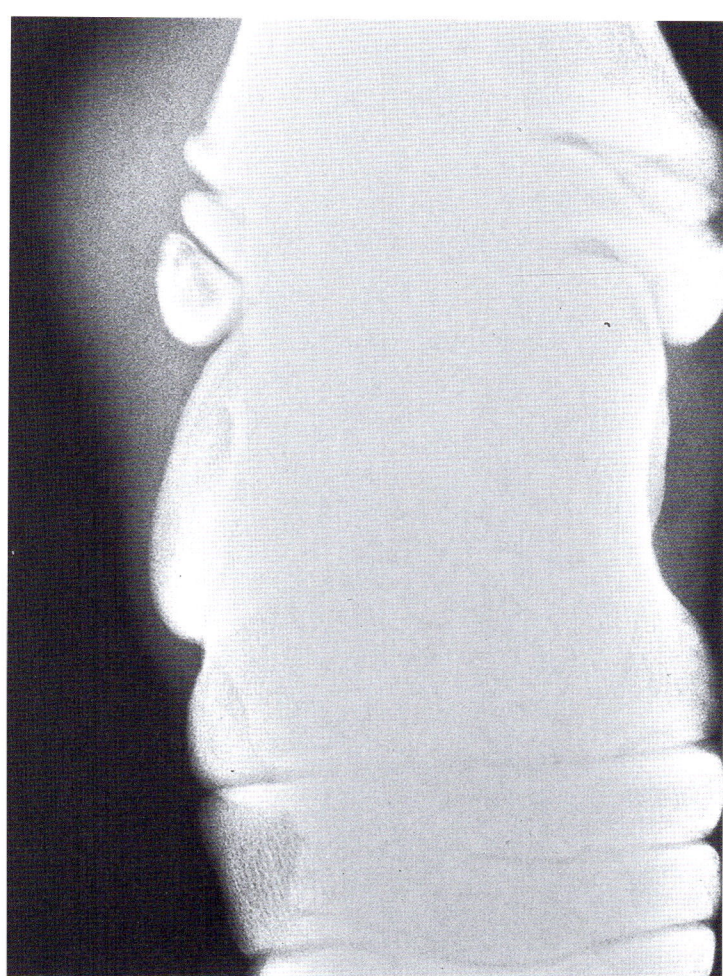

477 Right hock joint, dorsoplantar view: close-up.

Foal, 1 month.

Soft tissue swelling, most prominent lateral to the distal tibia, and a well defined radiolucent area in the lateral malleolus. The appearance mimics haemotogenous osteomyelitis type E, but in this foal resulted from soft tissue abscessation and subsequent infection of underlying bone.

The radiopaque center of the malleolar lesion indicates sequestrum formation.

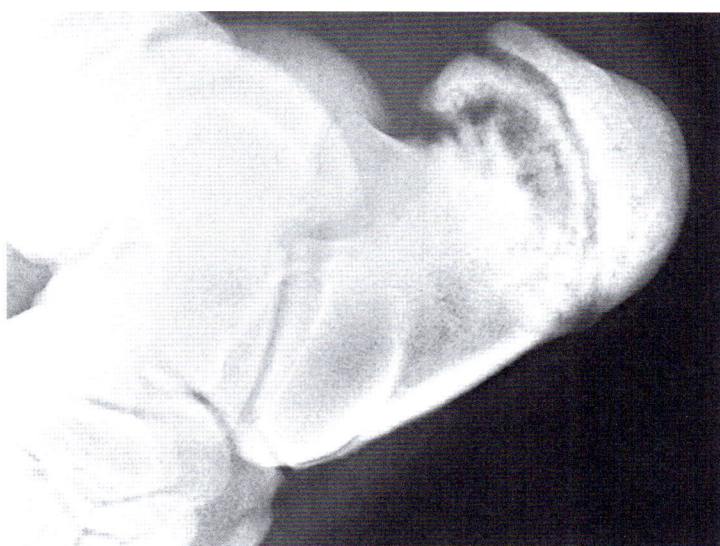

478 Right hock joint, lateromedial (flexed) view: close-up.

Foal, 3 months.

A zone of irregular radiolucency in the body of the fibular tarsal bone extending along the entire physis, resulting from osteomyelitis type P. The disruption of the dorsal cortex and radiolucency of the adjacent portion of the bone lesion indicate advanced bone lysis, implying the risk of pathological fracture.

Osteomyelitis

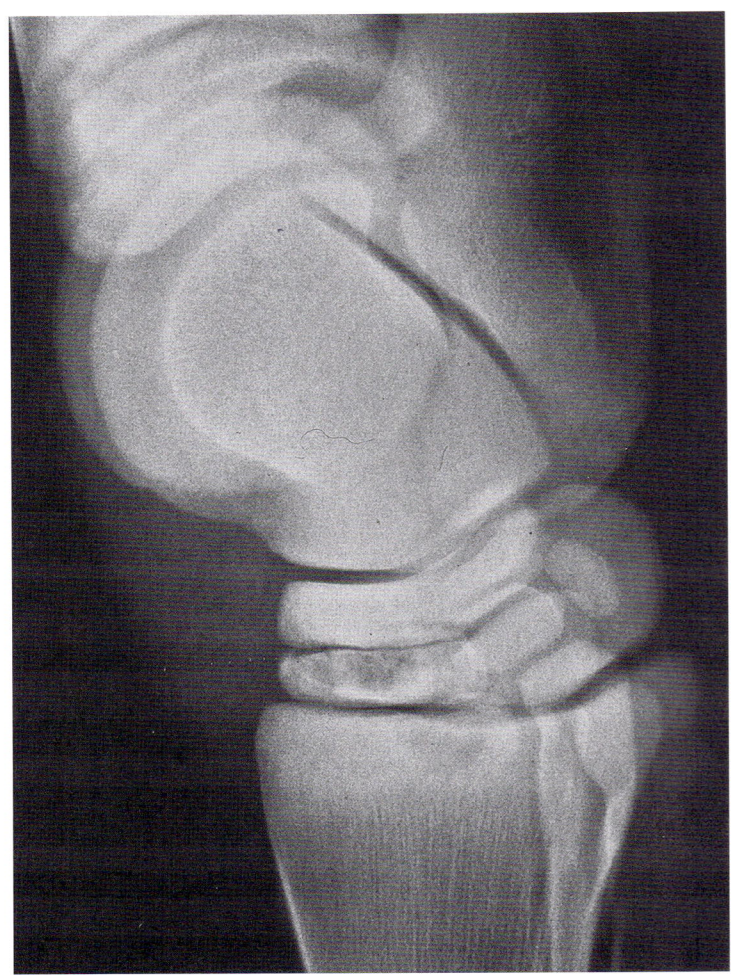

479

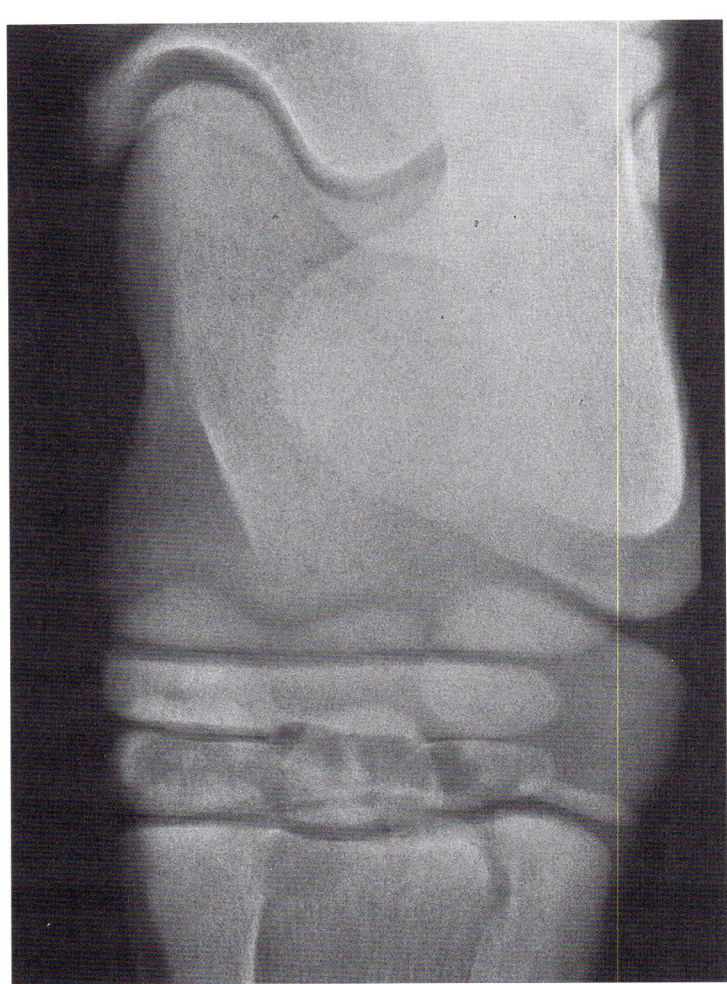

480

479/480/481/482 Left hock joint, serial lateromedial and dorsoplantar views.

Foal, 3 weeks.

The initial lateromedial (Fig. 479) and dorsoplantar view (Fig. 480) shows soft tissue swelling over the small tarsal bones, irregular radiolucency of the third tarsal bone, an ill bordered area of subchondral lucency in the proximomedial aspect of the third metatarsal bone and obvious narrowing of the distal intertarsal joint. Clinical and laboratory data revealed infectious arthritis/osteomyelitis. The radiographic appearance mimics tarsal bone collapse due to incomplete ossification (Fig. 454, 455, 456, 457), but the narrowing of the distal intertarsal joint and the absence of wedging of the central and/or third tarsal bone are in contradiction with this condition.

Follow-up examination 1½ year later (Fig. 481, 482) demonstrates subsequent osteoarthrosis, characterised by diffuse obliteration, i.e. ankylosis of the distal intertarsal joint and prominent spurring of the dorsoproximal aspect of the third metatarsal bone.

The subchondral area of radiolucency in the proximomedial aspect of the third metatarsal bone remains visible and is surrounded by a sclerotic rim. The irregular radiolucency of the third tarsal bone is blurred.

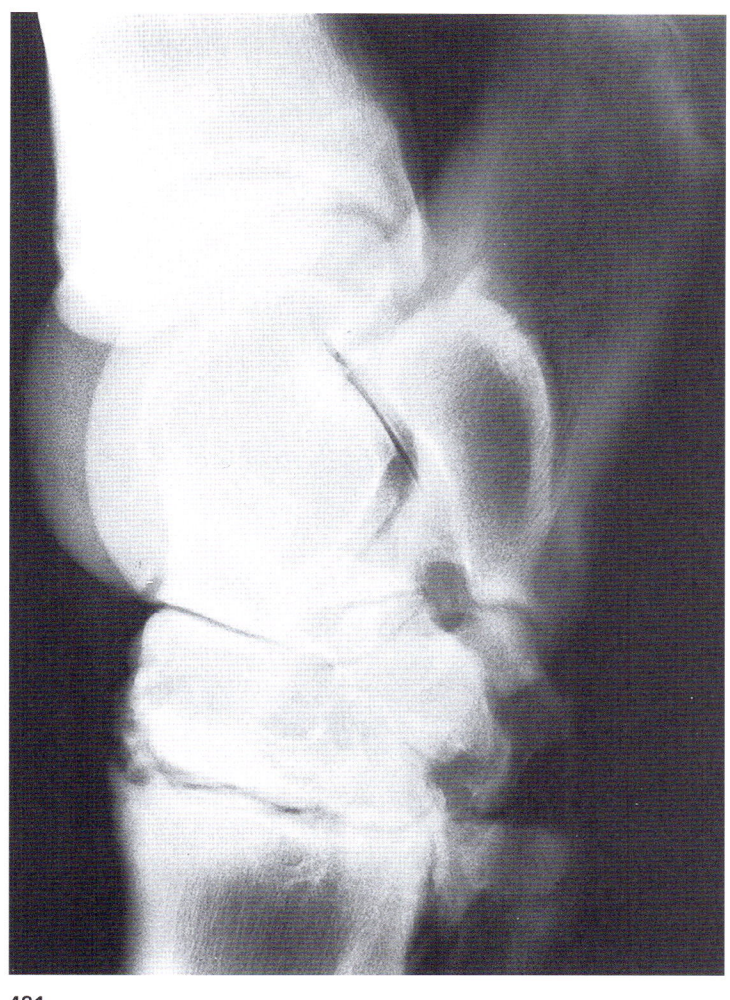

481

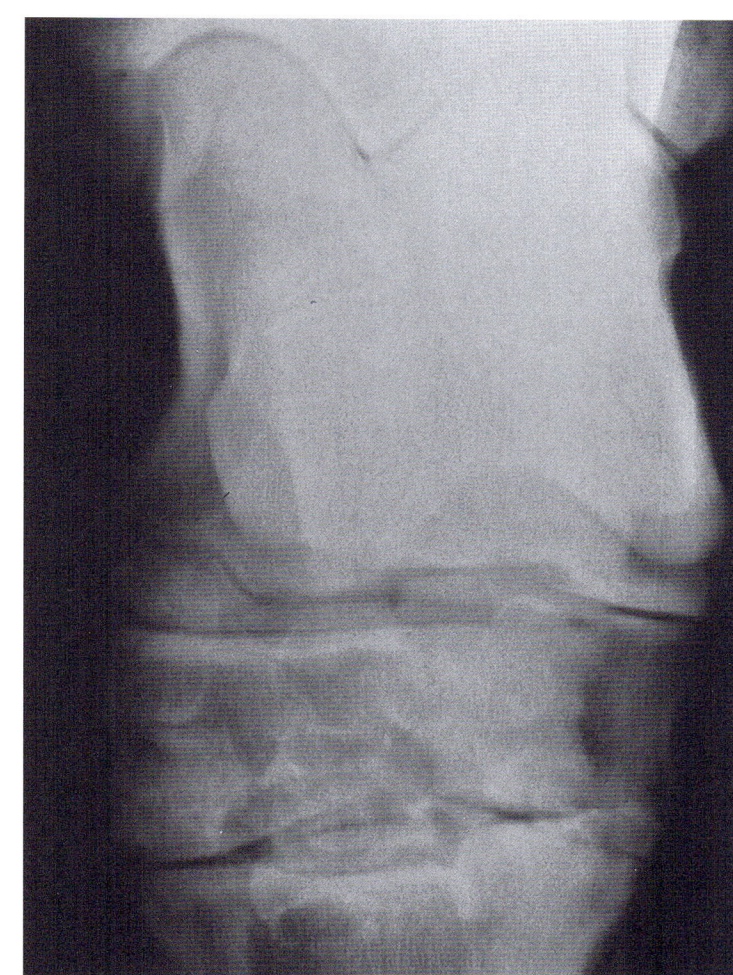

482

Osteomyelitis

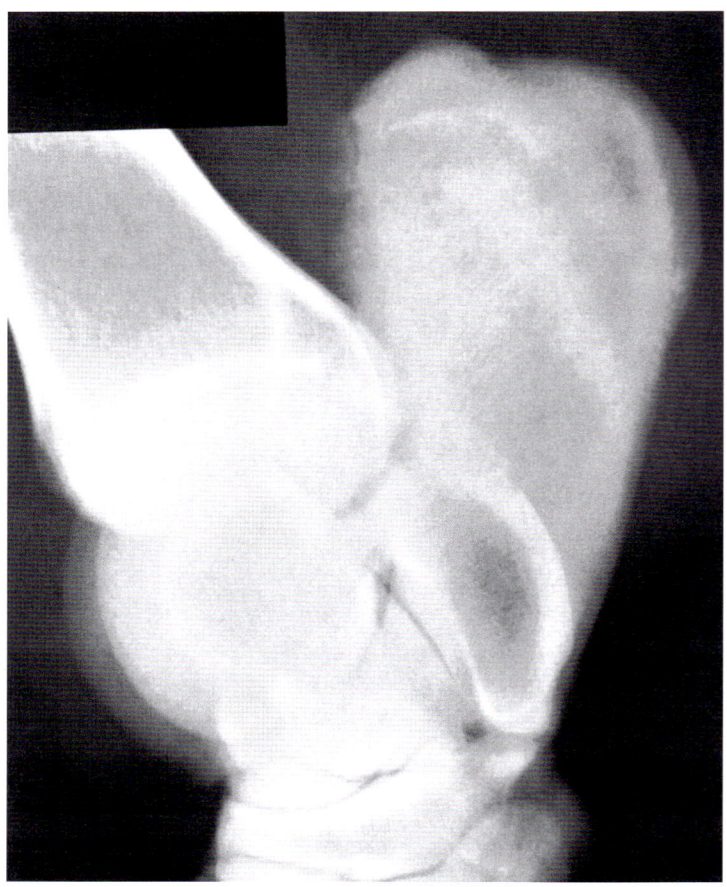

483

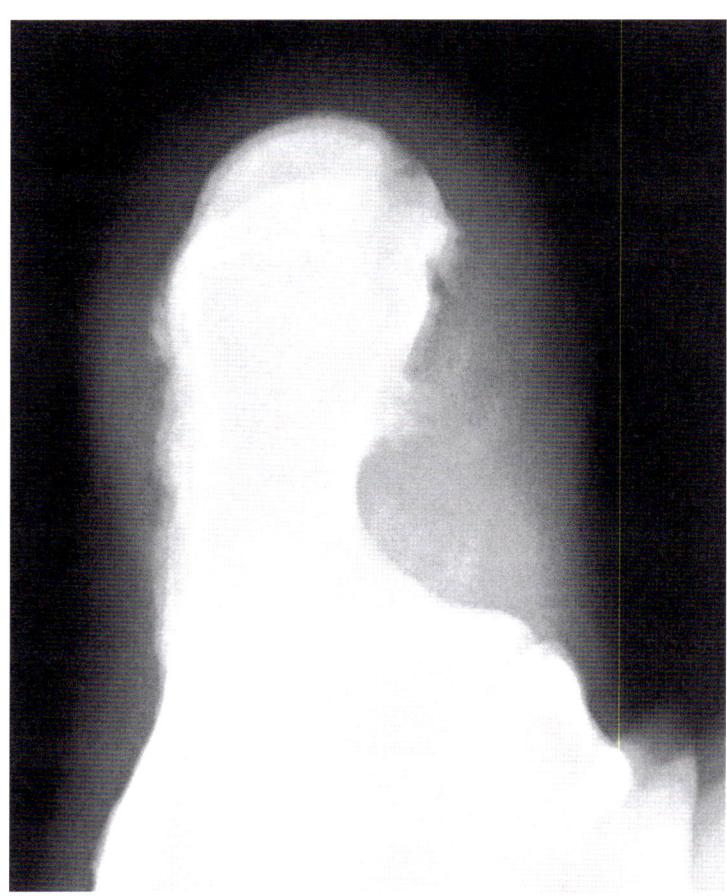

484

483/484 Right hock joint, lateromedial (Fig. 483) and dorsoplantar (flexed) "skyline" view (Fig. 484).

Warmblood, 11 years.

The soft tissue swelling over the fibular tarsal bone, the irregular layer of periosteal new bone on the dorsal, lateral and medial aspect of the fibular tarsal bone, and the obscure radiolucent area within the medial aspect of the tuber calcis are a consequence of osteomyelitis, introduced by a puncture wound 1 month prior to the examination.

The periosteal new bone is immature, as indicated by its ill defined border.

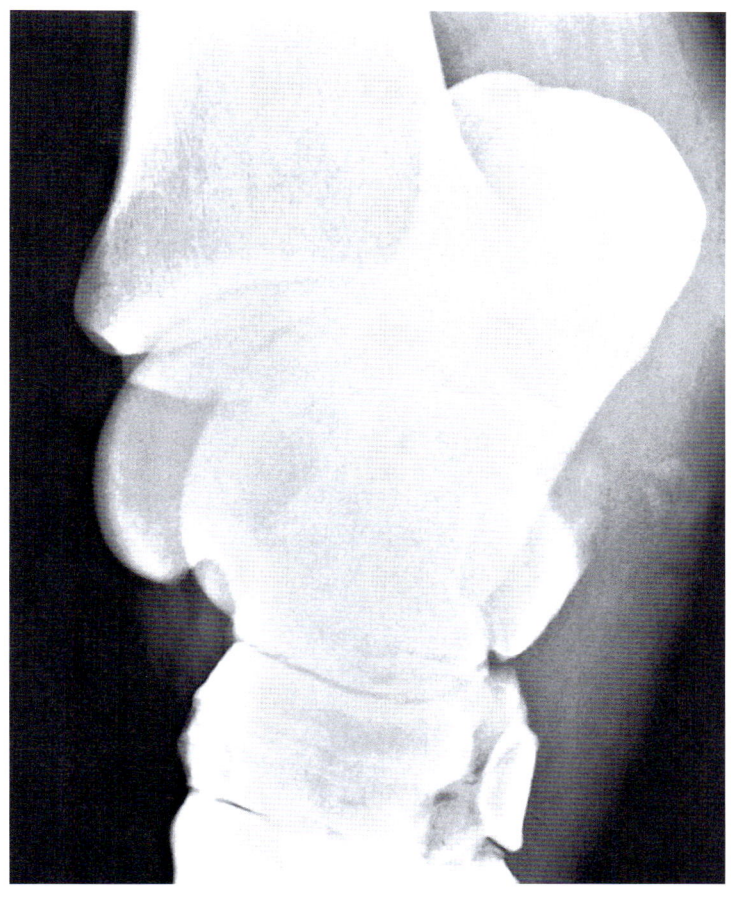

485 Right hock joint, dorsomedial-plantarolateral oblique view.
Warmblood, 16 years.

Soft tissue swelling plantar to the fibular tarsal bone, due to distension of the tarsal sheath, and a large irregularly radiolucent area in the proximomedial aspect of the sustentaculum are indicative of the presence of focal osteomyelitis induced by a perforating wound of the tarsal sheath, sustained 2 weeks previously.

The well defined irregular opacity plantar to the sustentaclulum is caused by scurf on the skin, resulting from the draining wound.

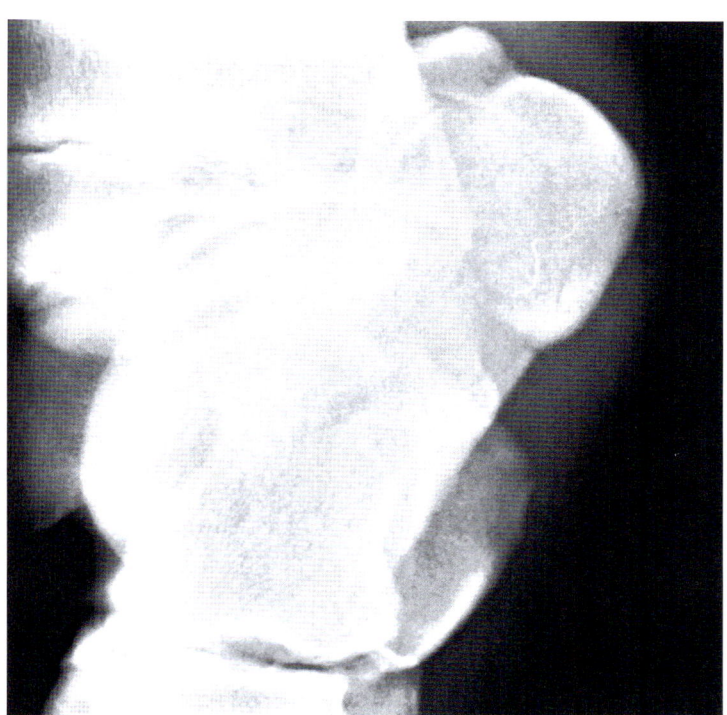

486 Left hock joint, dorsomedial-plantarolateral oblique view: close-up.
Warmblood, 1½ years.

Minimal soft tissue swelling plantar to the fibular tarsal bone, due to distension of the tarsal sheath, and an obscure radiolucency in the proximomedial aspect of the sustentaculum are indicative of the early stages of focal osteomyelitis of the sustentaculum induced by a perforating wound of the tarsal sheath, sustained 4 days prior to the examination.

Bone sequestration

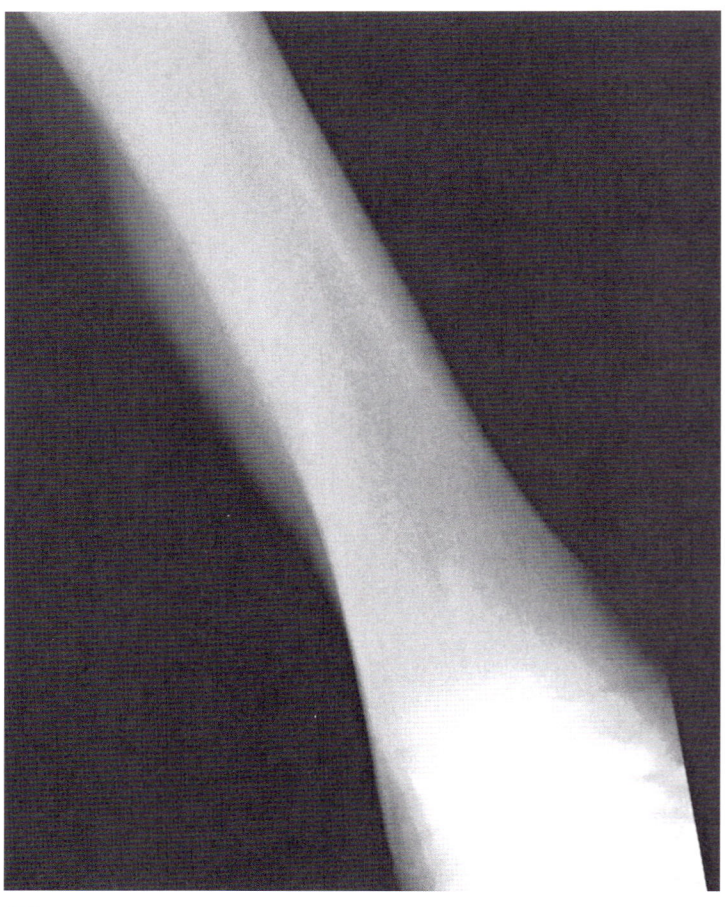

487

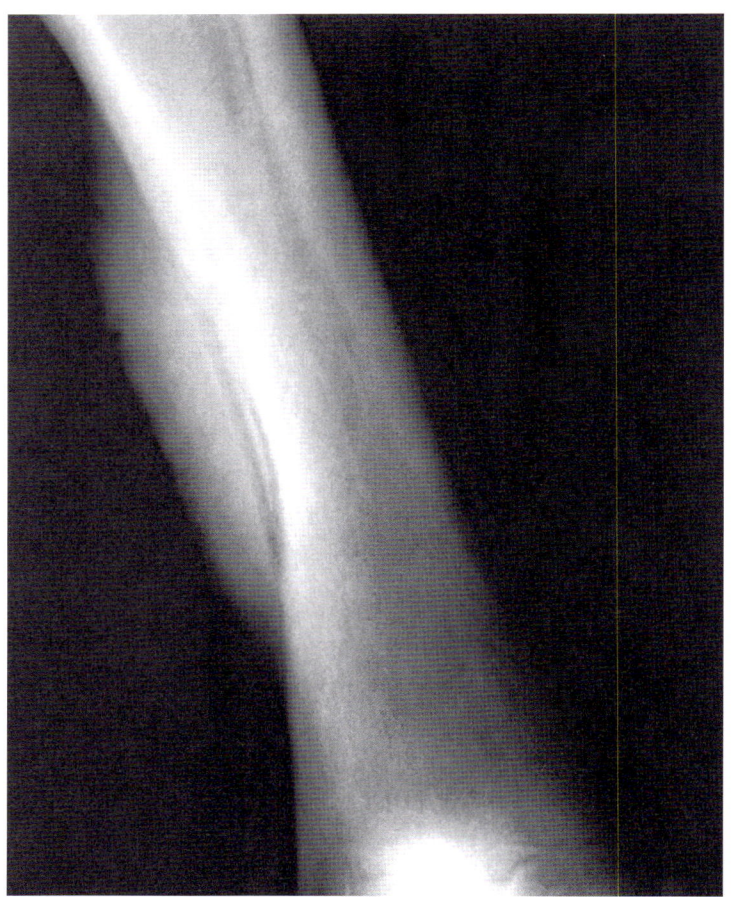

488

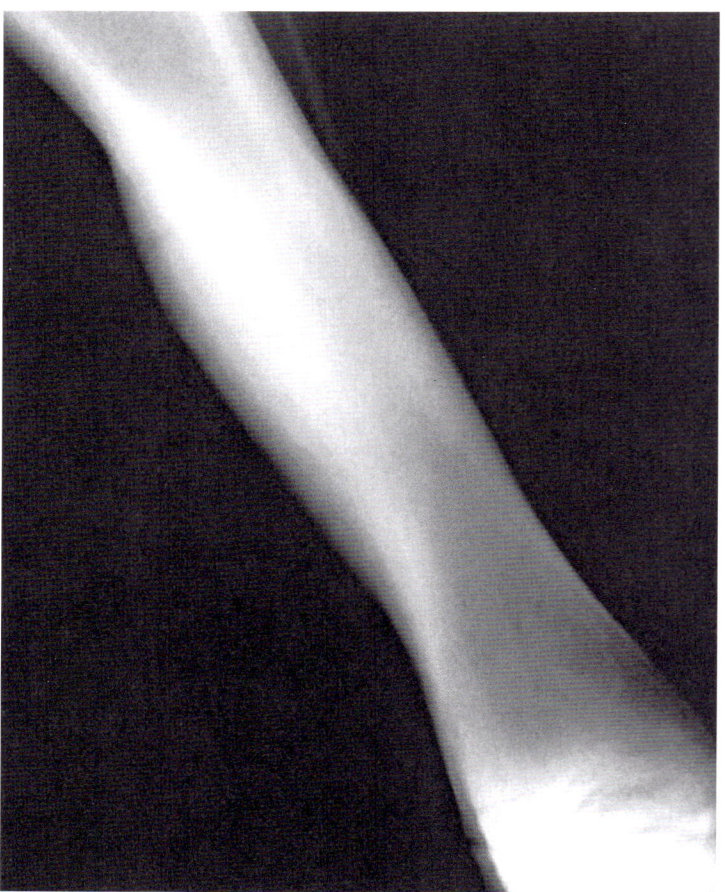

489

487/488/489 Left tibia, serial lateromedial views.

Warmblood, 1 year.

The initial examination (Fig. 487), 2 weeks after the onset of lameness of unknown origin, reveals an ill bordered layer of periosteal new bone on the mid-dorsal aspect of the tibia. Ten days later (Fig. 488) a long, thin bone fragment has separated from the underlying portion of the outer tibial cortex, indicating sequestration. The periosteal new bone, completely covering the sequestrum, is thicker and denser, but still immature, as indicated by its indistinct margin.

Two weeks later (Fig. 489), 38 days after the onset of lameness, the sequestrum has disappeared and the periosteal new bone formation has stopped, as indicated by its distinct margin.

N. B. Sequestration of the outer cortex is most frequently associated with a draining wound and is a consequence of severe injury and infection of the periosteum, resulting in disruption of the blood supply of the outer cortex of the bone. In most cases the necrotic piece of cortical bone no longer possesses a periosteal layer, and reactive periosteal new bone develops only on adjacent normal bone. Peripheral cortical sequestration following and completely covered by periosteal new bone without an accompanying draining wound is a rare phenomenon, which may result from separation of intact periosteum from the underlying cortex, probably due to subperiosteal haemorrhage.

Spontaneous resorption of a sequestrum, although possible, is seldom observed.

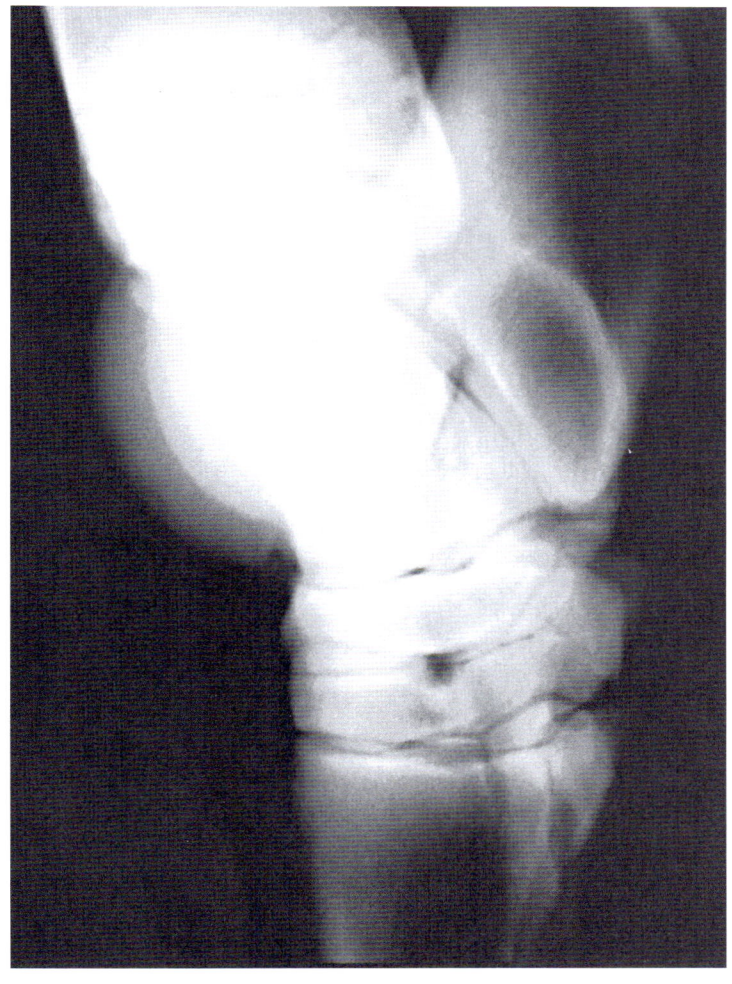

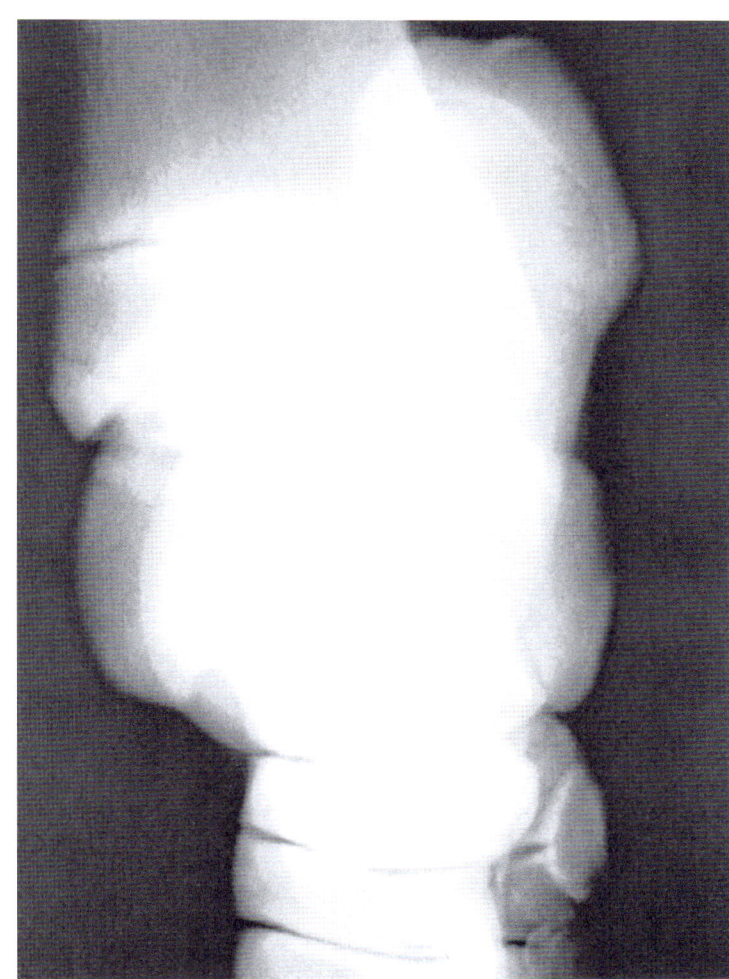

490

491

490/491 Left hock joint, lateromedial and dorsomedial-plantarolateral oblique view.

Standardbred, 1 year.

The lateromedial view (Fig. 490) shows an obscure bony fragment at the cranial aspect of the intermediate ridge of the tibia. Effusion of the tibiotarsal joint is not present. As usual the bony fragment is more obvious on a dorsomedial-plantarolateral oblique projection (Fig. 491). This view also reveals flattening and irregular radiolucency in the corresponding portion of the intermediate ridge.

N. B. One (or more) bony fragment(s) associated with a corresponding defect in the cranial aspect of the intermediate ridge of the tibia is the most common manifestation of osteochondrosis of the hock joint. Associated joint effusion and lameness may or may not be present.

A clinically asymptomatic form may become symptomatic with appropriate exercise.

Osteochondrosis

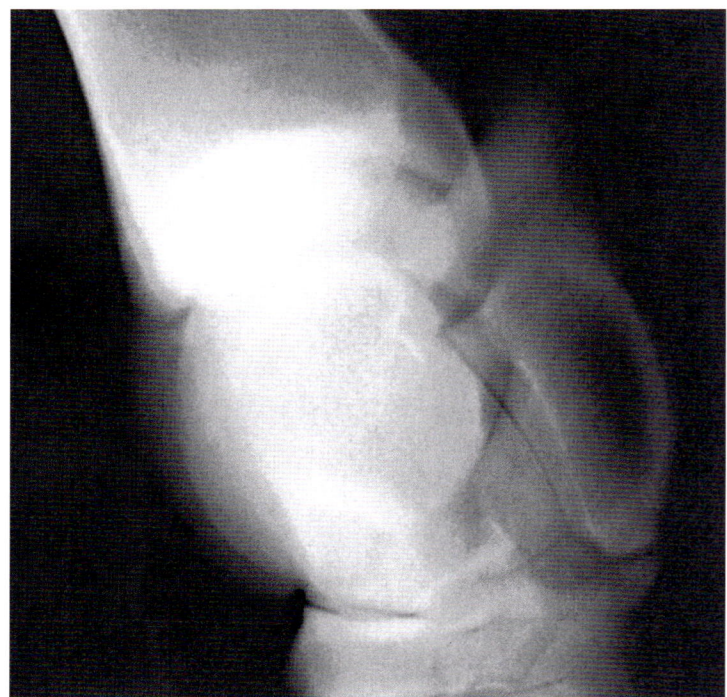

492

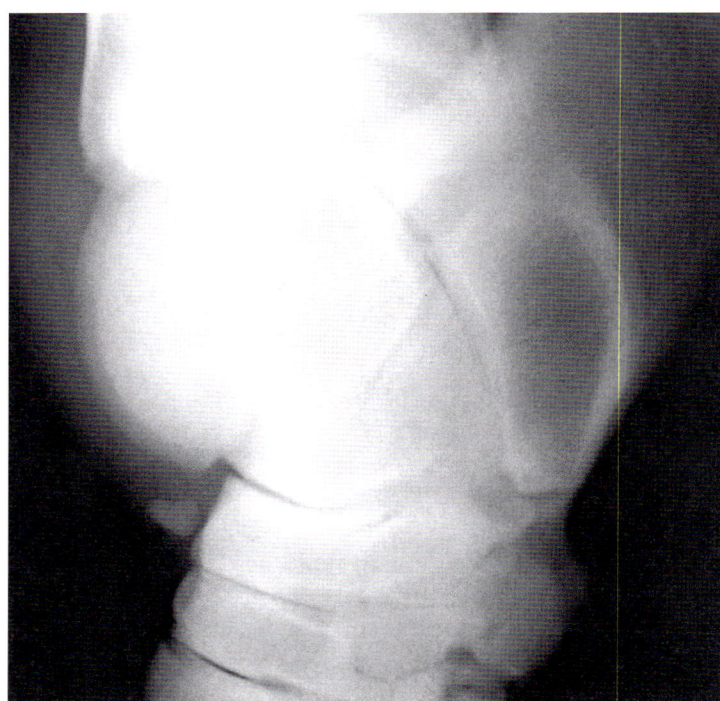

493

492/493 Left hock joint, serial lateromedial views: close-ups.

Warmblood, 3 years.

The initial lateromedial view (Fig. 492) reveals an obscure bony fragment at the cranial aspect of the intermediate ridge of the tibia. This could be referred to as an occult form of osteochondrosis, as indicated by the absence of joint effusion and lameness. The horse was put into training and 2 months later distension of the tibiotarsal joint and a moderate degree of lameness was observed.

On a second lateromedial view (Fig. 493), 2 weeks after the onset of lameness, the bony fragment is situated in the distal pouch of the tibiotorsal joint, indicating separation and displacement of the osteochondral fragment from the intermediate ridge.

The soft tissue swelling dorsal to the tibial tarsal bone represents associated joint effusion.

Additional finding: a small, insignificant, bony spur on the dorsoproximal aspect of the third metatarsal bone.

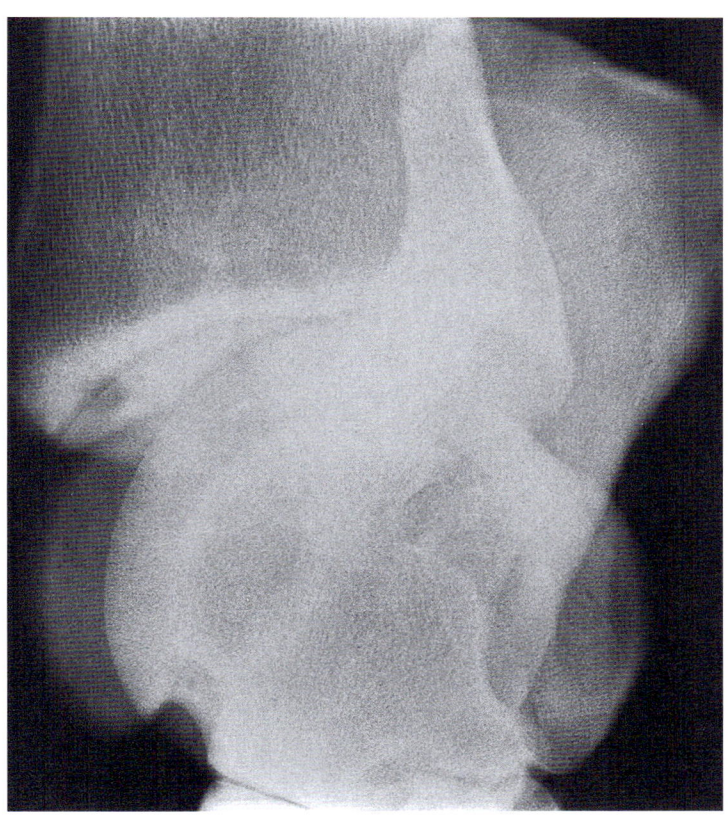

494 Left hock joint, dorsomedial-plantarolateral oblique view: close-up.

Warmblood, 3 years.

The rounded area of radiolucency in the cranial region of the intermediate ridge of the tibia mimics a subchondral bone cyst, but actually represents the remnant of an osteochondrosis lesion which has grown away from the joint surface (Fig. 506, 514). The differential diagnosis includes a cystic bone lesion in the proximal aspect of the lateral trochlear ridge of the tibial tarsal bone (Fig. 517, 518).

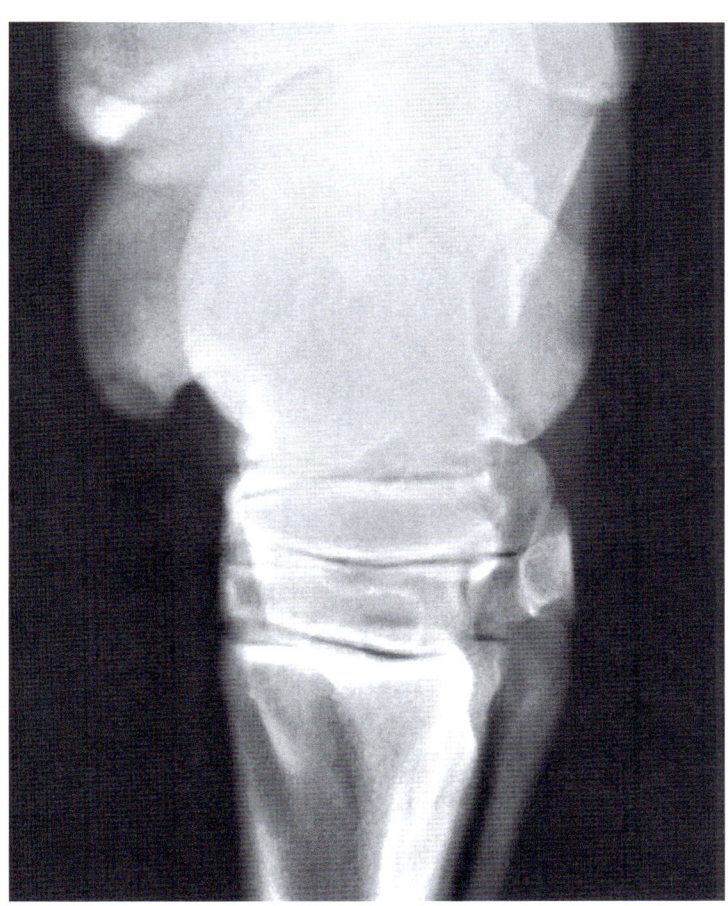

495 Right hock joint, dorsomedial-plantarolateral oblique view.

Standardbred, 1 year.

The bony fragment at the distal end of the lateral trochlear ridge of the tibial tarsal bone is a manifestation of osteochondrosis. The radiolucent zone between the fragment and the lateral trochlear ridge represents non-calcified tissue attaching the bony fragment to the tibial tarsal bone.

N. B. Osteochondrosis of the distal aspect of the lateral trochlear ridge occurs less frequently than osteochondrosis of the intermediate ridge of the tibia, but is more often associated with joint effusion and lameness.

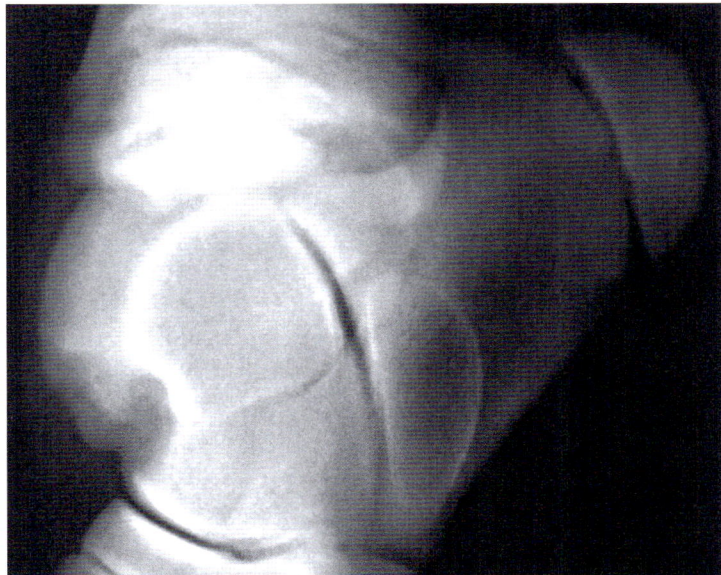

496 Left hock joint, lateromedial view: close-up.

Foal, 1 month.

The flattening and extensive irregular radiolucency of the distal aspect of the trochlea of the tibial tarsal bone represent the early stage of osteochondrosis.

Obscure soft tissue swelling dorsal to the tibial tarsal bone indicates minimal joint effusion.

The lesion is too large and too irregular to represent a (spontaneous healing) delayed ossification of the distal aspect of the trochlea of the tibial tarsal bone (Fig. 461). The absence of lameness, joint effusion and appropriate synovial fluid changes excluded a type E osteomyelitis (Fig. 460).

Osteochondrosis

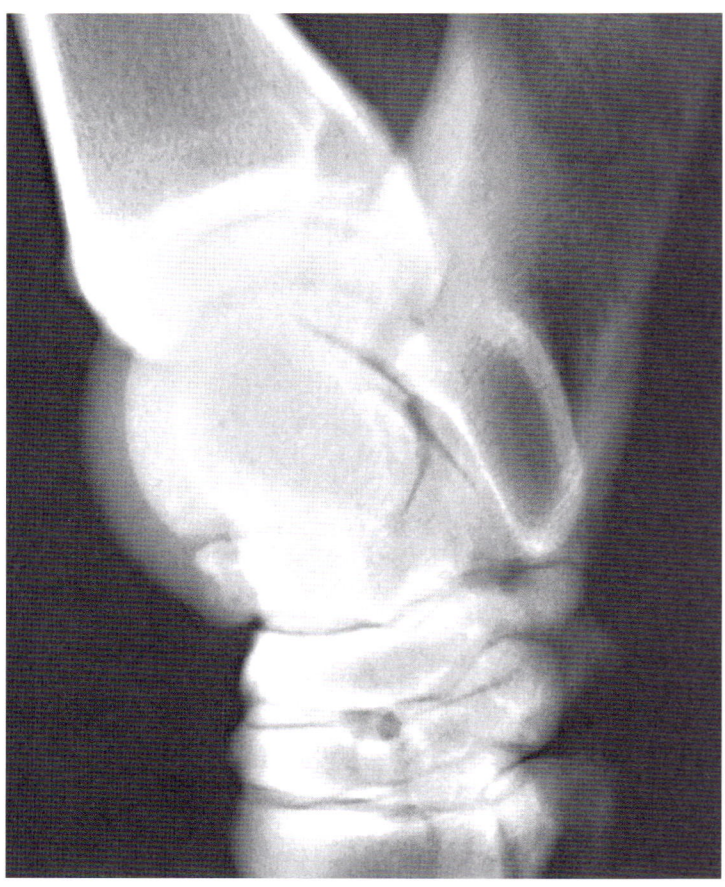

497

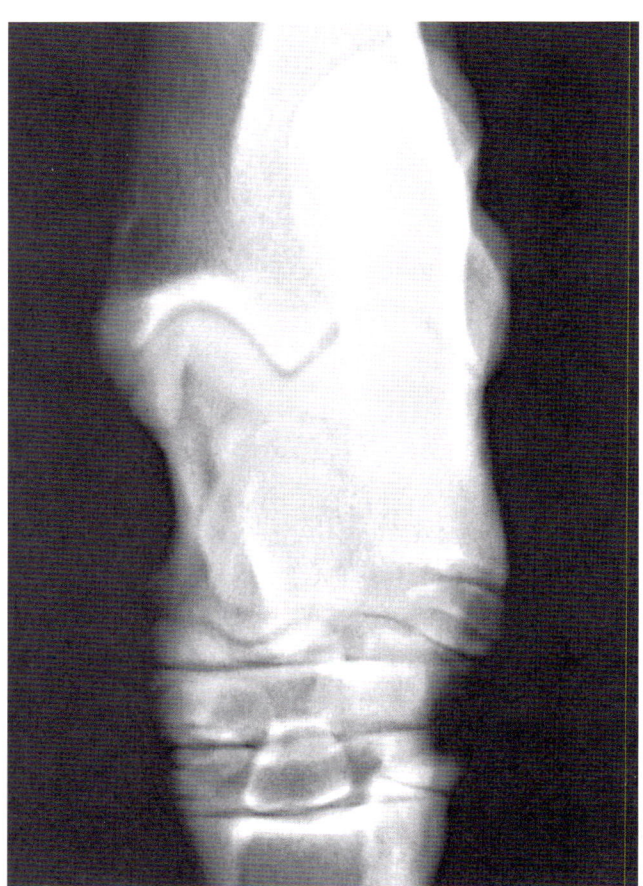

498

497/498 Left hock joint, lateromedial (Fig. 497) and dorsoplantar (Fig. 498) view.

Warmblood, 3 years.

The large bony fragment attached to the distal end of the lateral trochlear ridge of the tibial tarsal bone is a manifestation of osteochondrosis. Effusion of the tibiotarsal joint is not present.

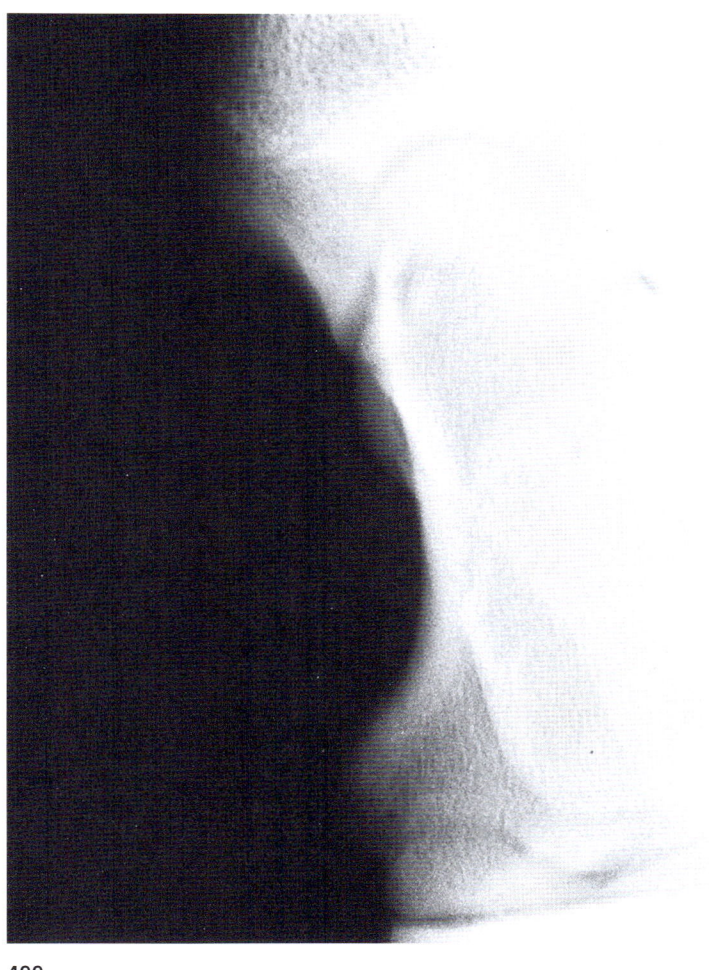

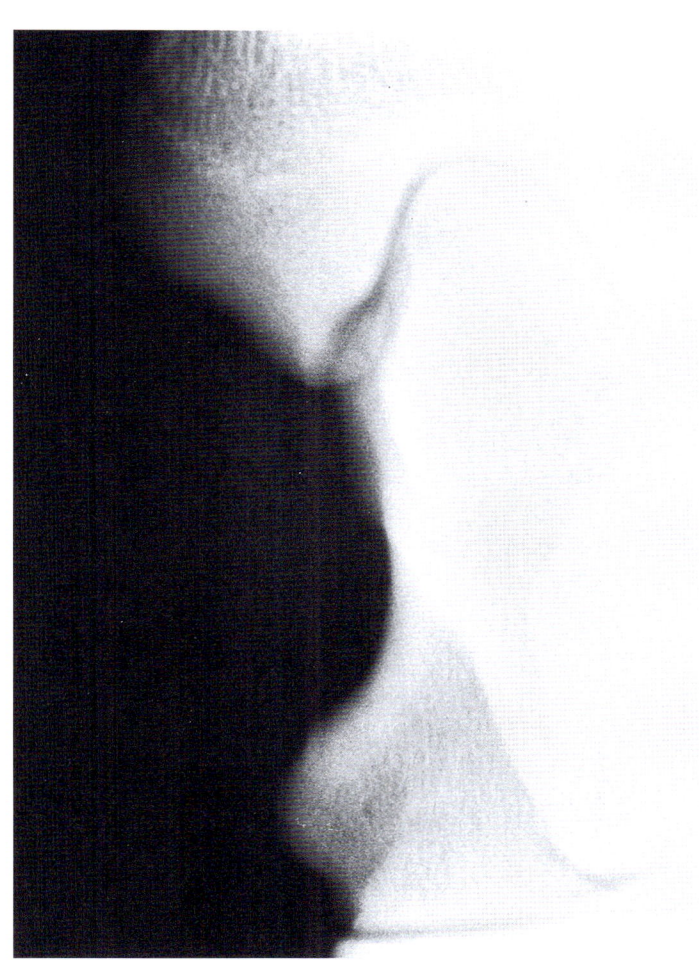

499

500

499/500 Left hock joint, dorsoplantar and slightly obliqued dorsoplantar view: close-ups.

Warmblood, 3 years.

The rounded fragment and corresponding contour defect involving the inner, i.e. articular surface of the medial malleolus represent a characteristic, but less common manifestation of osteochondrosis, and must not be confused with an avulsion fracture (Fig. 401). The fragment is most obvious on the dorso 20° lateral-plantaromedial oblique view (Fig. 500). On the standard dorsoplantar projection (Fig. 499) the lesion is obscured by superimposition of the medial trochlear ridge of the tibial tarsal bone.

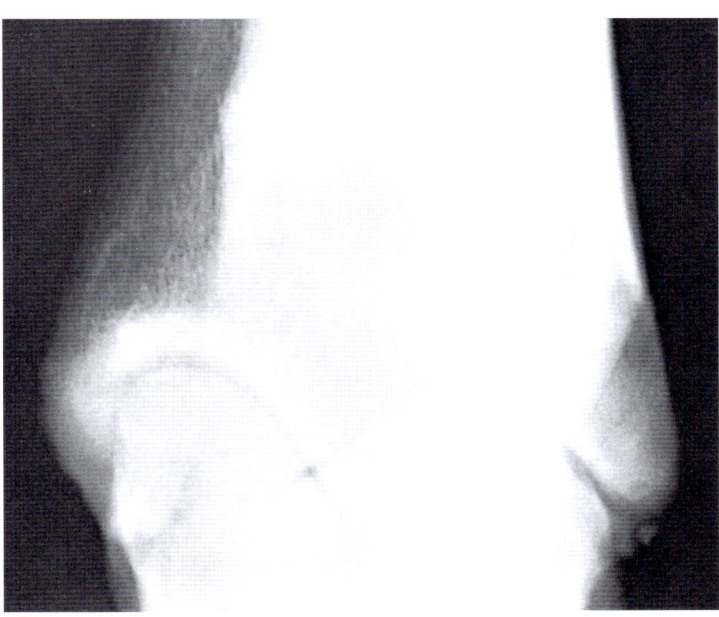

501 Left hock joint, dorsoplantar view: close-up.

Warmblood, 3 years.

The small, triangular, bony fragment at the distal end of the lateral malleolus is a seldom occurring manifestation of osteochondrosis, often unassociated with joint effusion and lameness.

Differential diagnosis includes fracture of the lateral malleolus (Fig. 399) and ligamentous calcification (Fig. 432).

Osteochondrosis

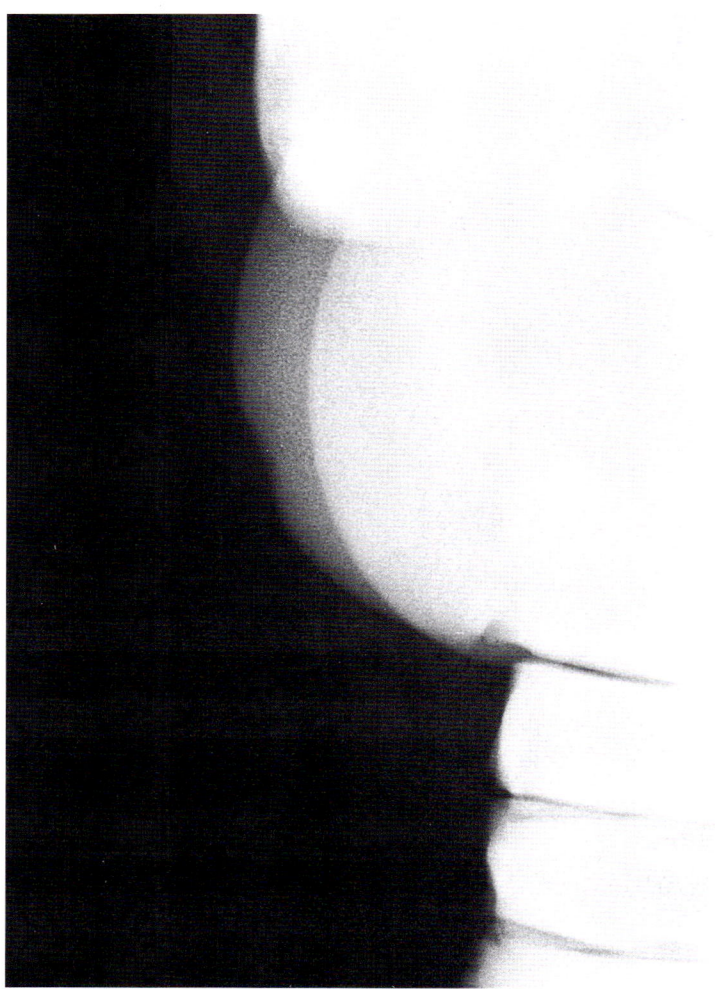

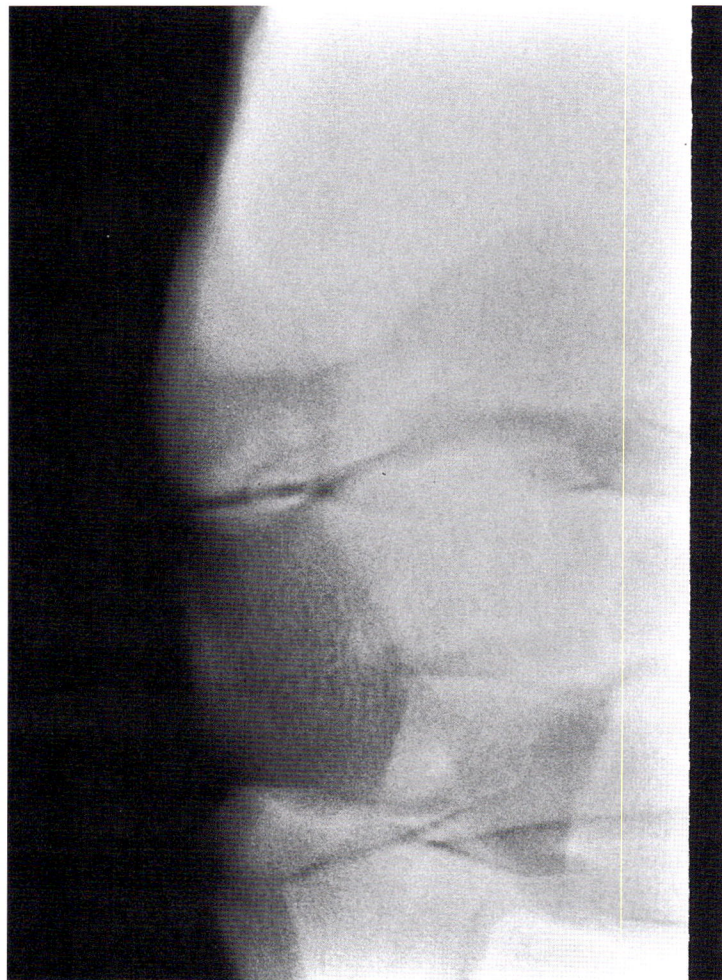

502 Left hock joint, lateromedial view: close-up.
Warmblood, 3 years.

The prominent flattening of the mid-distal contour of the medial trochlear ridge of the tibial tarsal bone is a less common form of osteochondrosis.

503 Right hock joint, dorsoplantar view: close-up.
Warmblood, 2 years.

The rounded bony fragment near the distolateral border of the tibial tarsal bone and superimposing the lateral region of the proximal intertarsal joint represents a seldom occuring manifestation of osteochondrosis.

Osteochondrosis development

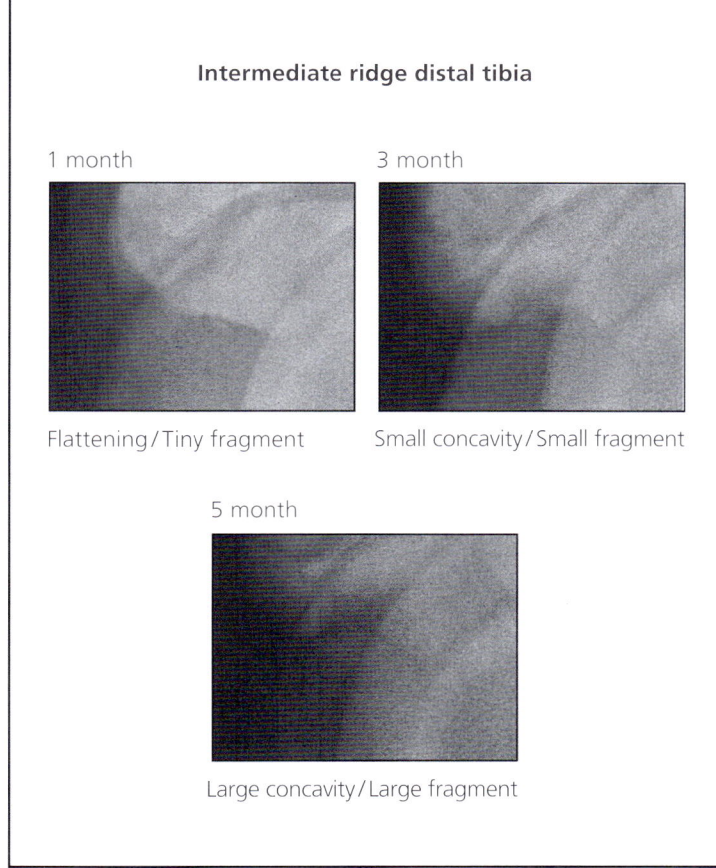

504

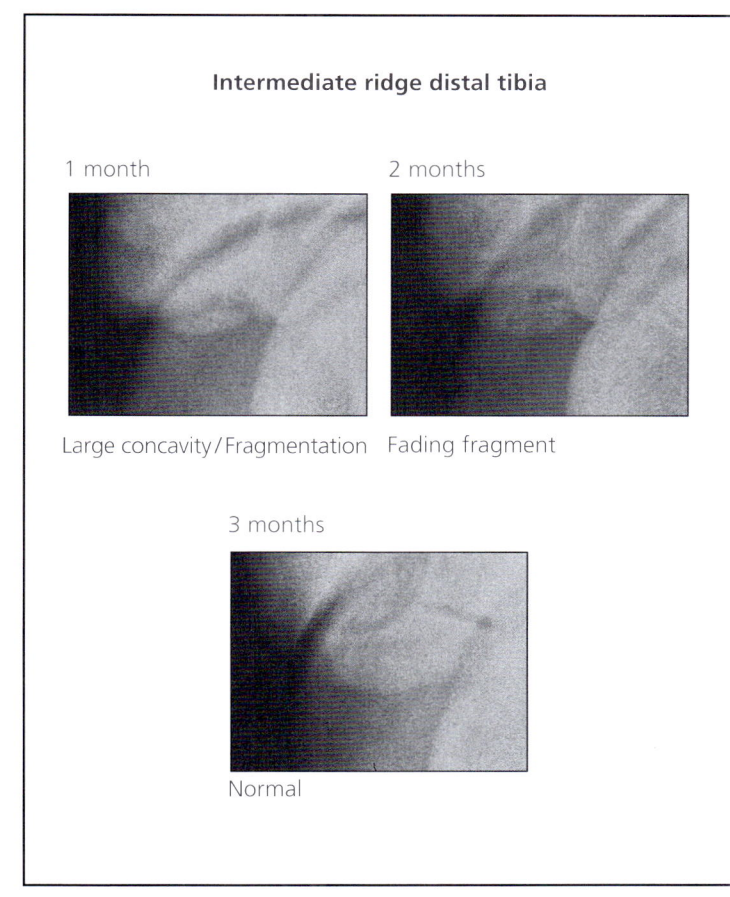

505

504/505 Intermediate ridge of the tibia, postnatal serial dorsomedial-plantarolateral oblique views: close-ups.

Abnormal appearances of the intermediate ridge of the tibia are relatively common at 1 month of age, the abnormalities varying from a smoothly or irregularly flattened bony contour to a small rounded or irregular concavity, with or without a corresponding bony fragment. Subsequently the majority of these lesions gradually disappear. However, progression is also possible and some of the initial abnormalities (± 25%) become permanent lesions. Normal initial appearances rarely develop into abnormal.

Lesions still existing at 5 months of age seldom resolve completely. The individual early development is variable and unpredictable. Initial flattening of the bony contour accompanied by a small bony fragment may be followed by progressive cavitation and fragmentation (Fig. 504). In contrast to this progression an initial concavity and a corresponding fragment may resolve completely (Fig. 505).

Osteochondrosis

Osteochondrosis development

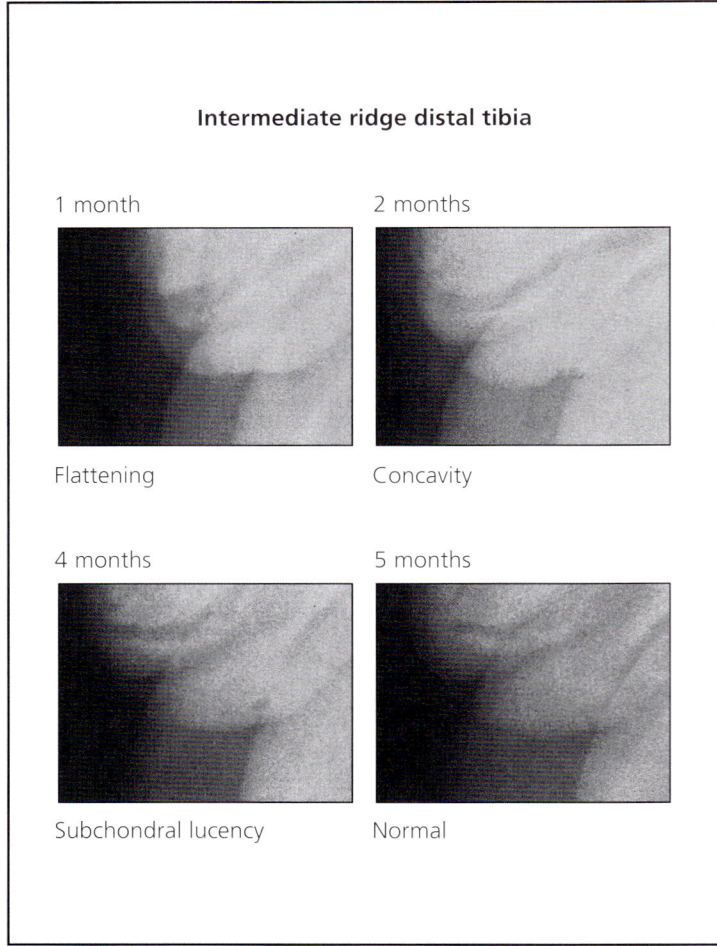

506

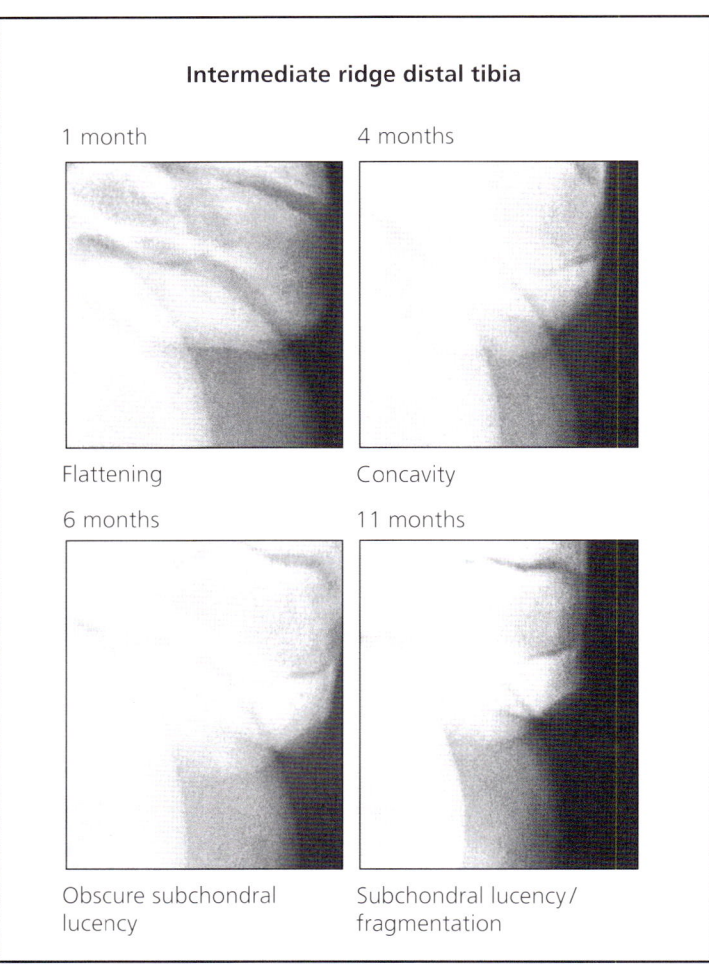

507

506/507 Intermediate ridge of the tibia, postnatal serial dorsomedial-plantarolateral oblique views: close-ups.

Initial flattening of the bony contour may also progress to a concavity which grows away from the joint surface thus becoming a rounded area of subchondral radiolucency mimicking a subchondral bone cyst, that may be permanent (Fig. 494) or resolves completely (Fig. 506).

From the age of 5 months permanent lesions may be stationary or develop further. This development may fluctuate, thus resulting in misleading instantaneous appearances, like initial flattening progressing to a concavity, followed by regression to obscure subchondral lucency, subsequently turning into fragmentation. (Fig. 507).

Osteochondrosis development

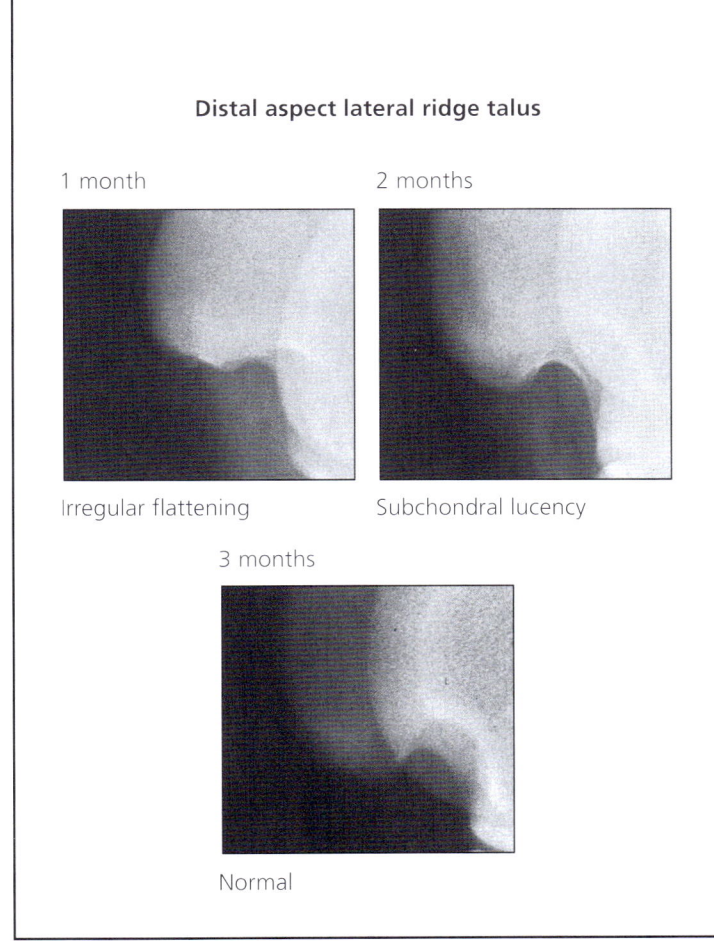

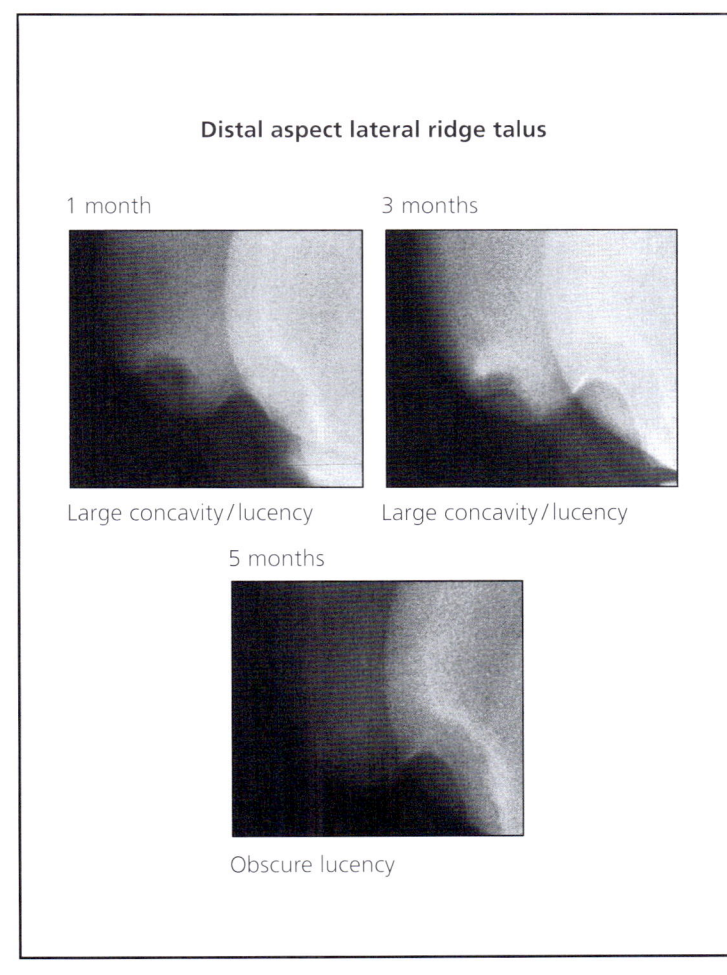

508

509

508/509 Distal aspect of the lateral trochlear ridge of the tibial tarsal bone, postnatal serial dorsomedial-plantarolateral oblique views: close-ups.

Abnormal appearances of the distal aspect of the lateral trochlear ridge of the tibial tarsal bone are far from uncommon at 1 month of age, but less common than on the intermediate ridge of the tibia.

These abnormalities vary from smooth or irregular flattening of the bony contour to large rounded or irregular concavities.

Almost all initial abnormalities (± 90%) gradually disappear, not only minor lesions such as irregular flattening (Fig. 508), but also large concavities (Fig. 509). Normal initial appearances rarely turn into abnormal.

Lesions still existing at 5 months of age usually become permanent.

Osteochondrosis

Osteochondrosis development

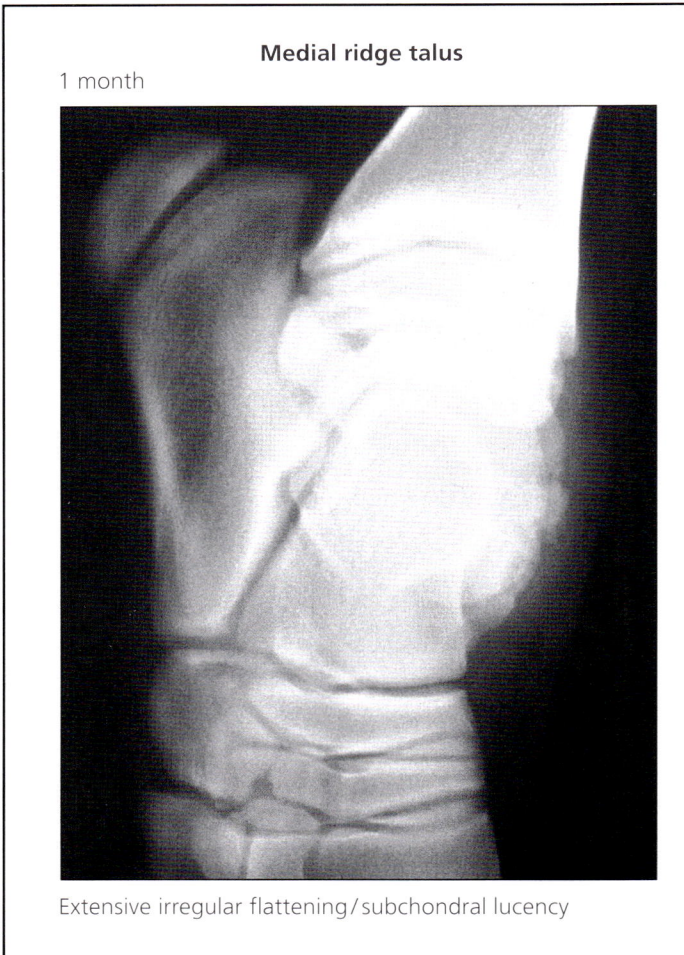

Medial ridge talus

1 month

Extensive irregular flattening/subchondral lucency

510

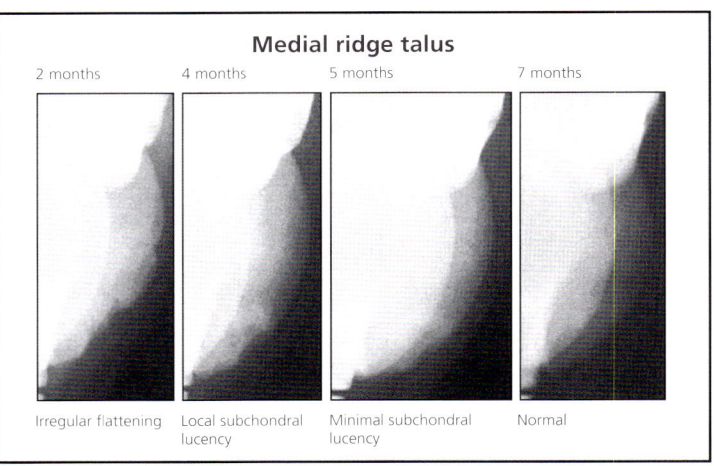

Medial ridge talus

2 months | 4 months | 5 months | 7 months

Irregular flattening | Local subchondral lucency | Minimal subchondral lucency | Normal

511

510/511 Medial trochlear ridge of the tibial tarsal bone, postnatal serial lateromedial views: initial survey and subsequent close-ups.

Abnormal appearances of the medial trochlear ridge of the tibial tarsal bone are seldom present at 1 month of age. Occasionally prominent irregular flattening is observed (Fig. 510). These lesions also show a clear tendency to regress and resolve completely (Fig. 511).

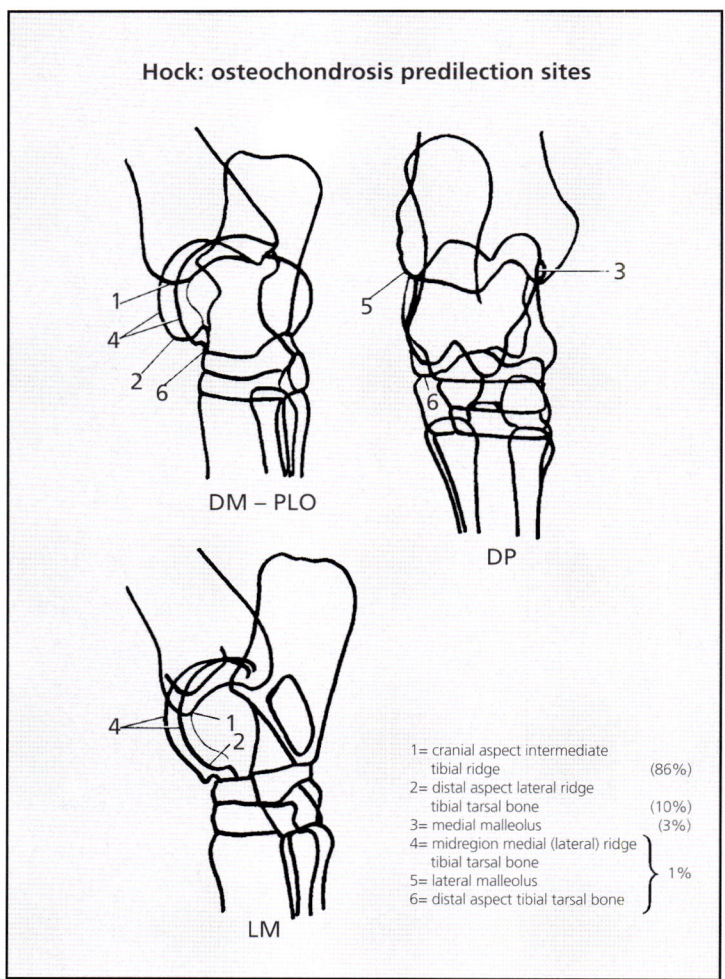

Hock: osteochondrosis predilection sites

DM – PLO

DP

LM

1= cranial aspect intermediate tibial ridge (86%)
2= distal aspect lateral ridge tibial tarsal bone (10%)
3= medial malleolus (3%)
4= midregion medial (lateral) ridge tibial tarsal bone
5= lateral malleolus } 1%
6= distal aspect tibial tarsal bone

512 Schematic drawing of the osteochondrosis predilection sites in the equine hock. The most common osteochondrosis locations are the cranial aspect of the intermediate ridge of the tibia and the distal aspect of the lateral trochlear ridge of the tibial tarsal bone. Less common sites are the inner, i.e. articular aspect of the medial malleolus, the mid region of the medial (or lateral) trochlear ridge of the tibial tarsal bone, the distal aspect of the lateral malleolus and the distolateral aspect of the tibial tarsal bone.

Osteochondrosis development

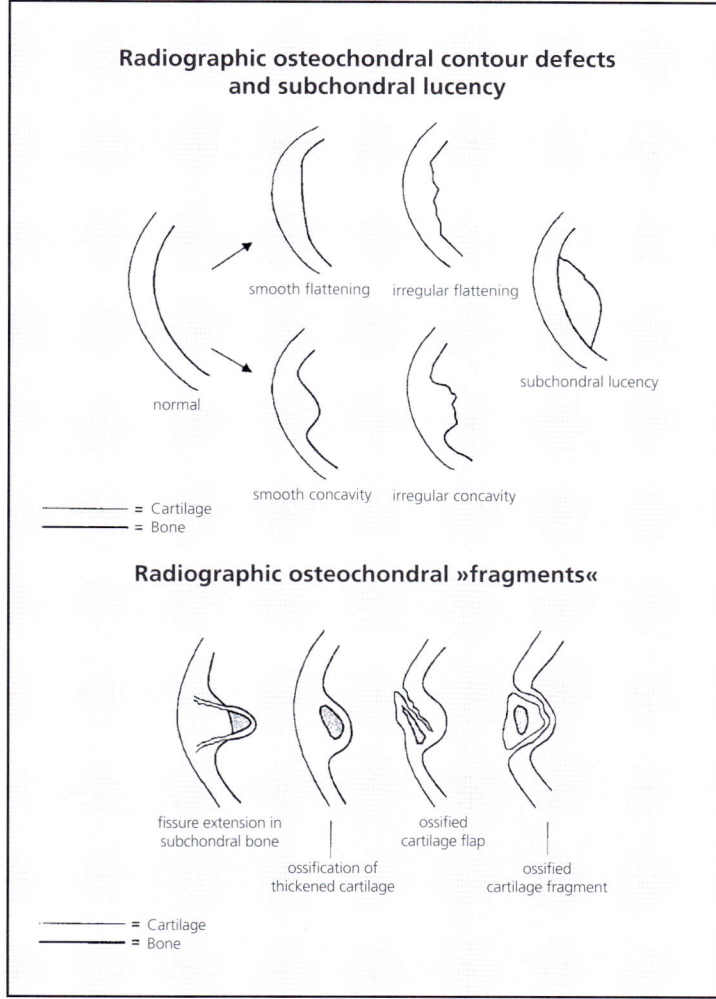

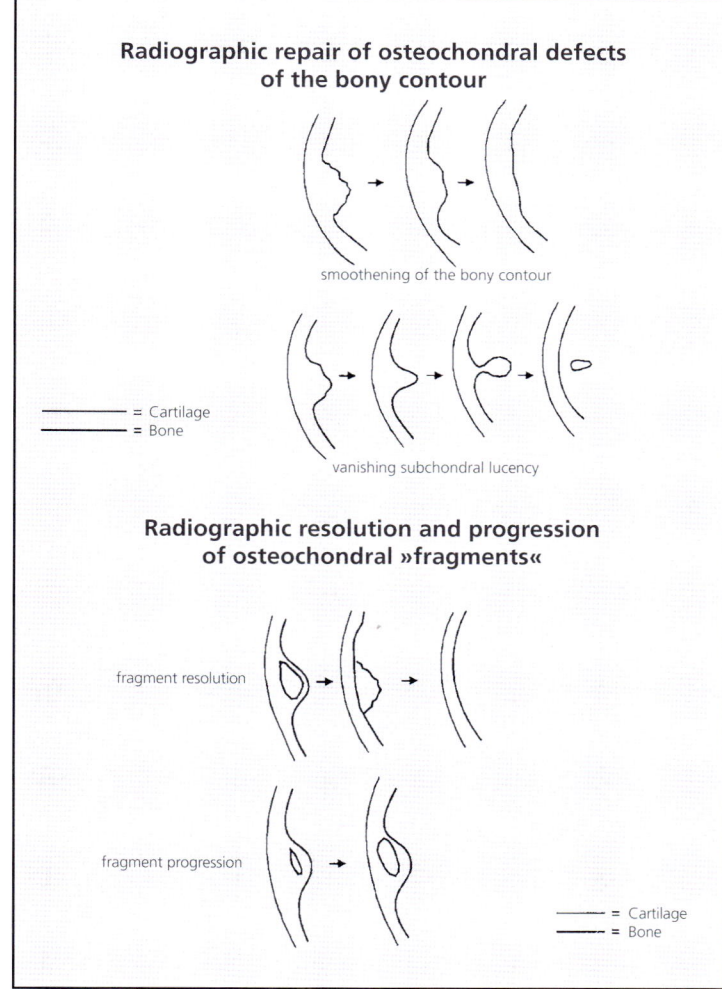

513 Schematic representation of the various radiographic contour defects and "bony fragments" associated with osteochondrosis.

Osteochondrosis is primarily a disease of ossifying cartilage, characterised by temporary or permanent focal failure of enchondral ossification, thus causing focal thickening of articular (or physeal) cartilage.

Cartilage is not visible on survey radiographs. Therefore, radiographically focal thickening of articular cartilage results in smooth or irregular flattening or cavitation of the underlying bony contour.

Retained cartilage within or superimposed on subchondral bone causes radiolucency of the subchondral bone texture.

Due to biomechanical loading of the articular surface, fissures may develop in deeper necrotic layers of the retained cartilage, thus causing formation of flaps and fragments. Radiographically these flabs and fragments are only visible if they contain bone, either by extension of fissures into underlying bone, or by secondary ossification within thickened cartilage, cartilage flaps or fragments.

514 Schematic representation of radiographic repair of osteochondrosis contour defects and resolution or progression of osteochondrosis "fragments".

Due to repair and/or secondary ossification focal thickening of articular cartilage may gradually disappear.

Associated defects of the bony contour become smaller and less irregular, and may resolve completely, or grow away from the joint surface thus becoming a temporary or permanent cyst-like subchondral radiolucency.

Secondary ossification of thickened cartilage may also result in resolution, i.e. fusion, or enlargement of radiographic "fragments".

Villonodular synovitis

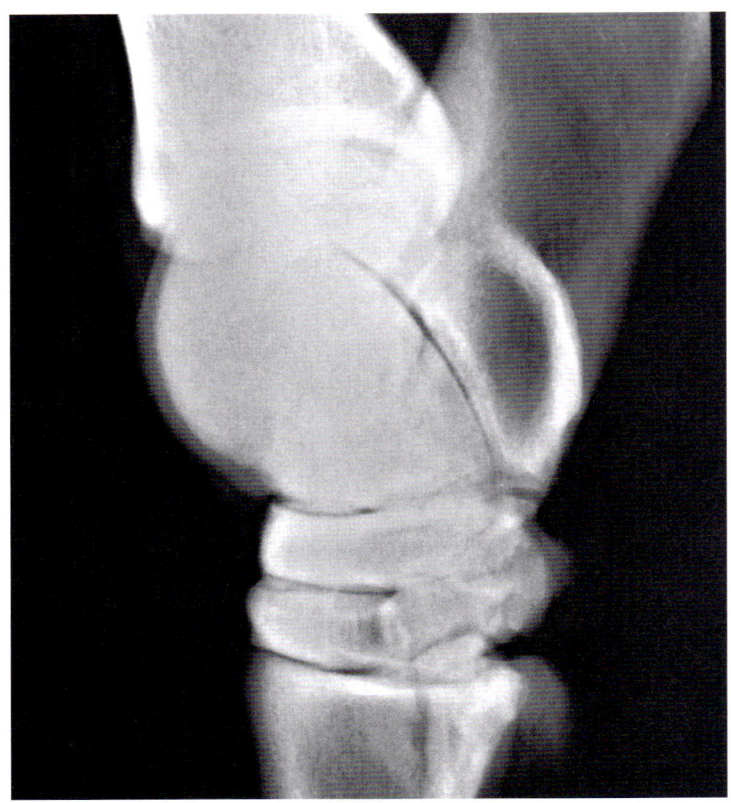

515

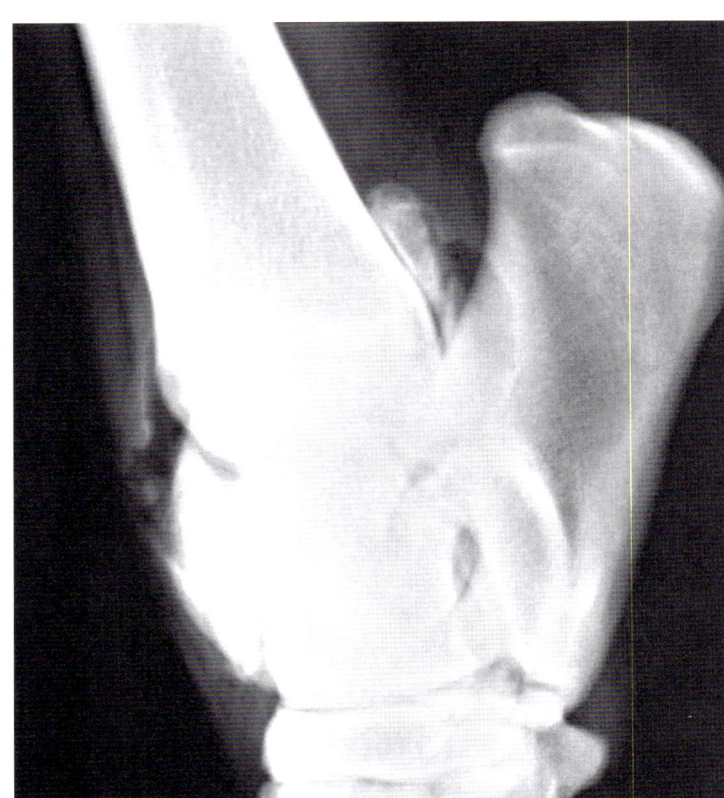

516

515/516 Right hock joint, lateromedial survey and double-contrast study.

Warmblood, 4 ½ years.

The lateromedial survey radiograph (Fig. 515) reveals slight flattening **(1)** of the mid-proximal contour of the medial trochlear ridge of the tibial tarsal bone.

Six ml positive contrast material and 60 ml room air injected into the tibiotarsal joint (Fig. 516) outlines a small nodular synovial mass **(2)** at the level of the bony flattening, which is probably caused by localised increased pressure induced by the villondular mass.

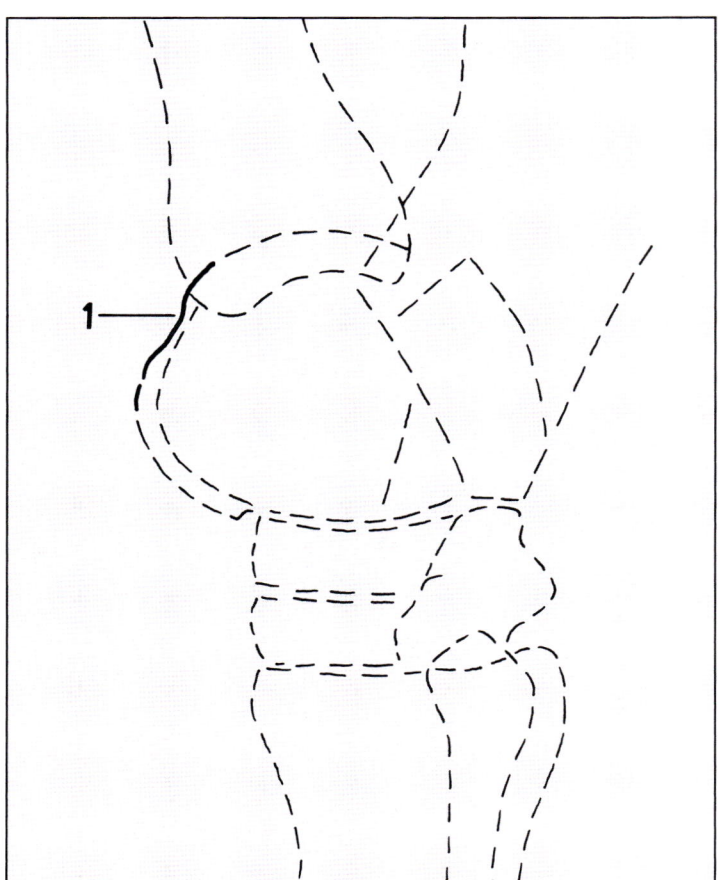

515 a

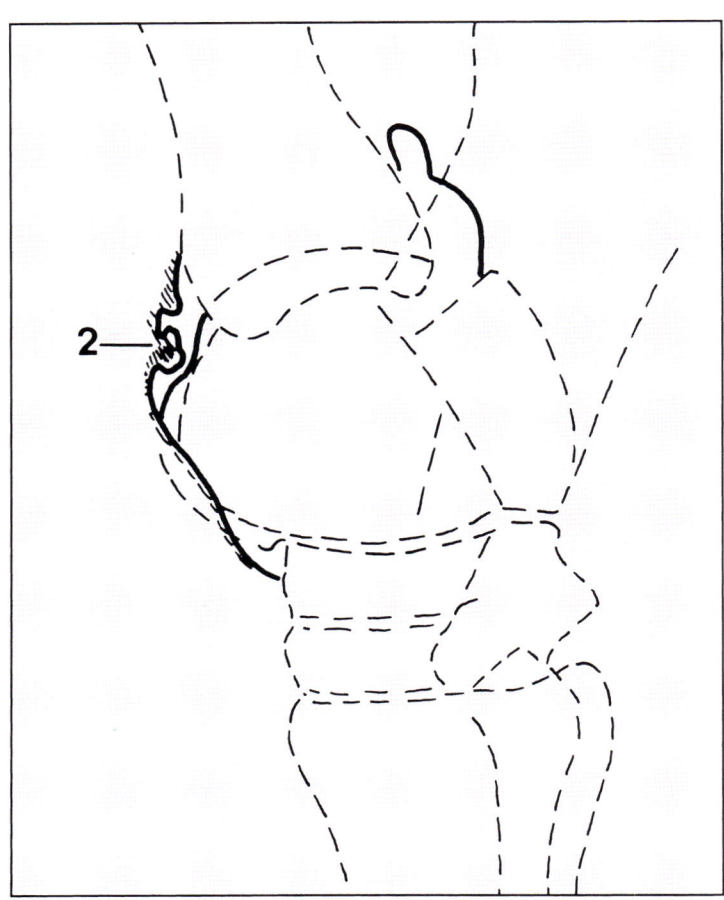

516 a

515 a/516 a Schematic drawings

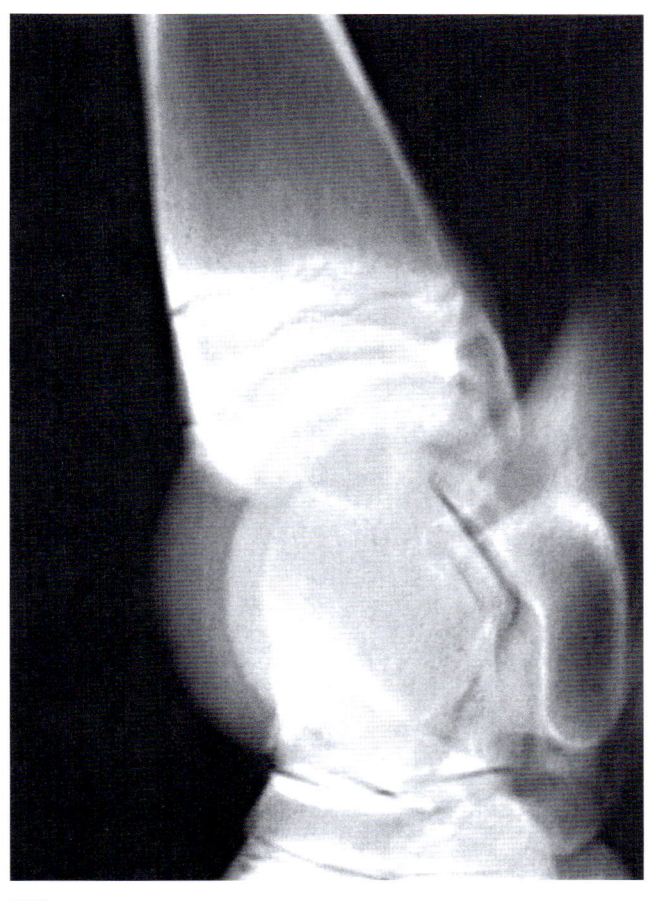

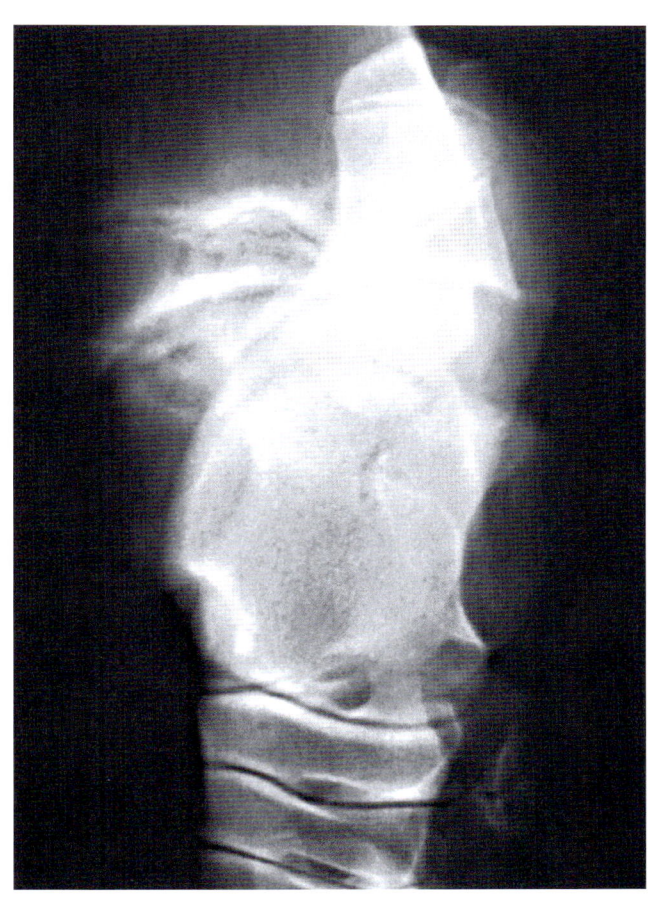

517

518

517/518 Right hock joint, lateromedial (Fig. 517) and dorsomedial-plantarolateral oblique (Fig. 518) view: close-ups.

Warmblood, 1 year.

A large, solitary, clearly defined, cystic area of diffuse radiolucency within the proximal aspect of the lateral trochlear ridge of the tibial tarsal bone, indicating a bone cyst, surrounded by a thin sclerotic zone.

The precise location of the lesion is defined by the dorsomedial-plantarolateral oblique view. There is no visible communication between the cyst lumen and the tibiotarsal joint.

N. B. Cysts are generally of clinical significance, particularly in young horses.

Cyst-like radiolucent lesions in the hock joint may also be the result of osteoarthrosis of particularly the small tarsal joints (Fig. 519, 520), osteochondrosis (Fig. 494) or osteomyelitis type E.

Bone cyst

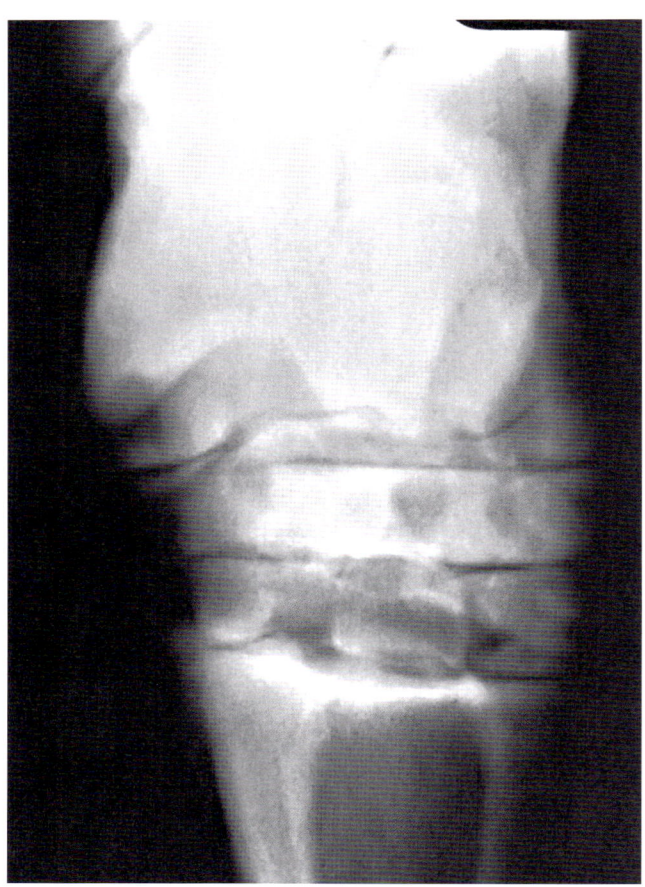

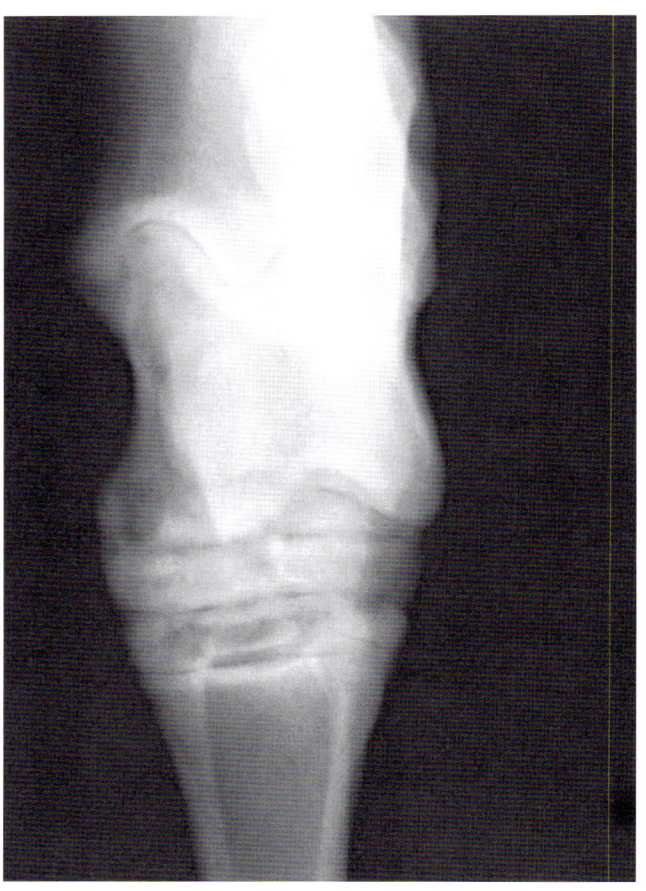

519 Right hock joint, dorsoplantar view: close-up.

Warmblood, 14 years.

Multiple, large, cystic areas of diffuse radiolucency surrounded by a thin, ill defined, sclerotic border, within the central tarsal bone and the distomedial aspect of the tibial tarsal bone, communicating with the proximal intertarsal joint space.

The cystic lesions are associated with osteoarthrosis of the proximal intertarsal joint, indicated by the irregular subchondral radiolucency of the distocentral region of the tibial tarsal bone.

520 Left hock joint, dorsoplantar view.

Pony, 2 years.

A large solitary cystic area of diffuse radiolucency within the distomedial aspect of the tibial tarsal bone, communicating with the proximal intertarsal joint space. The cystic lesion is associated with osteoarthrosis of the proximal intertarsal joint, indicated by the hazy appearance and minimal irregularity of the joint space.

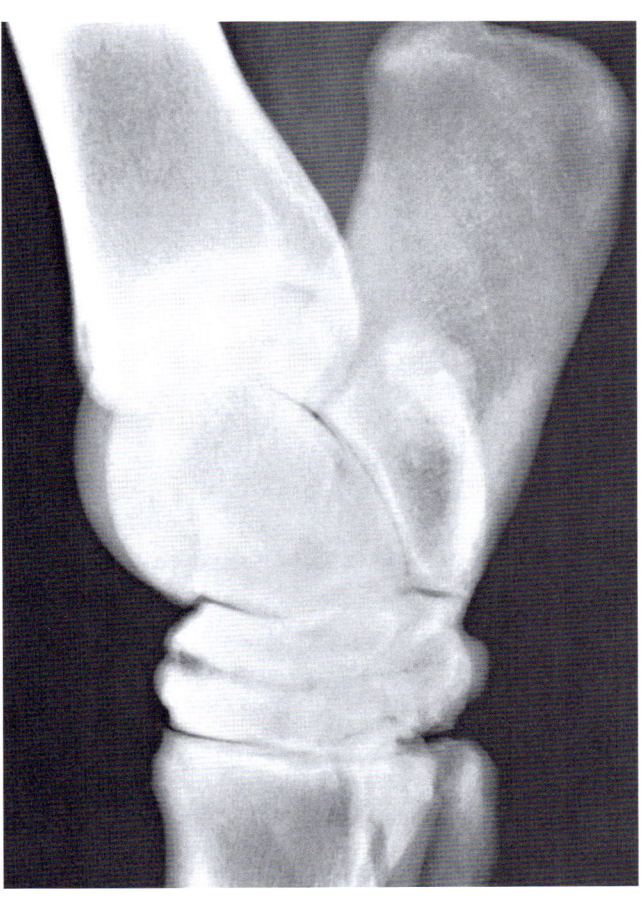

521

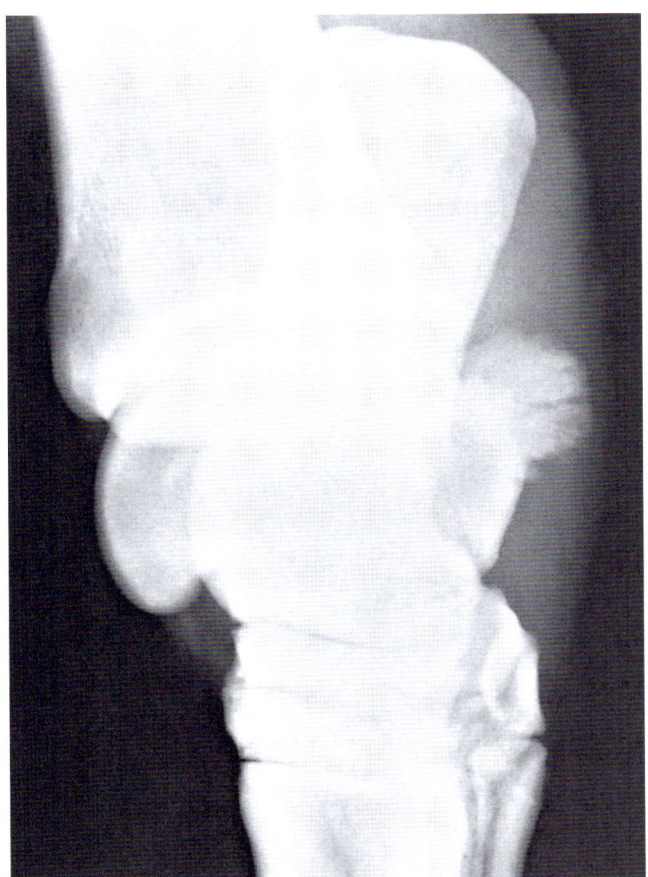

523

522

521/522/523 Right hock-joint, lateromedial dorsoplantar and dorsomedial-plantarolateral oblique view.

Warmblood, 9 years.

Extensive, irregular bony proliferation on the proximomedial aspect of the sustentaculum tali, associated with distension of the tarsal sheath. The bony changes are best demonstrated on the dorsomedial-plantarolateral oblique view (Fig. 523), are les obvious on the dorsoplantar view (Fig. 522) and are difficult to identify on the lateromedial projection (Fig. 521).

Additional finding: osteoarthrosis of the distal intertarsal joint characterized by a mixture of destructive and proliferate changes.

Thoroughpin
(with associated bony lesions of the sustentaculum tali)

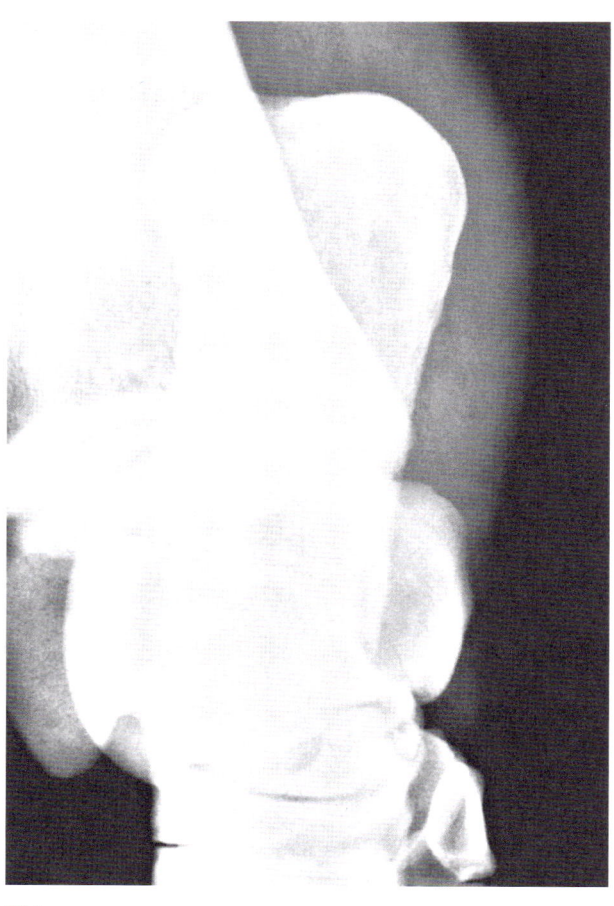

524

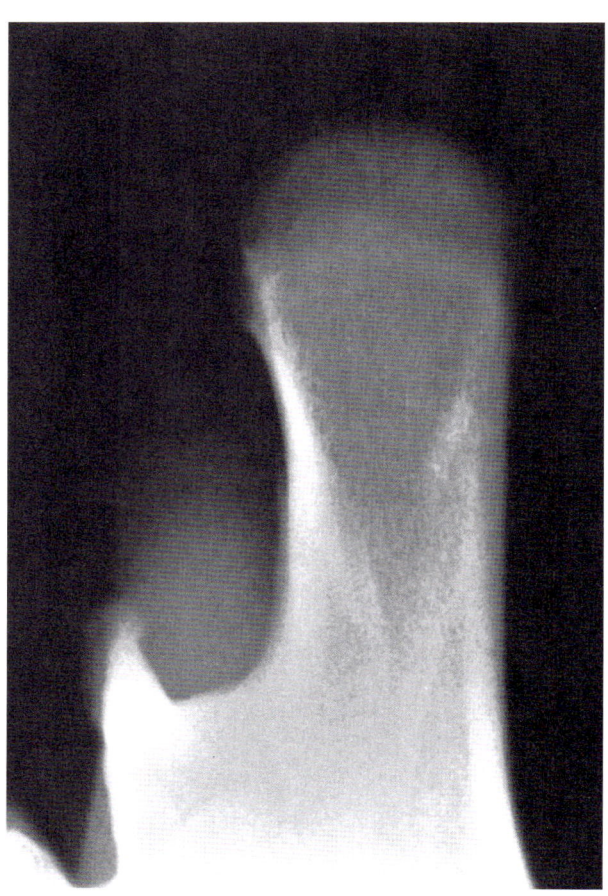

525

524/525/526/527 Left hock joint, dorsomedial-plantarolateral oblique and dorsoplantar (flexed) "skyline" survey: close-ups; dorsomedial-plantarolateral oblique tarsal sheath positive contrast study, and lateromedial positive contrast study of a normal tarsal sheath: close-up.

Standardbred, 5 years.

The survey radiographs reveal a large ridge of new bone on the medial border of the sustentaculum tali. The extension of the bony ridge is best demonstrated on the "skyline" projection (Fig. 525) and less obvious on the dorsomedial-plantarolateral oblique view (Fig. 524). Twenty ml positive contrast material injected into the distended tarsal sheath (Fig. 526) shows moderate distension and minimal folding of the proximal and distal end of the sheath. An additional longitudinal band-like filling defect, resulting from bulging of the deep digital flexor tendon over the bony ridge on the sustentaculum, is demonstrated in the central portion of the sheath. The radiographic findings were confirmed by surgical exploration of the sheath.

The usual configuration of the proximal and central portion of the tarsal sheath is demonstrated by the positive contrast radiograph of a normal tarsal sheath (Fig. 527).

N. B. Other bony lesions of the sustentaculum tali associated with distension of the tarsal sheath are fracture (Fig. 403, 404, 405) and osteomyelitis (Fig. 485, 486).

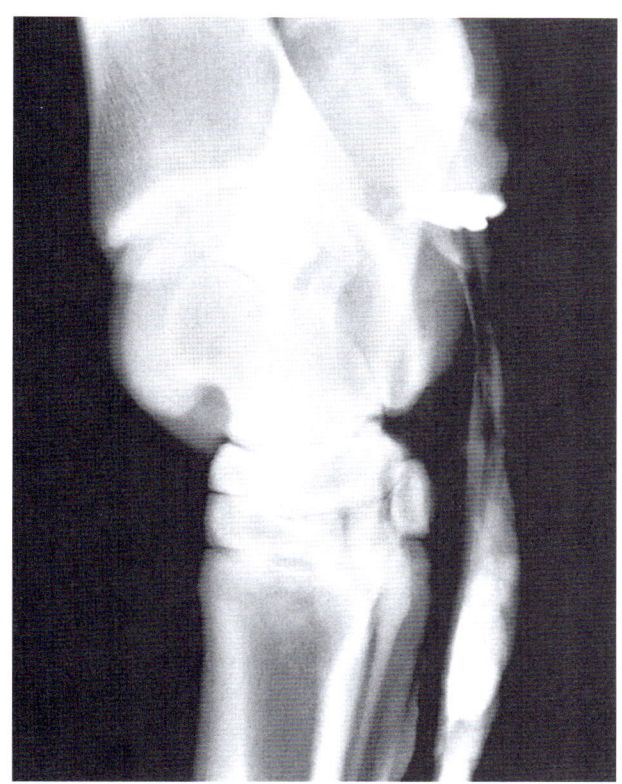

526

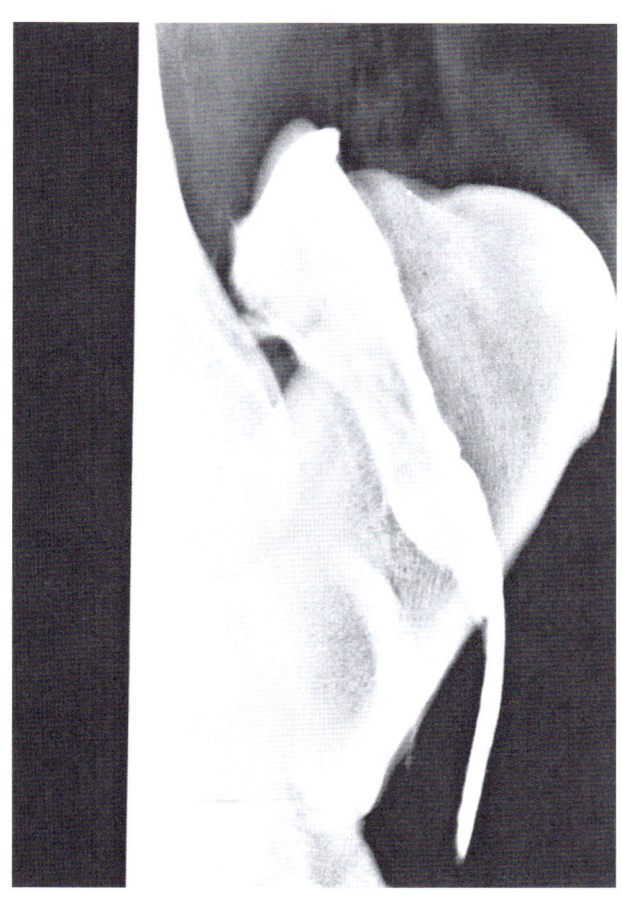

527

Thoroughpin
(without associated bony lesions of the sustentaculum tali)

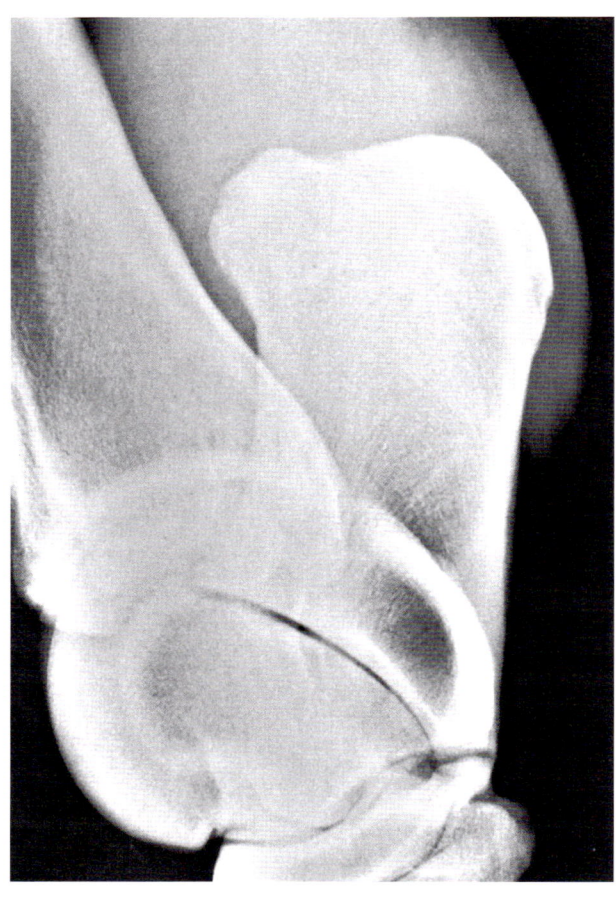

528

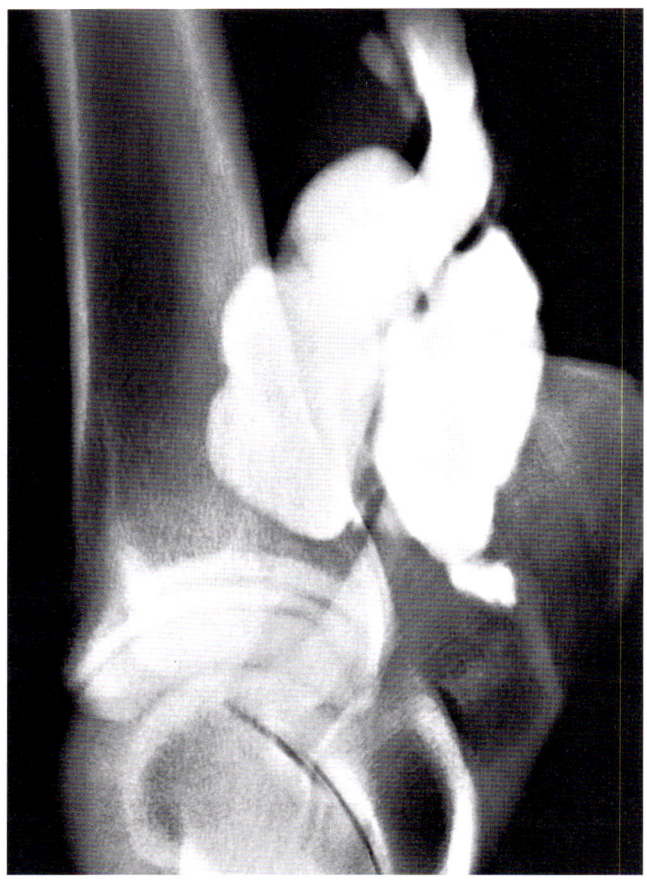

529

528/529/530 Left hock joint, lateromedial survey, positive and double contrast study of the tarsal sheath: close-ups.

Warmblood, 18 years.

The lateromedial survey radiograph (Fig. 528) reveals soft tissue swelling proximal to the tuber calcis, resulting from distension of the proximal aspect of the tarsal sheeth. Twenty ml positive contrast material injected into the distended portion of the tarsal sheath (Fig. 529) shows marked dilatation and excessive folding of the proximal end of the sheath.

An additional double contrast study (Fig. 530), obtained by removal of most of the positive contrast material, followed by injection of 20 m. room air, outlines a normal synovial membrane **(1)** which is smooth, thin and without villi and allows the deep digital flexor tendon **(2)** to be visualized.

N. B. Therapy of tarsal sheath distension without bony lesions of the sustentaculum tali is more successful than in cases associated with bony lesions.

Tarsal sheath contrast examination is of value in determining the aetiology, particularly of tarsal sheath distension without associated bony lesions, and in deciding whether to treat the case conservatively or surgically.

Differential diagnosis: Distension of the proximal aspect of the tarsal sheath may be confused with an extratendovaginal (fluid filled) swelling (Fig. 535, 536).

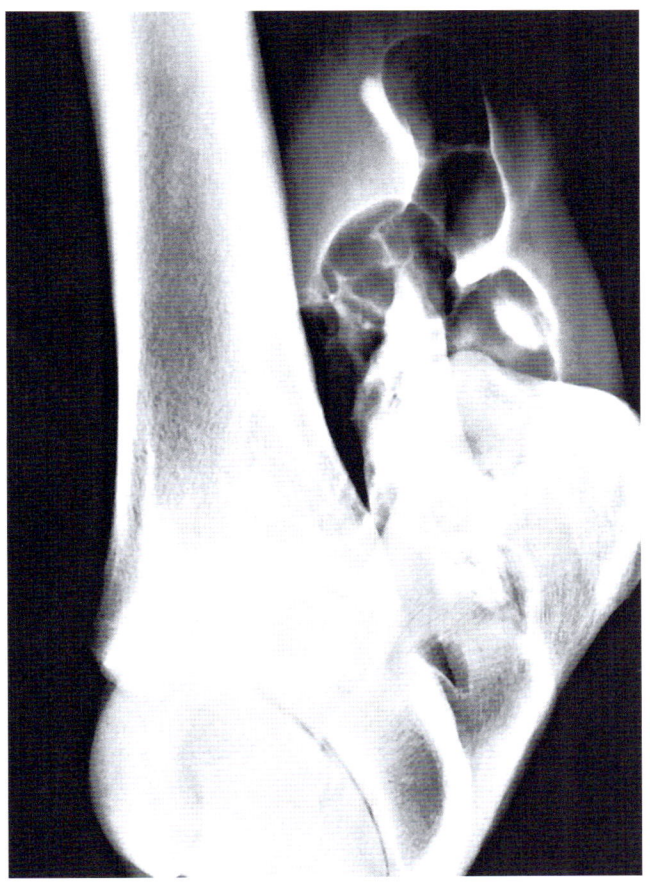

530

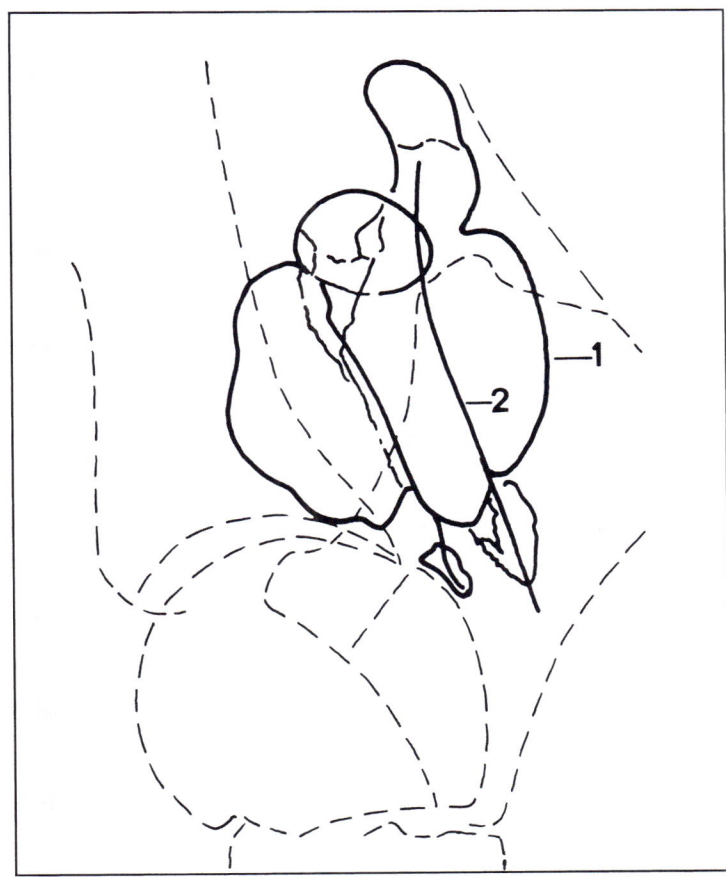

530 a Schematic drawing

Thoroughpin
(without associated bony lesions of the sustentaculum tali)

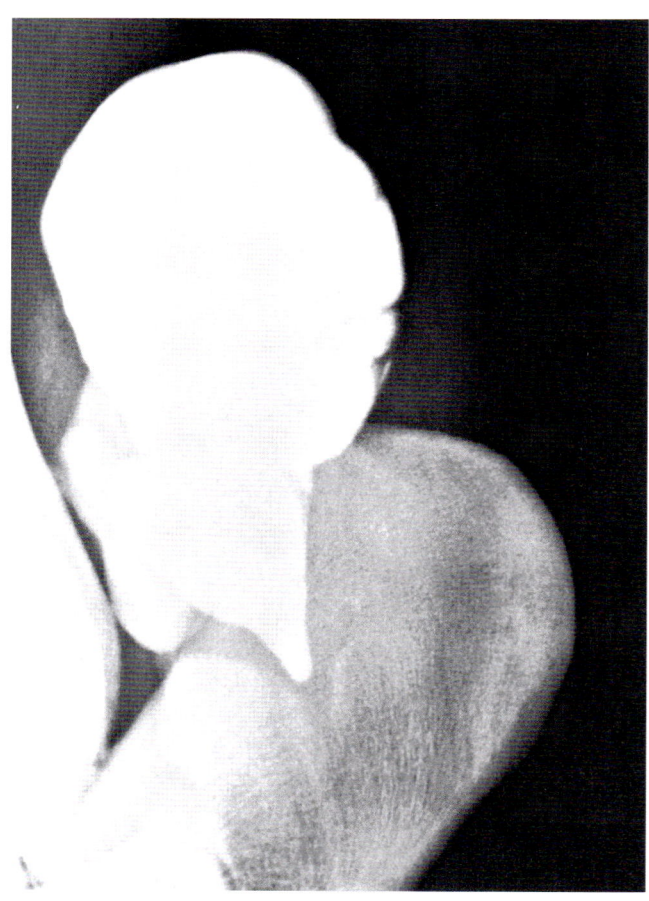

531

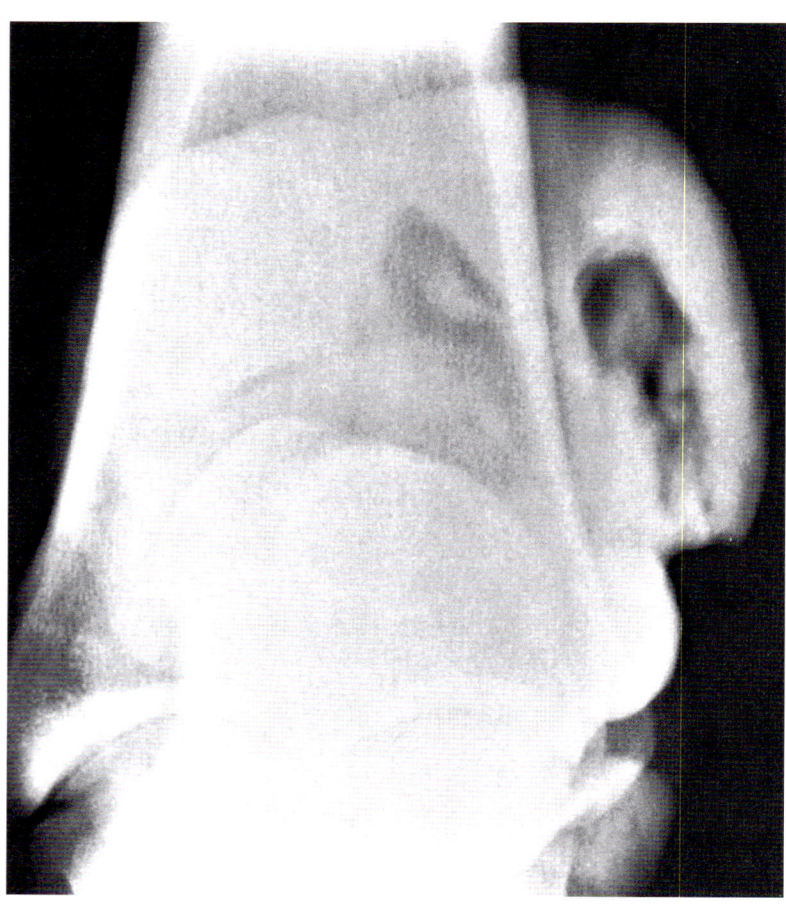

532

531/532 Left hock joint, lateromedial and dorsomedial-plantarolateral oblique tarsal sheath positive contrast study: close-ups.

Warmblood, 4 ½ years.

The lateromedial contrast radiograph (Fig. 531), taken immediately after injection of 20 ml positive contrast material into the distended proximal portion of the sheath, shows only marked dilatation and minimal folding. The dorsomedial-plantarolateral oblique projection (Fig. 532) reveals an additional thin horizontal band-like and a triangular filling defect in the central area of the distended sheath portion and a large nodular filling defect in the medial part of the sheath. The affected sheath was surgically explored.

The band-like and triangular filling defect resulted from folding of the sheath. The nodular filling defect appeared to be a nodular outgrowth of the sheath, resembling fibrous tissue and blood clots covered by synovial villi. Histological examination of the nodular mass showed it to be chronic reactive inflammation tissue, probably arising from trauma.

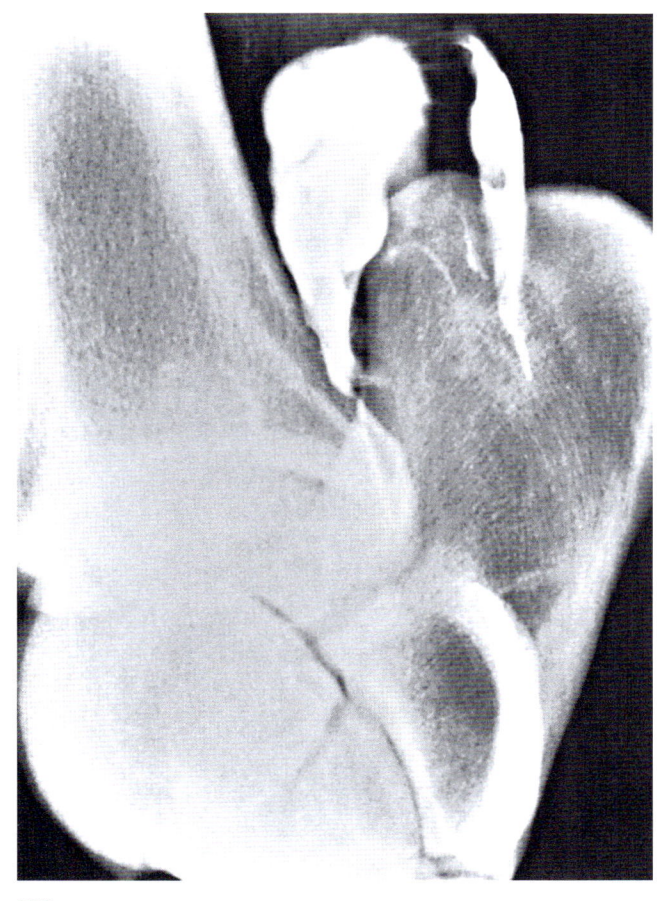

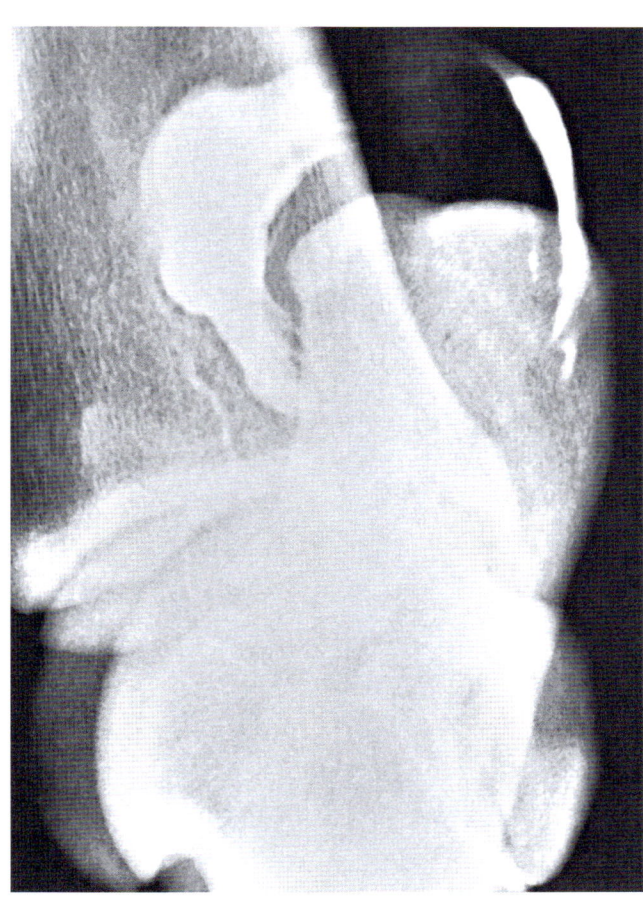

533

534

533/534 Left hock joint, lateromedial (Fig.533) and dorsomedial-plantarolateral oblique (Fig. 534) tarsal sheath positive contrast study: close-ups. Warmblood, 6 years.

Fifteen ml contrast material injected into the distended proximal portion of the sheath outlines a semicircular dilatation of the proximal sheath aspect. The "collar shape" of the dilatation is best demonstrated on the dorsomedial-plantarolateral oblique view and suggests incomplete rupture of the sheath.

False thoroughpin

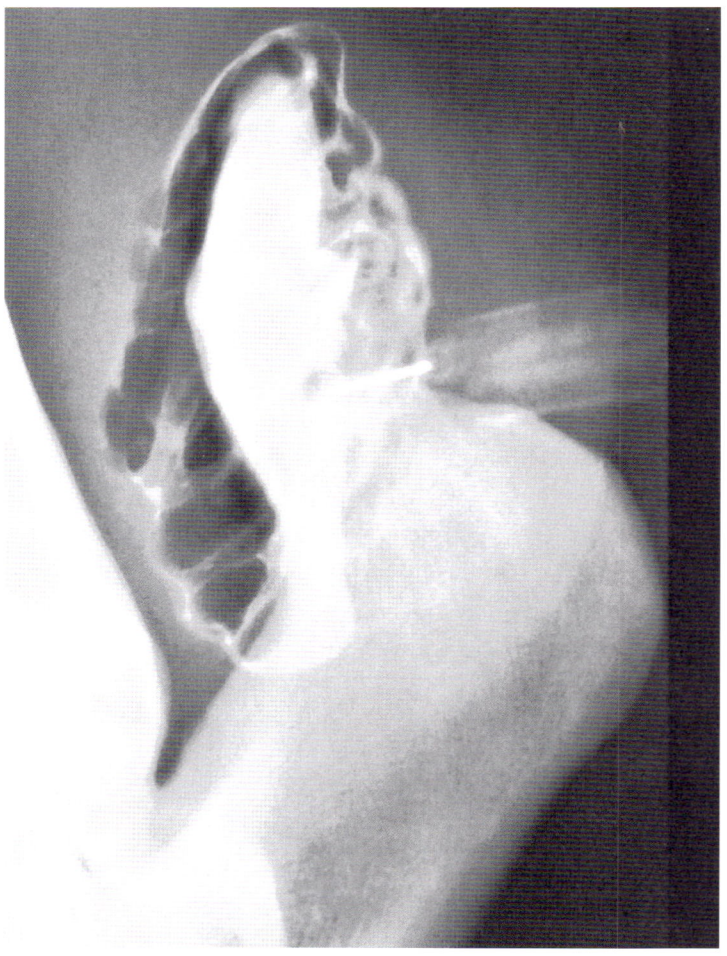

535

536

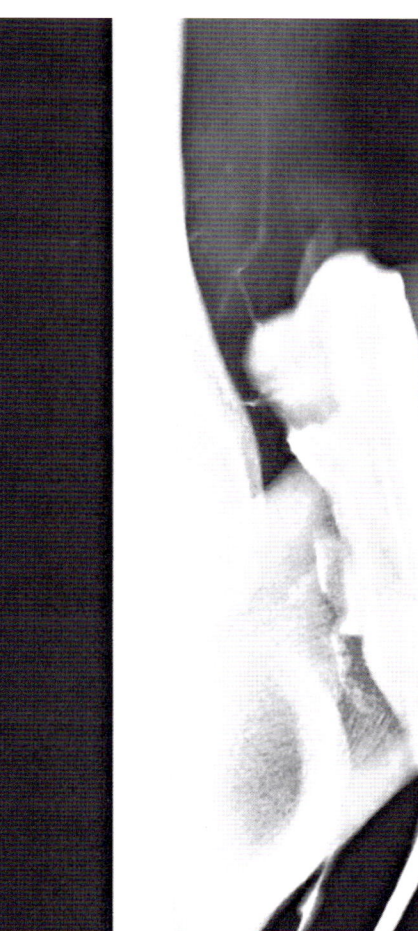

537

535/536/537 Right hock joint, lateromedial double contrast study of a false thoroughpin and additional lateromedial positive tarsal sheath contrast studies: close-ups.

Warmblood, 3 years.

The lateromedial double contrast radiograph (Fig. 535), taken after injection of 5 ml positive contrast material and 40 ml room air into a fluctuating soft tissue swelling proximal to the tuber calcis, suggests cystic dilatation and marked folding of the proximal end of the tarsal sheath, although the deep digital flexor tendon is not visualized despite the excellent double contrast. Additional puncture of the central part of the sheath where it lies on the sustentaculum tali, followed by injection of 10 ml positive contrast material demonstrates the deep digital flexor tendon and central aspect of the tarsal sheath (Fig. 536), superimposed on, or communicating with, the cystic lesion.

A repeated tarsal sheath contrast study, after spontaneous absorption of the contrast material, shows a normal tarsal sheath (Fig. 537), and the cystic lesion is not visible. These findings indicate that the fluctuating soft tissue swelling is not a dilatation of the proximal aspect of the tarsal sheath. It probably represents the remnant of an extra-tendovaginal haematoma.

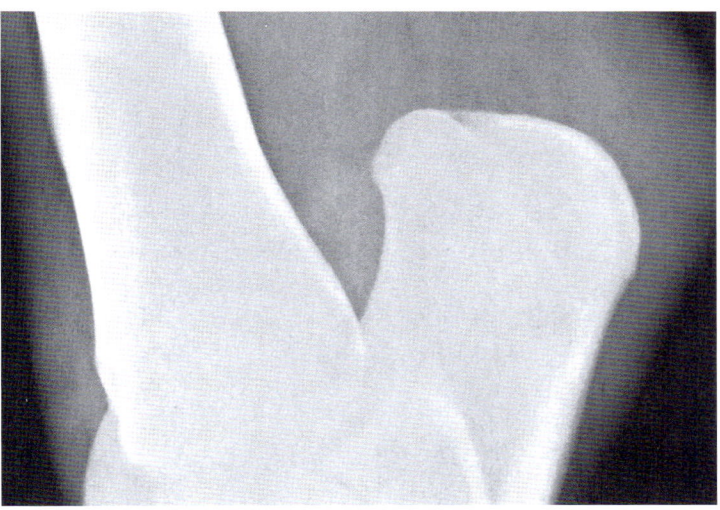

538

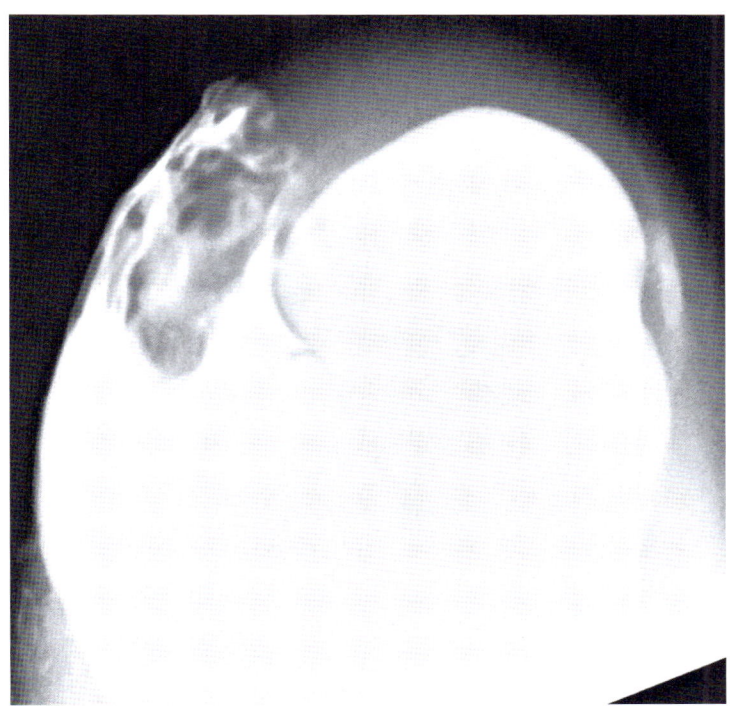

539

538/539 Left hock joint, lateromedial survey and dorsoplantar (flexed) "skyline" positive contrast study: close-ups.

Warmblood, 11 years.

The lateromedial survey radiograph (Fig. 538) shows soft tissue swelling over the tuber calcis, resulting from recent slippage of the superficial digital flexor tendon off the point of the hock. The radiograph was taken to rule out concomitant fracture of the calcaneal tuber. The "skyline" contrast radiograph (Fig. 539), taken after injection of 20 ml positive contrast material into the subtendinous calcaneal bursa, demonstrates marked dilatation and medial displacement of the bursa **(1)**. The large filling defect **(2)** represents the medial displaced superfical digital flexor tendon.

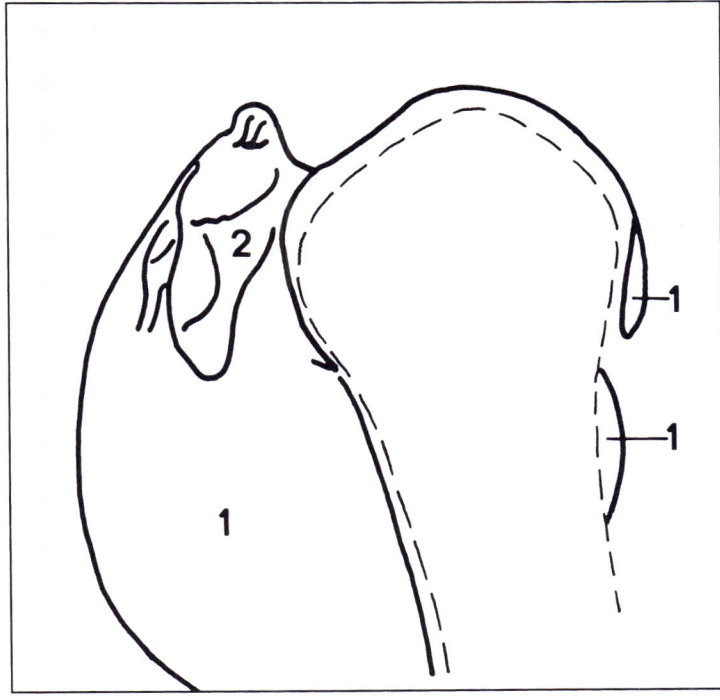

539 a Schematic drawing

Superficial digital flexor tendon luxation

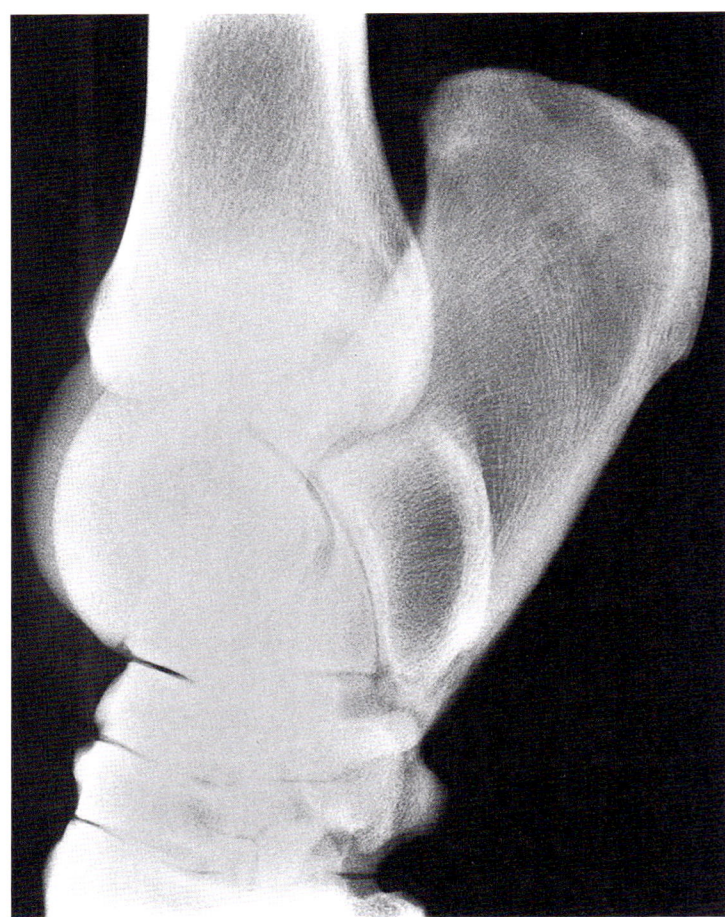

540

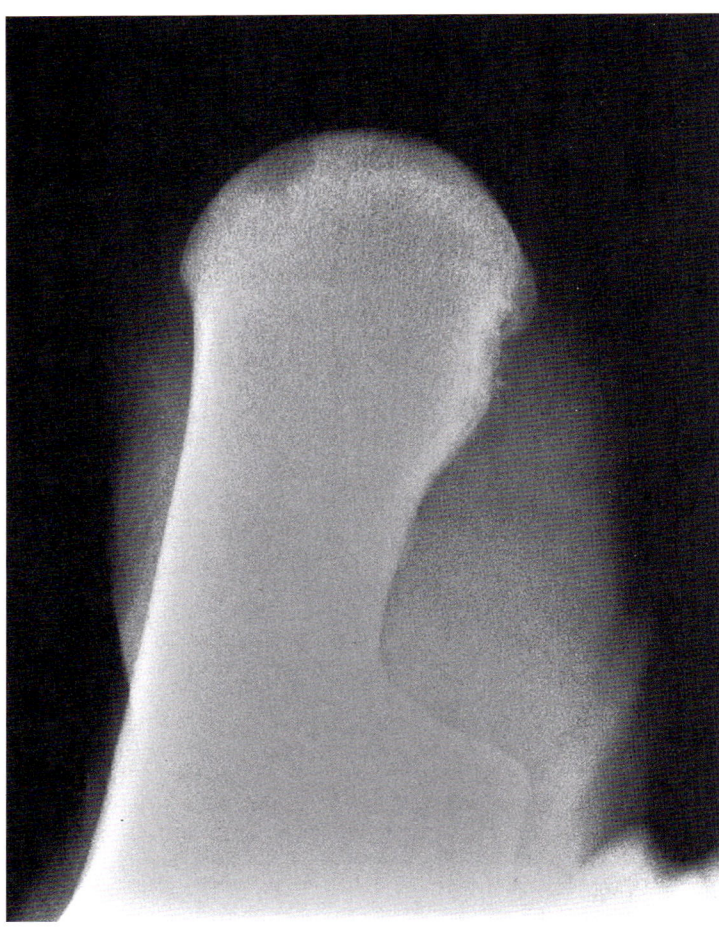

541

540/541 Right hock joint, lateromedial and dorsoplantar (flexed) "skyline" view.

Frisian horse, 15 years.

The lateromedial view (Fig. 540) shows a rounded area of radiolucency in the plantar aspect of the tuber calcis and irregular radiopacity of the proximal aspect of the fibular tarsal bone, associated with chronic lateral luxation of the superficial digital flexor tendon.

On the additional dorsoplantar flexed "skyline" projection (Fig. 541) the rounded defect, probably resulting from concurrent avulsion injury of the gastrocnemius tendon, appears situated in the plantarolateral aspect of the tuber calcis. This view also demonstrates irregular periosteal new bone formation along the proximomedial aspect of the fibular tarsal bone in the region of the ruptured attachment of the superficial digital flexor tendon, thus causing the irregular radiopacity of this region on the lateromedial radiograph.

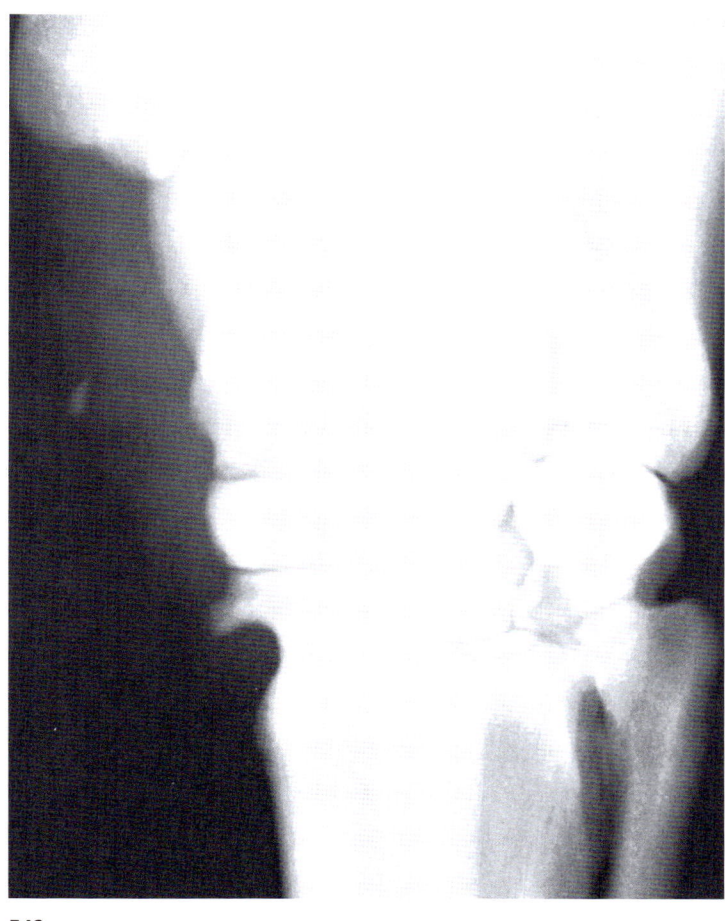

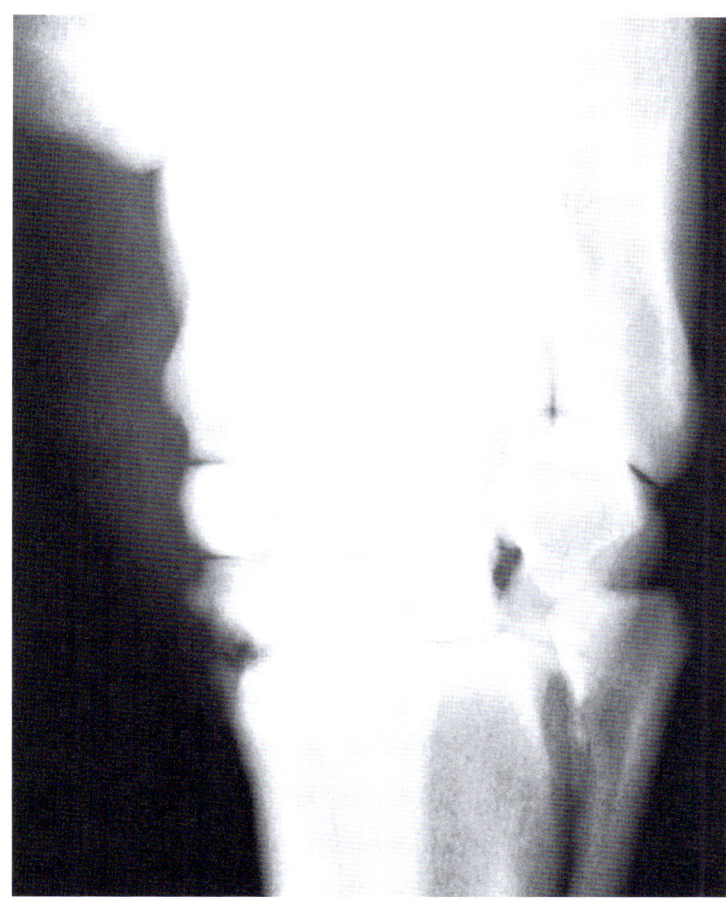

542

543

542/543 Right hock joint, serial dorsolateral-plantaromedial oblique views: close-ups.

Warmblood, 7 years.

The semicircular defect in the dorsomedial border of the third tarsal bone on the initial view (Fig. 542) is characteristic of a recent wire cut through the outer cortex of the bone. The small well defined opacity dorsal to the distal aspect of the tibial tarsal bone probably represents a bone fragment separated from the third tarsal bone by the wire cut. The small, ill defined opacity dorsal to the central aspect of the tibial tarsal bone results from scurf on the skin. Four weeks later (Fig. 543) part of the cortical defect is filled with new bone, bridging the tarsometatarsal joint. The small, displaced bone fragment is no longer present.

Puncture wound

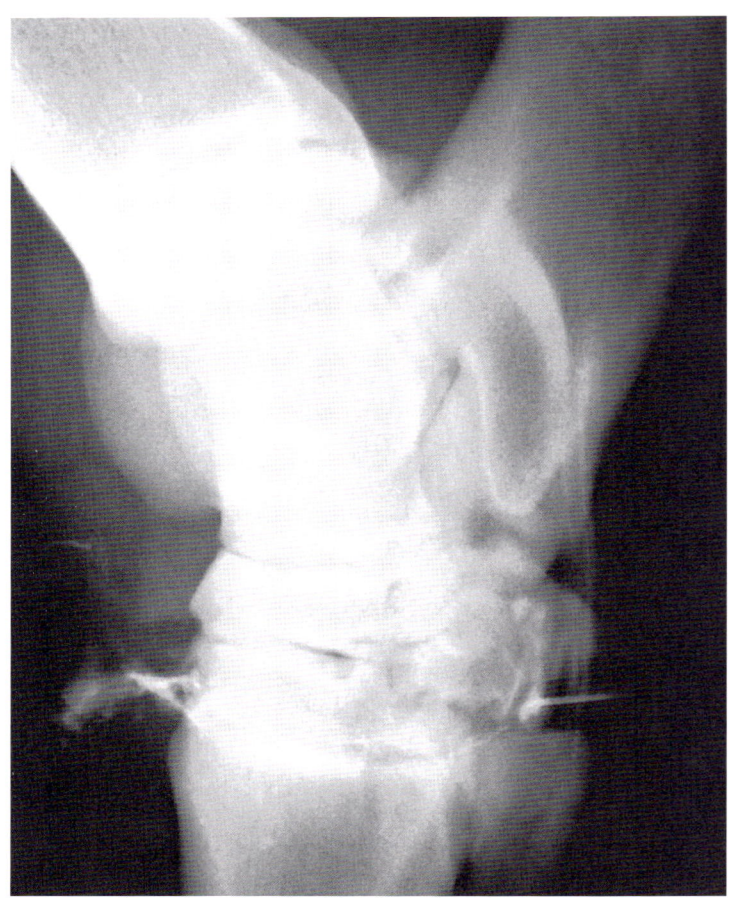

544

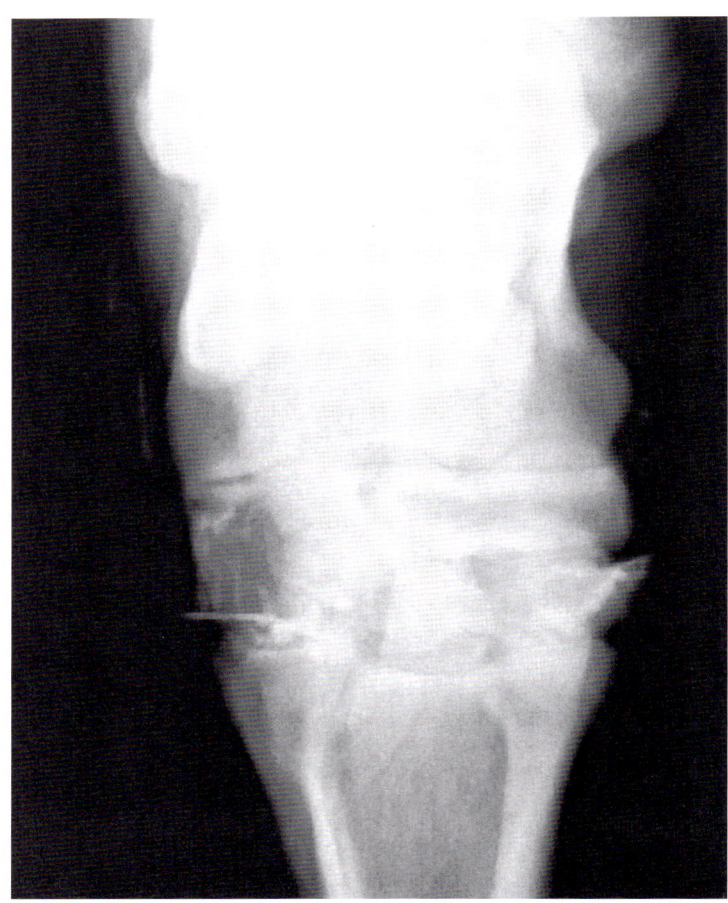

545

544/545 Right hock joint, lateromedial (Fig. 544) and dorsoplantar (Fig. 545) costrast study.

Warmblood, 2 years.

A recent stab wound to the dorsal aspect of the hock, without associated radiographic bone or joint lesions. Five ml positive contrast material injected into the plantarolateral aspect of the tarsometatarsal joint demonstrates a direct communication between joint and stab wound.

The linear opacities over the plantarolateral aspect of the hock result from leakage of contrast material through the needle puncture hole.

N. B. Arthrography instead of fistulography to demonstrate communication between a joint and a puncture wound is indicated if a wound is too extensive for contrast material injection under pressure directly into the wound.

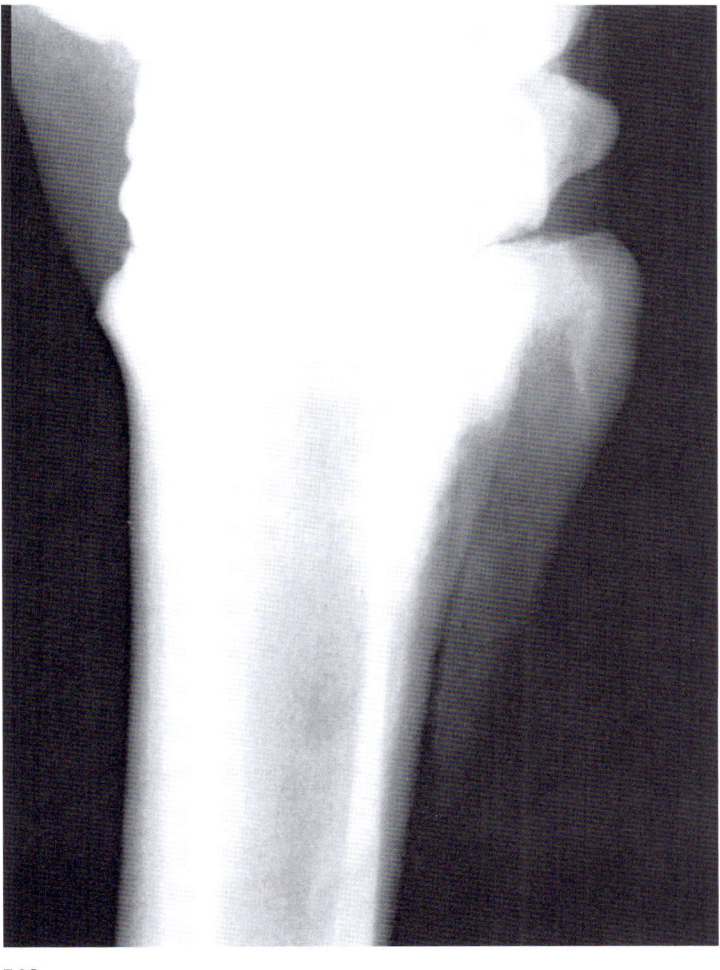

546

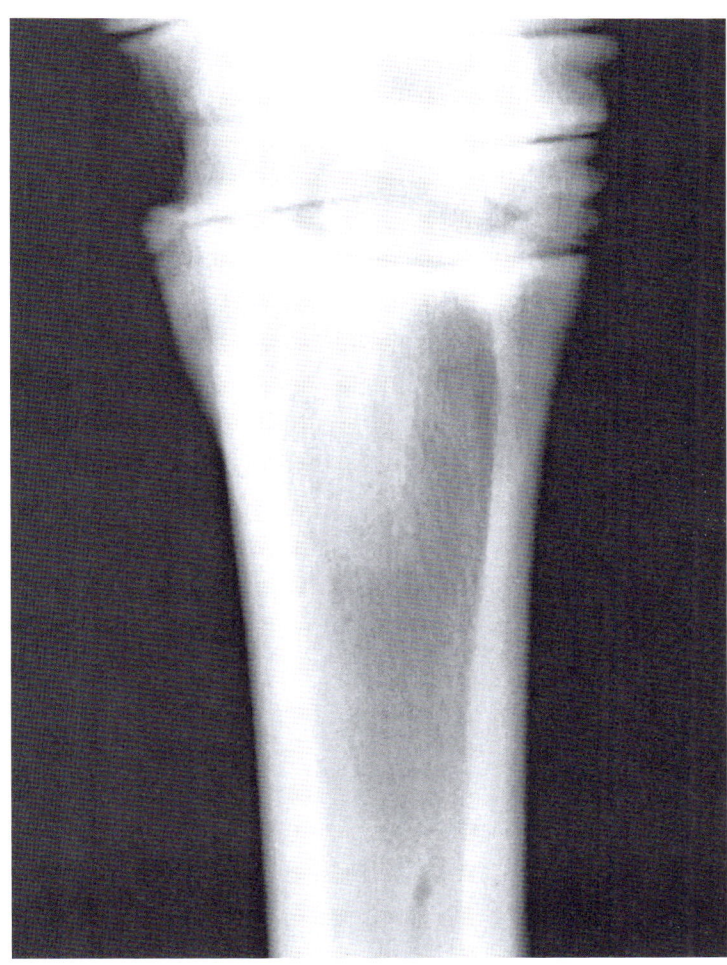

547

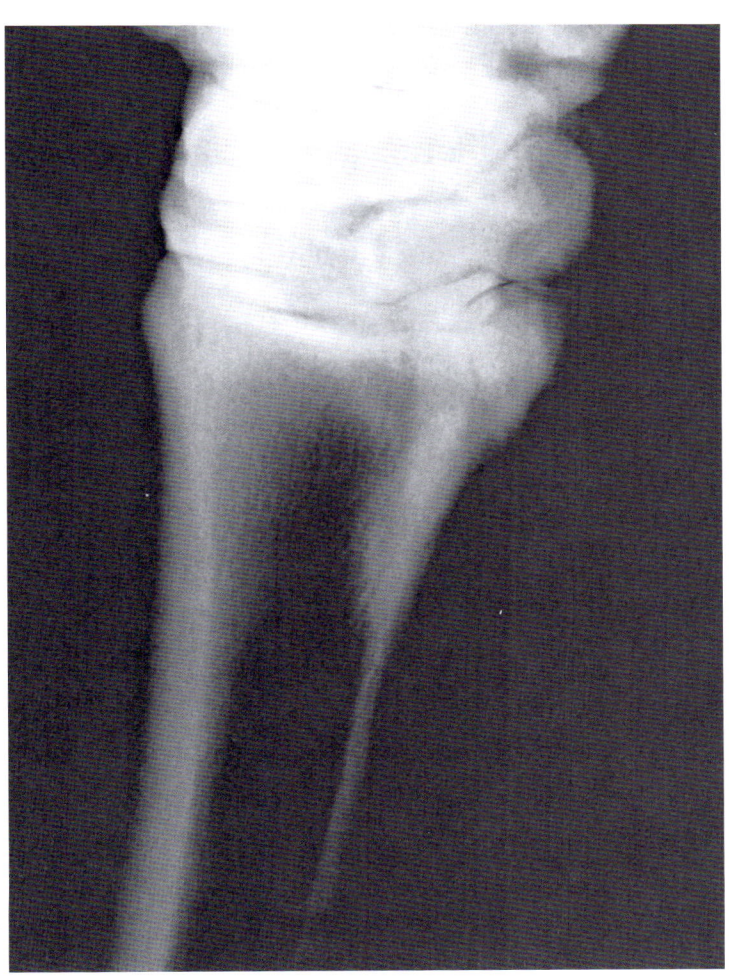

548

546/547/548 Right hock joint, lateromedial and dorsoplantar views: close-ups of the proximal half of the cannon bone.

Warmblood, 4 years.

Sclerosis of the trabecular pattern of the proximolateral aspect of the third metatarsal bone, associated with chronic desmites of the proximal attachment of the suspensory ligament.

The increased trabecular radiopacity is best demonstrated on a deliberately overexposed lateromedial view (Fig. 548), less obvious on the dorsoplantar projection (Fig. 547) and difficult to identify on the routine lateromedial exposure (Fig. 546).

Local infiltration of analgesic solution confirmed the diagnosis of high suspensory desmitis.

The Stifle Joint

Fracture

Luxation

Ligamentous injury

Normal postnatal ossification pattern

Infectious arthritis

Puncture wound

Osteomyelitis

"Epiphysitis"

Osteochondrosis

Bone cyst

Bone sequestration

Calcified haematoma

Ossifying myopathy

Tumoral calcinosis (Calcinosis circumscripta)

Infarction

Osteoclastoma

Fracture

Femur

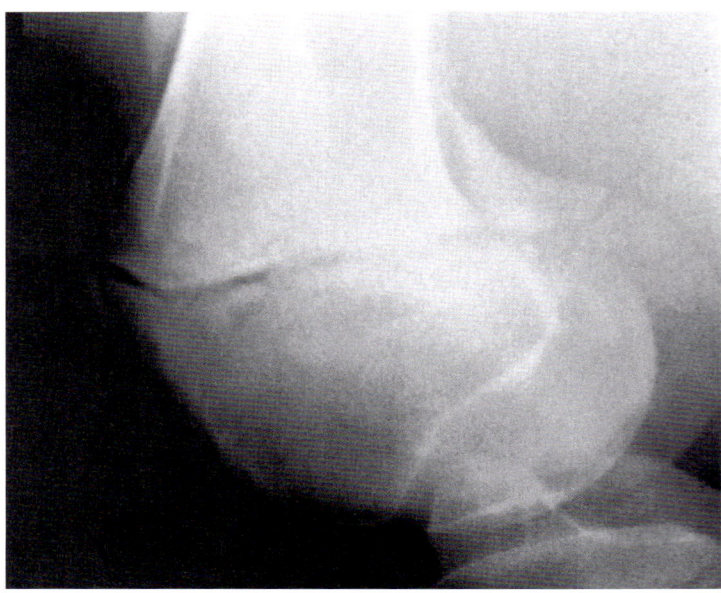

549

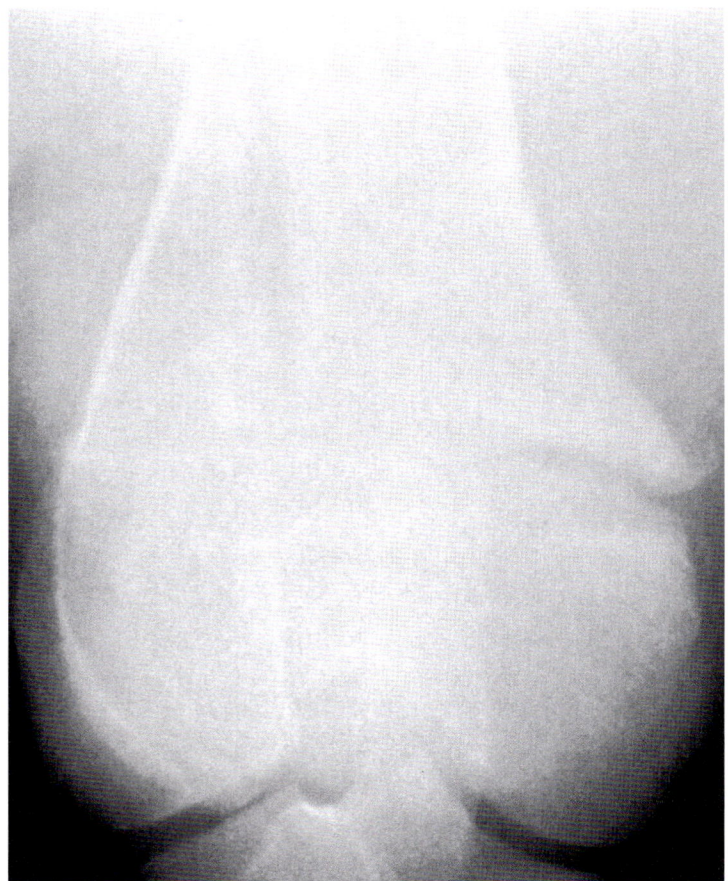

550

549/550 Left stifle joint, lateromedial (Fig. 549) and caudocranial (Fig. 550) view: close-ups.

Foal, 2 months.

The vertical radiolucent zone **(1)** through the caudolateral portion of the metaphysis of the distal femur, extending from the physis to the caudolateral cortex and interrupting the continuity of the proximal cortical bone **(2)**, indicates the presence of a Salter-Harris type 2 physeal fracture. Additional small obscure fragments **(3)** superimposed on the caudal aspect of the metaphysis are visible on the slightly oblique lateromedial view. This projection also reveals ill defined new bone **(4)** on the caudal surface of the femur proximal to the fracture, indicating that the fracture occurred several weeks prior to the examination.

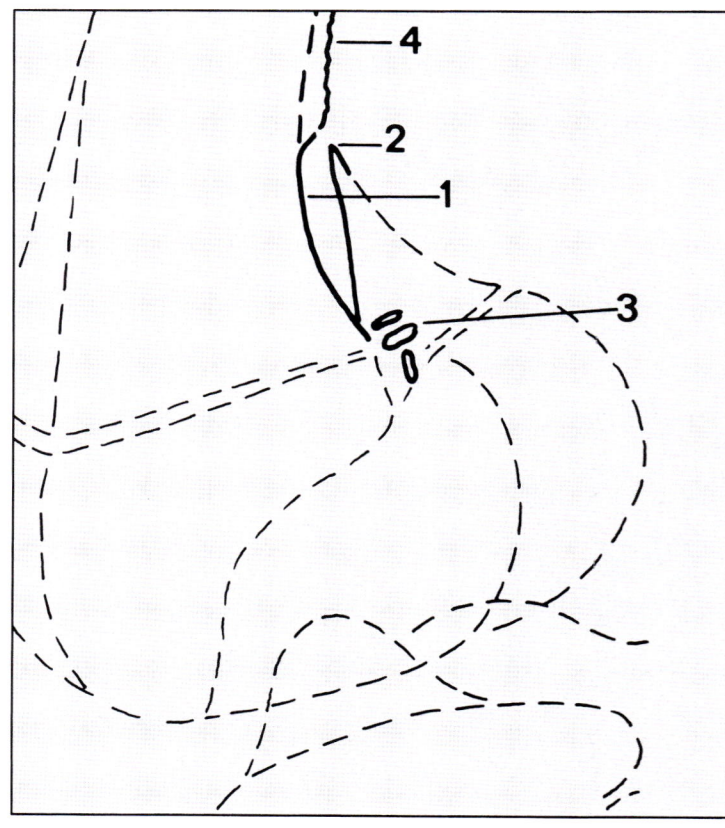

549 a

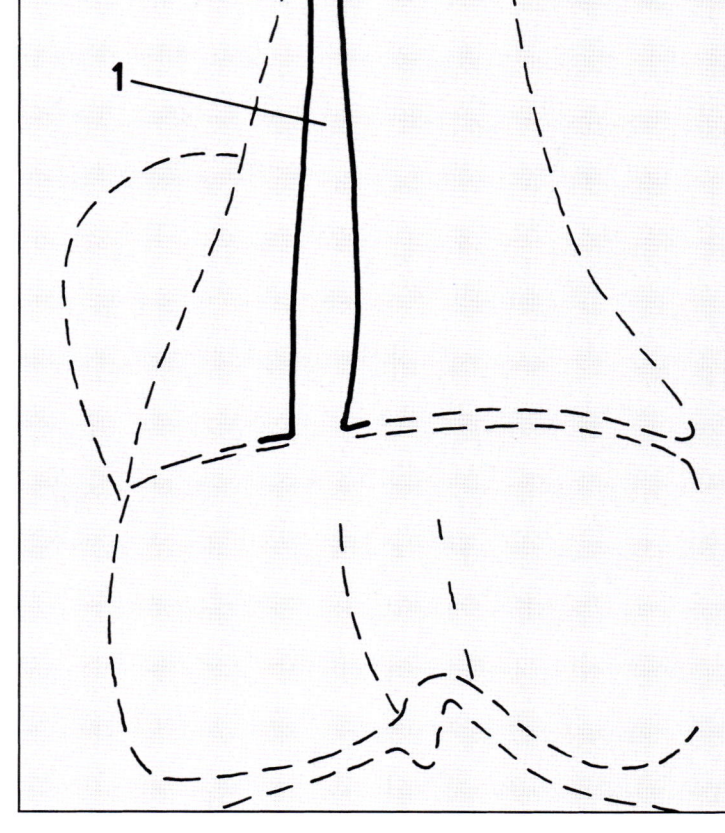

550 a

549 a/550 a Schematic drawings

Femur

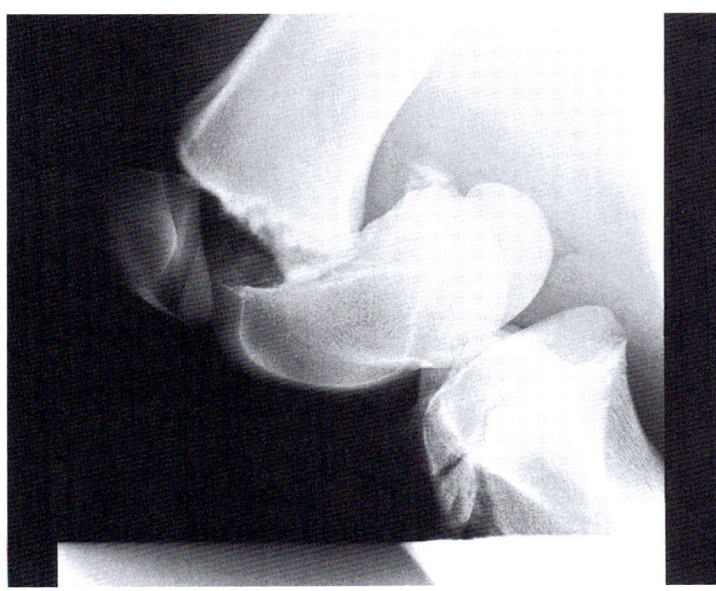

551 Left stifle joint, lateromedial view.

Pony, 1 year.

Prominent caudal displacement and rotation of the distal femoral epiphysis due to a recent physeal fracture combined with minimal caudal metaphyseal fragmentation.

Considering the combined proximal attachment of the peroneus tertius / long digital extensor tendons on the extensor fossa of the distal femoral epiphysis, epiphyseal detachment enables extension of the hock without extending the stifle, thus mimicking rupture of the peroneus tertius.

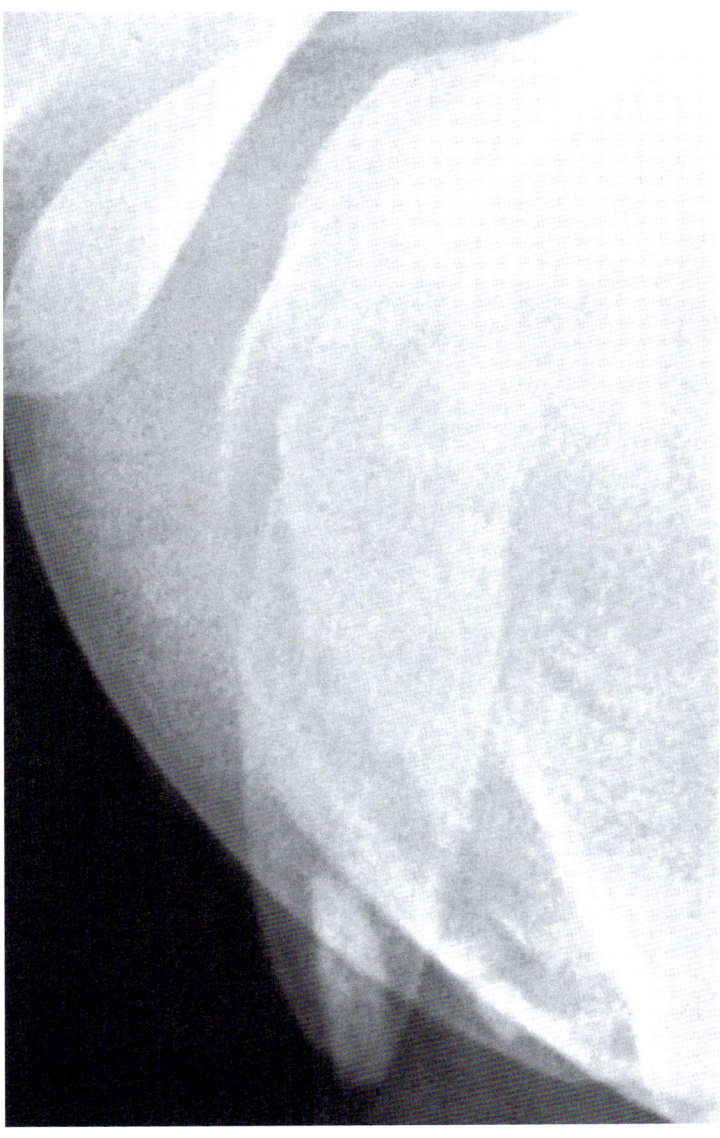

552 Left stifle joint, lateromedial view: close-up.

Warmblood, 4 ½ years.

The large elliptical bone fragment superimposed on the femoral trochlea and the clearly defined radiolucency of the distal half of the lateral trochlear ridge result from a fracture of the major part of the lateral trochlear ridge.

Small additional fracture fragments are visible over the distal aspect of the major fragment and femoral trochlea. The diagnosis was confirmed by histological examination. The differential diagnosis includes osteochondrosis (Fig. 622, 623).

Fracture

Femur

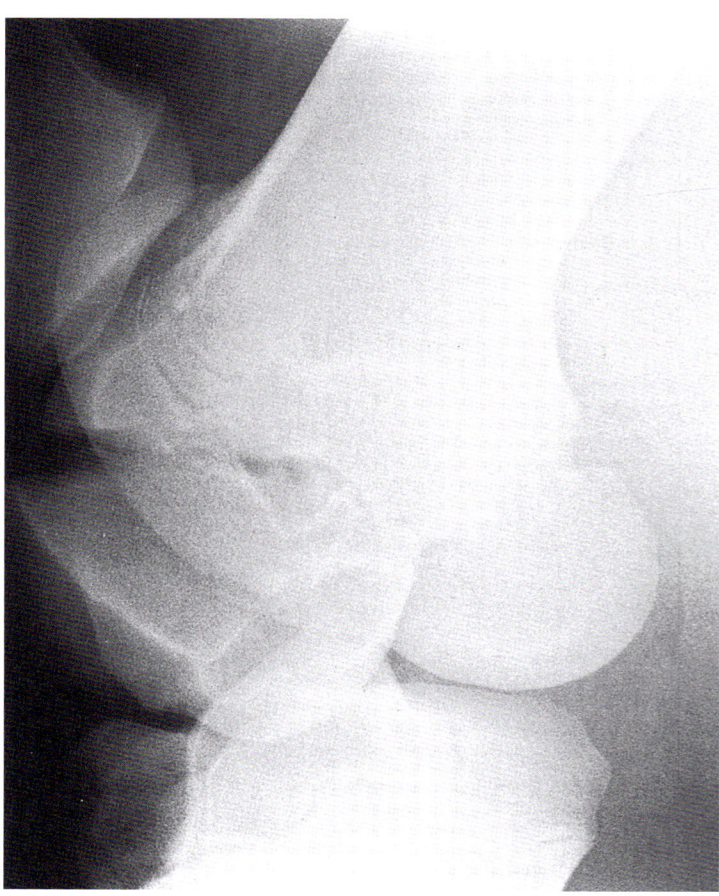

553 Left stifle joint, lateromedial view.

Arabian, 1 ½ years.

The well defined horizontal radiolucent zone cranioproximally disrupting the continuity of the lateral ridge of the femoral trochlea and obvious cranial displacement of the lateral femoral condyle indicate a recent simple horizontal fracture involving the lateral condyle and the corresponding portion of the femoral trochlea. The separated lateral half of the distal femoral extremity includes the combined proximal attachment of the peroneus tertius/long digital extensor tendons, thus mimicking peroneus tertius rupture.

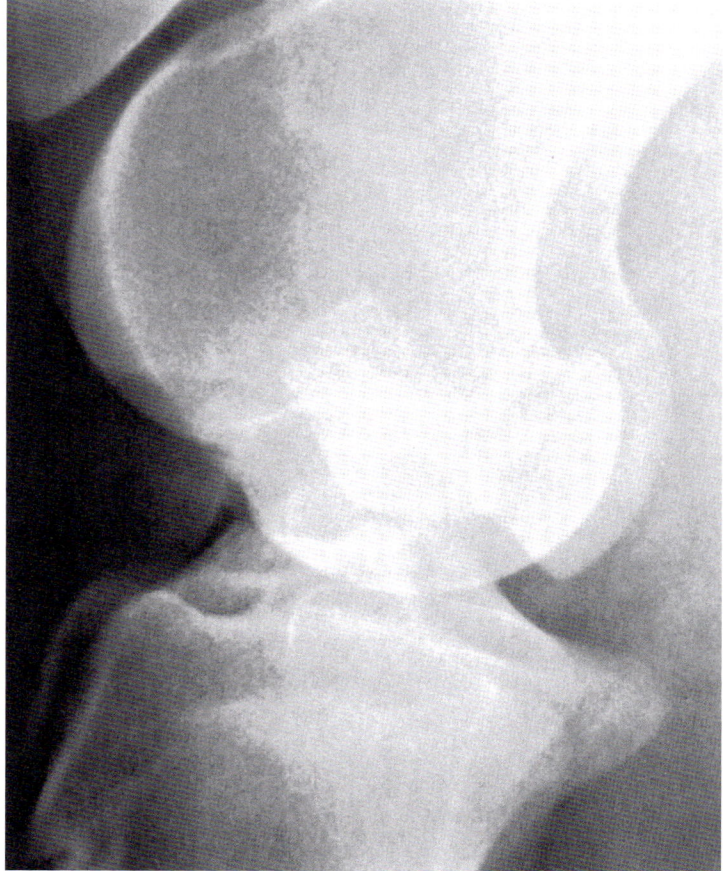

554

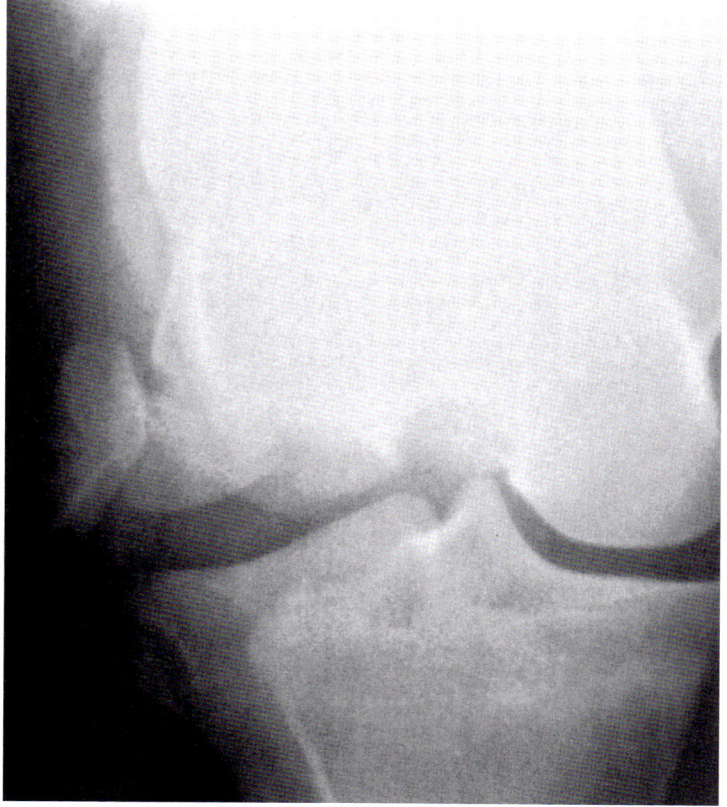

554/555 Left stifle joint, lateromedial and caudocranial view.

Warmblood, 2 years.

Several large bone fragments lateral to the distal femur and a large corresponding defect in the distal aspect of the lateral trochlear ridge and cranial aspect of the lateral femoral condyle are indicative of an avulsion fracture. This probably resulted from extreme tension on the proximal attachment of the peroneus tertius and long digital extensor tendons. The bone fragments are clearly visible on the caudocranial projection (Fig. 555). The fracture "bed" is more easily noticed on the lateromedial view (Fig. 554).

The diagnosis was confirmed by histological examination.

555

Femur

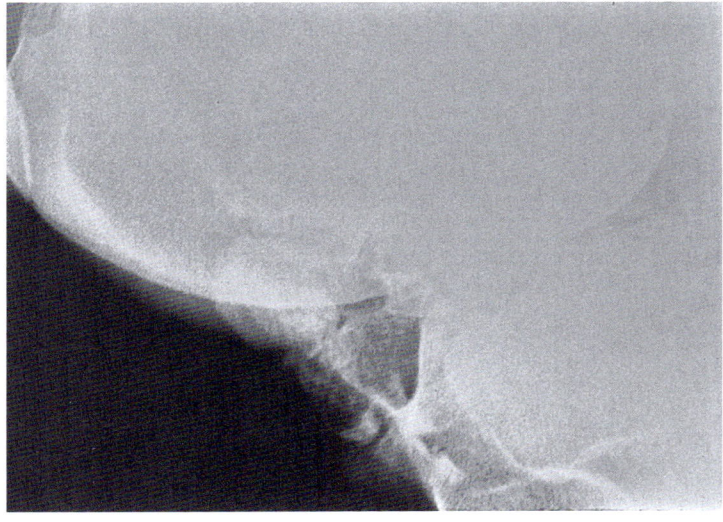

556

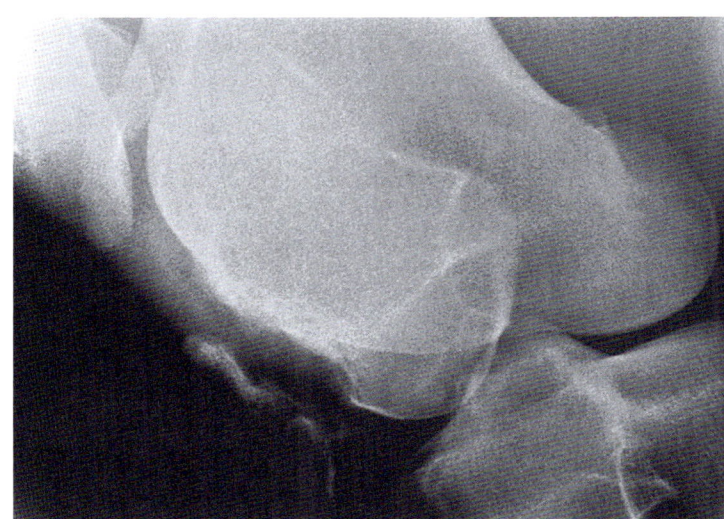

557

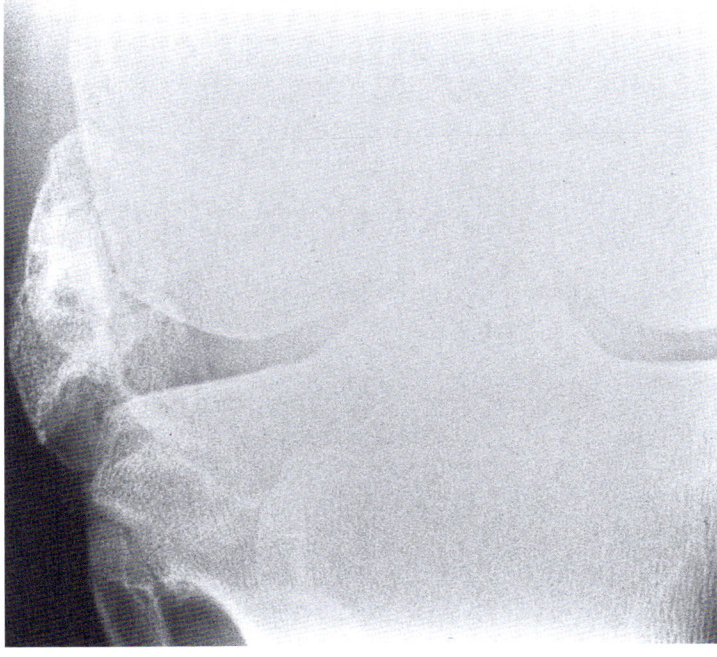

558

556/557/558 Right stifle joint, lateromedial, caudolateral-craniomedial oblique and caudocranial view: close-ups.

Warmblood, 8 years.

Several large bone fragments lateral to the distal femur and proximal tibia and a corresponding irregular contour defect of the extensor fossa is characteristic of avulsion fracture of the combined origin of the peroneus tertius/long digital extensor. The fracture "bed", i.e. the irregular contour defect of the extensor fossa is outlined on the lateromedial view (Fig. 556), but more easily seen on the caudolateral-craniomedial oblique projection (Fig. 557). The fragmentation is most obvious on the caudocranial view (Fig. 558) and appears larger than the corresponding fracture "bed".

Additional ultrasonography demonstrated associated peroneus tertius/long digital extensor calcification.

Fracture

Femur

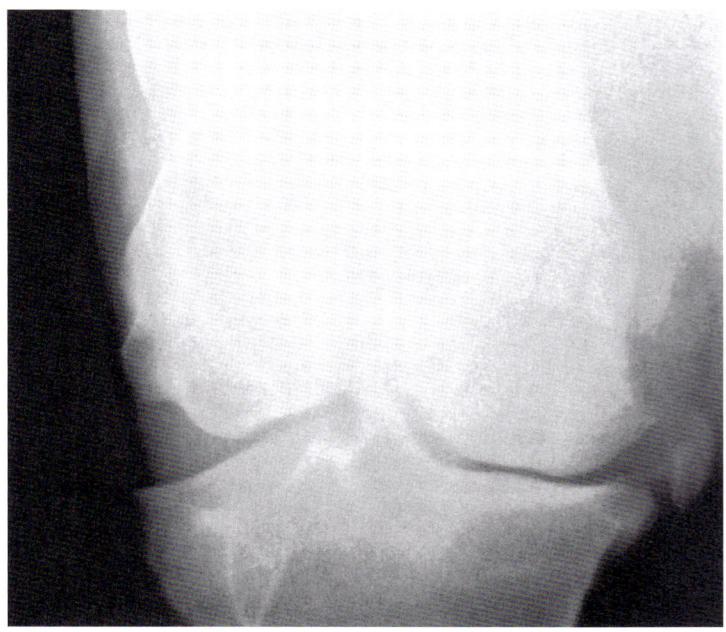

559 Left stifle joint, caudocranial view.

Warmblood, 22 years.

The bone fragment medial to the femorotibial joint and excavation and irregularity of the concave contour of the medial femoral condyle result from a recent avulsion fracture at the proximal insertion of the medial collateral ligament.

Additional finding: the minimal marginal lipping and narrowing of the medial femorotibial joint indicate osteoarthrosis, probably associated with medial meniscal injury.

Patella

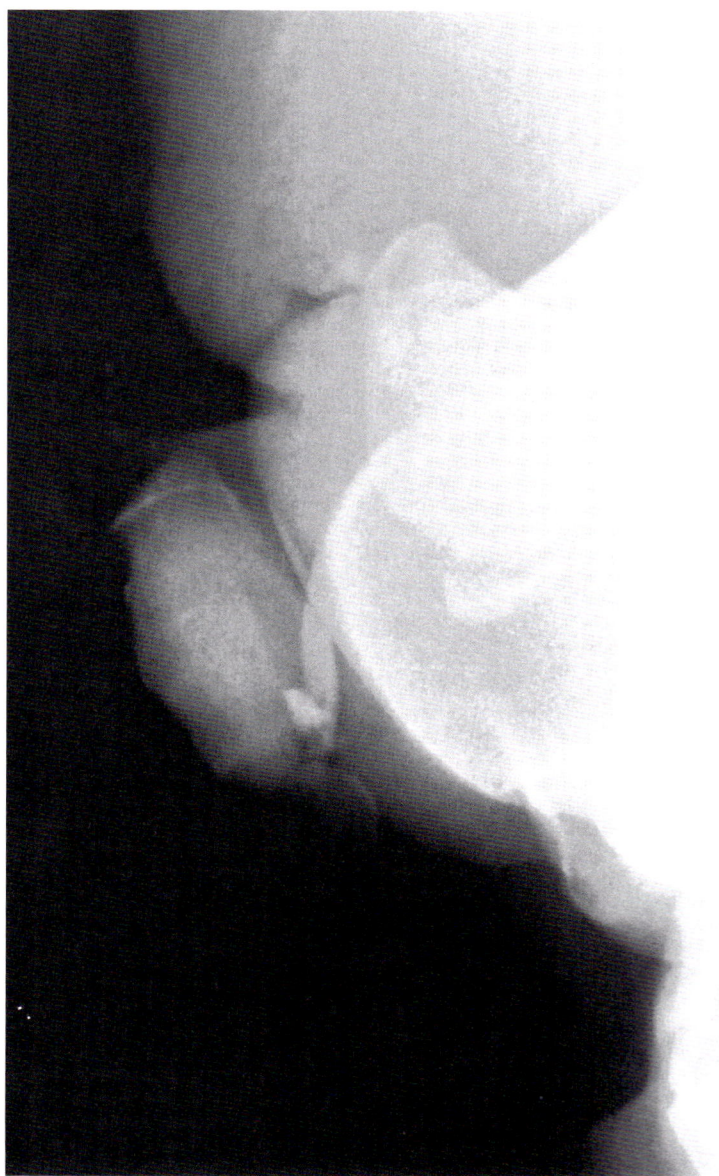

560 Right stifle joint, lateromedial view: close-up.

Warmblood, 6 years.

Separation of the patella into two large displaced fragments, due to a longitudinal fracture. Additional smaller fragments are visible in the apical and basilar regions of both major fragments. The fluid level proximal to the cranial major patellar fragment results from air accumulation in the proximal aspect of the femoropatellar joint cavity. This indicates that the fracture is an open one, associated with a wound penetrating the femoropatellar joint.

Patella

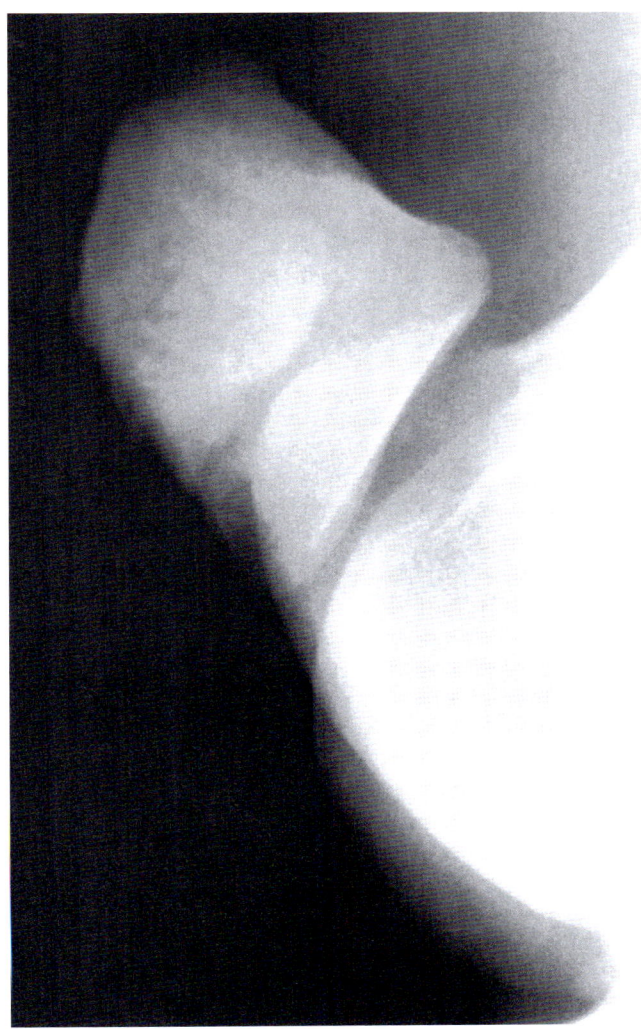

561

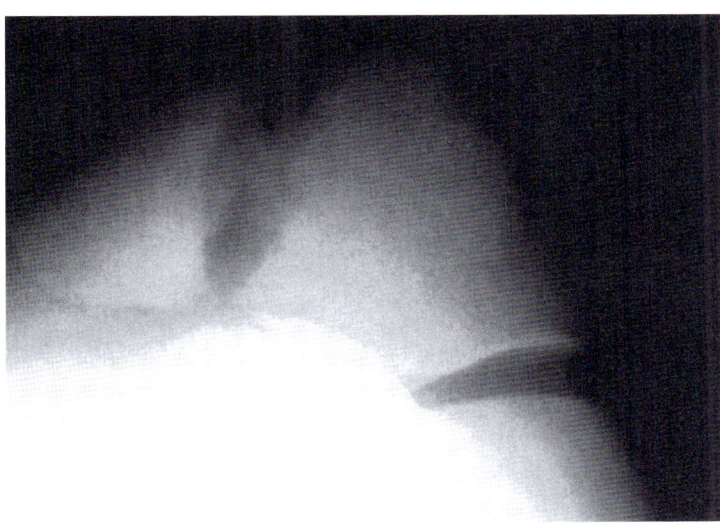

562

561/562 Right stifle joint, lateromedial and cranioproximal-craniodistal "skyline" view: close-ups.

Warmblood, 2 years.

The lateromedial view (Fig. 561) presents only an irregular radiolucent pattern **(1)** in the cranial aspect of the patella. The "skyline" projection (Fig. 562) clearly demonstrates a sagittal radiolucent zone through the central aspect of the patella, interrupting the articular surface and the cranial border. This indicates the presence of a complete longitudinal fracture with slight displacement of the fragments.

N. B. "Skyline" projections of the stifle are especially indicated if a patellar injury has occurred and lateromedial views ar not diagnostic.

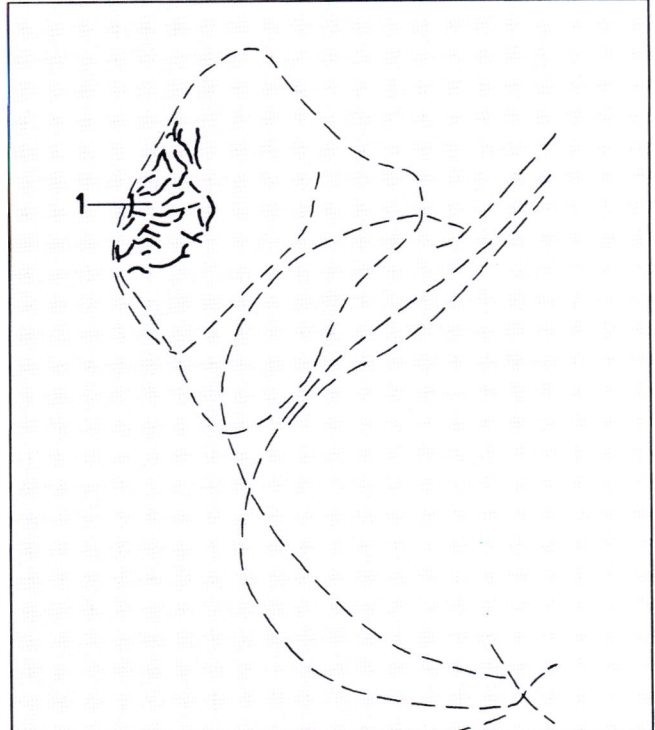

561 a Schematic drawing

Fracture

Patella

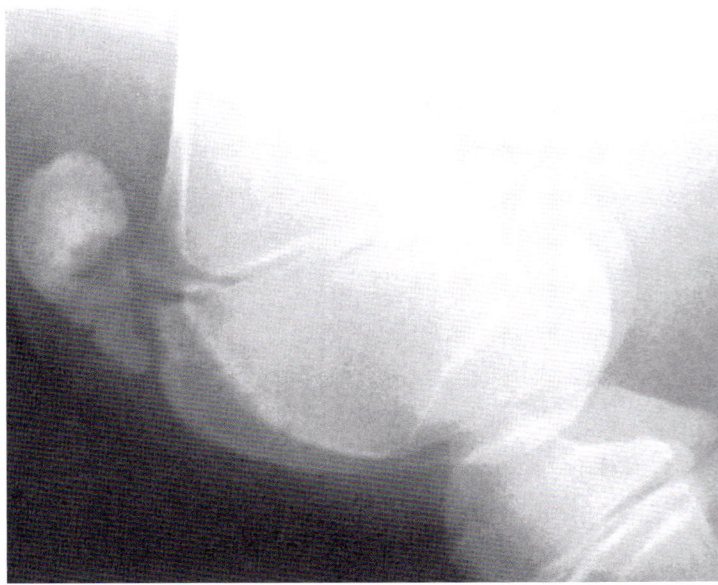

563 Left stifle joint, lateromedial view.

Foal, 1 month.

The fragmentation of the distal half of the patella results from a committed fracture with slight displacement.

N. B. The irregularity of the borders of the femoral trochlea and the patella represents the normal irregular subchondral ossification pattern in sites not completely ossified at birth. These irregularities disappear after the rapid phase of ossification is completed (Fig. 590–593).

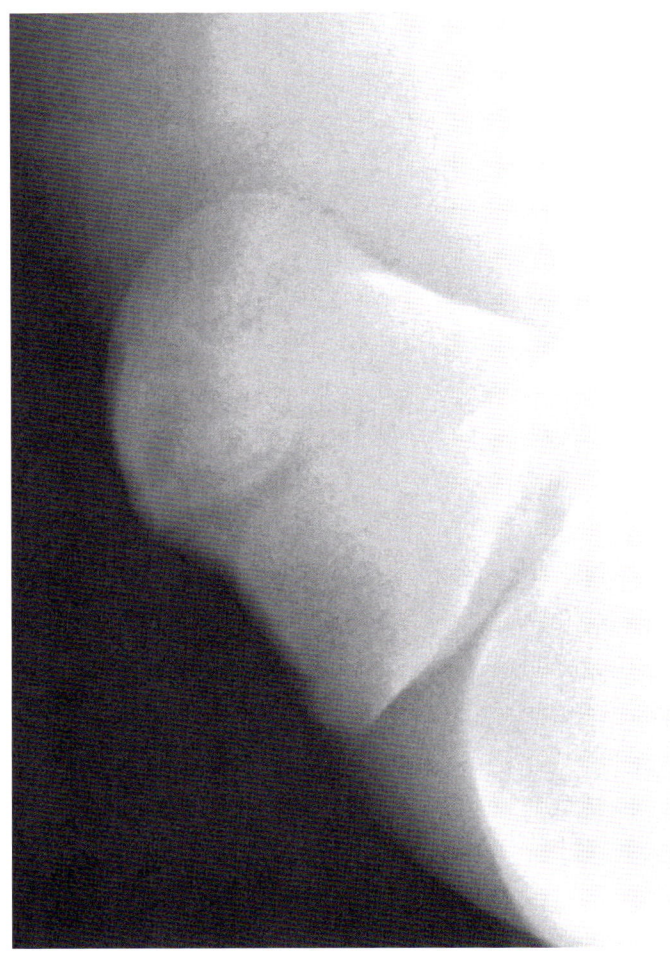

564

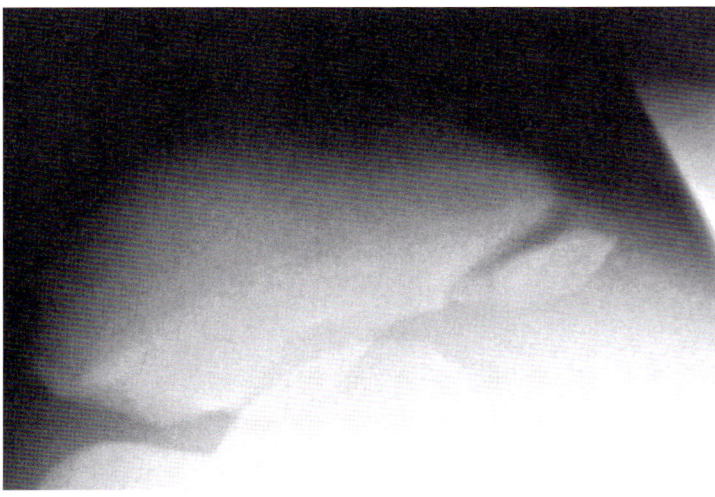

565

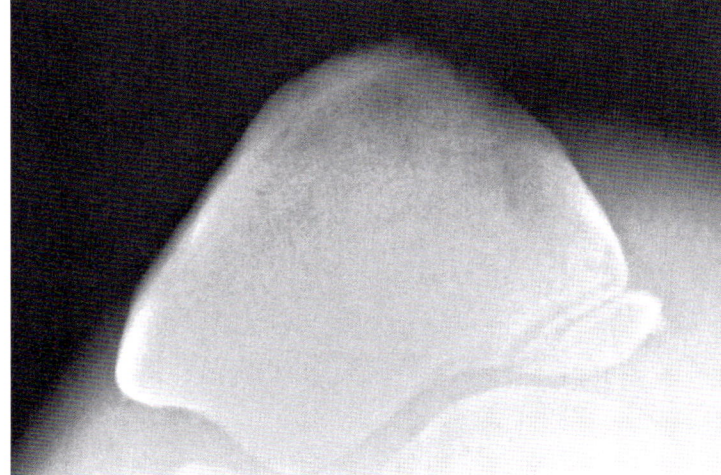

566

564/565/566 Left stifle joint, lateromedial and serial cranioproximal-craniodistal skyline views: close-ups.

Warmblood, 8 years.

The initial "skyline" view (Fig. 565) clearly demonstrates an isolated bone fragment at the medial patellar angle, resulting from a simple intra-articular avulsion fracture due to extreme tension on the attachment of the medial patellar ligament to the accessory fibrocartilage of the medial patellar angle. The lateromedial view (Fig. 564) shows only an obscure radiolucent pattern in the cranial aspect of the patella.

On a follow-up "skyline" projection 1½ years later (Fig. 566), the fragment remains visible despite clinical recovery. The fracture plane is not parallel with the proximodistally directed central beam and therefore two radiolucent lines are visible. Healing of the fracture by fibrous callus, not visible on survey radiographs, may explain the discrepancy between the clinical and radiographic findings.

Patella

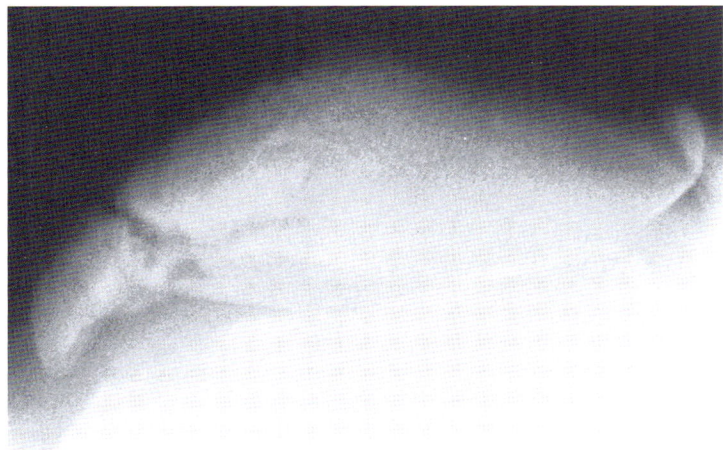

567 Left stifle joint, cranioproximal-craniodistal "skyline" view: close-up.

Standardbred, 11 months.

An isolated bone fragment at the lateral patellar angle and a concomitant radiolucent line in the adjacent portion of the patellar base resulting from avulsion fracture due to extreme tension on the attachment of the lateral femoropatellar ligament. These fractures are less common than those at the medial patellar angle. The ill bordered fracture zone suggests a fracture of some duration. However, due to potential healing of patellar angle fractures by fibrous callus (Fig. 564–566), the delineation of fracture zone and bone fragment is not a good criteria of fracture duration.

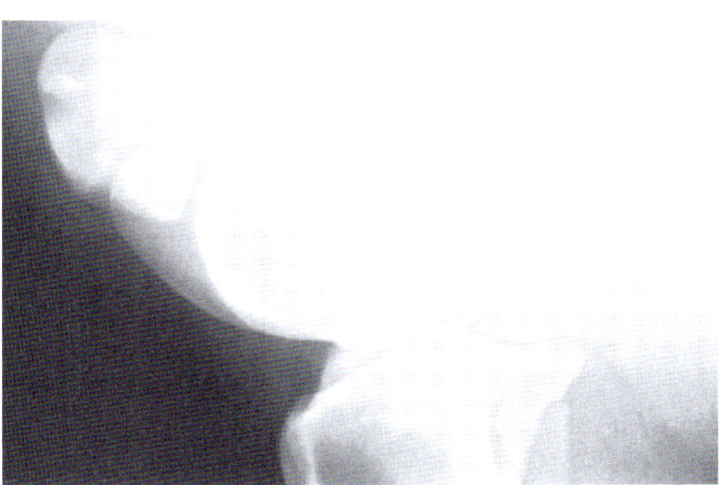

568 Right stifle joint, lateromedial view.

Pony, 11 years.

The ill defined bone fragment proximal to a corresponding radiolucent defect in the cranial part of the patella results from a chip fracture caused by a kick from another horse 2 weeks prior to the examination.

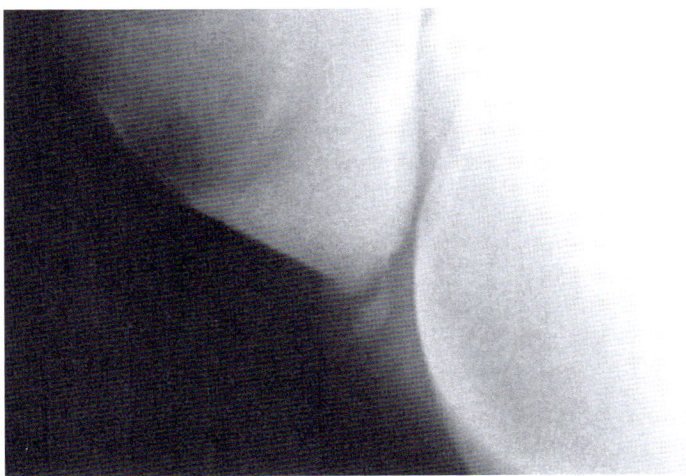

569 Right stifle joint, lateromedial view: close-up.

Warmblood, 8 years.

The well defined bone fragment distal to the apex of the patella represents an apical avulsion fracture. This seldom occurring fracture followed medial patellar desmotomy.

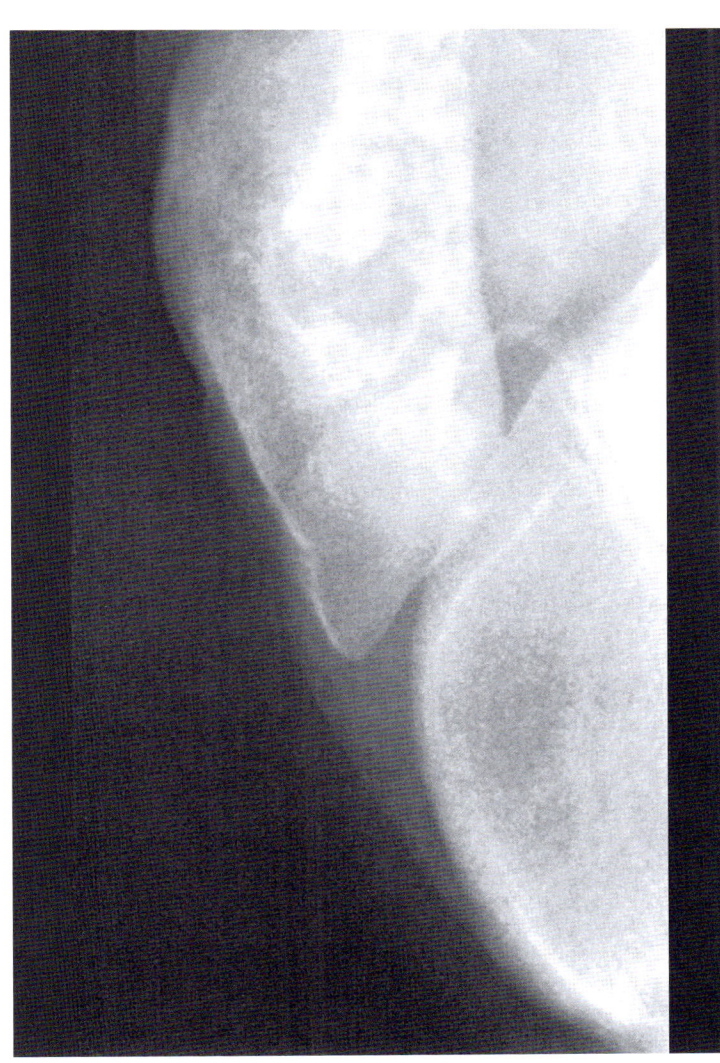

570 Left stifle joint, lateromedial view: close-up.

Foal, 6 months.

The deformation and irregular radiopacity of the caudoproximal aspect of the patella result from a traumatic injury 4 weeks prior to the examination. The differential diagnosis includes osteochondrosis (Fig. 626).

Fracture

Tibia

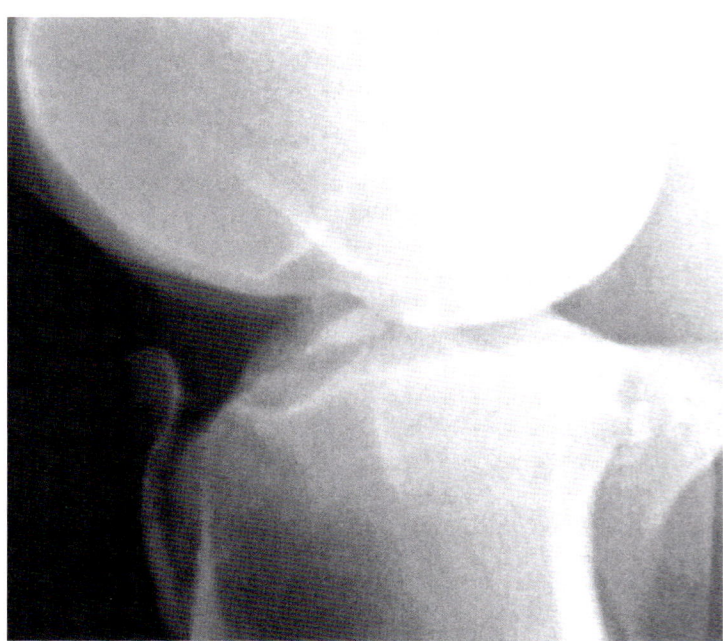

571

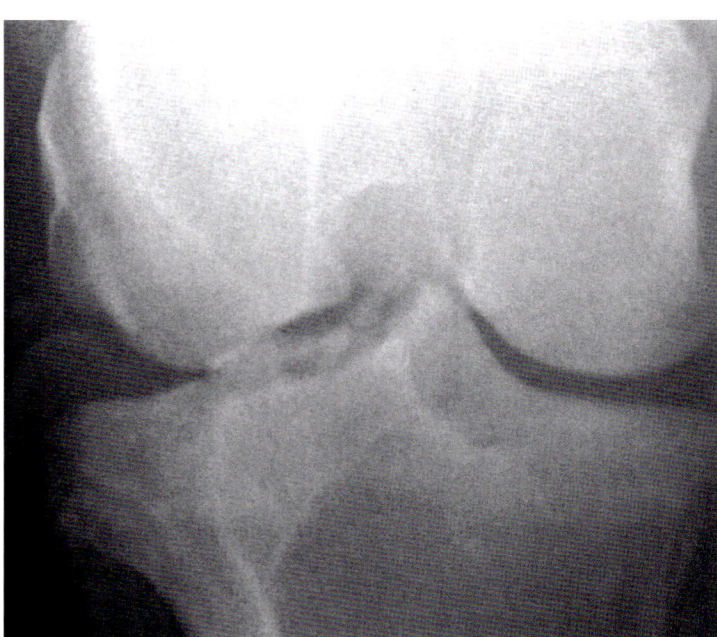

572

571/572 Left stifle joint, lateromedial and caudocranial view: close-ups.

Warmblood, 7 years.

The large bone fragment cranial to the proximal tibia, clearly visualized on the lateromedial view (Fig. 571), results from a fracture of the lateral part of the tibial tuberosity. The caudocranial projection (Fig. 572) reveals additional fragmentation of the articular surface of the lateral tibial condyle and tibial spine.

The radiographic changes indicate severe injury of the patellar and cranial cruciate ligaments and considerable associated damage to the lateral compartment of the femorotibial joint.

Tibia

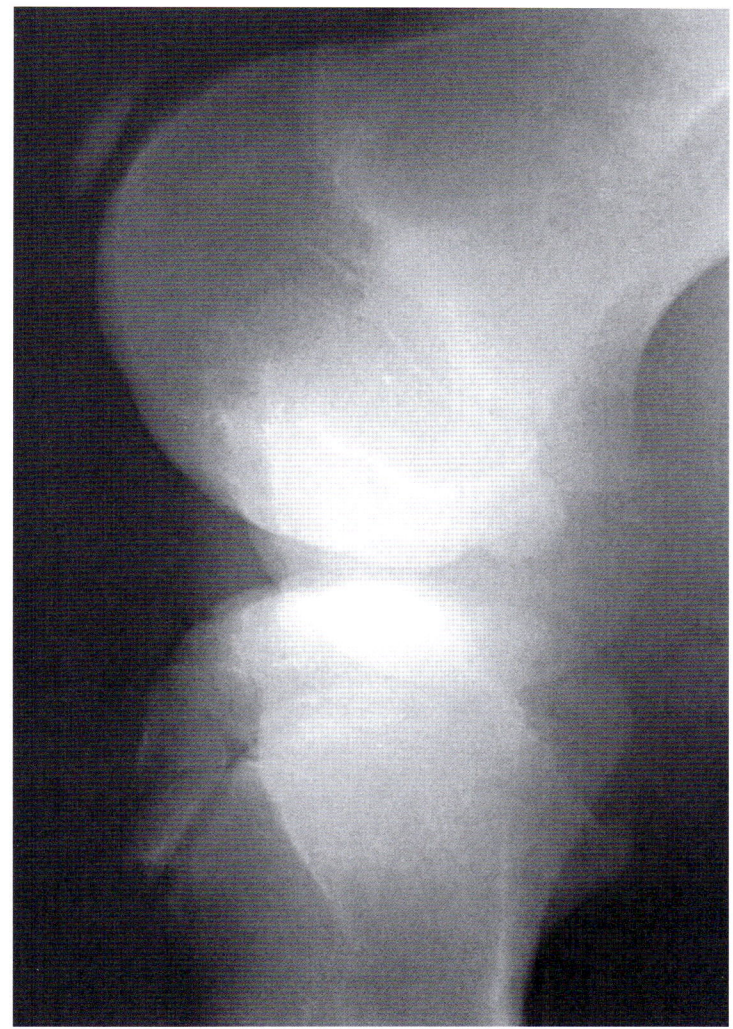

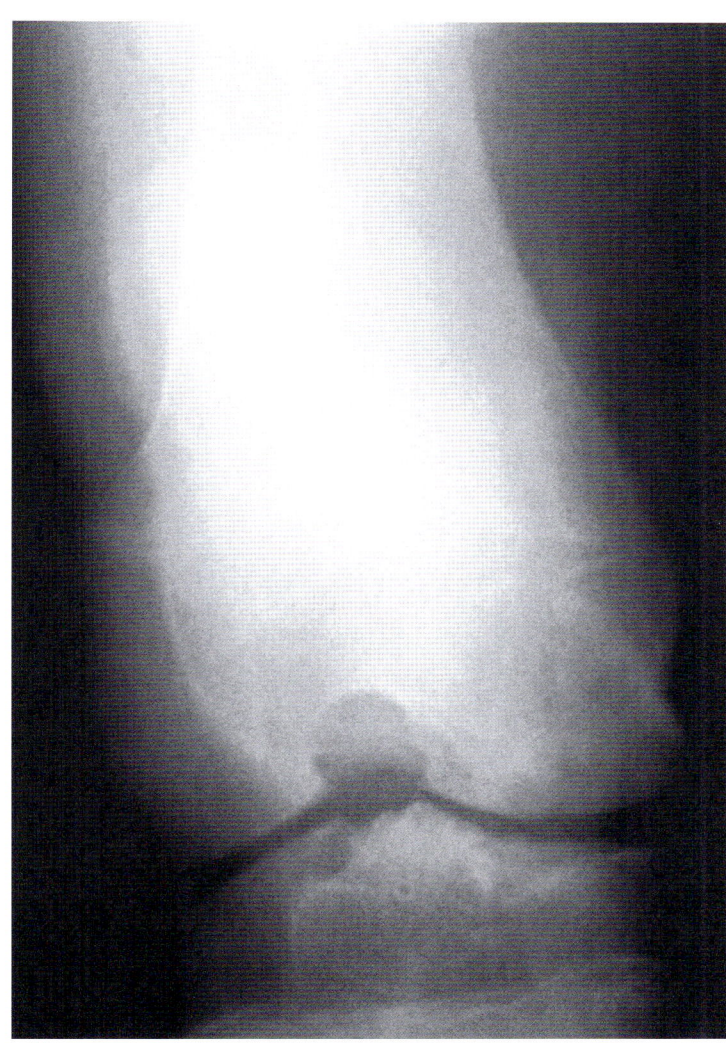

573

574

573/574 Left stifle joint, lateromedial and caudocranial view.

Warmblood, 14 months.

The slightly oblique lateromedial view (Fig. 573) reveals flattening and irregularity of the caudoproximal aspect of the medial femoral condyle, and the tibial spine appears to be absent.

On the caudocranial view (Fig. 574) the tibial spine is visible but not as prominent as it should be, and the articular surface of the medial tibial condyle is slightly irregular.

The radiographic changes, indicating osteoarthrosis of the medial compartment of the femorotibial joint associated with severe chronic injury of the cruciate ligaments, resulted from a traumatic injury 1 year prior to examination.

Fracture

Tibia

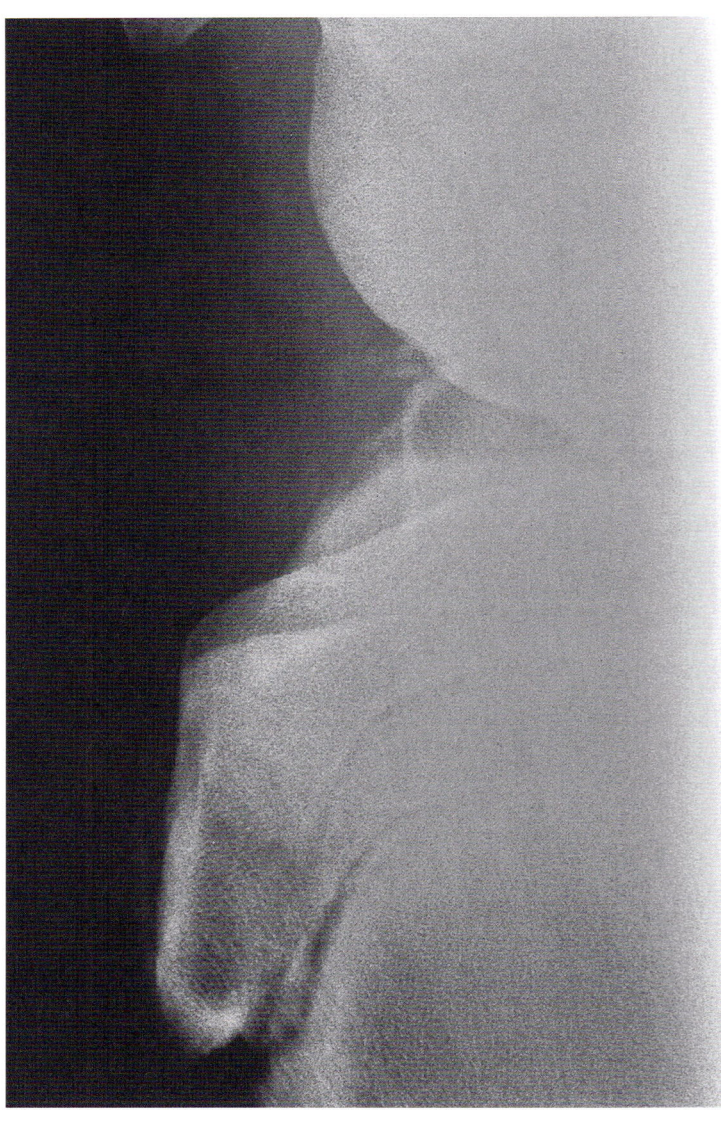

575 Right stifle joint, flexed lateromedial view: close-up.

Warmblood, 1 ½ years.

Small bone fragments cranial to the craniomedial part of the intercondylar eminence, indicating trauma to the tibial insertion of the cranial cruciate ligament. In this horse this was caused by a recent puncture wound and not resulting from an avulsion injury.

Tibia

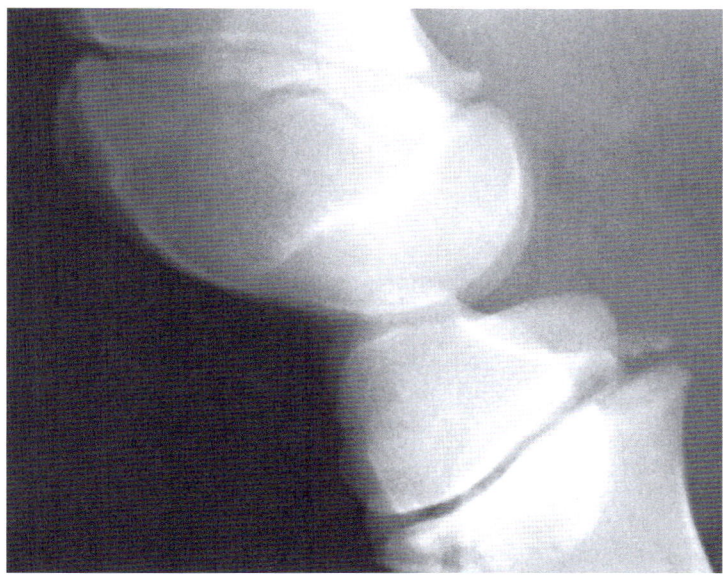

576

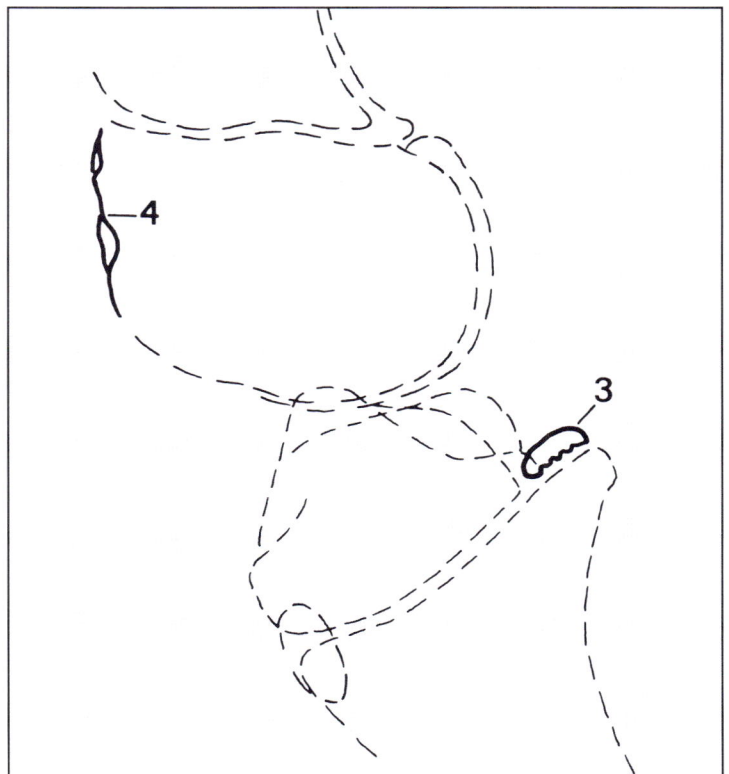

576 a

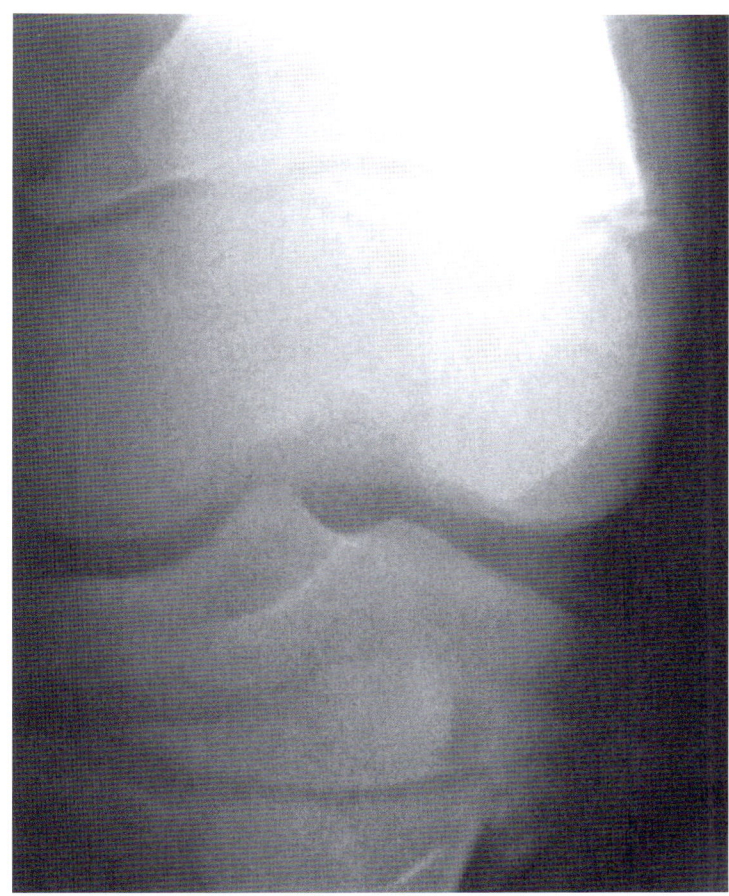

577

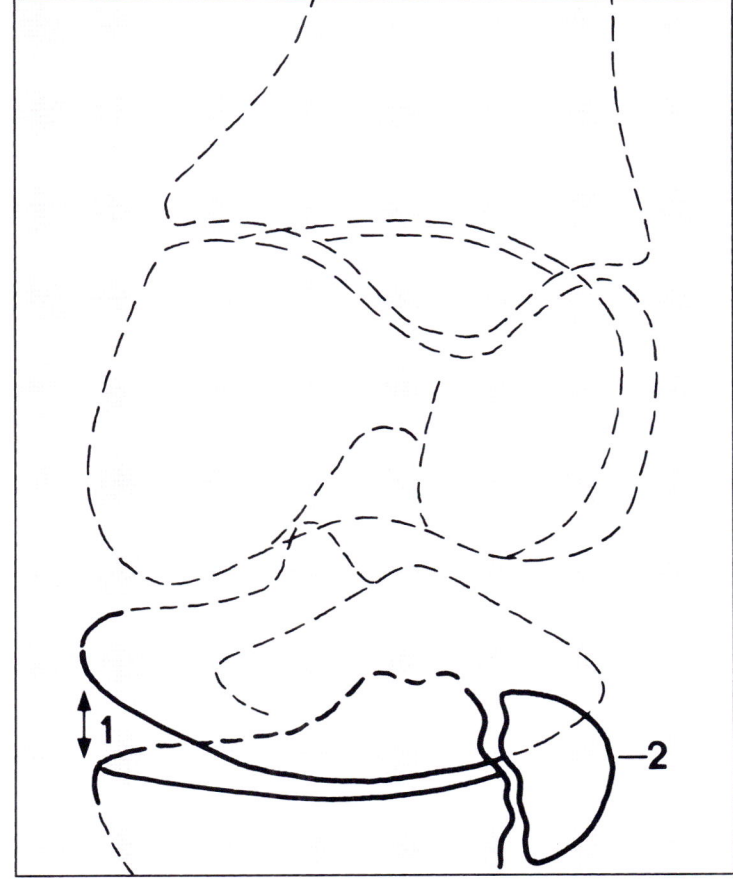

577 a

576/577 Right stifle joint, lateromedial and caudocranial view.

Foal, 2 weeks.

The widening of the medial aspect of the proximal tibial physis **(1)** and fragmentation of the lateral part of the corresponding metaphysis **(2)** on the caudocranial view (Fig. 577), indicate a Salter-Harris type 2 physeal fracture.

The lateromedial projection (Fig. 576) shows only an irregular, slightly displaced (metaphyseal) fracture fragment **(3)** caudal to the tibial physis. The proximal tibial growth plate appears to be normal.

N. B. The irregularity of the borders of the femoral trochlea **(4)** represents the normal irregular ossification pattern in the distal femoral epiphysis in young foals (Fig. 590 – 593).

576 a/577 a Schematic drawings

Fracture

Tibia

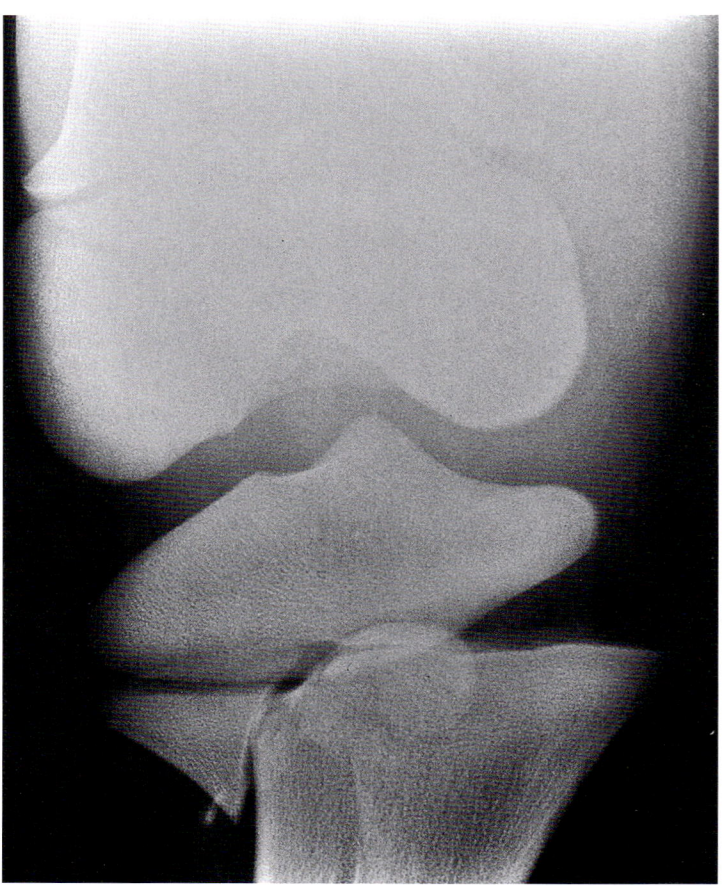

578 Left stifle joint, caudocranial view.

Foal, 1 day.

Prominent widening of the medial aspect of the proximal tibial physis, as well as a large triangular bone fragment and superimposing small bone fragments involving the lateral part of the corresponding metaphysis consistent with a recent Salter-Harris type 2 physeal fracture.

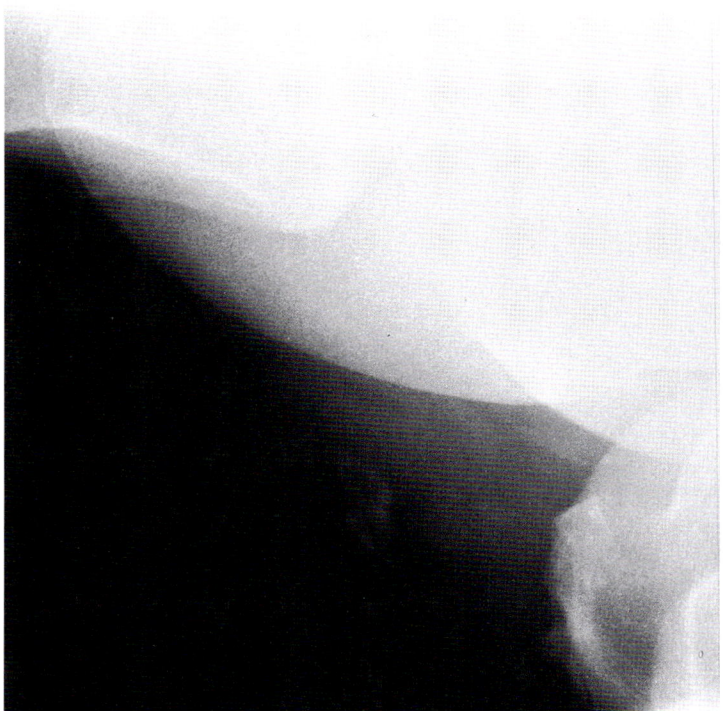

579 Right stifle joint, craniolateral-caudomedial oblique view: close-up. Standardbred, 7 years.

The ill defined radiopacity cranial to the femoral trochlea combined with the irregular contour of the proximomedial border of the tibial tuberosity suggest avulsion injury of the tibial insertion of the medial patellar ligament, the radiopacity representing the avulsed tibial bone fragment.

Additional imaging with ultrasonography confirmed the diagnosis.

Tibia

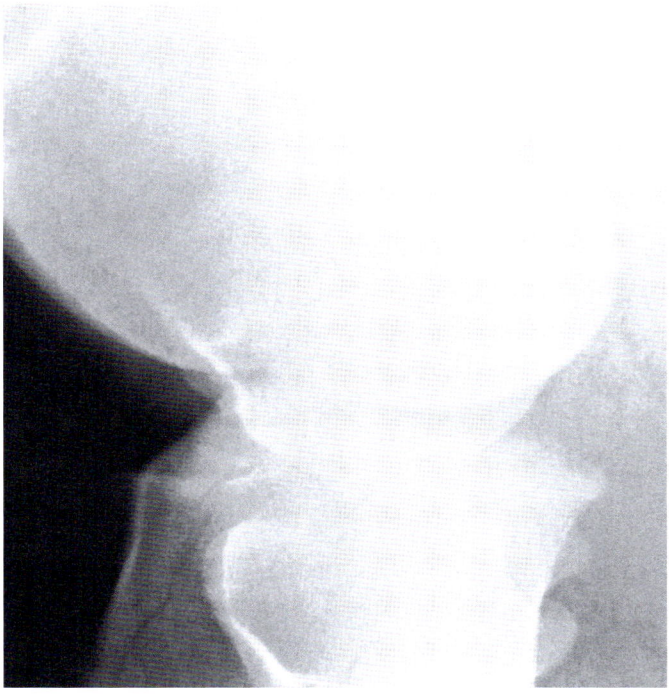

580

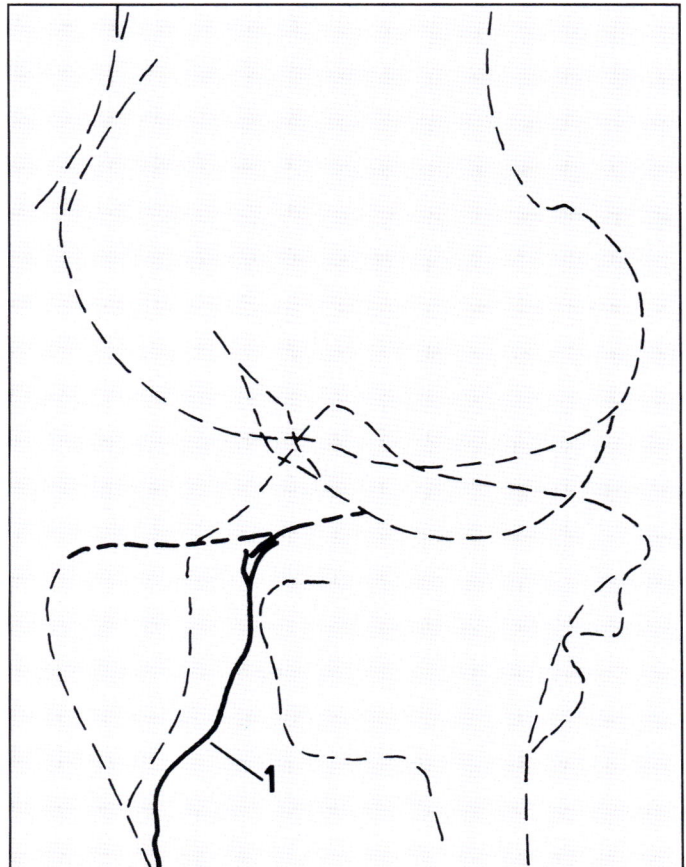

580 a

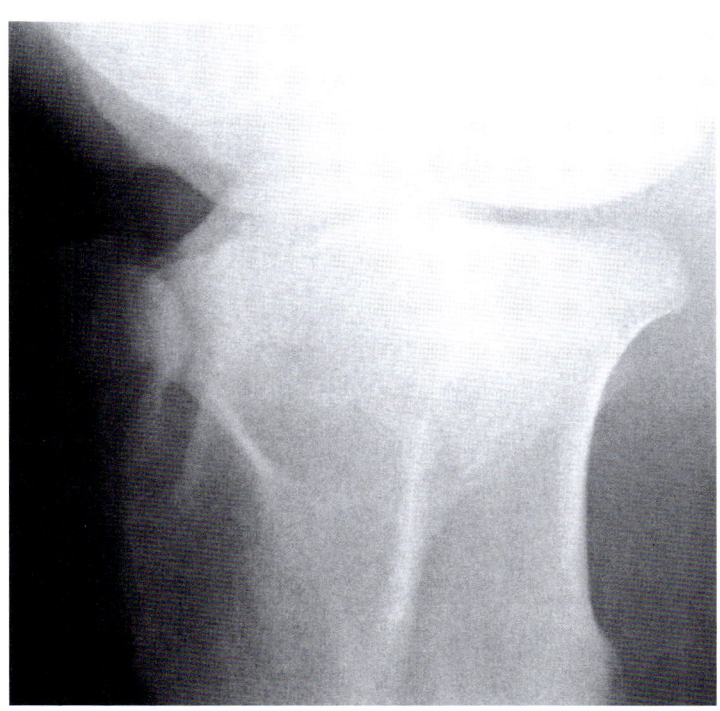

581

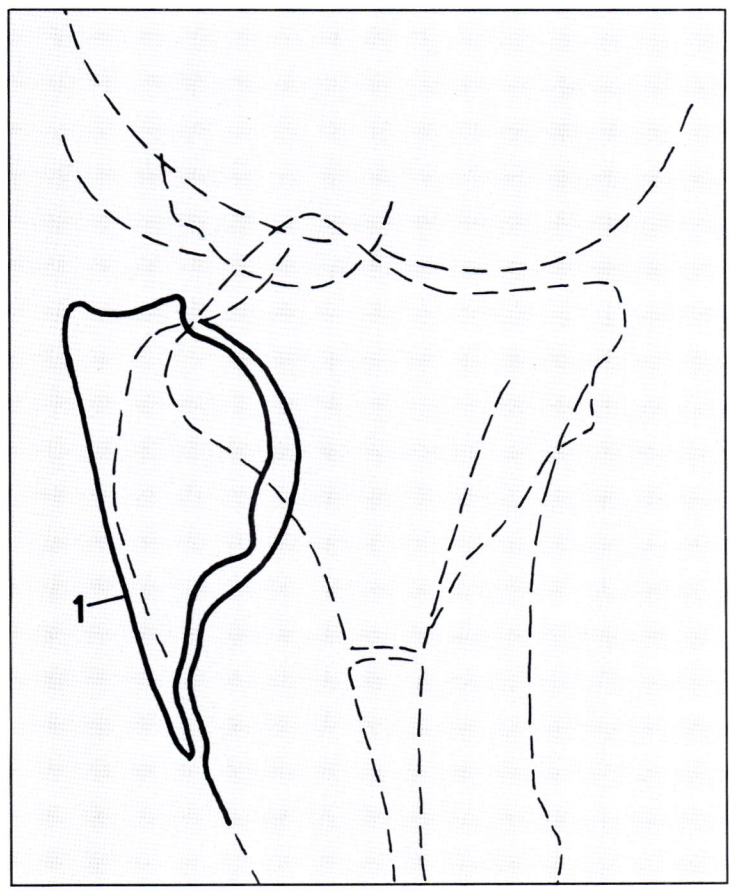

581 a

580 Right stifle joint, lateromedial view.

Warmblood, 8 years.

The vertical-oblique sharply bordered radiolucent line **(1)** through the lateral part of the tibial tuberosity represents a recent, complete, non-displaced, extra-articular avulsion fracture. The fracture probably resulted from extreme tension on the attachment of the patellar ligaments to the tibial tuberosity.

(The radiograph is deliberately underexposed to highlight the fracture.)

580 a Schematic drawing

581 Left stifle joint, caudolateral-craniomedial oblique view: close-up.

Warmblood, 9 years.

The large, sharply bordered bone fragment **(1)** superimposed on the cranial aspect of the tibial tuberosity indicates a complete, slightly displaced, extra-articular avulsion fracture of the lateral part of the tibial tuberosity.

The sharply bordered fracture zone suggests a recent fracture, although injury occurred 3 weeks prior to examination.

581 a Schematic drawing

Luxation

Patella

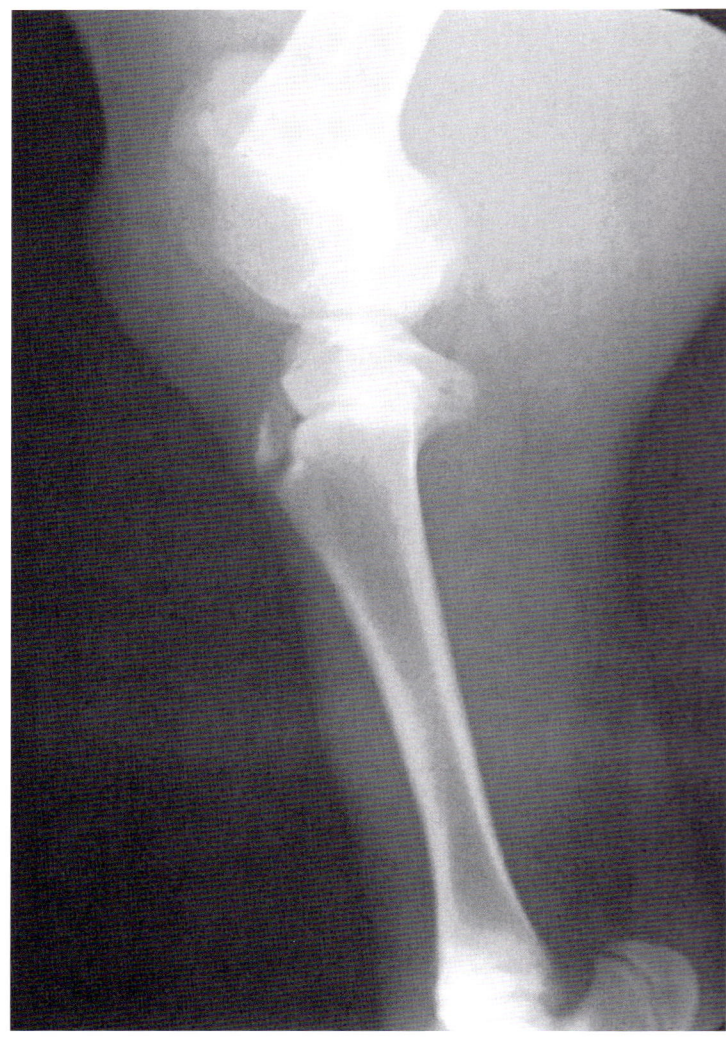

582

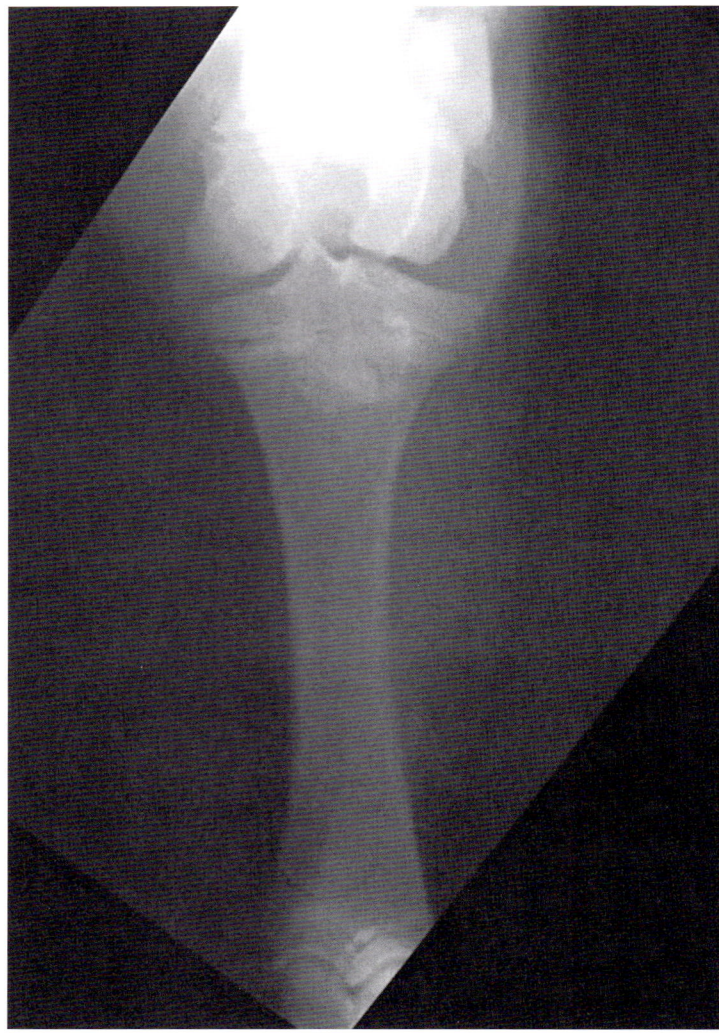

583

582/583 Right stifle joint, lateromedial and caudocranial view.

Shetland pony, 3 months.

On the lateromedial view (Fig. 582) the patella is difficult to identify due to superimposition of the femur, and has a rounded instead of triangular shape. This is the result of (congenital) lateral patellar luxation, clearly demonstrated on the caudocranial projection (Fig. 583).

The soft tissue swelling cranial to the femoral trochlea, visible on the lateromedial view, results from concomitant effusion of the femoropatellar joint.

Patella

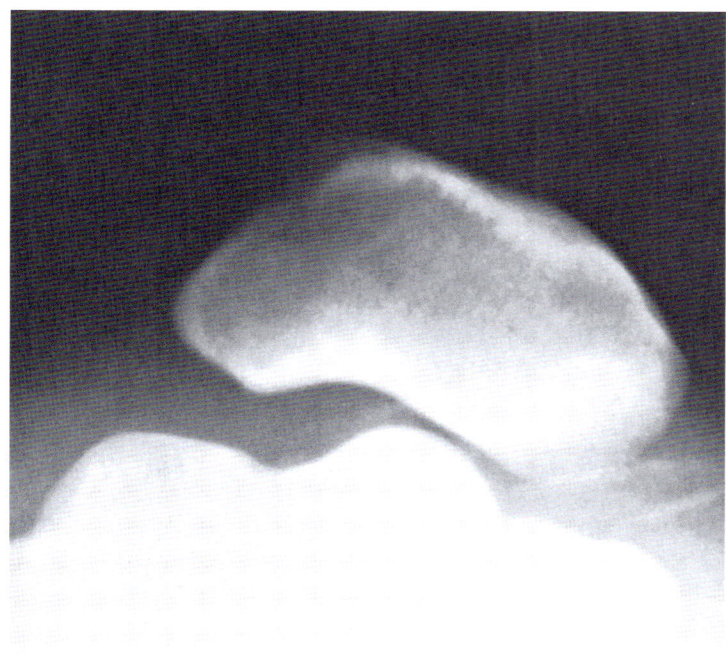 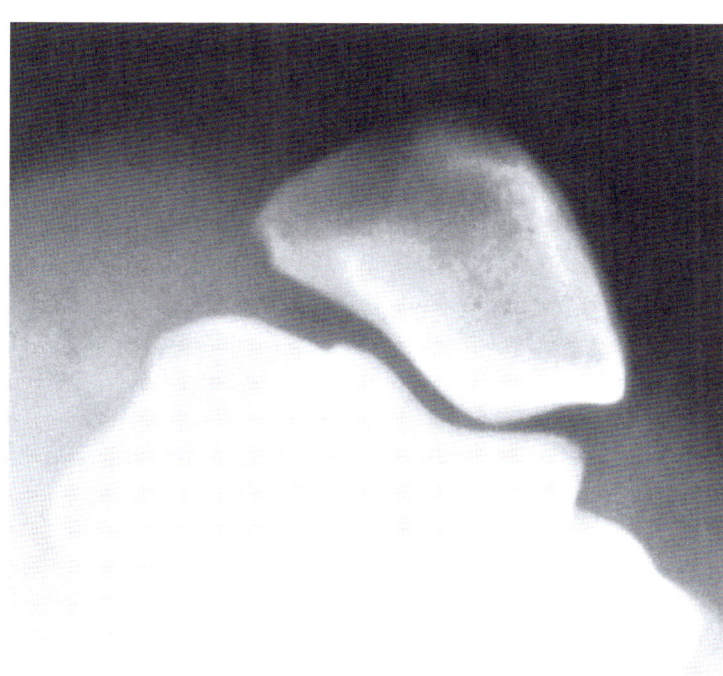

584   585

584/585 Right stifle joint, cranioproximal-craniodistal "skyline" view of an abnormal and a normal patella: close-ups.
Shetland pony, 2 years (abnormal patella).

(Congenital, intermittent) lateral subluxation of the patella (Fig. 584). The "skyline" view permits accurate assessment of the degree of displacement. The abnormal patellar shape suggested by this projection is a false finding, resulting from distortion due to the patellar displacement.

The normal patellar shape is demonstrated by the "skyline" view of a non-displaced patella (Fig. 585).

Tibia

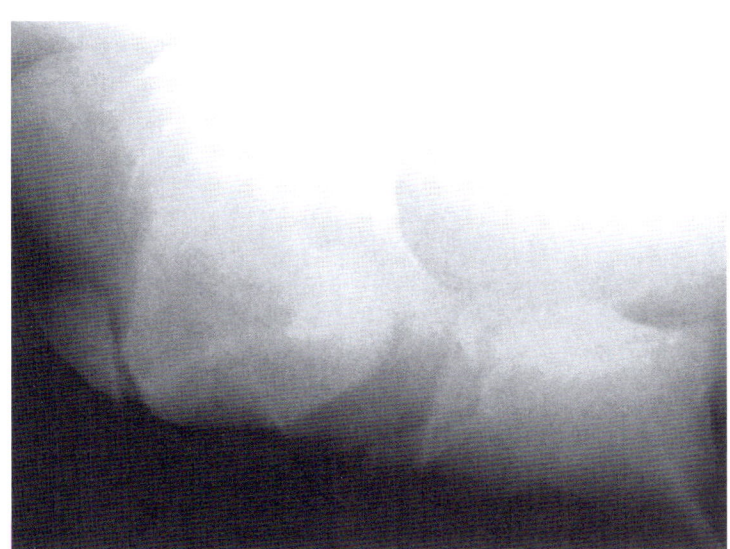

586 Right stifle joint, lateromedial view.
Warmblood, 10 years.

Complete luxation of the femorotibial joint with caudoproximal displacement of the tibia and overriding of the lateral femoral condyle, indicating complete rupture of the caudal cruciate ligament.

Ligamentous injury

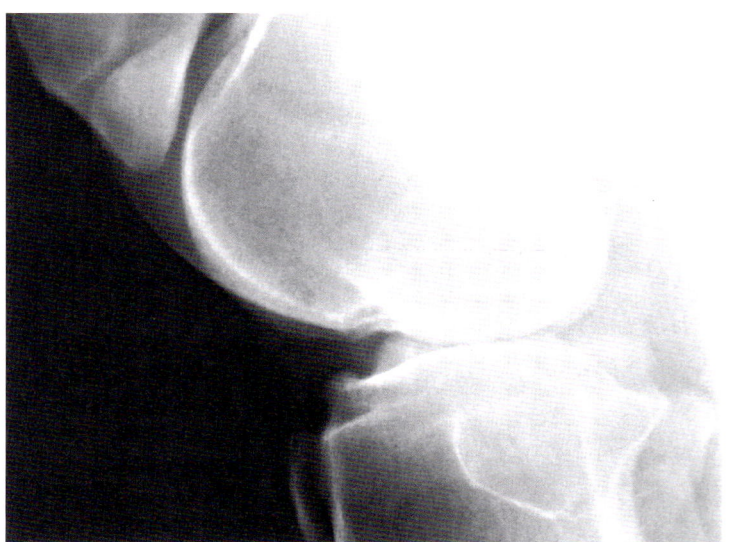

587

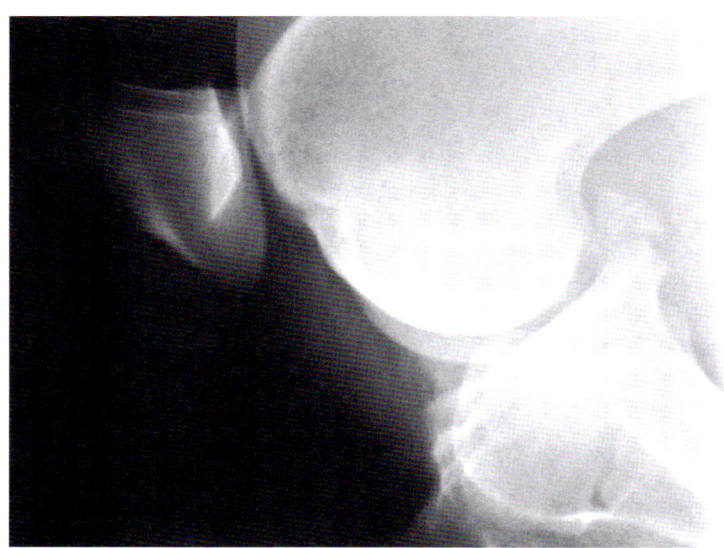

588

587/588 Right stifle joint, weight-bearing and flexed lateromedial view.

Warmblood, 22 years.

The routine weight-bearing lateromedial view (Fig. 587) shows considerable narrowing of the femorotibial joint space, an obscure bone fragment caudal to the articular surface of the femoral condyles, and bony proliferation at the proximal aspect of the tibia cranial to the tibial spine. The radiographic changes indicate osteoarthrosis of the femorotibial joint associated with meniscal damage. On an additional flexed lateromedial view (Fig. 588) cranial displacement and irregularity of the tibial spine (normally positioned between the femoral condyles) indicate injury to the cranial cruciate ligament, along with the meniscal damage. This view reveals spur formation on the caudoproximal aspect of the tibia, and more clearly demonstrates the bone fragment caudal to the femoral condyles, which resulted from either calcification of the damaged meniscus or detachment from the intercondyloid fossa.

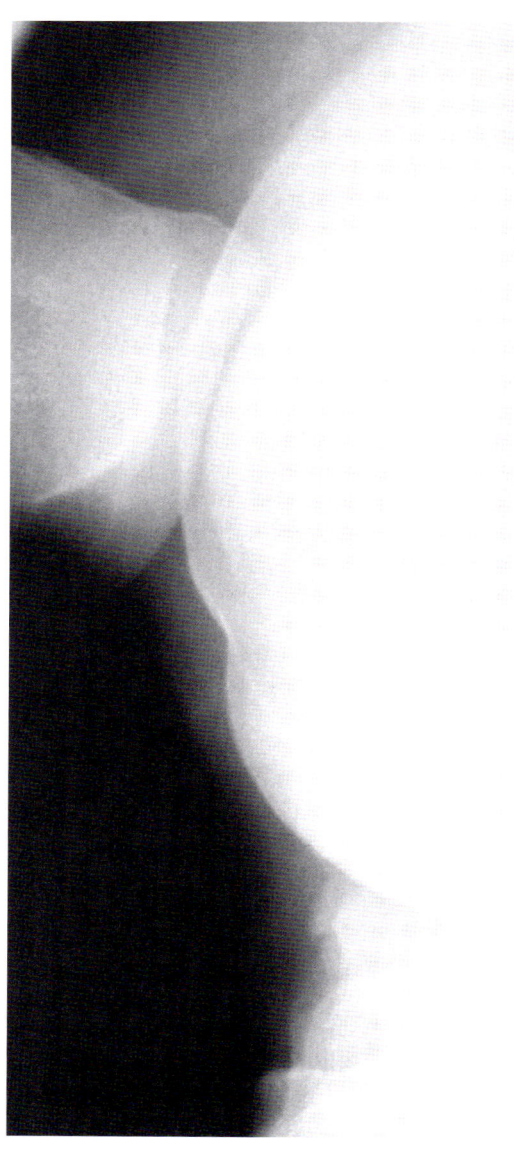

589 Right stifle joint, flexed lateromedial view: close-up.

Warmblood, 10 years.

Cranial displacement and a radiolucent defect in the cranial aspect of the tibial spine characteristic of injury to the cranial crucial ligament.

N. B. Cranial displacement of the tibial spine, i. e. the tibia, is frequently visible only on a flexed lateromedial view of the stifle and not clearly demonstrated on a standard weight-bearing lateromedial projection.

589

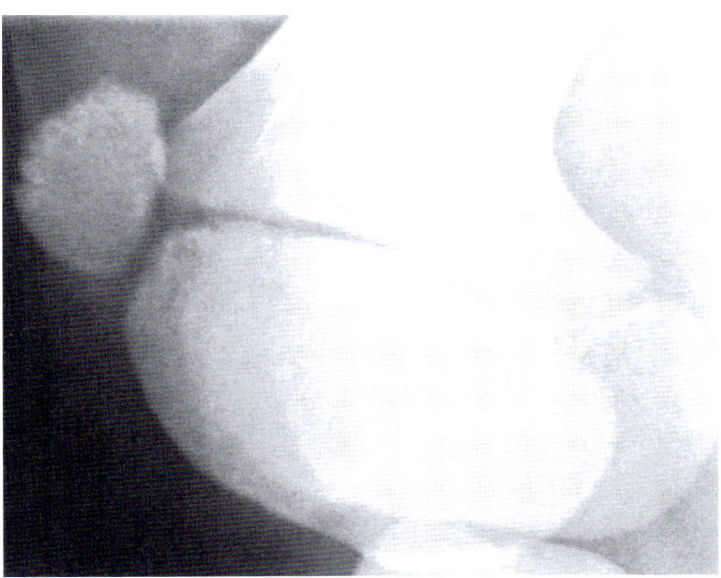

590 Right stifle joint, lateromedial view: close-up.

Foal, 2 days.

The mottled radiolucency and irregular border of the patella and femoral trochlea on this (slightly oblique) lateromedial view represent the normal irregular postnatal ossification pattern. At this age the bony patella is semicircular and the lateral trochlear ridge is not yet apparent radiographically.

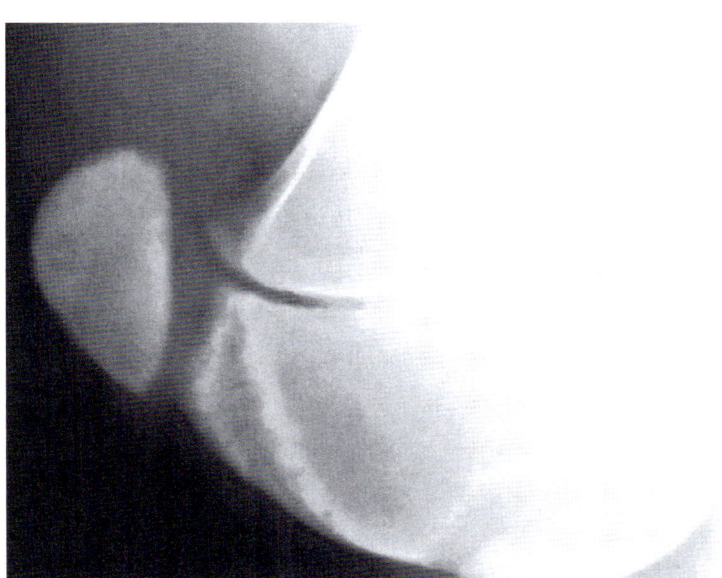

591 Right stifle joint, lateromedial view: close-up.

Foal, 24 days.

The irregularity of the femoral trochlea, due to the irregular postnatal ossification, is very prominent. The irregularity of the patella is slightly less obvious than it is directly after birth. Gradually the shape of the patella becomes more triangular. At this age both the medial and lateral trochlear ridges are visible radiographically.

The proximal aspect of the medial trochlear ridge is still narrower than the corresponding metaphysis, and the discrepancy in size between the trochlear ridges is small.

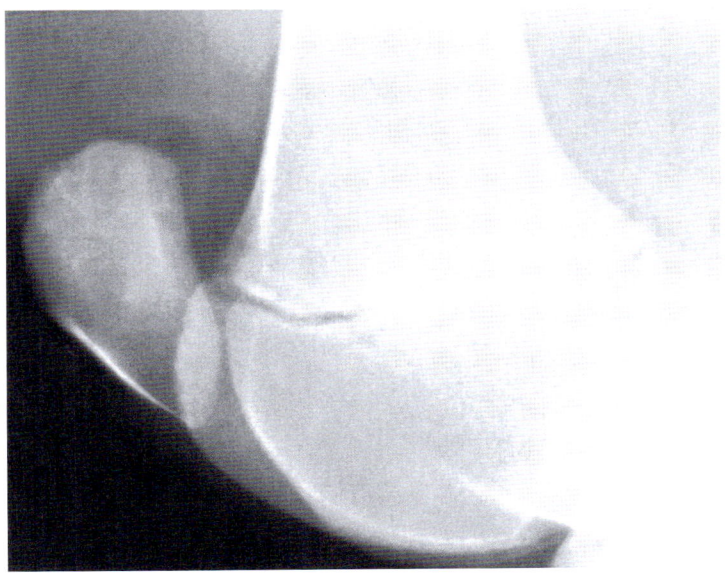

592 Right stifle joint, lateromedial view: close-up.

Foal, 3 months.

Minimal irregularity limited to the cranioproximal aspect of the patella and proximal aspect of the medial trochlear ridge indicates that the rapid phase of postnatal ossification of these sites is nearly completed.

As this age the patella has reached its definitive shape. The proximal aspect of the medial trochlear ridge has become wider than the corresponding metaphysis, but the discrepancy in size between the trochlear ridges is not yet very prominent..

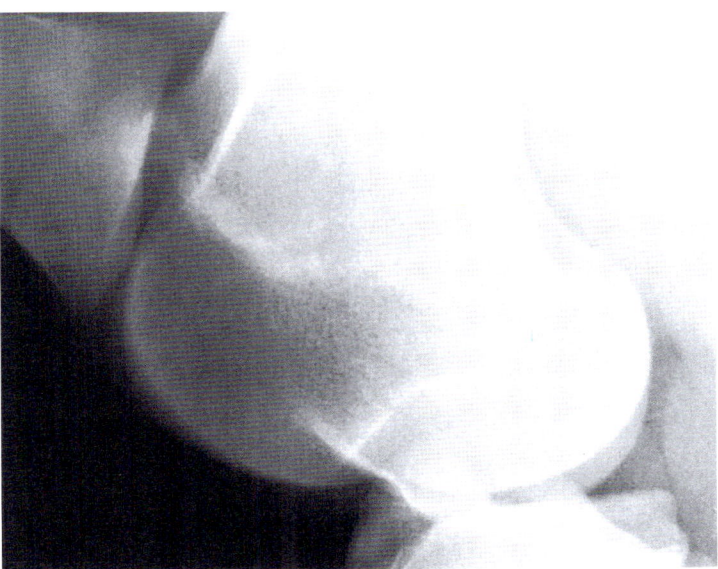

593 Right stifle joint, lateromedial view.

Warmblood, 2 years.

The medial trochlear ridge is much larger, especially proximally, than the lateral ridge. The ossification of the patella and trochlear ridges is completed between 3 and 6 months of age, and "ossification irregularities" are therefore no longer present at these sites.

Infectious arthritis

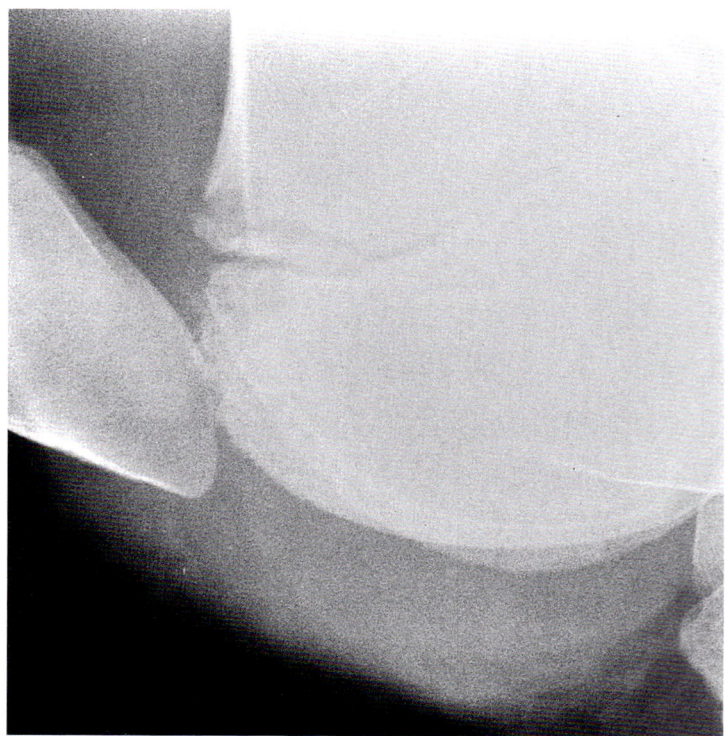

594

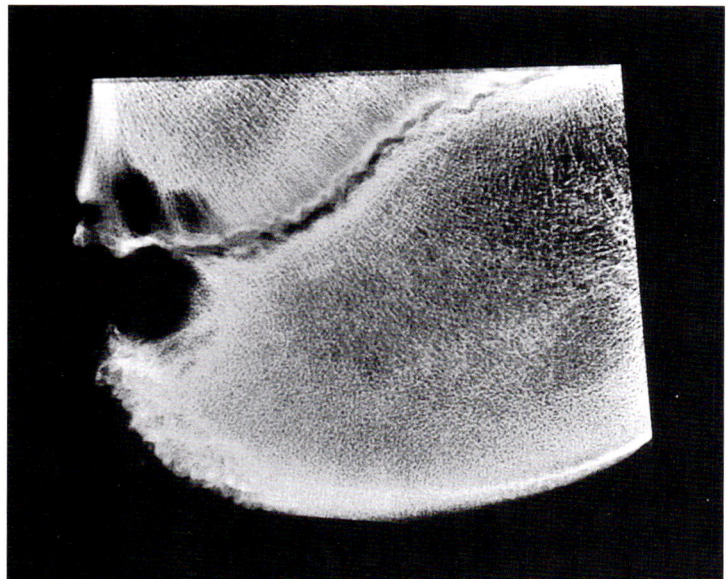

595

594/595 Left stifle joint, lateromedial view: close-up, in vivo and post mortem study.

Foal, 5 weeks.

The in vivo radiograph (Fig. 594) reveals prominent soft tissue swelling cranial to the femoral trochlea, and ill defined radiolucency of the proximal aspect of the femoral trochlea as well as the corresponding metaphyseal region of the distal femur. These findings are consistent with haematogeneous osteomyelitis type P and concomitant effusion of the femoropatellar joint.

The rounded, radiolucent osteomyelitic bone lesions close to and eroding the distal femoral physis are more clearly demonstrated on the post mortem radiograph (Fig. 595). The roughening of the proximal contour of the medial trochlear ridge represents the normal postnatal ossification pattern.

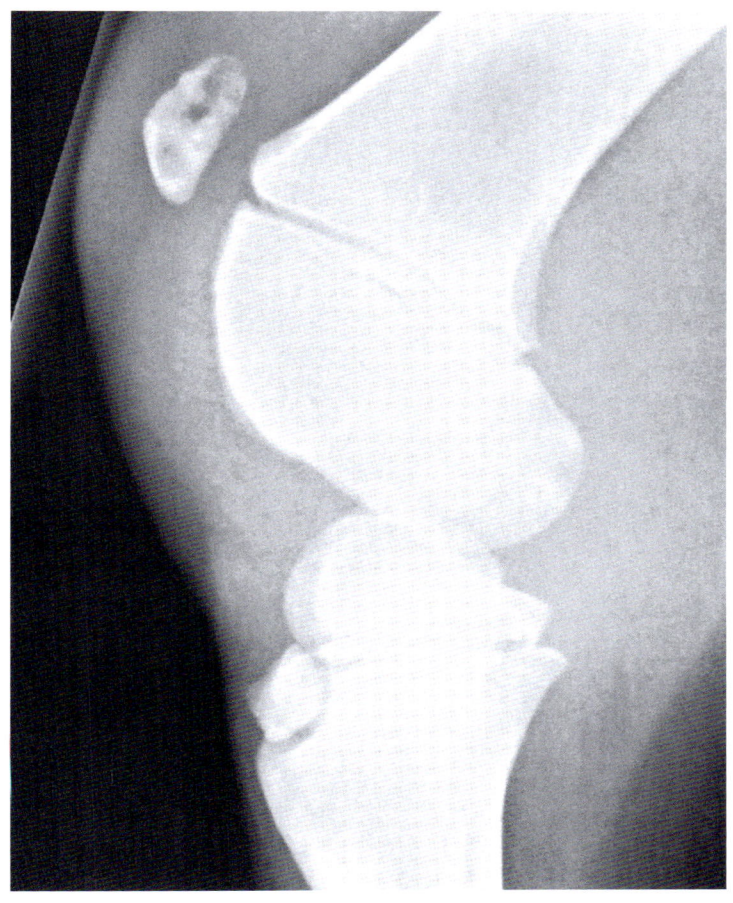

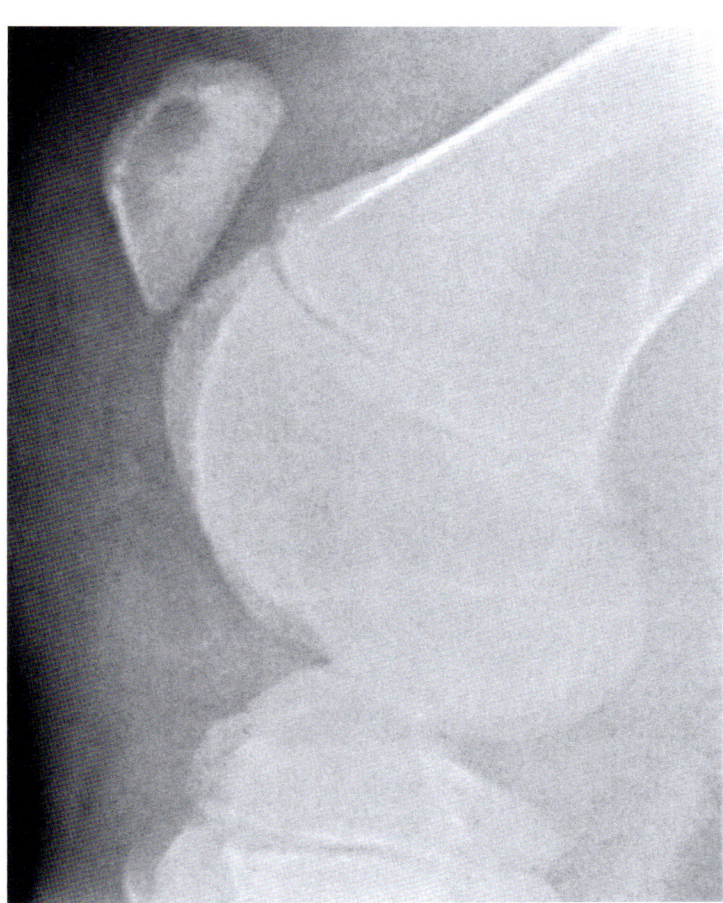

596 Left stifle joint, lateromedial view.

Foal, 3 weeks.

The soft tissue swelling cranial to the femoral trochlea and the irregular mottled radiolucent appearance of the patella are a consequence of haematogenous osteomyelitis type E, with associated infectious arthritis of the femoropatellar joint.

Additional finding: the obscure radiolucency within the caudoproximal aspect of the medial femoral condyle and the soft tissue swelling caudal to the femoral condyles represents the early stages of another type E osteomyelitic lesion with associated infectious arthritis of the femorotibial joint.

597 Left stifle joint, lateromedial view.

Foal, 5 weeks.

The large, clearly defined area of slightly irregular radiolucency within the cranial aspect of the patella represents a more advanced stage of type E osteomyelitis.

Extensive irregular soft tissue swelling cranial to the femoral trochlea and caudal to the femoral condyles results from concomitant infectious arthritis of the femoropatellar and femorotibial joint. Roughening of the contour of the proximal aspect of the medial trochlear ridge represents the normal irregular postnatal ossification pattern.

Infectious arthritis

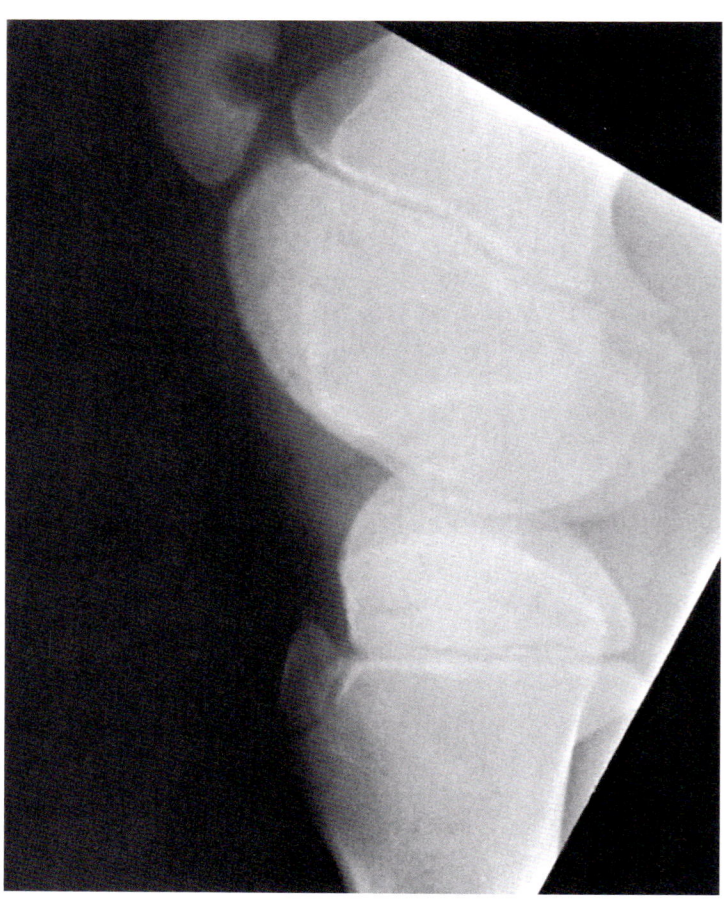

598 Right stifle joint, lateromedial view.

Foal, 2 weeks.

The subchondral cystic area of diffuse radiolucency **(1)** surrounded by a sclerotic rim and disrupting the articular surface of the patella, represents the end stage of a type E osteomyelitic lesion.

Additional finding: the ill defined radiolucent areas within the caudal aspect of the medial femoral condyle **(2)** and the distal aspect of the femoral trochlea **(3)** indicate the presence of other type E osteomyelitis lesions.

The mottled appearance of the femoral trochlea **(4)** represents the normal irregular postnatal ossification pattern.

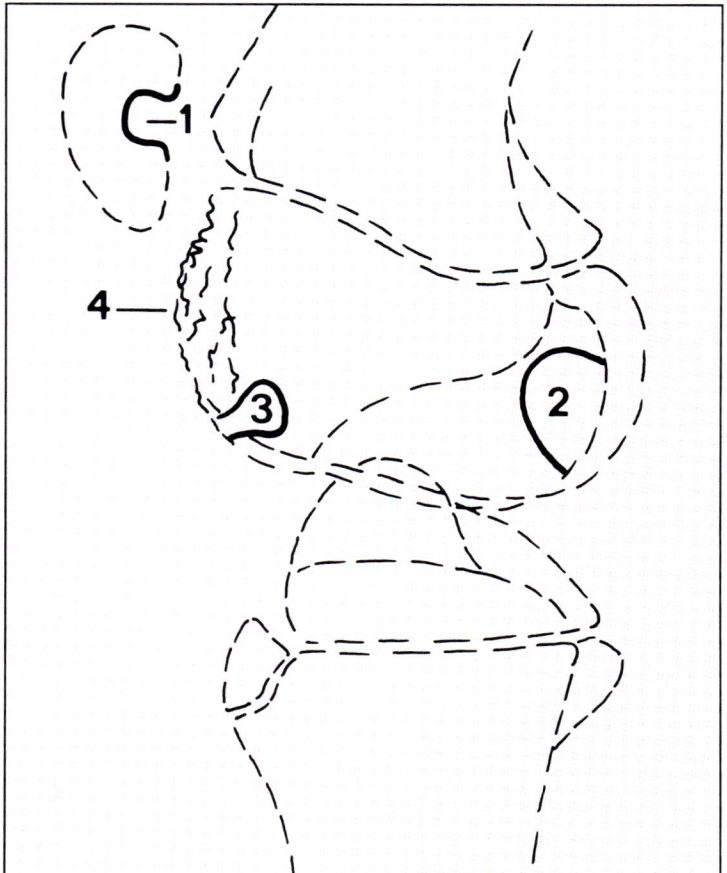

598 a Schematic drawing

599 Left stifle joint, lateromedial view.

Foal, 4 weeks.

The large, ill bordered radiolucent area within the subchondral bone of the distal part of the femoral trochlea represents an osteomyelitic type E lesion. Roughening of the corresponding trochlear border is the result of normal postnatal ossification. Marked soft tissue swelling cranial to the femoral trochlea and caudal to the femoral condyles indicates effusion of the femoropatellar and femorotibial joint, due to concomitant infectious arthritis.

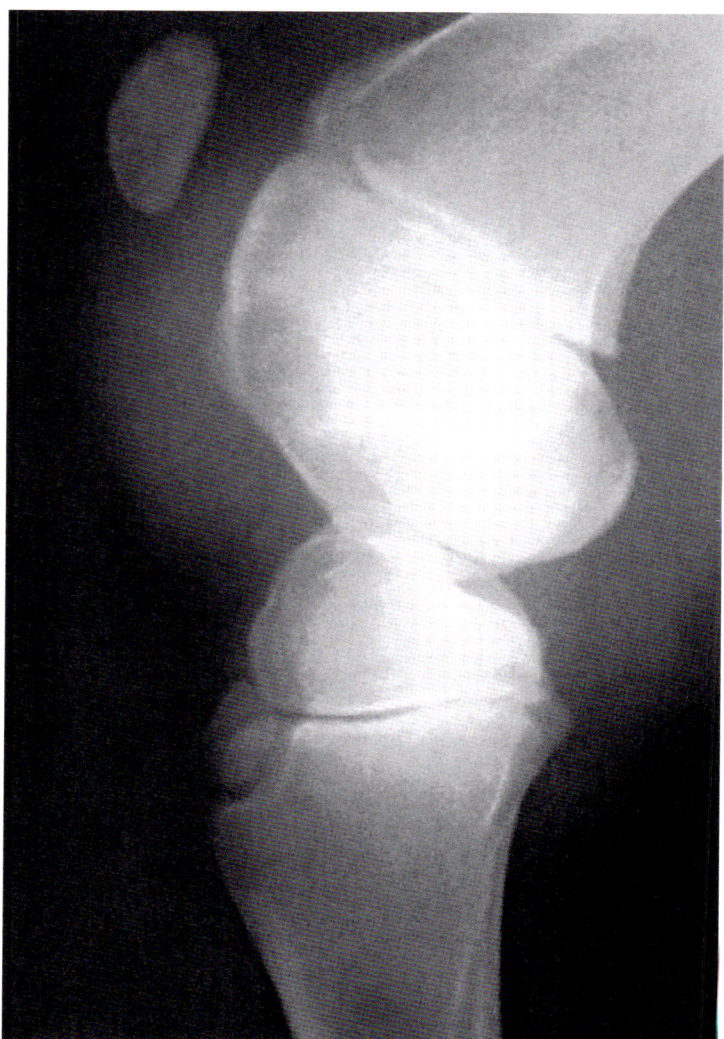

599

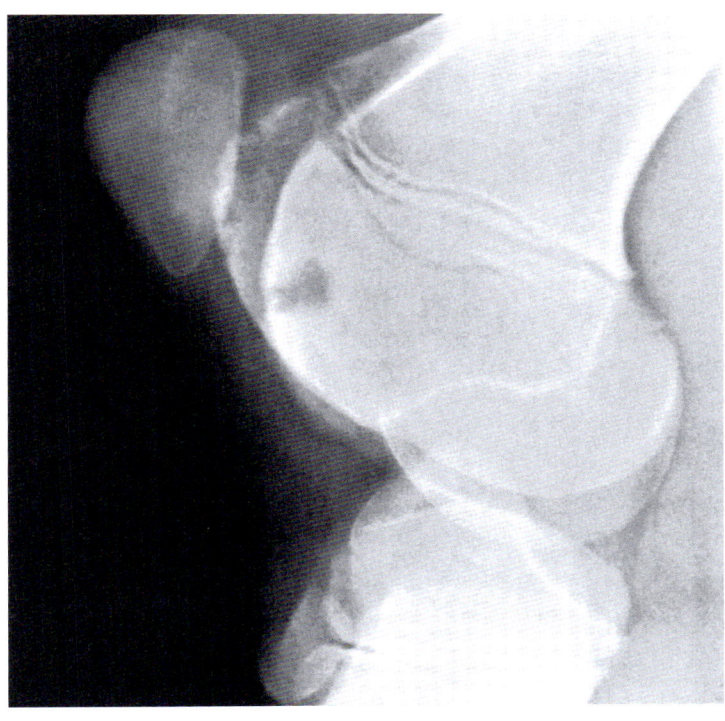

600

600/601 Right stifle joint, lateromedial survey and double contrast study. Foal, 7 weeks.

The lateromedial survey radiograph (Fig. 600) reveals a clearly defined radiolucent area within the subchondral bone of the middle portion of the lateral trochlear ridge, resulting from type E osteomyelitis. The extensive irregularity of the proximal aspect of the medial trochlear ridge, roughening of the middle and distal part of the lateral trochlear ridge, and mottled appearance of the patella represent the normal postnatal ossification pattern of these sites.

Type E lesions develop at the junction of bone and articular cartilage, and they frequently break through the cartilage to communicate with the joint cavity. Ten ml positive contrast material and 30 ml room air injected into the femoropatellar joint (Fig. 601) outlines the joint capsule **(1)**, articular cartilage of the patella **(2)**, and medial **(3)** and lateral **(4)** trochlear ridges. The bone lesion **(5)** is covered by articular cartilage and not filled with contrast material, indicating that the osteomyelitic focus does not communicate with the joint cavity. The radiograph was obtained in dorsal recumbency. Surplus positive contrast material **(6)** remains in the suprapatellar pouch, thereby allowing examination of the entire trochlea. Histological examination confirmed the arthrographic findings.

N. B. The existence of communication between a type E lesion and the joint cavity cannot be established by clinical or synovial fluid examination, because of the concomitant infectious synovitis present in all cases.

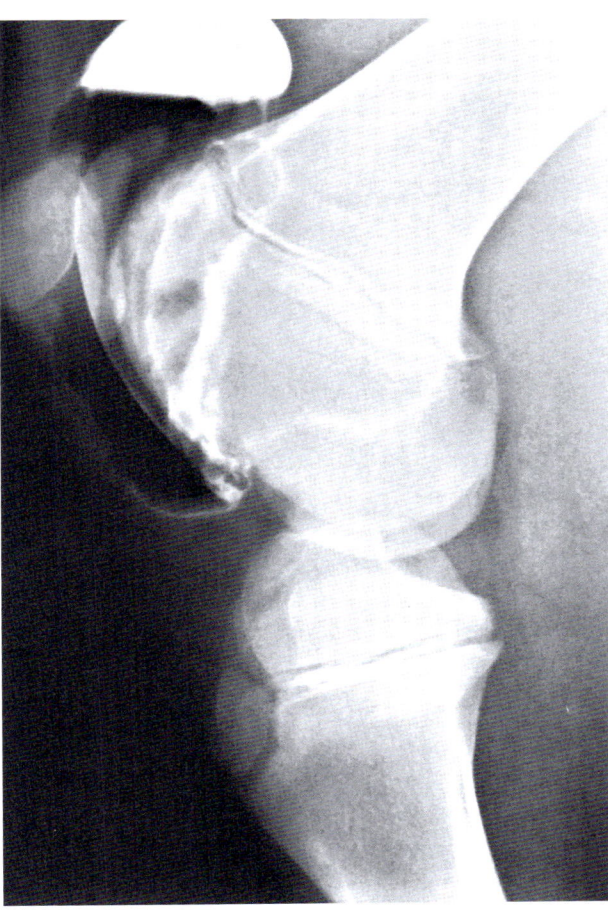

601

601 a Schematic drawing

Infectious arthritis

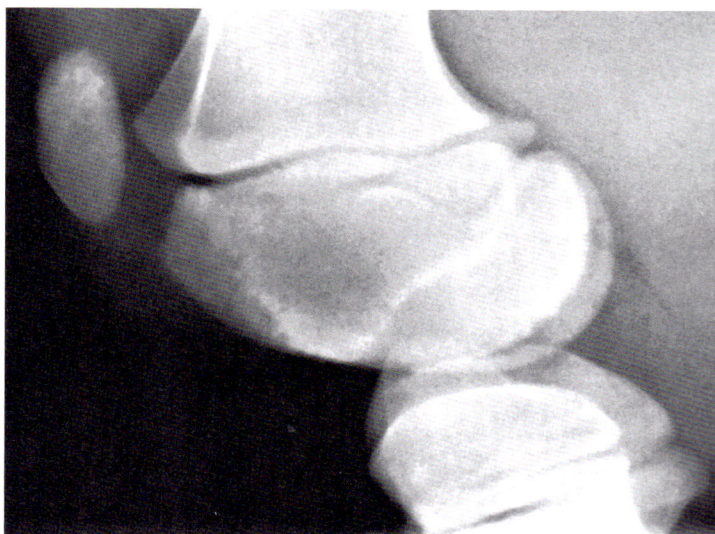

602 Left stifle joint, lateromedial view.

Foal, 4 weeks.

The roughening of the medial femoral condyle should be interpreted as pathologic and represents the early stage of type E osteomyelitis.

The patchy radiolucency of the patella and femoral trochlea represent the normal irregular postnatal ossification pattern of these sites. Such irregularities are not present in the femoral condyles.

Histological examination confirmed the diagnosis.

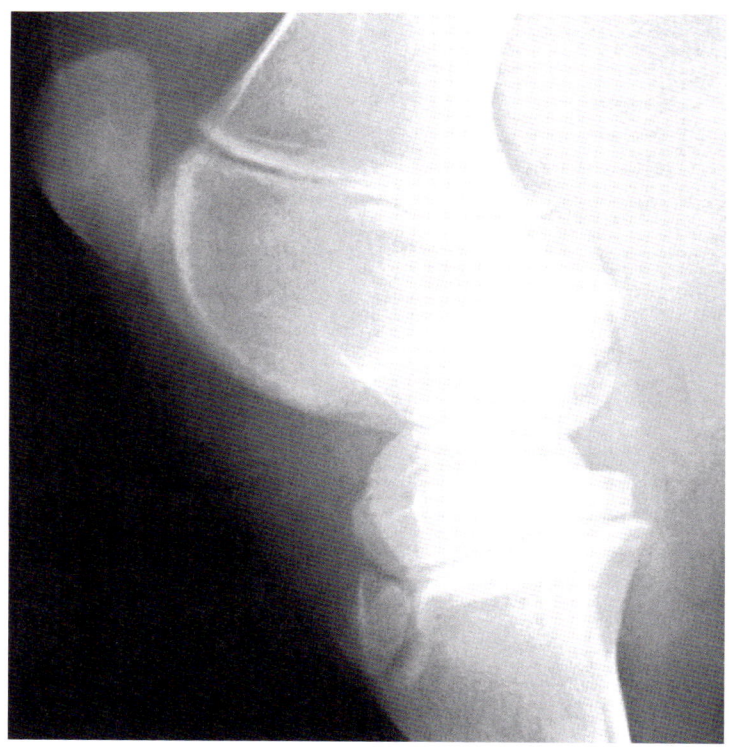

603 Right stifle joint, lateromedial view.

Foal, 2 months.

Soft tissue swelling cranial and caudal to the femur and tibia indicates effusion of the femorotibial joint. Roughening of the proximal aspect of the femoral trochlea represents normal irregular ossification. The cystic area of irregular radiolucency within the caudal aspect of the medial femoral condyle represents a type E osteomyelitic lesion. Disruption of the corresponding condylar border suggests extension of the osteomyelitic focus into or through, the articular cartilage. Histological examination demonstrated extensive cartilage destruction and communication of the osteomyelitic lesion with the joint cavity.

N. B. The medial femoral condyle is a predilection site for this type of lesion.

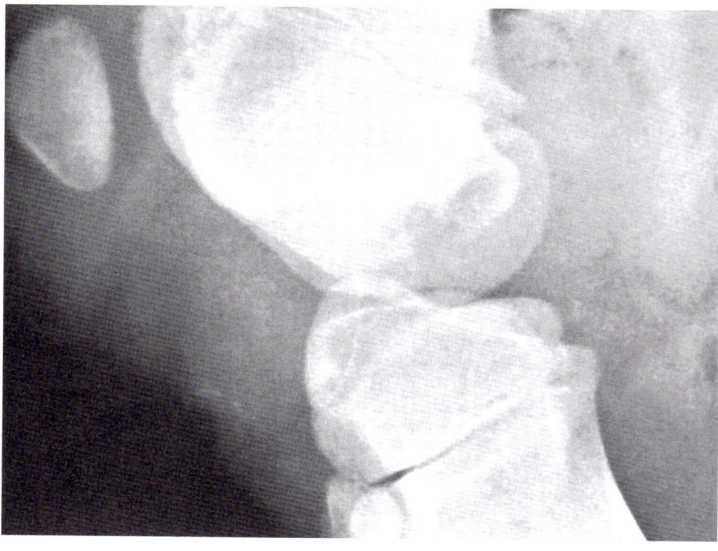

604

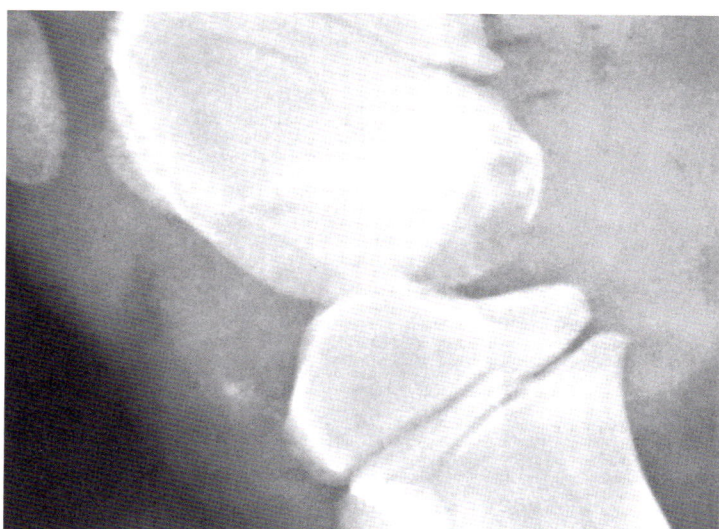

605

604/605 Right stifle joint, lateromedial (Fig. 604) and caudolateral-craniomedial oblique (Fig. 605) view: close-ups.

Foal, 4 weeks.

Marked soft tissue swelling and some calcification cranial to the femur and tibia, extensive soft tissue swelling, multiple small, irregular, radiolucent areas extending along the caudal aspect of the femur and tibia, and a large area of irregular radiolucency within the caudal aspect of the medial femoral condyle. This is a more advanced case of osteomyelitis type E, with concomitant infectious arthritis, calcification of the joint capsule and (peri-)articular abscess formation.

On the caudolateral-craniomedial oblique view the projection of the lateral femoral condyle is shifted cranially, resulting in clearer visualization of the lesion in the medial femoral condyle. The irregularity and patchy radiolucency of the proximal aspect of the femoral trochlea and patella represent the normal ossification pattern in these sites.

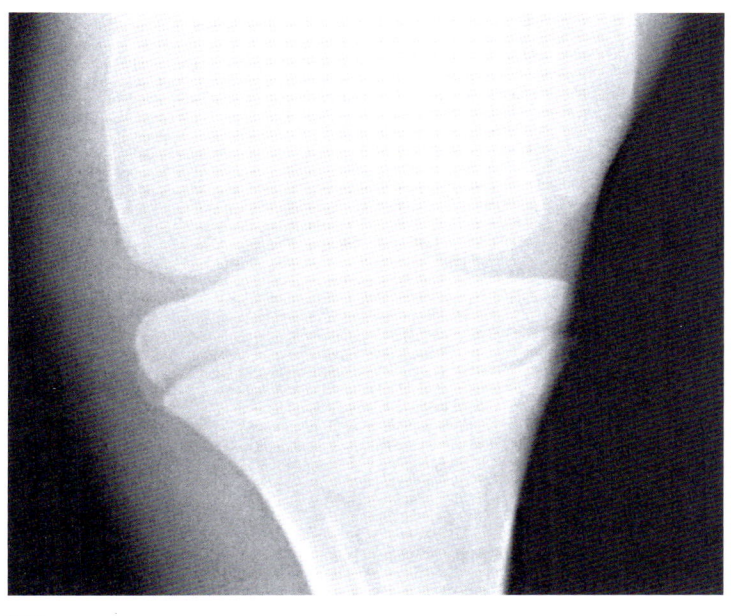

606

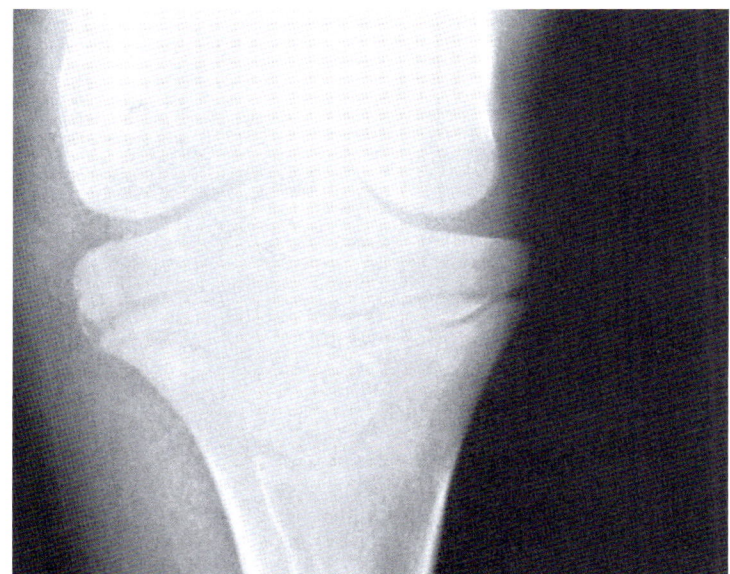

607

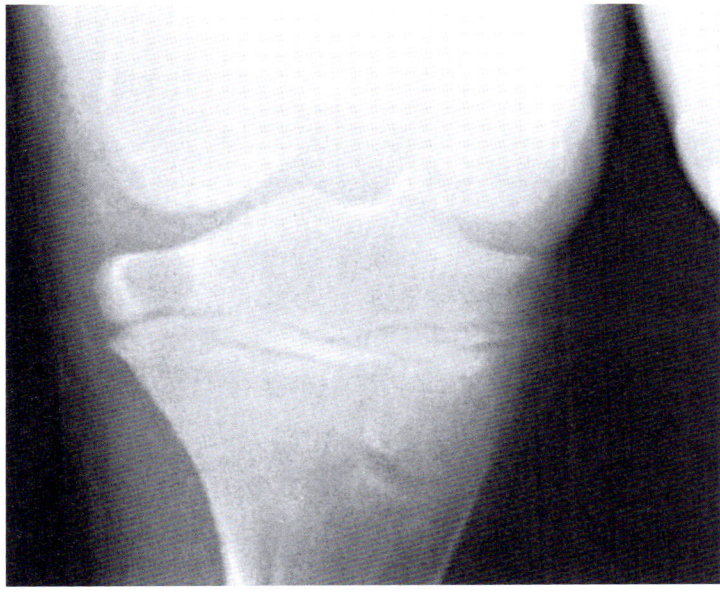

608

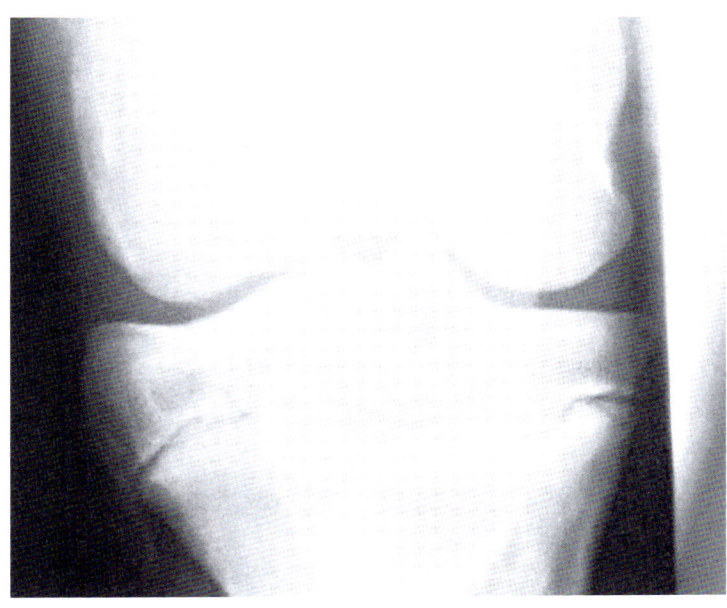

609

606/607/608/609 Left stifle joint, serial caudocranial views.

Foal, 4 weeks.

The initial view (Fig. 606), 1 week after the onset of lameness, reveals moderate soft tissue swelling lateral to the distal femur and proximal tibia, due to effusion of the lateral femorotibial joint.

Clinical and laboratory data indicated an infectious arthritis. A second examination 2 weeks later (Fig. 607) shows a very obscure radiolucent area within the proximolateral aspect of the tibial epiphysis, representing the early stage of a type E osteomyelitic focus.

Two weeks later (Fig. 608) the bone lesion is larger, more lucent, round and surrounded by a sclerotic rim. Communication between the bone lesion and the femorotibial joint is not apparent radiographically. On a follow-up examination 6 months later (Fig. 609) the cystic bone lesion remains visible, despite clinical recovery. Due to continuing growth and ossification of the tibial epiphysis, the lesion has moved away from the joint surface.

Puncture wound

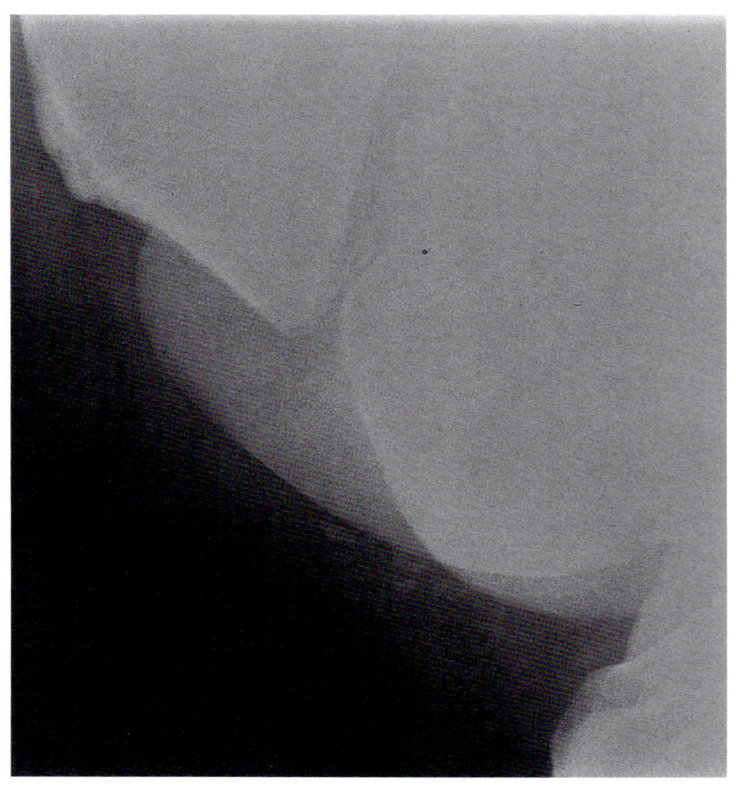

610 Left stifle joint, lateromedial view.

Warmblood, 8 years.

Effusion of the femoropatellar joint combined with multiple well defined radiopacities close to the femoral trochlea, representing pieces of metal which perforated the joint 2 weeks prior to the examination. The differential diagnosis includes artefactual densities created by scurf on the skin and osteochondrosis. Artefactual densities should no longer be visible after cleaning the skin. Osteochondrosis fragments should be accompagnied by irregularity or cavitation of the underlying bony contour (Fig. 628, 629).

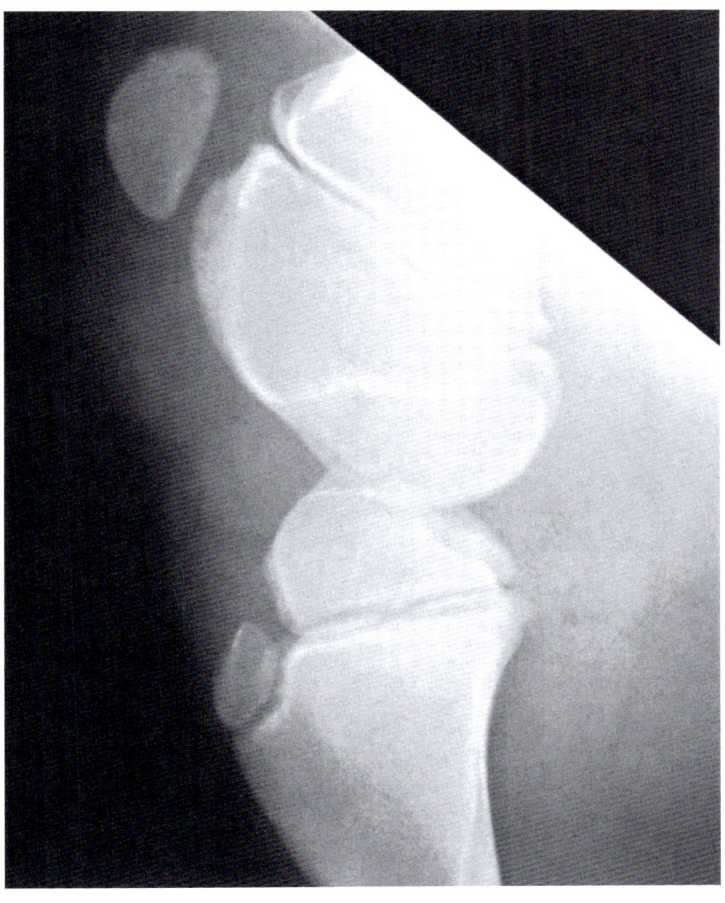

611

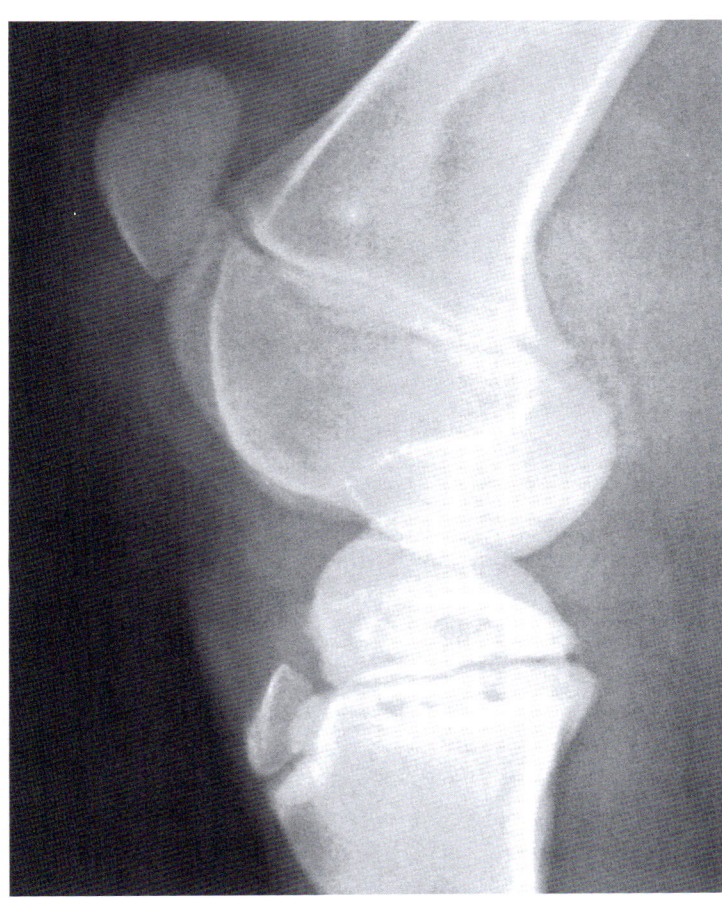

612

611/612 Left stifle joint, serial lateromedial views.

Foal, 4 weeks.

The initial view (Fig. 611), 2 days after the onset of lameness, shows soft tissue swelling cranial to the femoral trochlea and tibial epiphysis and caudal along the femur and tibia, indicating effusion of the femoropatellar and femorotibial joints. Clinical and laboratory data indicated infectious arthritis. The irregularity of the patella and femoral trochlea represents the normal ossification pattern in these sites.

Three weeks later (Fig. 612) an irregular zone of radiolucency in the epi- and metaphysis of the proximal tibia, extending along the physis, indicates haematogenous osteomyelitis type P. The lesion in the epiphysis shows an irregular radiopaque pattern surrounded by a radiolucent zone, suggestive of sequestrum formation.

The well defined, slightly sclerotic border of the bone lesions indicates a more advanced stage of osteomyelitic bone destruction.

"Epiphysitis"

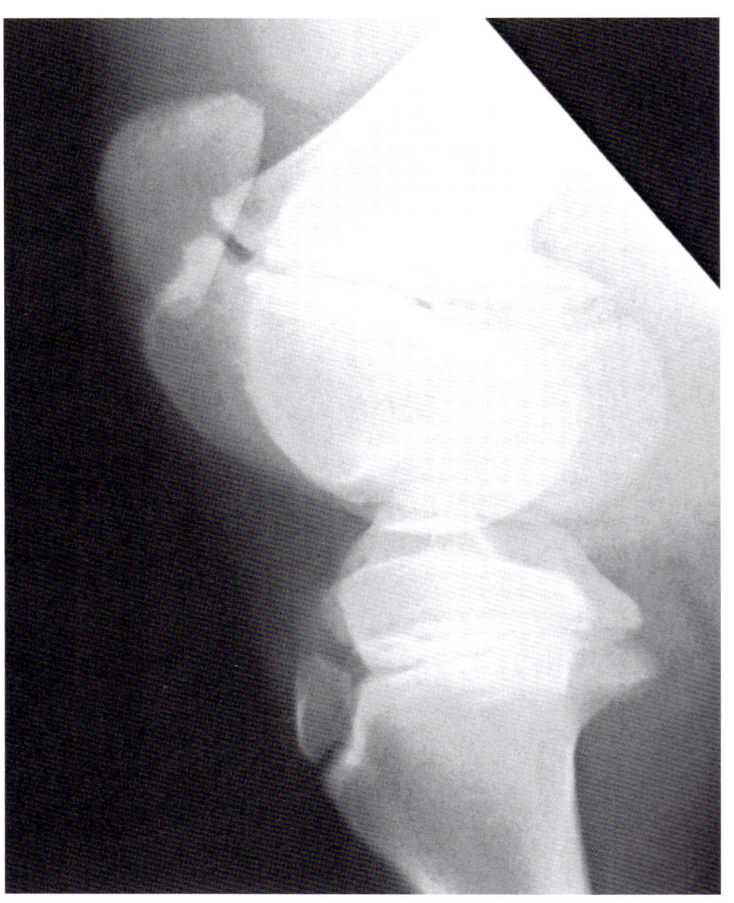

613 Right stifle joint, lateromedial view.

Foal, 6 weeks.

The (slightly oblique) lateromedial view shows minimal widening and tipping on the caudal side of the distal femoral growth plate, characteristic of "epiphysitis". The roughening of the proximal aspect of the patella and medial trochlear ridge represents the normal ossification pattern.

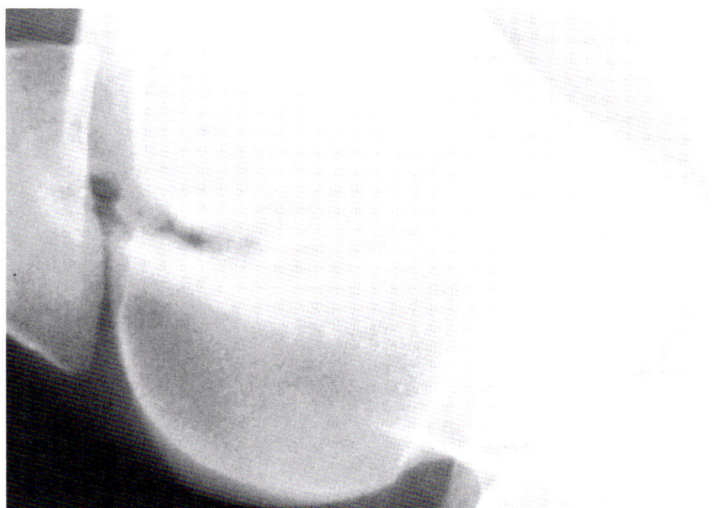

614 Left stifle joint, lateromedial view: close-up.

Foal, 1 year.

Marked irregular widening on the cranial side of the distal femoral growth plate due to "epiphysitis".

N. B. Compared with the distal radial growth plate, the incidence of epiphysitis at this site is very low.

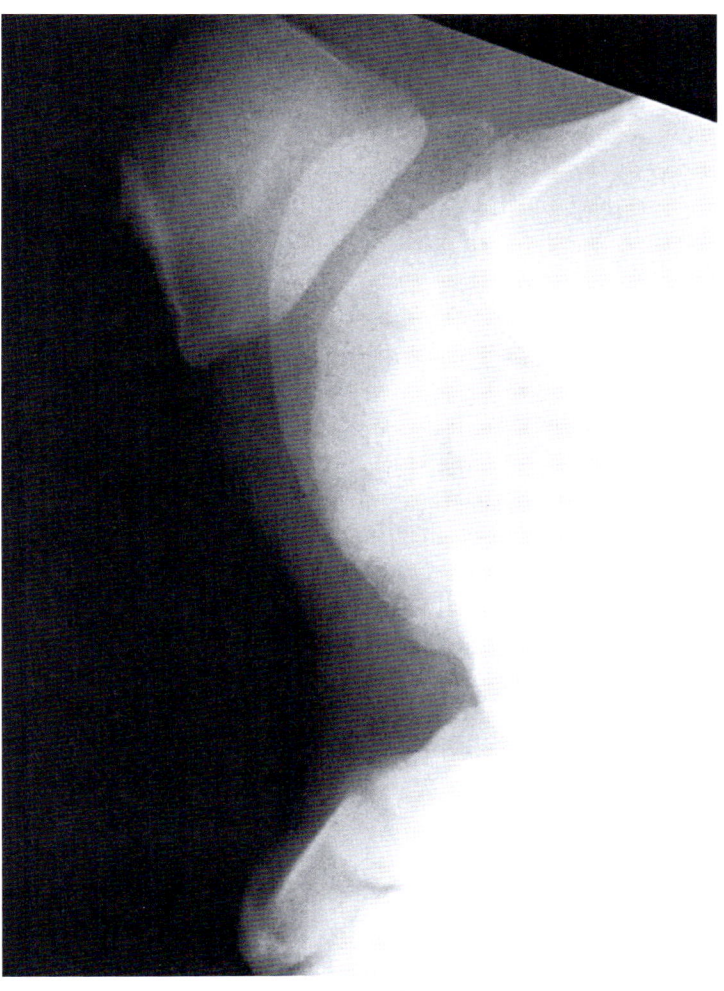

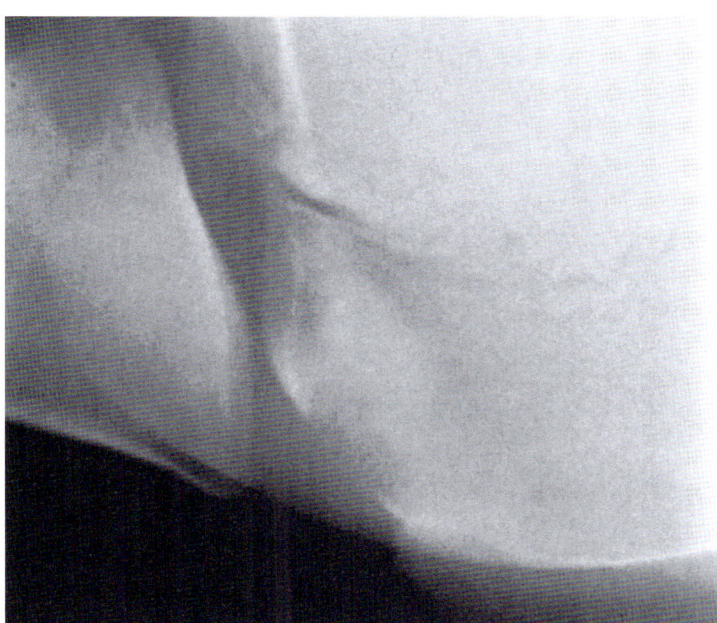

616 Left stifle joint, lateromedial view: close-up.

Foal, 9 months.

Marked flattening of the middle aspect of the lateral trochlear ridge, radio-lucency and local sclerosis of the corresponding subchondral bone, indicate less extensive, more localized osteochondrosis.

615 Left stifle joint, lateromedial view: close-up.

Foal, 6 months.

The flattening of the contour of the distal half of the lateral trochlear ridge and the irregular subchondral radiolucency surrounded by a sclerotic zone are a manifestation of extensive severe osteochondrosis. Soft tissue swelling cranial to the femoral trochlea indicates associated effusion of the femoro-patellar joint.

N. B. The lateral trochlear ridge is a predilection site for osteochondrosis of the equine stifle.

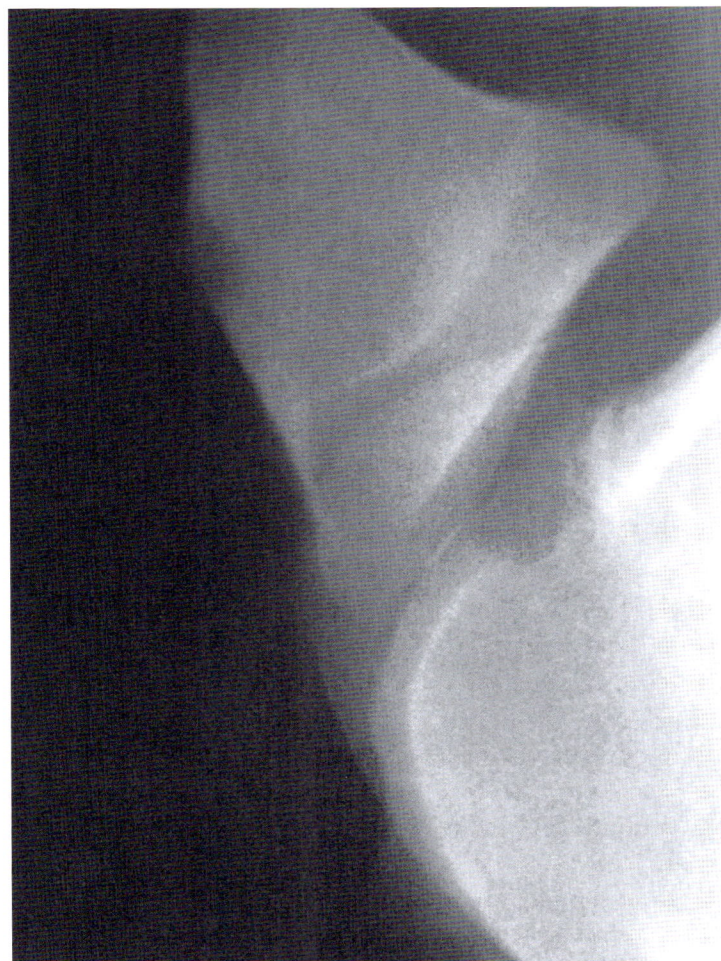

617 Right stifle joint, lateromedial view: close-up.

Warmblood, 1 ½ years.

The "dished-out" area in the mid-contour of the lateral trochlear ridge represents a small, localised osteochondral lesion.

N. B. The extension and severity of osteochondral lesions of the lateral tro-chlear ridge tend to be age-related; extensive, severe lesions are most fre-quently encountered in foals, and more localized, circumscribed, less exten-sive lesions in older horses. Osteochondrosis of the stifle is more often asso-ciated with joint effusion and lameness than osteochondrosis of the hock joint. The more extensive the radiographic changes are, the more pro-nounced the clinical signs are and the worse the prognosis is.

The normal indentation proximally between the trochlear ridges should not be confused with an osteochondral lesion.

617

Osteochondrosis

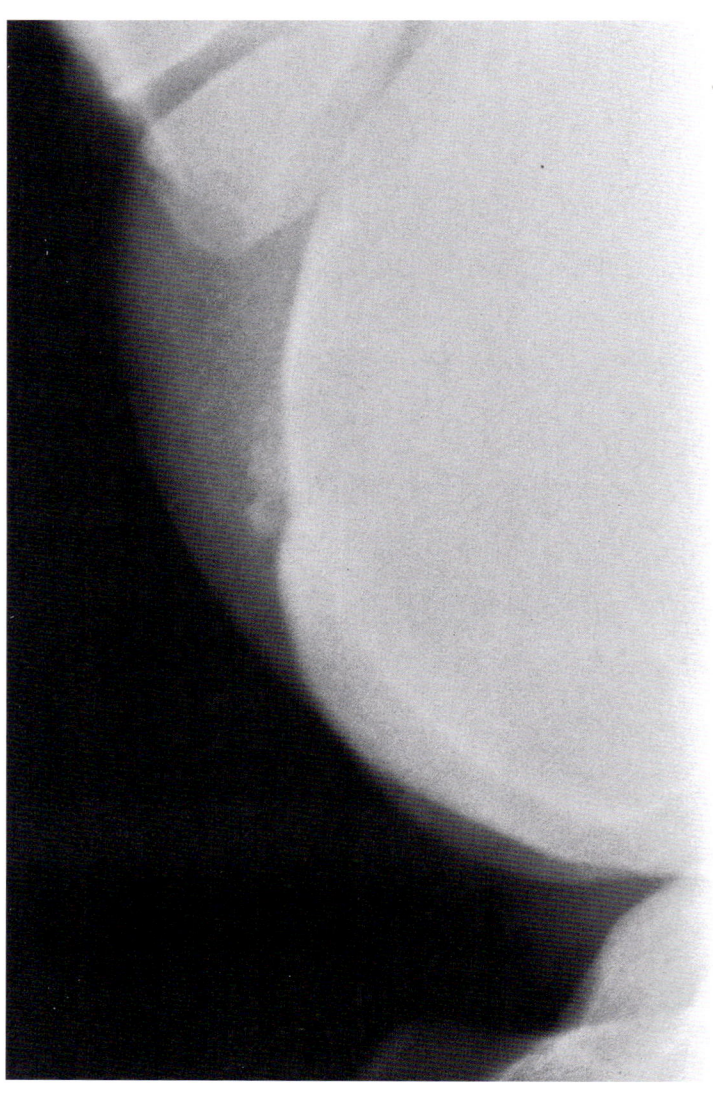

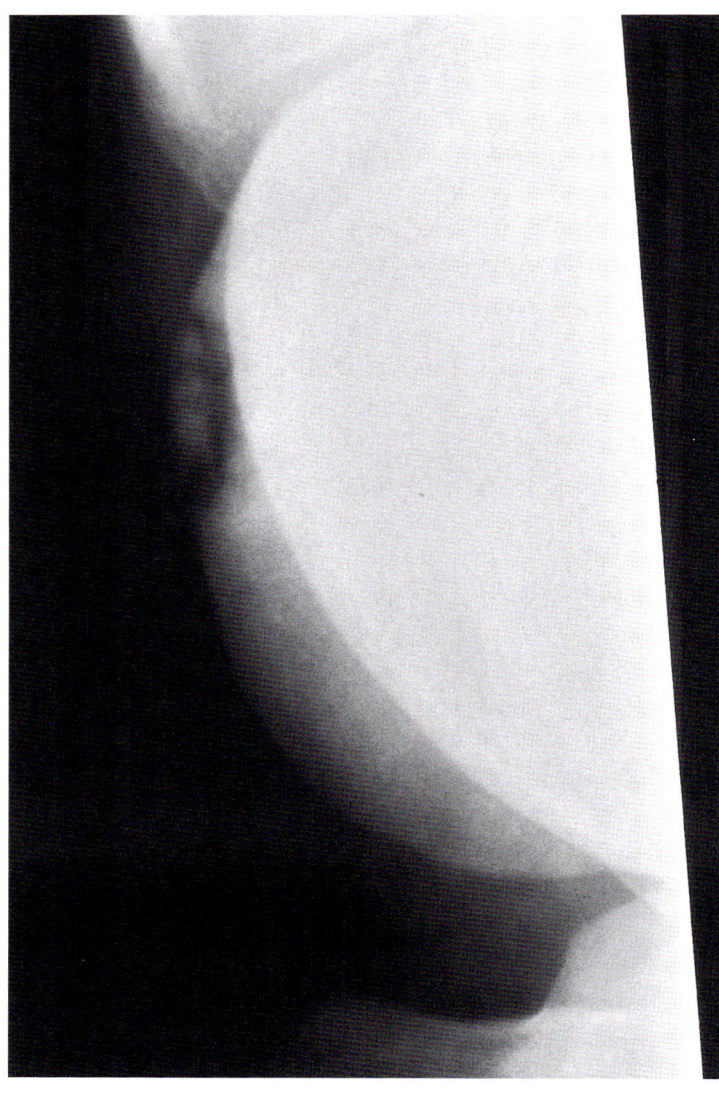

618

619

618/619 Left stifle joint, lateromedial and caudolateral-craniomedial oblique view: close-ups.

Warmblood, 3 years.

The bony fragment and underlying defect in the mid contour of the lateral trochlear ridge represent a characteristic and common manifestation of osteochondrosis. As usual the lesion is most obvious on the caudolateral-craniomedial oblique projection (Fig. 619) and less clearly seen on the lateromedial view (Fig. 618) due to superimposition of the medial trochlear ridge.

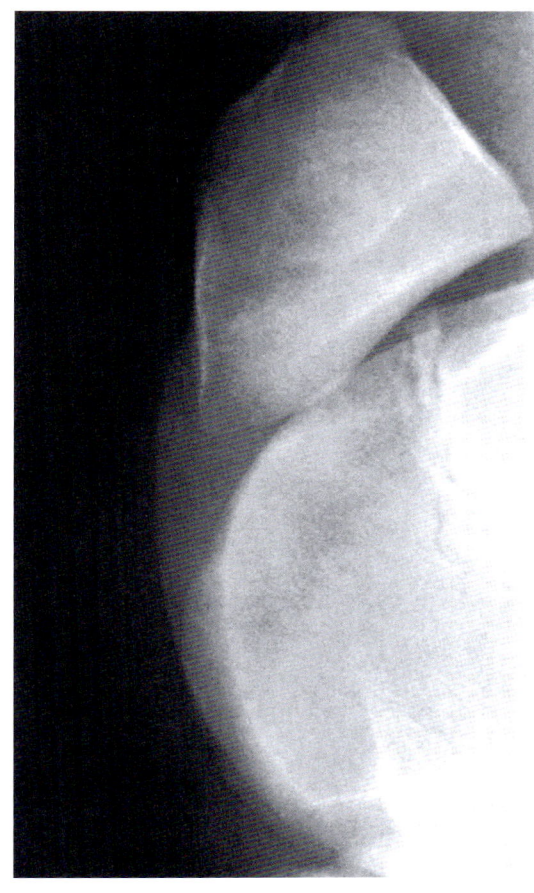

620

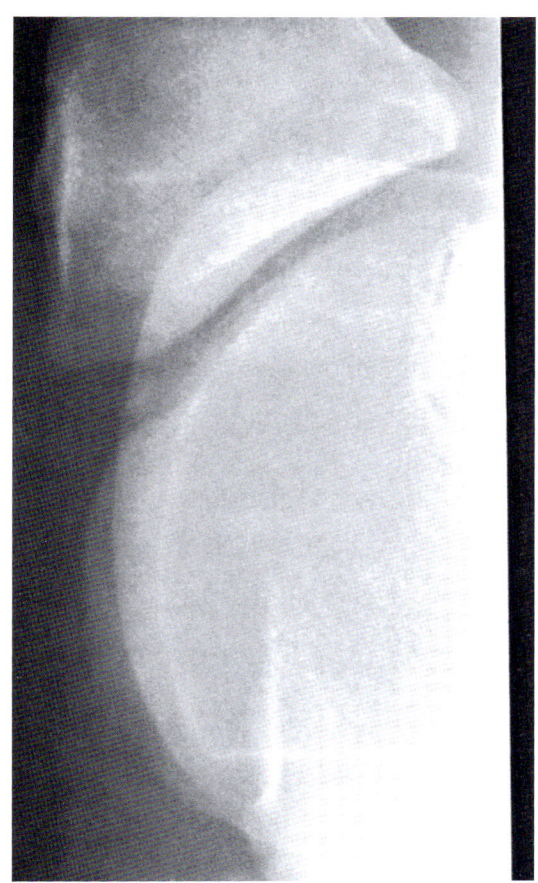

621

620/621 Left stifle joint, serial lateromedial views: close-ups.

Foal, 6 months.

The initial examination (Fig. 620) shows minimal flattening of the middle aspect of the lateral trochlear ridge, due to osteochondrosis. Four months later (Fig. 621) linear opacities opposite the defect of the lateral trochlear ridge indicate secondary ossification within the osteochondral lesion.

Osteochondrosis

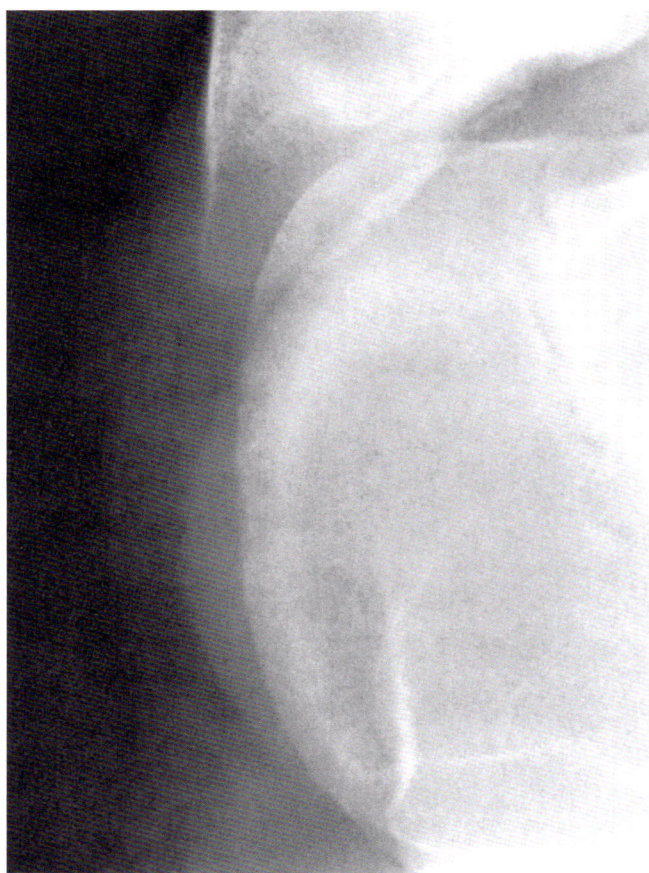

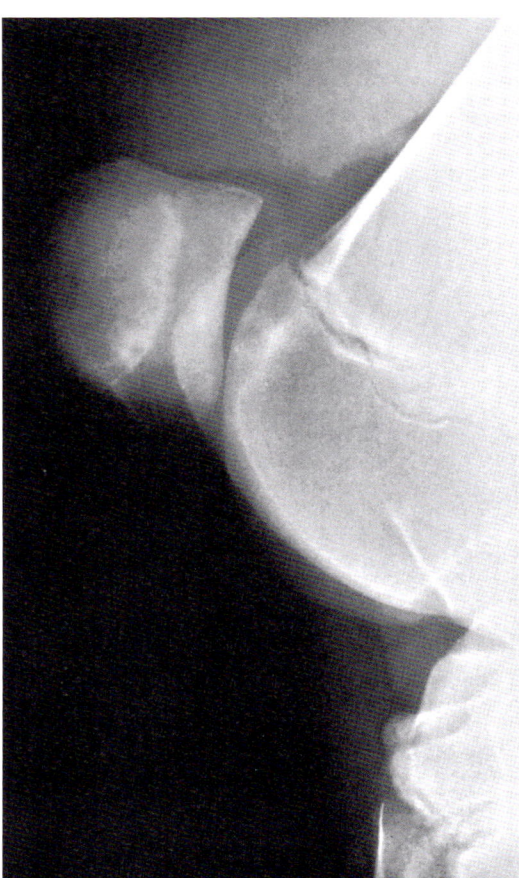

622 Right stifle joint, lateromedial view: close-up.

Foal, 10 months.

The clearly defined patchy subchondral radiolucency in the midproximal articular surface of the patella and indistinct mixed radiolucency and radiopacity of the subchondral bone of the entire lateral trochlear ridge are manifestations of osteochondrosis affecting the femoral trochlea and patella. Soft tissue swelling cranial to the femoral trochlea indicates associated effusion of the femoropatellar joint.

623 Right stifle joint, lateromedial view: close-up.

Foal, 10 months.

The small cystic area of radiolucency, surrounded by a sclerotic rim, within the subchondral bone of the distomedial aspect of the articular surface of the patella is a manifestation of osteochondrosis.

N. B. In most cases the major radiographic changes of osteochondrosis are in the lateral trochlear ridge; the articular cartilage of the patella is less frequently affected. Radiographic changes of only the patella are rare.

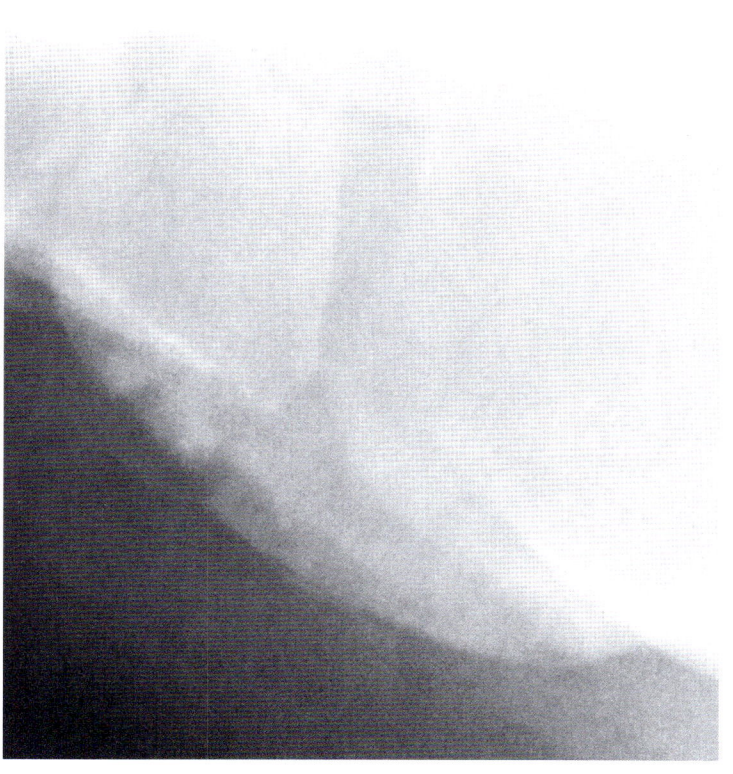

624

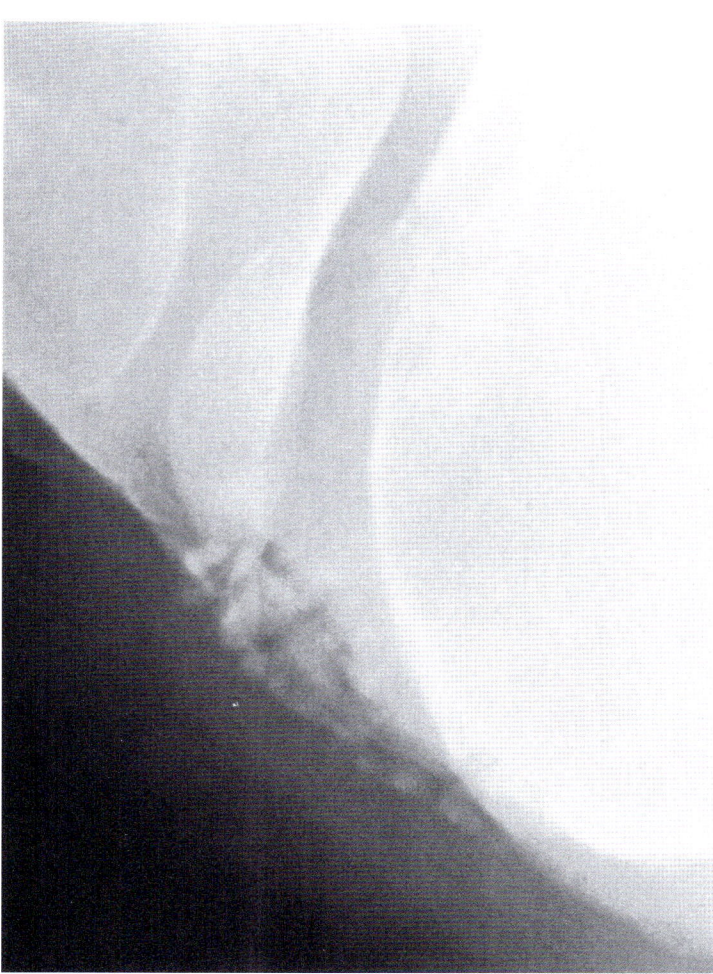

625

624/625 Left stifle joint, serial lateromedial views: close-ups.

Foal, 7 months.

The irregularity of the contour of the distal half of the medial trochlear ridge, ill defined linear opacities adjacent to the articular surface of the medial ridge, and mottled radiopacity of the underlying bone on the initial radiograph (Fig. 624) represent the early stages of disruption and fragmentation of cartilage and underlying subchondral bone, associated with osteochondrosis. Sixteen months later (Fig. 625) the bony fragments, still attached to the trochlear ridge, are more spherical, dense and sharply delineated, due to secondary ossification within the osteochondral lesion.

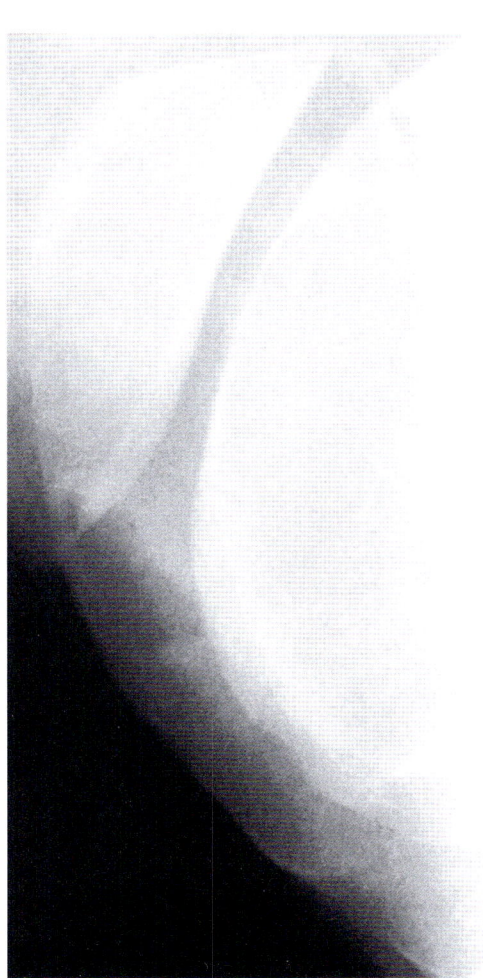

626 Right stifle joint, lateromedial view: close-up.

Foal, 8 months.

The well defined radiolucent area, surrounded by a sclerotic rim, within the midportion of the medial trochlear ridge is a manifestation of osteochondrosis.

N. B. The medial trochlear ridge is an infrequent site of occurence of osteochondrosis in the equine stifle.

Osteochondrosis

Osteochondrosis development

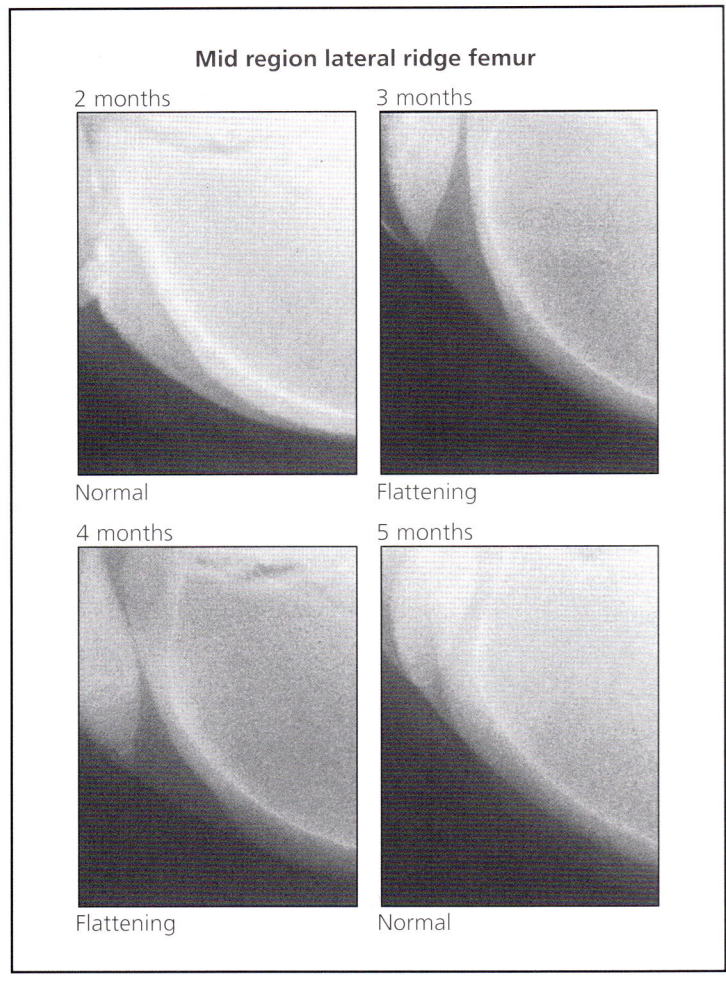

Mid region lateral ridge femur

2 months — Normal

3 months — Flattening

4 months — Flattening

5 months — Normal

627

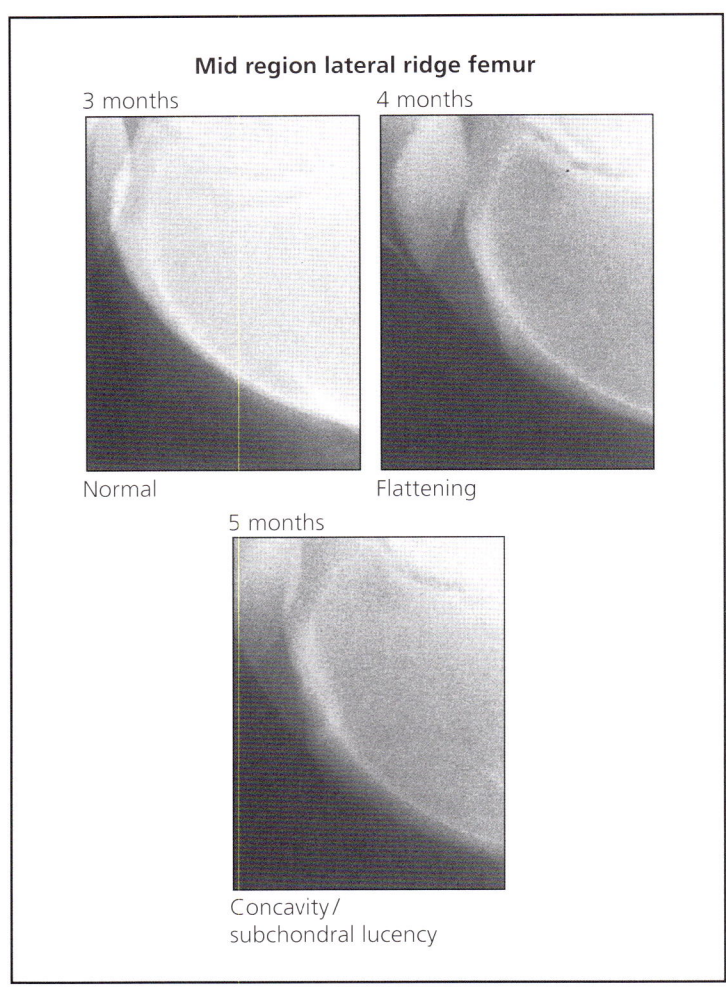

Mid region lateral ridge femur

3 months — Normal

4 months — Flattening

5 months — Concavity/subchondral lucency

628

Mid region lateral ridge femur

4 months — Normal

5 months — Subchondral lucency

6 months — Concavity/subchondral lucency

629

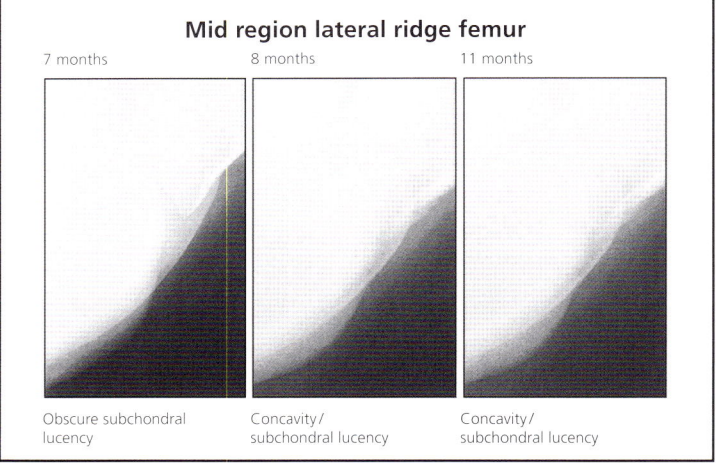

Mid region lateral ridge femur

7 months — Obscure subchondral lucency

8 months — Concavity/subchondral lucency

11 months — Concavity/subchondral lucency

630

627/628/629/630 Midregion of the lateral ridge of the femoral trochlea, postnatal serial lateromedial views: close-ups.

Abnormal appearances of the midregion of the lateral trochlear ridge commonly become obvious at 3 – 4 months of age.

At this age the abnormalities are usually limited to smooth or irregular flattening of the bony contour (Fig. 627). In almost all cases subsequent progression, like cavitation (Fig. 628), is followed by regression. Therefore the majority (± 90%) of these abnormalities is temporary and returns to normal before the age of 8 months.

Lesions still existing at 8 months usually become permanent. The development of permanent lesions may fluctuate, like initial flattening progressing to a concavity, followed by regression to obscure subchondral radiolucency, subsequently returning to cavitation (Fig. 629, 630), thus resulting in misleading temporary appearances.

Osteochondrosis development

631 Articular surface of the patella, postnatal serial lateromedial views: close-ups.

Osteochondrosis of the articular surface of the patella also becomes visible relatively late and, like lesions of the midregion of the lateral trochlear ridge, progression of patellar lesions may be followed by regression, e.g. initial subchondral lucency progressing to prominent cavitation, subsequently regressing to minimal indentation.

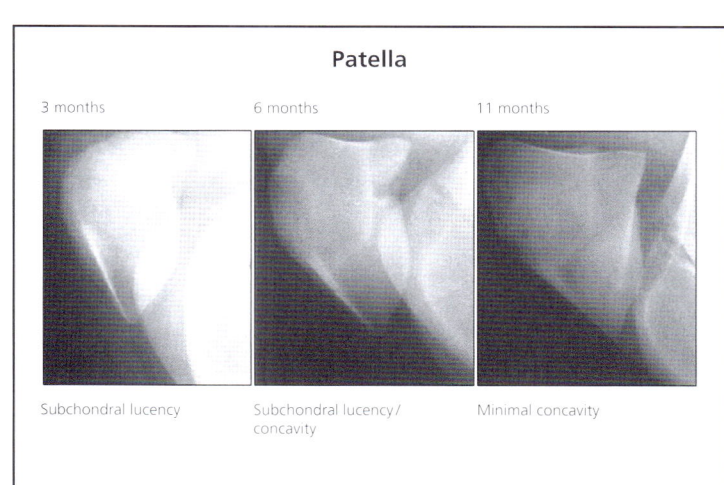

631

632/633 Medial ridge of the femoral trochlea, serial lateromedial views: close-ups.

Osteochondrosis manifestations of the medial trochlear ridge follow the same pattern of development as observed for the other praedilection sites in the equine stifle. Initial lesions, like indentation of the mid proximal aspect of the medial ridge become obvious at 3 – 4 months of age. Progression may be followed by regression and the repair may result in linear horizontal sclerosis.

These osteochondral "scars" are occasionally observed in adult horses.

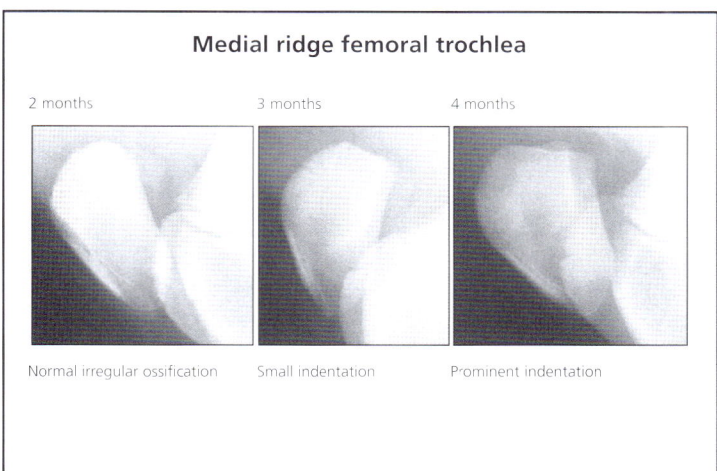

632

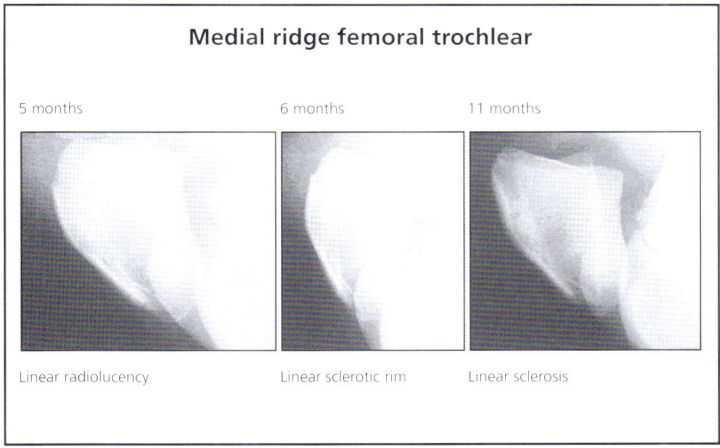

633

Osteochondrosis development

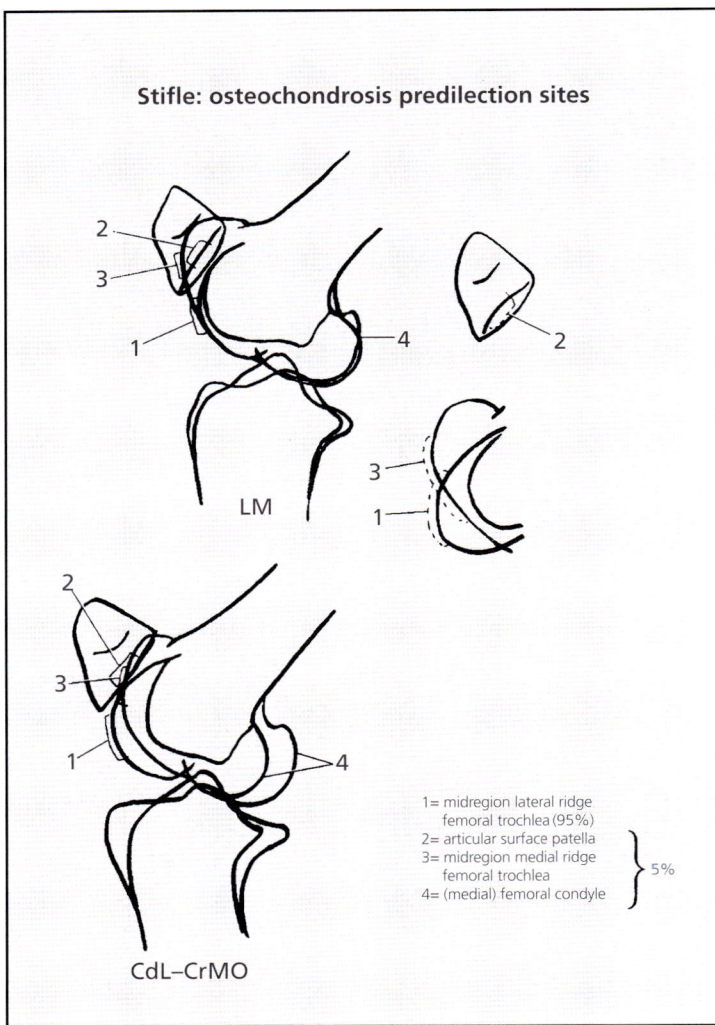

Stifle: osteochondrosis predilection sites

LM

CdL–CrMO

1 = midregion lateral ridge
femoral trochlea (95%)
2 = articular surface patella
3 = midregion medial ridge
femoral trochlea
4 = (medial) femoral condyle
} 5%

634 Schematic drawing of osteochondrosis praedilection sites in the equine stifle. The predominant location is the midregion of the lateral ridge of the femoral trochlea. Rare sites are the articular surface of the patella and the midregion of the medial trochlear ridge. Abnormalities of the (medial) femoral condyle such as cystic lesions are considered by some veterinarians to be part of the osteochondrosis syndrome, but actually have a traumatic origin (Fig. 635, 636), or result from osteomyelitis type E (Fig. 598, 603 – 605).

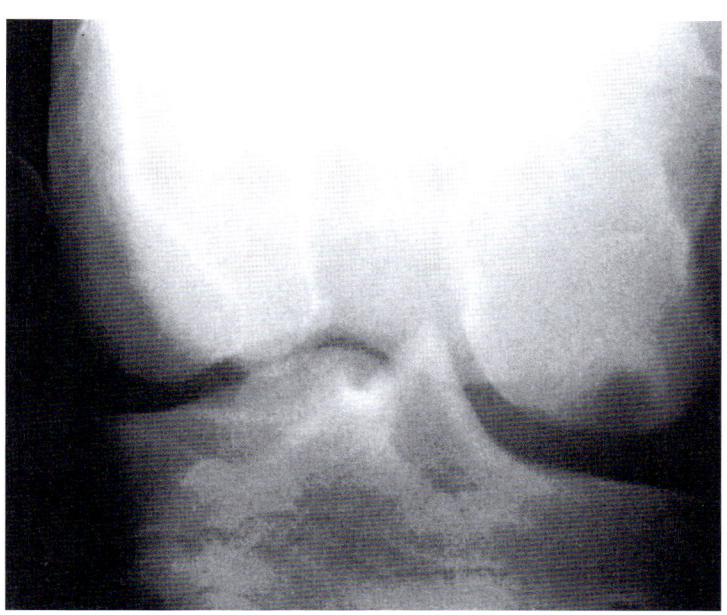

635 Left stifle joint, caudocranial view: close-up.

Foal, 8 months.

A solitary, clearly defined, cystic area of diffuse radiolucency within the distal aspect of the medial femoral condyle, characteristic of a bone cyst.

The subchondral bone in the corresponding area is disrupted, suggesting direct communication between the cyst and the femorotibial joint, or separation of the lesion from the joint by only a thin layer of articular cartilage.

N. B. The medial femoral condyle is the commonest site of cyst occurence in the equine stifle.

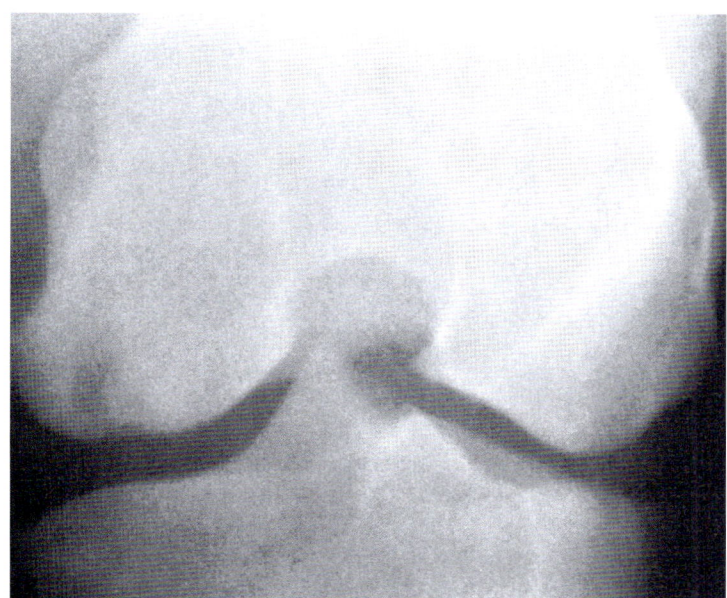

636 Right stifle joint, caudocranial view: close-up.

Pony, 5 years.

A solitary, indistinct, oval-shaped area of diffuse radiolucency within the distal aspect of the medial femoral condyle, indicating the presence of a bone cyst.

The corresponding articular surface of the femoral condyle is slightly irregular, but direct communication between the cystic lesion and the joint is not visible.

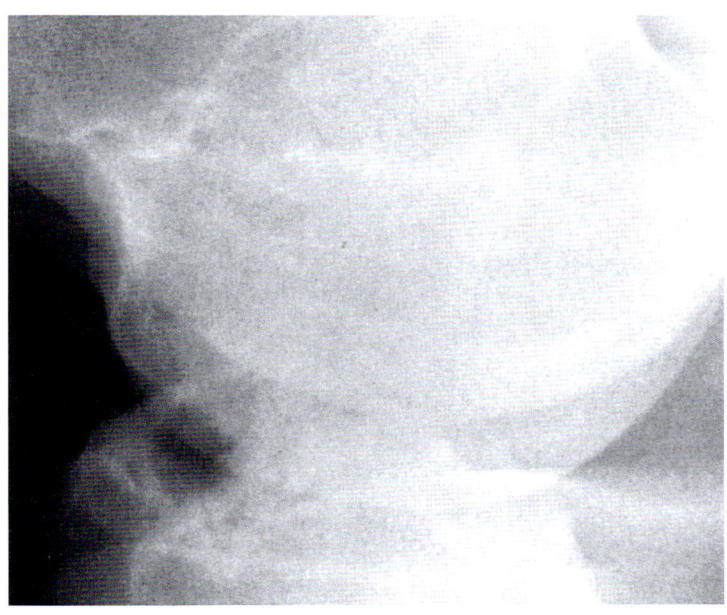

637 Right stifle joint, lateromedial view: close-up.

Warmblood, 6 years.

A solitary, clearly defined, irregularly shaped area of diffuse radiolucency within the cranial aspect of the tibial spine, indicative of a bone cyst. There is no visible connection between the cyst lumen and the femorotibial joint.

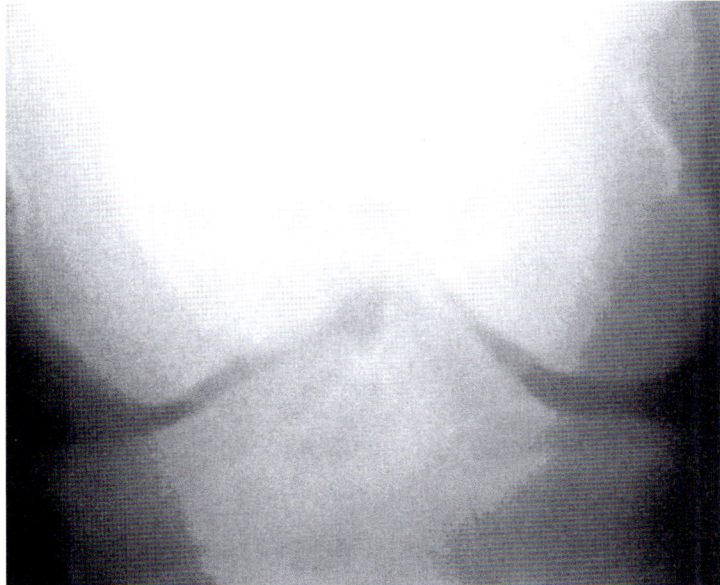

638 Left stifle joint, caudocranial view: close-up.

Warmblood, 1 ½ years.

A solitary indistinct circular area of radiolucency, surrounded by a sclerotic zone, in the lateral tubercle of the tibial spine, indicative of a bone cyst. There is no visible connection between the cyst lumen and the femorotibial joint.

N. B. Cystic lesions within the tibial spine (or lateral femoral condyle, adjacent to the intercondyloid fossa) occur less frequently and have a less favourable prognosis than a bone cyst within the centre of the medial femoral condyle.

Bone sequestration

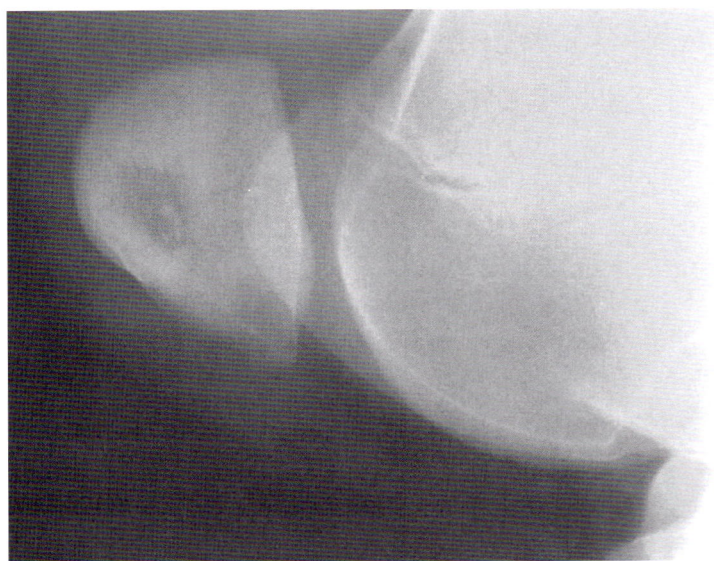

639

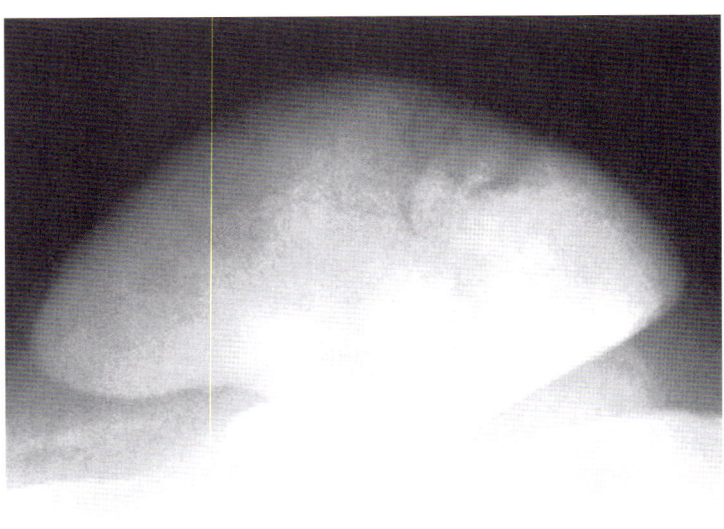

640

639/640 Right stifle joint, lateromedial and cranioproximal-craniodistal "skyline" view: close-ups.

Foal, 5 months.

The lateromedial view (Fig. 639) reveals a small, dense, irregularly shaped bone fragment in a radiolucent pocket, surrounded by a sclerotic zone, within the craniocentral aspect of the patella. The radiographic changes are characteristics of a mature bone sequestrum, bathed in a pocket of pus, surrounded by sclerotic bone tissue. The lesion resulted from a puncture wound to the cranial aspect of the patella, 3 weeks prior to the examination.

On the additional "skyline" projection (Fig. 640) several less clearly defined sequestra are visible and the surrounding radiolucent area opens widely onto the craniolateral aspect of the patella. The combination of the two projections enables evaluation of the full extent and precise location of the sequestration process.

Additional finding: minimal roughening of the proximal aspect cf the medial trochlear ridge and the cranioproximal border of the patella (Fig. 639) represents the normal, nearly completed, irregular, postnatal ossification pattern in these sites.

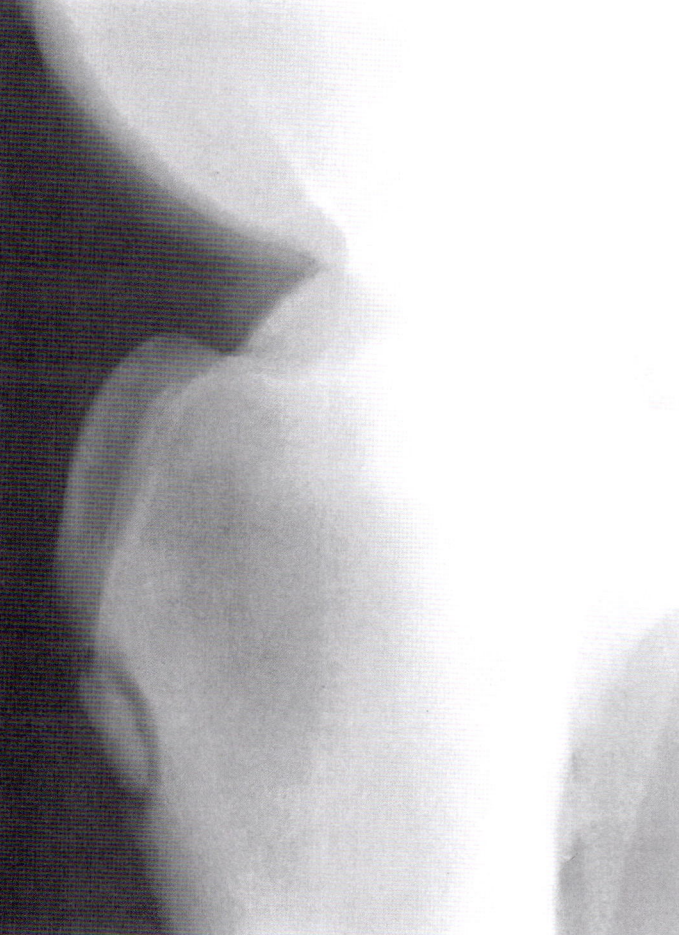

641

641 Right stifle joint, lateromedial view: close-up.

Warmblood, 3 ½ years.

The well demarcated bone fragment in the centre of a semicircular defect in the cranioproximal border of the tibia represents a bone sequestrum completely separated from the cortex. The lesion resulted from a puncture wound 3 weeks prior to the examination. Associated periosteal new bone formation proximal and distal to the cortical defect is not present.

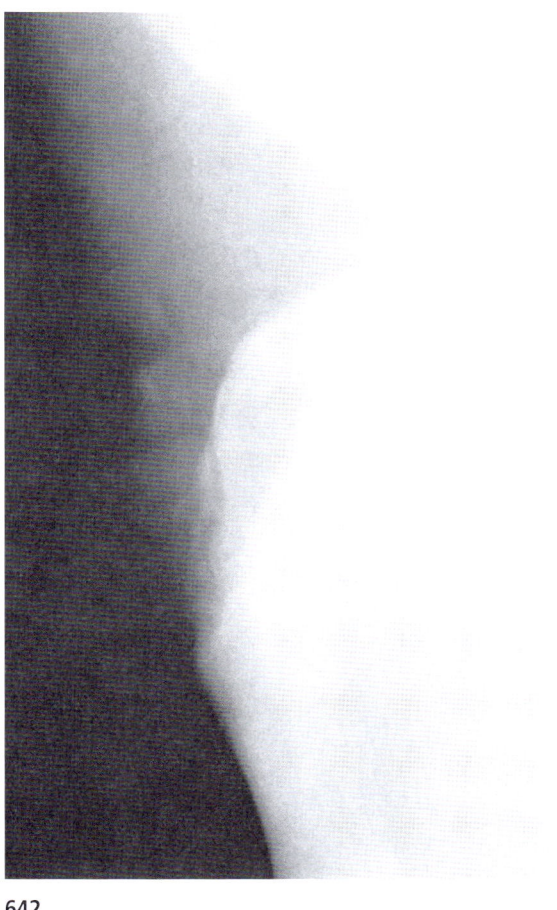

642

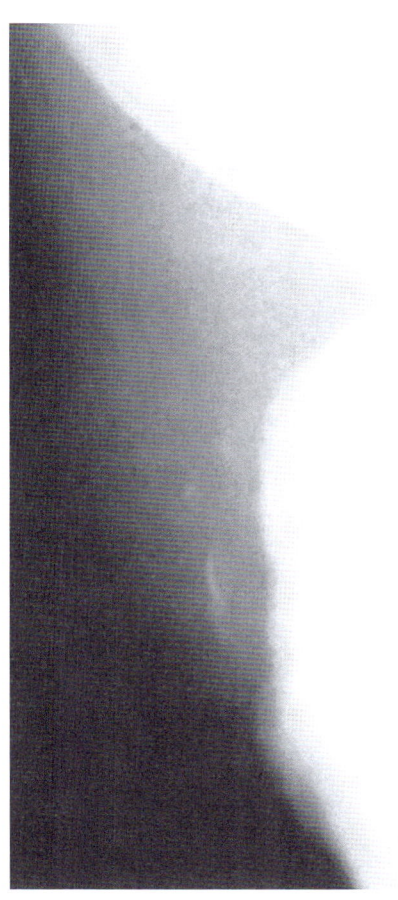

643

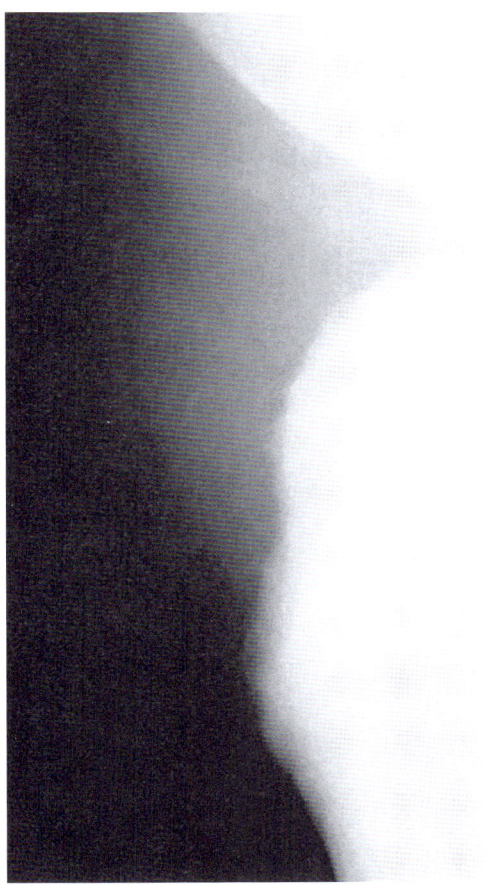

644

642/643/644 Left stifle joint, serial lateromedial views: close-ups.

Warmblood, 7 years.

The initial examination (Fig. 642), 2 weeks after a puncture wound to the cranial aspect of the proximal tibia, reveals a fine radiolucent band beneath the outer cortex of the lateral part of the tibial tuberosity, separating a superficial layer of bone from the cortex. The radiographic changes represent an intermediate stage of bone sequestration, the sequestrum not yet being completely separated from the cortex. The irregular soft tissue opacities cranial to the proximal tibia result from the same trauma. Two weeks later (Fig. 643) several bone sequestra of various sizes are visible completely separated and at some distance from the underlying cortex.

The corresponding irregularity of the cranial surface of the tibial tuberosity results from separation of the thin sequestra from the cortex and minimal periosteal new bone formation on adjacent normal bone.

Three weeks later (Fig. 644) only one small indistinct bone fragment remains. This fragment has moved further away from the underlying cortex. The other sequestra are no longer visible. The periosteal new bone is slightly thicker and denser.

The increasing distance between bone fragment and underlying cortex and disappearance of other fragments indicate spontaneous resolution of sequestration, which occurs only seldom.

Calcified haematoma

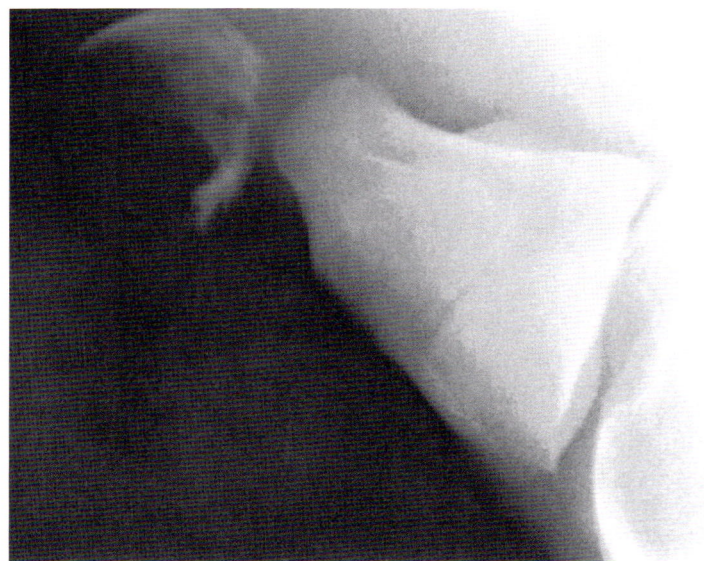

645 Right stifle joint, lateromedial view.

Warmblood, 10 years.

The well defined soft tissue opacity cranial to the proximal aspect of the patella represents focal calcification of a nodular soft tissue mass. The semi-circular configuration of the radiopaque zone suggests partial (dystrophic) calcification of a cyst wall, probably the remnant of a haematoma.

Ossifying myopathy

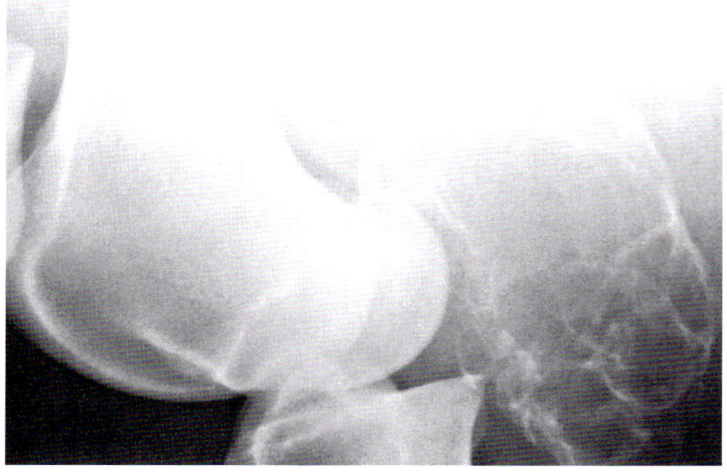

646

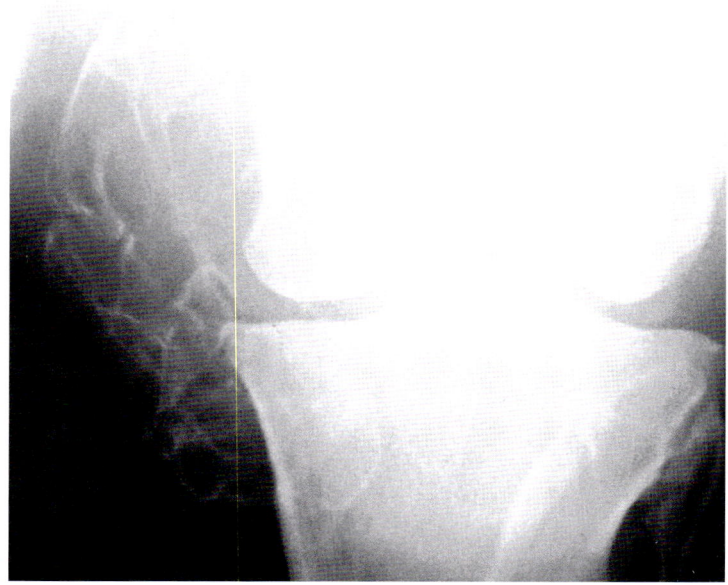

647

646/647 Right stifle joint, lateromedial and caudocranial view.

Hackney, 14 years.

A cystic, thin walled, multiloculated soft tissue opacity, adjacent to the caudomedial aspect of the distal femur and proximal tibia, due to ossification within the gastrocnemius muscle and probably arising from trauma.

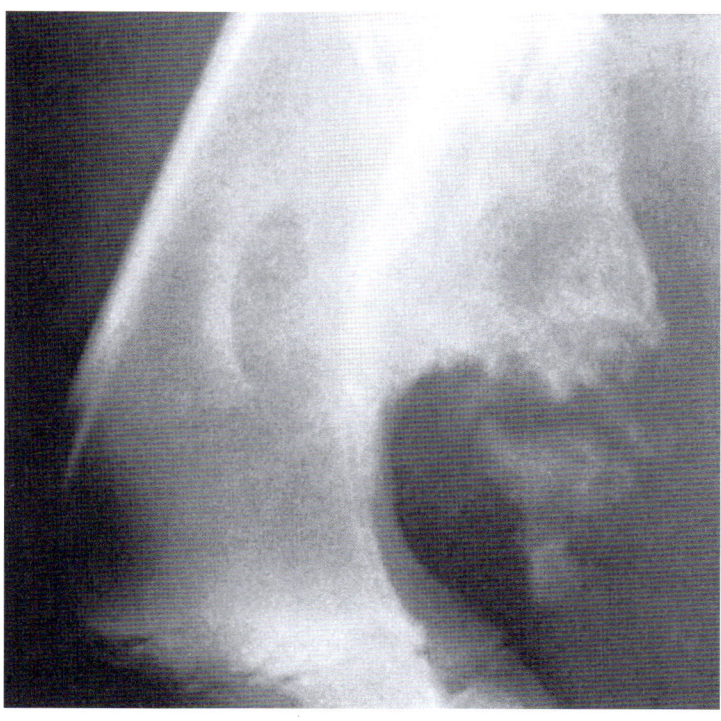

648

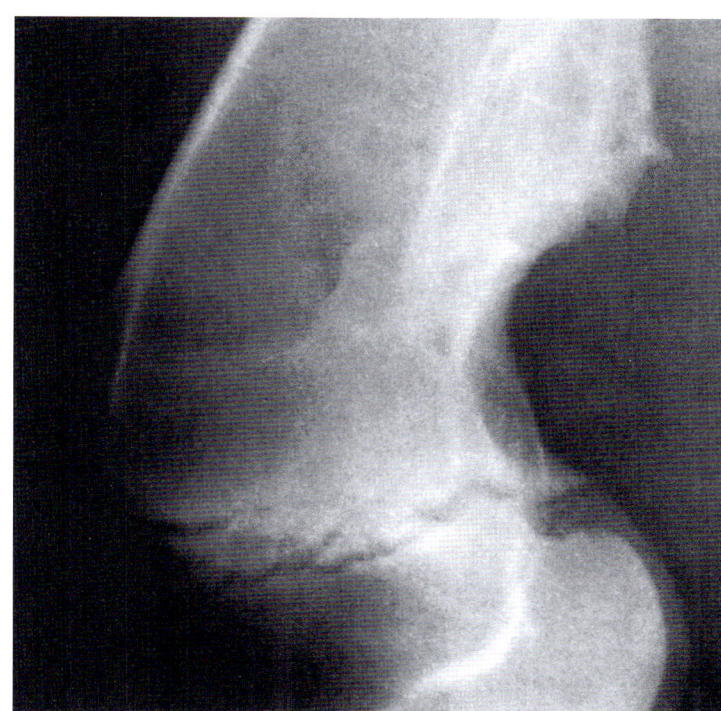

649

648/649 Right and left distal femur, lateromedial views: close-ups.

Foal, 5 months.

Triangular-shaped new bone formation on the caudodistal aspect of the right (Fig. 648) and left (Fig. 649) femur, and additional isolated soft tissue ossification adjacent to the exostosis on the right femur. The radiographic changes indicate ossification of the gastrocnemius muscle at the site of attachment to the femur. Muscle ossification resulted from a congenital form of fibrotic myopathy.

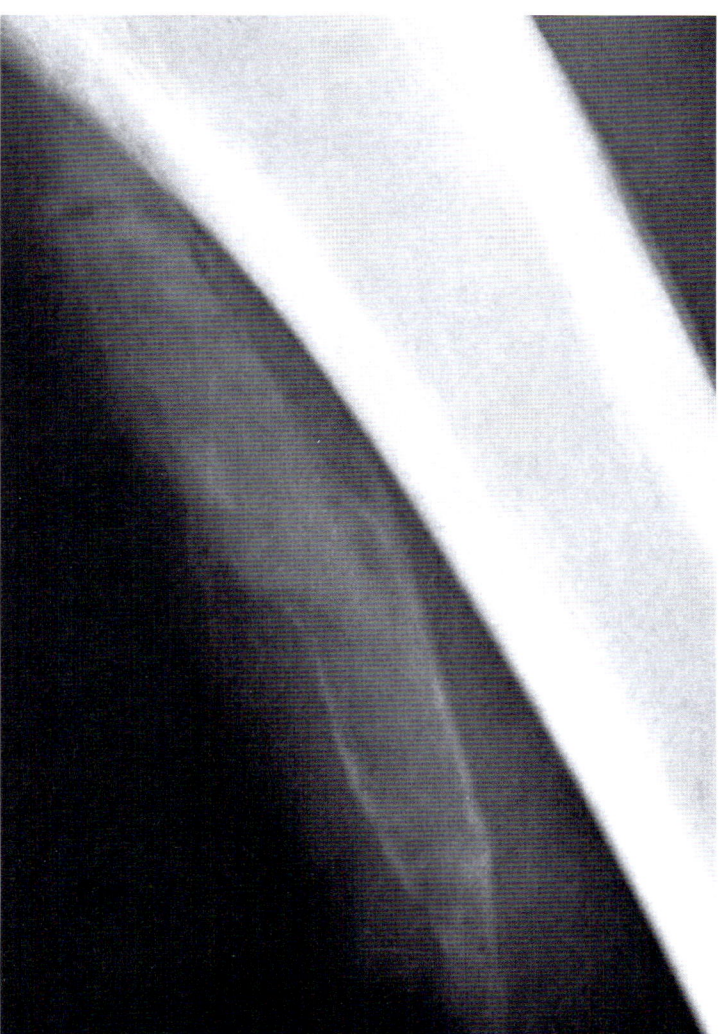

650 Left proximal tibia, lateromedial view: close-up.

Warmblood, 4 years.

The large, well defined soft tissue opacity, parallel with the cranial aspect of the midproximal tibia, represents ossification within a ruptured peroneus tertius muscle.

Tumoral calcinosis
(Calcinosis cirumscripta)

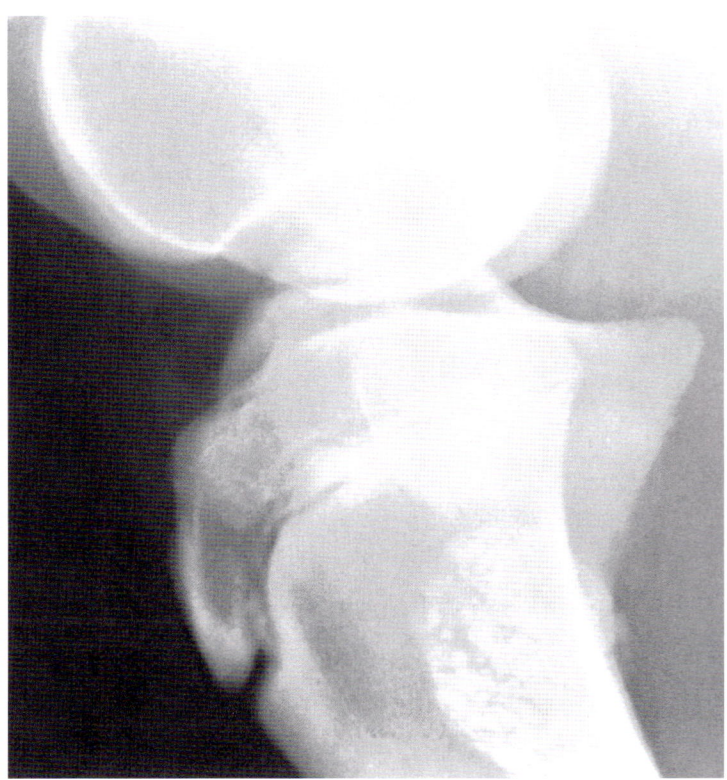

651

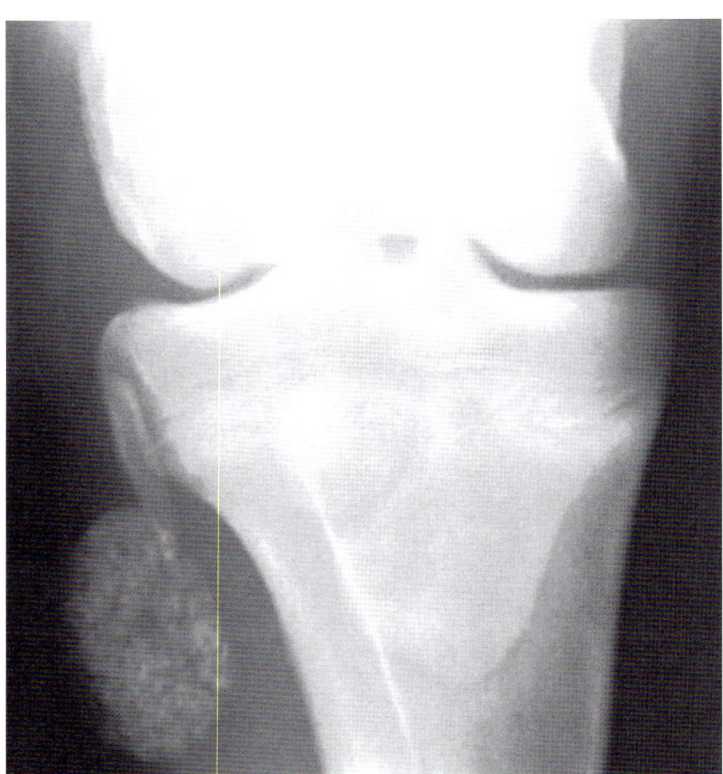

652

651/652 Left stifle joint, lateromedial (Fig. 651) and caudocranial (Fig. 652) view.

Pony, 1 year.

A well defined, rounded, granular soft tissue opacity lateral to the proximal tibia, characteristic of tumoral calcinosis.

N. B. In the horse the lateral aspect of the proximal tibia is a predilection site for this condition, the nodular calcified mass being near or firmly attached to the stifle joint capsule.

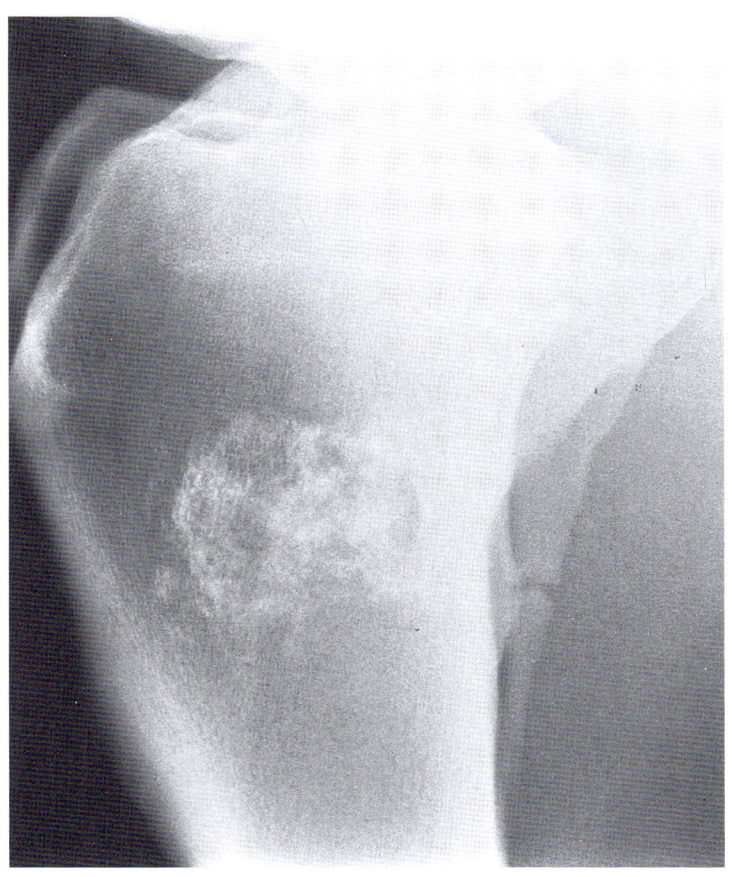

653 Left stifle joint, lateromedial view: close-up.

Warmblood, 11 years.

The well defined area of irregular calcification within the proximal tibia is consistent with bone infarction.

These infarcts may be extensive, multiple and bilateral.

Frequently the calcification at the periphery is more prominent than in the center of the lesion. Clinically such lesions may be completely asymptomatic, or lameness is apparent 1 – 2 months prior to the radiographic manifestation.

Osteoclastoma

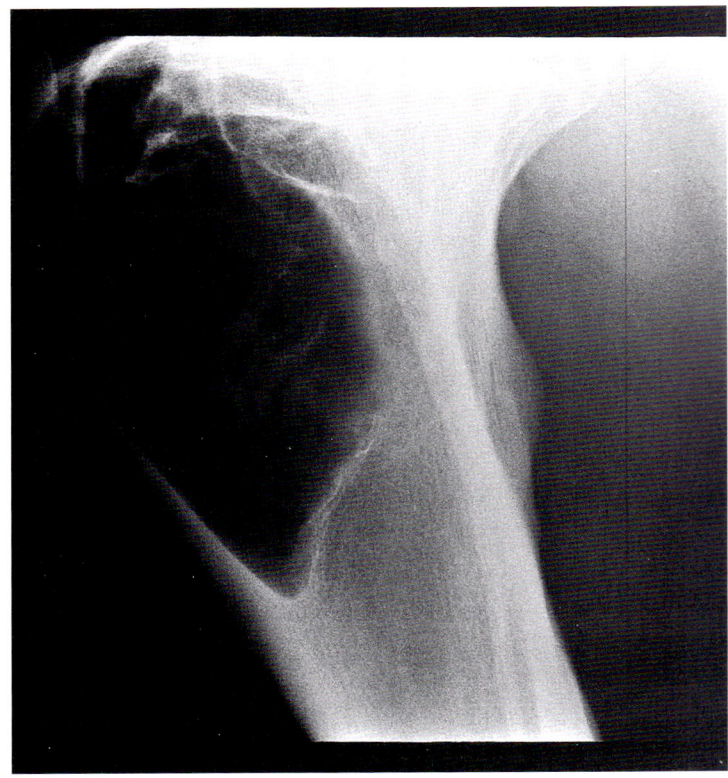

654

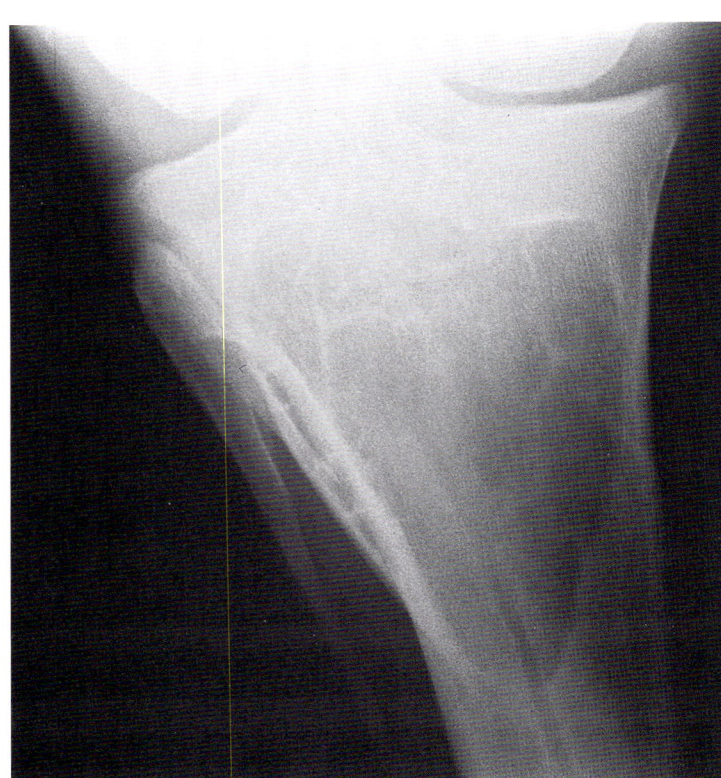

655

654/655 Left stifle joint, lateromedial and caudocranial view: close-ups.

Thoroughbred, 10 years.

A large, clearly delineated radiolucent lesion in the cranioproximal end of the tibia. Cranially the lesion is bordered by a ballooning, thin, uninterrupted layer of bone. Thin bone septa are present within the radiolucent mass.

The radiographic appearance is consistent with a benign expansile bone tumor. Histological examination revealed osteoclastoma.

The Pelvis

Fracture

Luxation

Osteoarthrosis

Infectious arthritis

Osteomyelitis

Osteochondrosis

Femoral head necrosis

Hip dysplasia

Fracture

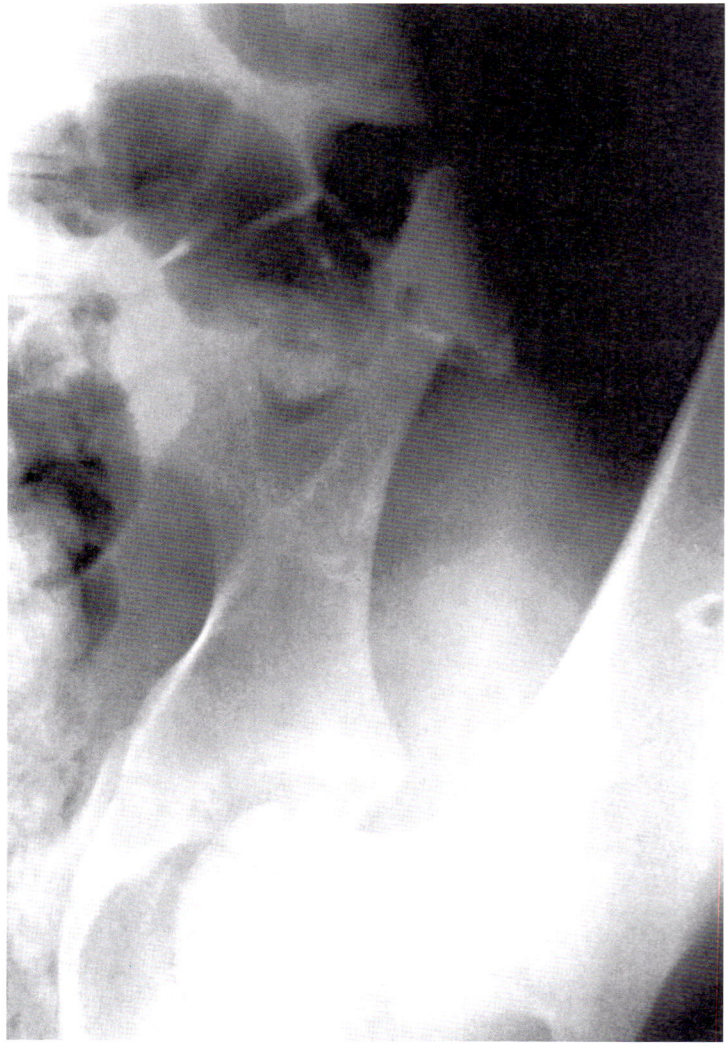

656

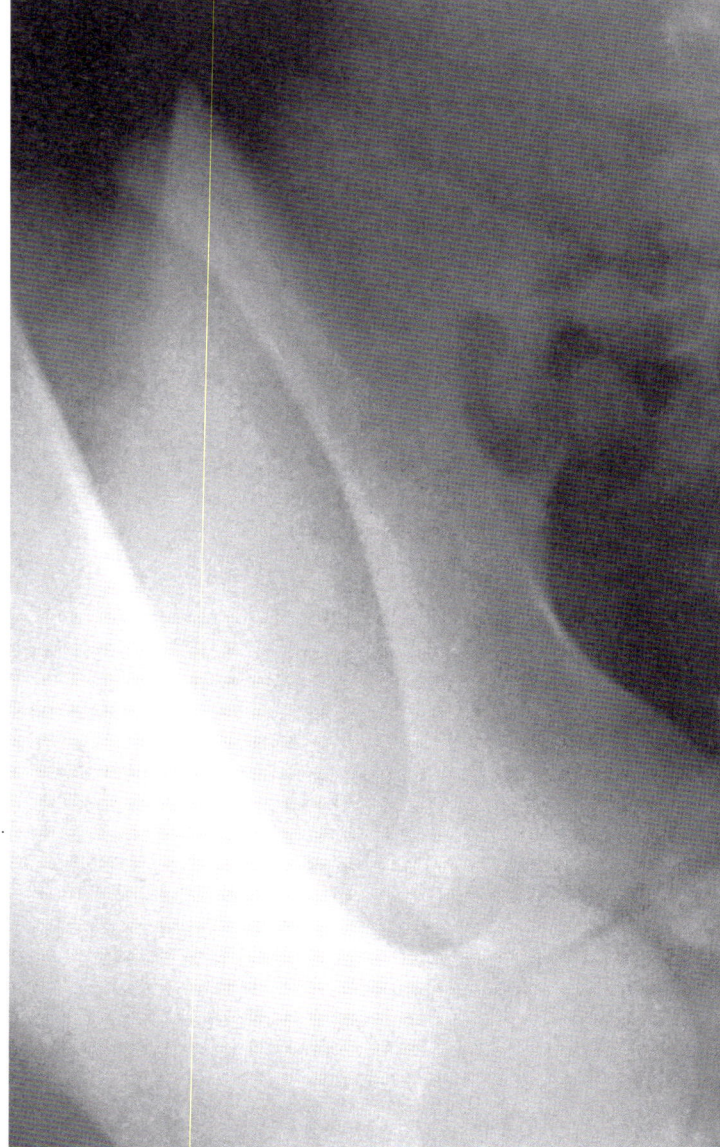

657

656/657 Left and right tuber coxae, ventrodorsal views: close-ups.

Foal, 1 week.

Lateral shifting of the left tuber coxae (Fig. 656) resulting in a "step" defect in the craniolateral surface of the wing of the ilium, due to a recent simple fracture of the tuber coxae. The fracture zone is obscured by the radiolucent contents of superimposed intestine and minimal overriding of fracture fragments. The normal radiographic tuber coxae configuration is demonstrated by the ventrodorsal projection of the right tuber coxae (Fig. 657).

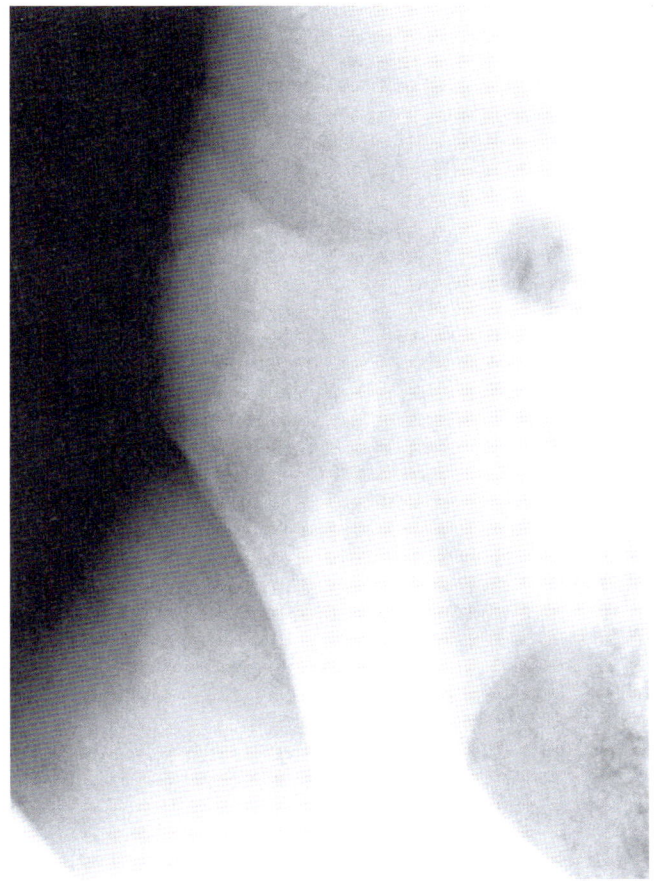

658

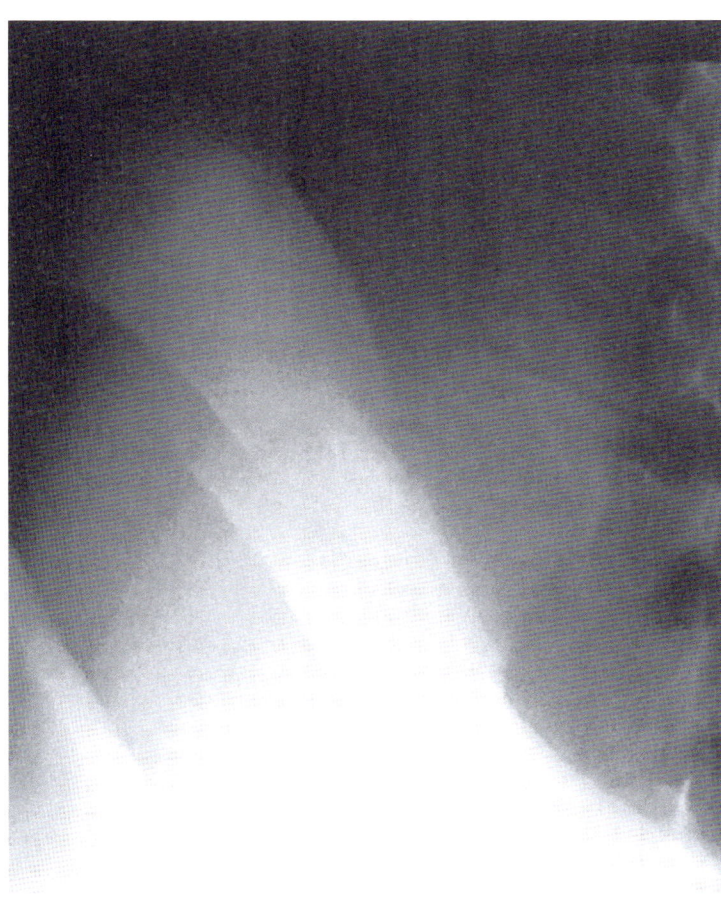

659

658/659 Right tuber coxae, ventrodorsal and right ventral-left dorsal oblique view: close-ups.

Foal, 6 months.

The two oblique, wide radiopaque zones through the cranial aspect of the wing of the right ilium, visible on the ventrodorsal view (Fig. 658), result from a simple, oblique fracture through the wing of the ilium, with overriding of the fracture fragments.

The additional ventrodorsal oblique view (Fig. 659), obtained by lowering the left hip, with the horse in dorsal recumbency and the vertical beam centred on the right elevated hip, clearly demonstrates a "step" defect in the craniolateral surface of the wing of the ilium, due to medial displacement of the cranial fracture fragment.

The oblique fracture plane is not parallel with the ventrodorsally directed central beam, and the fracture zone is therefore not visible.

N. B. The radiolucent zone through the craniolateral aspect of the ilium (Fig. 658) represents the apophyseal growth plate of the tuber coxae.

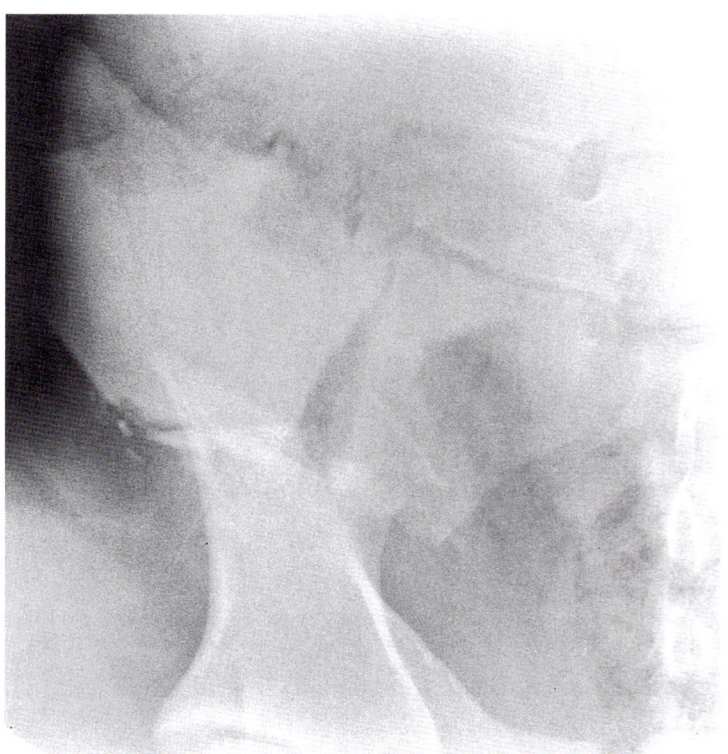

660 Right tuber coxae, ventrodorsal view: close-up.

Warmblood, 4 years.

An obvious longitudinal radiolucent zone through the midregion of the wing of the right ilium, combined with discontinuity of the midregion of the ilium shaft, indicating a recent multiple wing fracture. Cranial displacement of the ilium shaft results in slight overriding of fracture fragments, thus obscuring the transverse fracture zones and producing a prominent step defect in the lateral and medial contour of the ilium shaft.

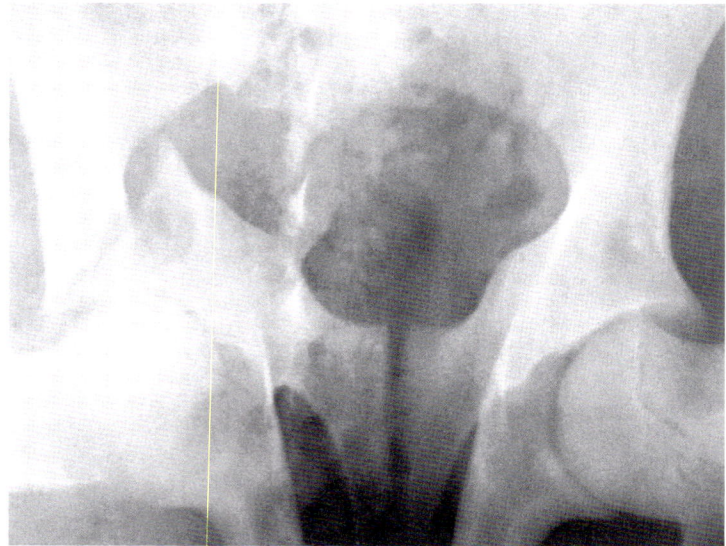

661

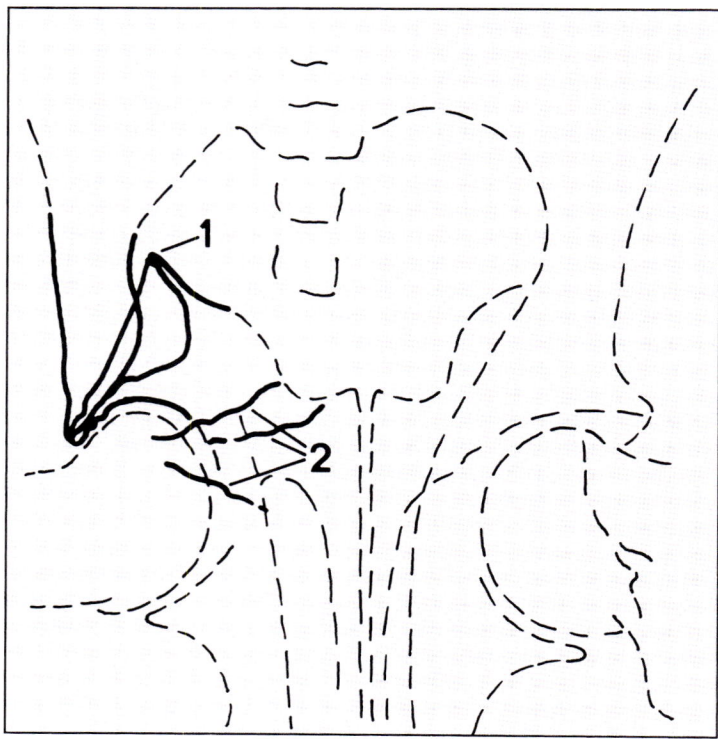

661 a

661 Pelvis, ventrodorsal view.

Foal, 10 months.

Discontinuity of the shaft of the right ilium **(1)**, due to a recent oblique fracture, with cranial displacement and slight overriding of fracture fragments, which also involves the craniolateral aspect of the acetabulum. The fracture plane is not parallel with the ventrodorsally directed central beam, and the fracture zone is therefore indistinct. Several additional ill defined fracture lines **(2)** superimposed on the cranial aspect of the femoral head are visible, running through the acetabular branch of the pubis and dorsal rim of the acetabulum.

661 a Schematic drawing

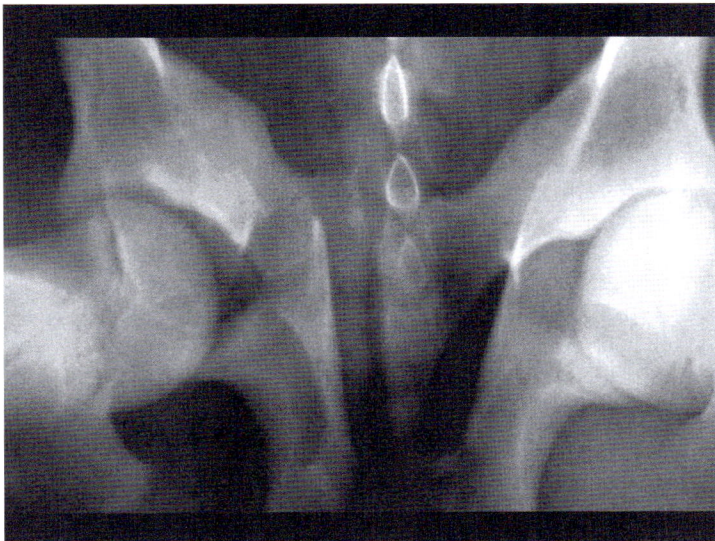

662

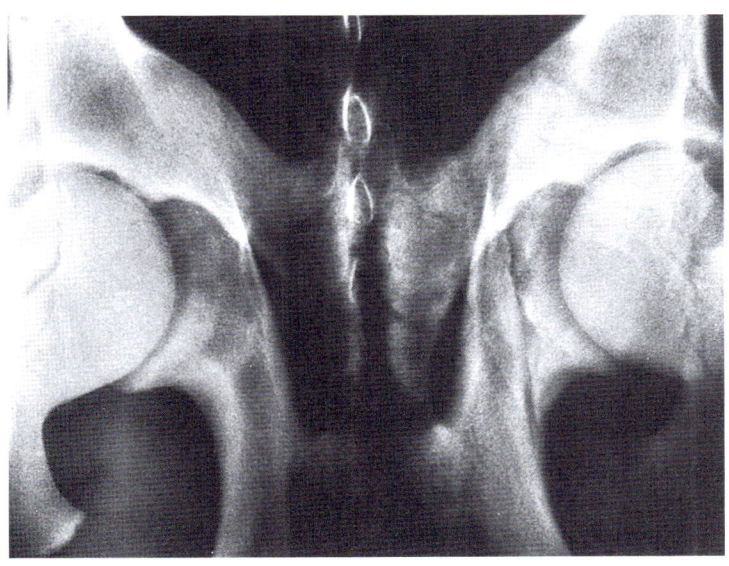

663 Pelvis, ventrodorsal view: close-up.

Foal, 7 months.

A well defined longitudinal radiolucent line extending through the acetabular branch of the left ischium and the dorsal rim of the left acetabulum, resulting from a simple acetabular fracture sustained 3 week prior to the examination.

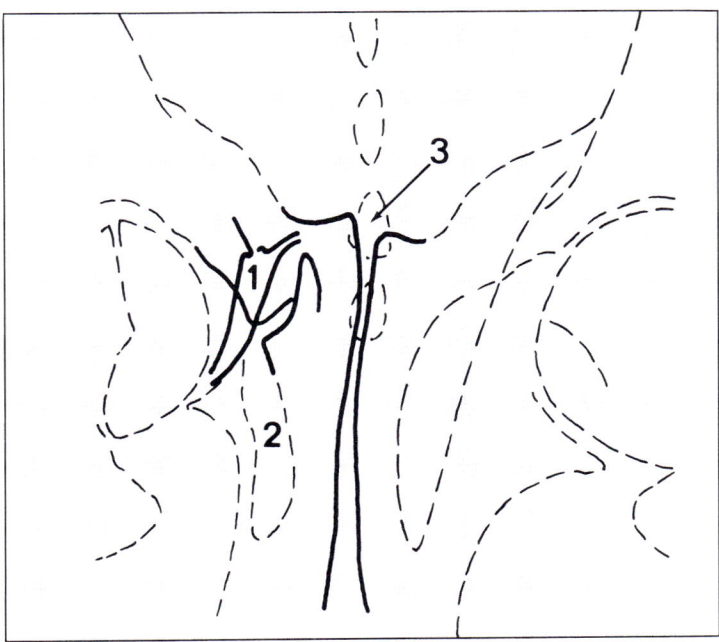

662 a

662 Pelvis, ventrodorsal view: close-up.

Foal, 8 months.

A clearly defined wide, oblique, radiolucent zone **(1)** through the acetabular branch of the right pubis and dorsal rim of the right acetabulum, indicating a recent, simple, oblique acetabular fracture. Moderate displacement of the acetabular branch of the ischium results in obliteration of the right obturator foramen **(2)**. A minimal "step" defect **(3)** between the cranial border of the right and left pubis indicates the presence of an additional fracture through the pelvic symphysis.

662 a Schematic drawing

The Pelvis

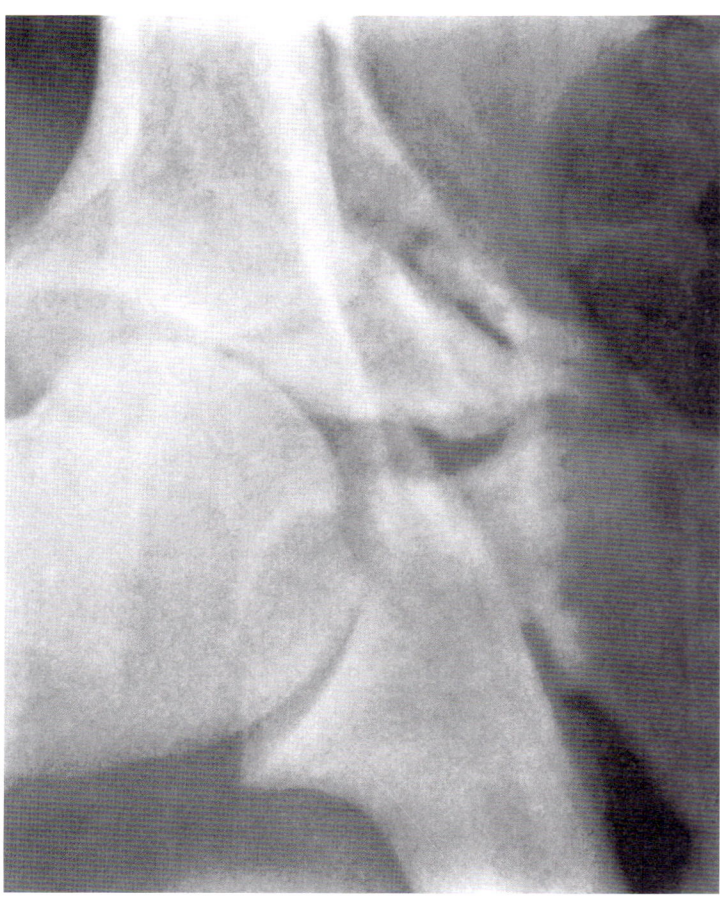

664

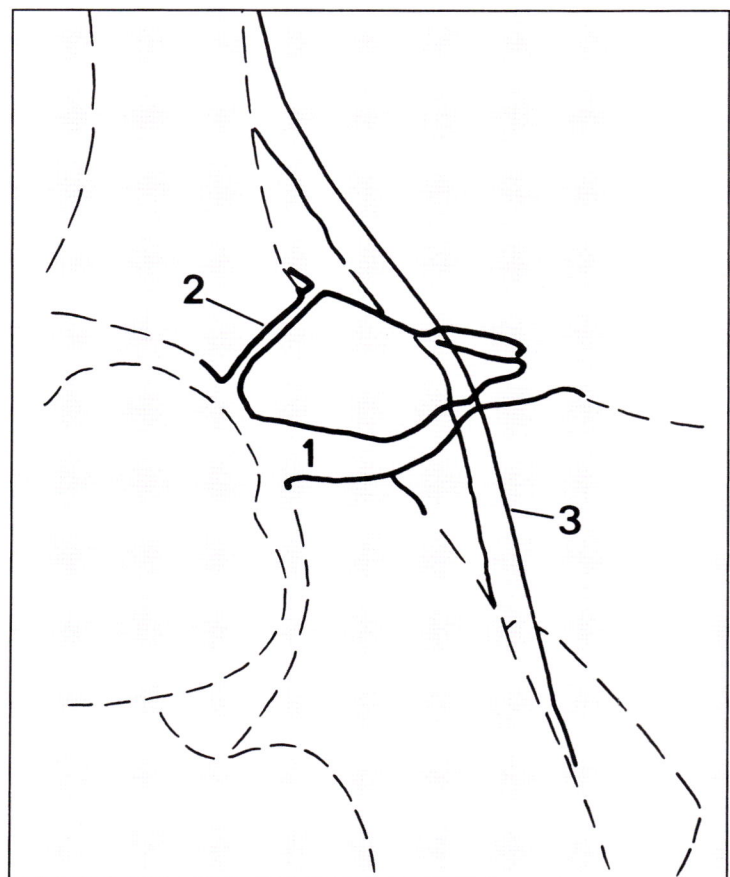

664 a Schematic drawing

664 Right hip joint, ventrodorsal view: close-up.

Warmblood, 2 years.

The clearly defined, transverse, V-shaped, radiolucent zone **(1)** through the acetabular branch of the pubis and dorsal rim of the acetabulum and the indistinct oblique radiolucent line **(2)** through the caudal aspect of the shaft of the ilium, disrupting the continuity of the ilium shaft and extending to the acetabulum, indicate a multiple acetabular fracture. The rather dense ill bordered layer of periosteal new bone **(3)** along the medial aspect of the acetabulum and the caudomedial aspect of the ilium indicate a fracture of some duration. The traumatic injury occurred 3 weeks prior to the examination.

665 Right hip joint, ventrodorsal view: close-up.

Warmblood, 3 years.

Several transverse and oblique, indistinct, irregular radiolucent lines through the acetabulum and acetabular branch of the ischium and rather dense periosteal new bone formation along the medial and caudal aspect of the acetabulum indicate a multiple acetabular fracture of some duration. The fracture lines are blurred by overlying callus formation. The traumatic damage was sustained 6 weeks prior to the examination.

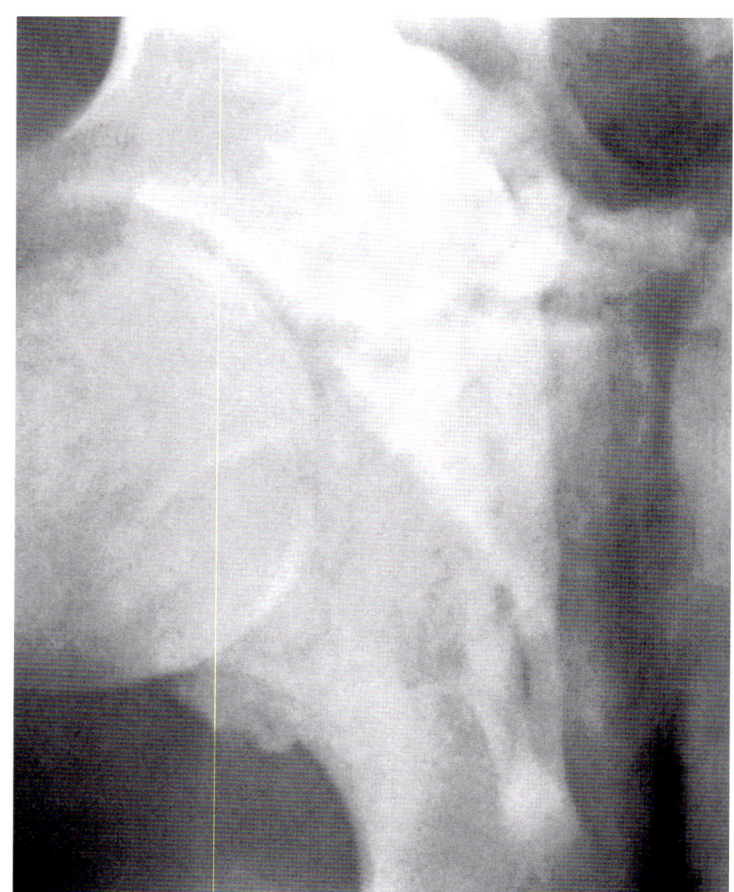

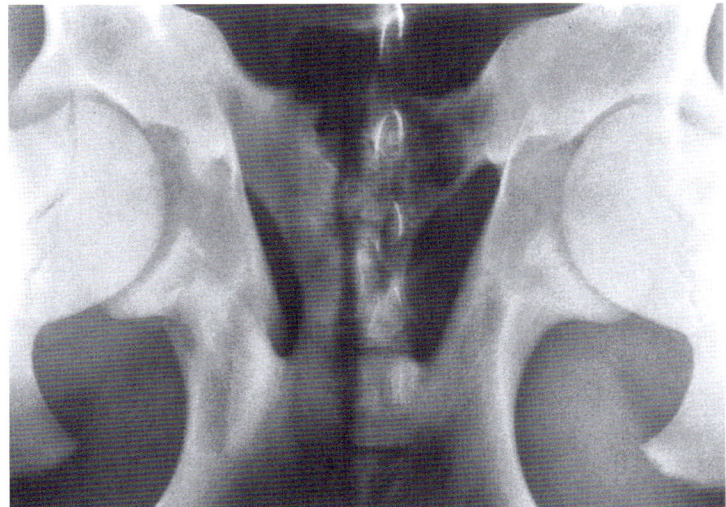

666 Pelvis, ventrodorsal view: close-up.

Warmblood, 1 year.

Prominent narrowing of the right obturator foramen with a slight step defect in the medial and lateral contour of the corresponding acetabular branch of the ischium is due to a recent simple extra-articular right ischium fracture.

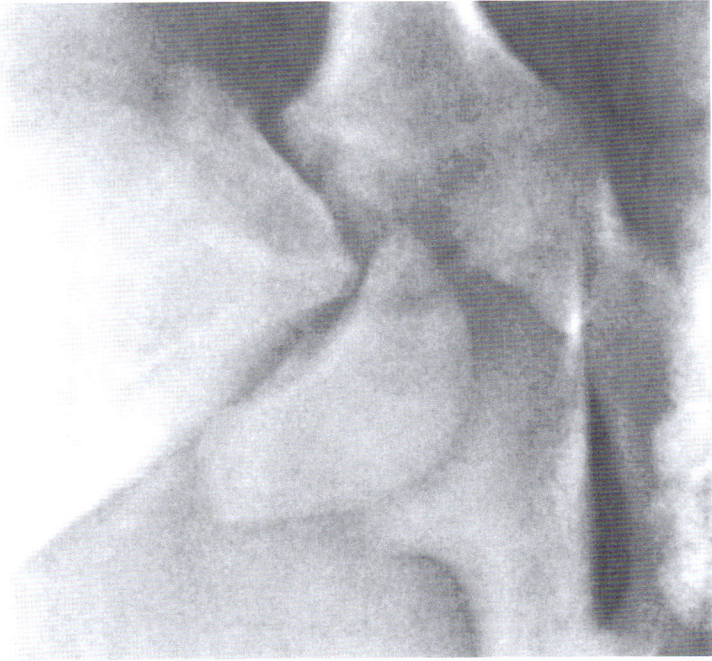

667 Right hip joint, ventrodorsal view: close-up.

Foal, 2 months.

The femoral epiphysis is completely separated from the metaphysis of the femoral neck, indicating the presence of a recent Salter-Harris type 1 physeal fracture (synonyms: epiphysiolysis or slipped femoral epiphysis). The femoral head is displaced caudally, its physeal surface lying on the caudal surface of the femoral neck.

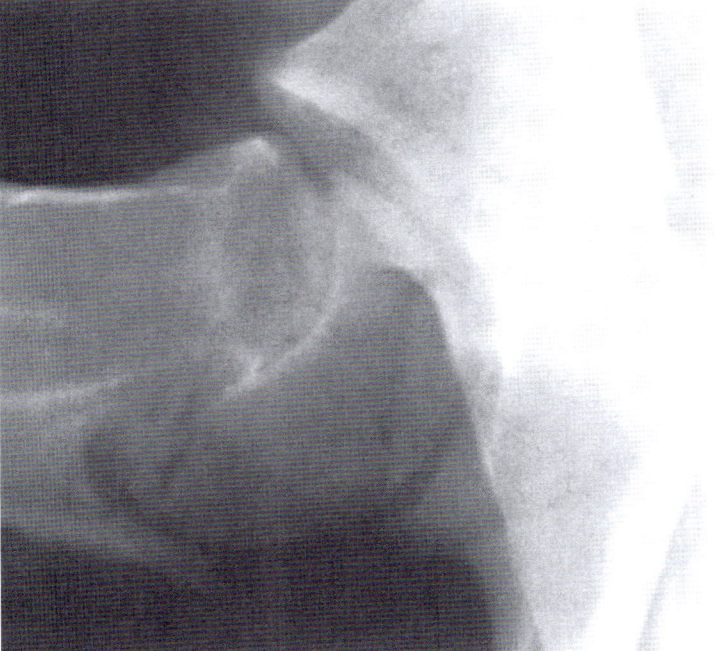

668 Right hip joint, ventrodorsal view: close-up.

Foal, 2 months.

The "step" defect cranially between the femoral epiphysis and metaphysis and the zone of irregular radiolucency in the metaphysis, extending along the entire growth plate, indicate a recent Salter-Harris type 2 physeal fracture, with minimal caudal displacement of the femoral head.

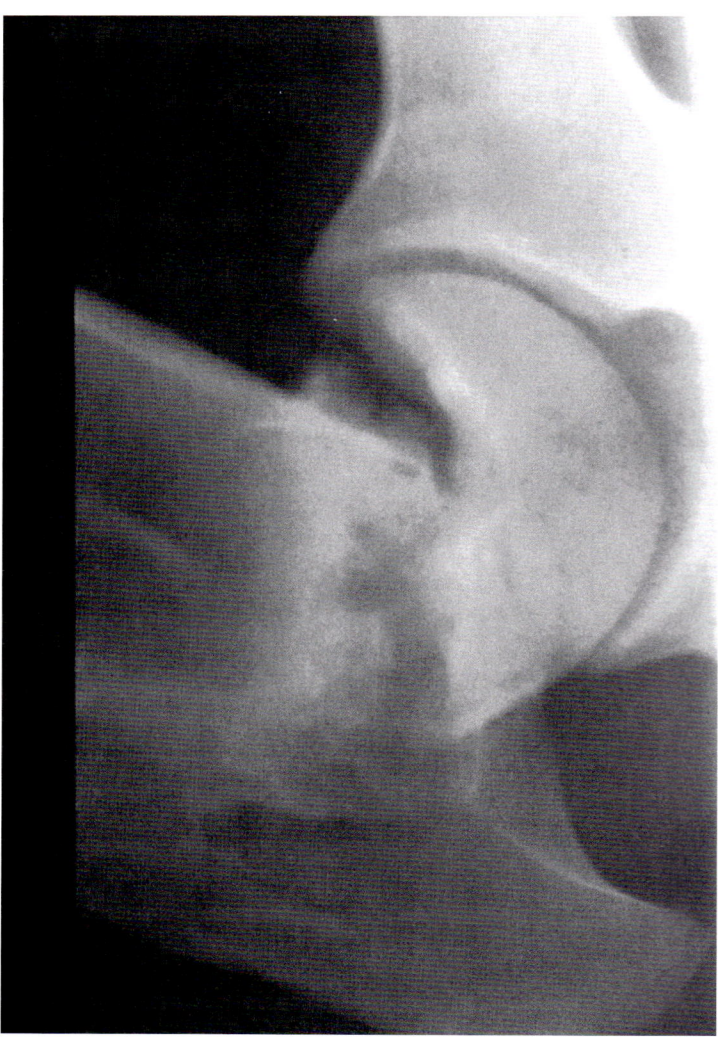

669 Right hip joint, ventrodorsal view: close-up.

Foal, 1 year.

The wide, irregular, sclerotic bordered, radiolucent zone between the femoral head and neck and periosteal new bone formation on the cranial metaphyseal surface indicate a chronic, non-union physeal fracture. Moderate caudal displacement of the femoral neck results in a "step" defect cranially between the epiphysis and metaphysis.

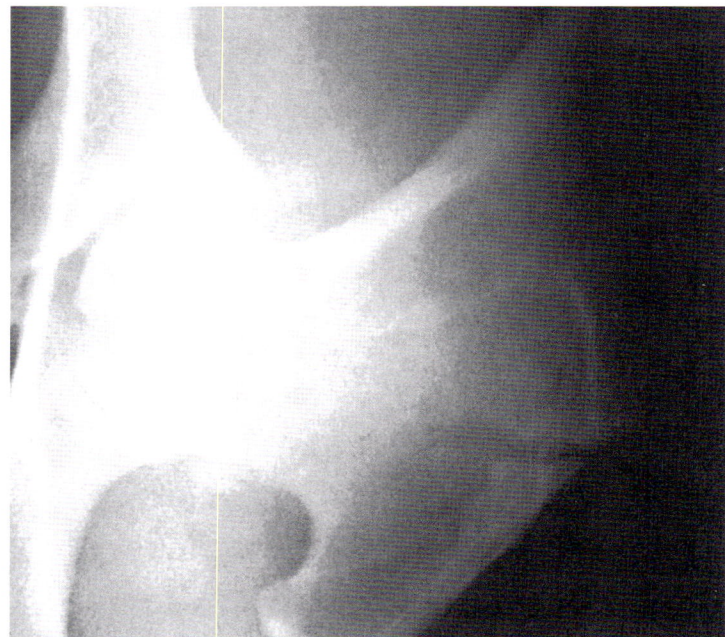

670 Left hip joint, ventrodorsal view: close-up.

Warmblood, 8 years.

The oblique, radiolucent zone disrupting the caudoproximal cortex of the femur indicates a recent fracture of the trochanter major. Proximal shifting results in a minimal "step" defect between the femoral neck and trochanter major.

The narrow, indistinct proximal aspect of the fracture and widening of the fracture zone distally indicate minimal rotation of the trochanter major.

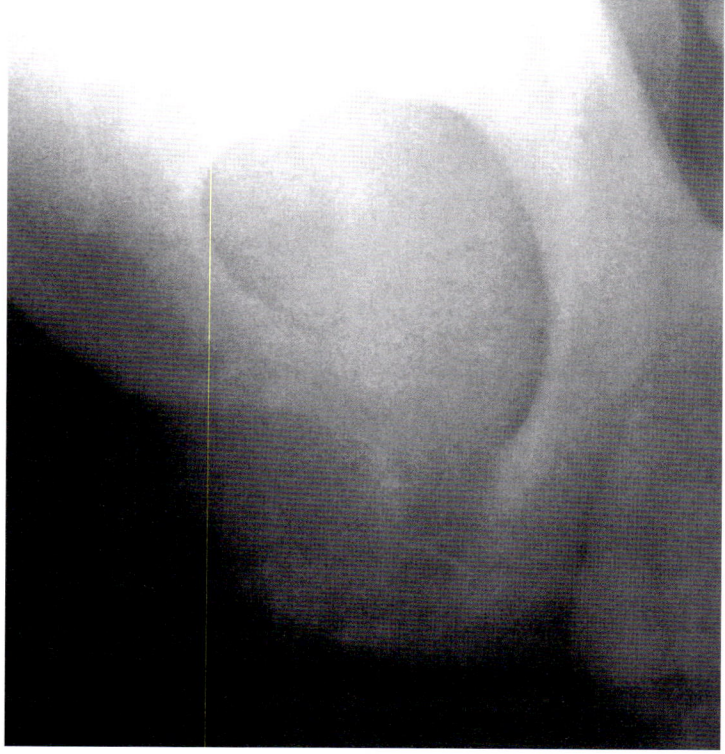

671 Right tuber ischii, ventrodorsal view: close-up.

Warmblood, 9 years.

Multiple, slightly displaced, bone fragments originating from the right tuber ischii, due to a recent comminuted fracture.

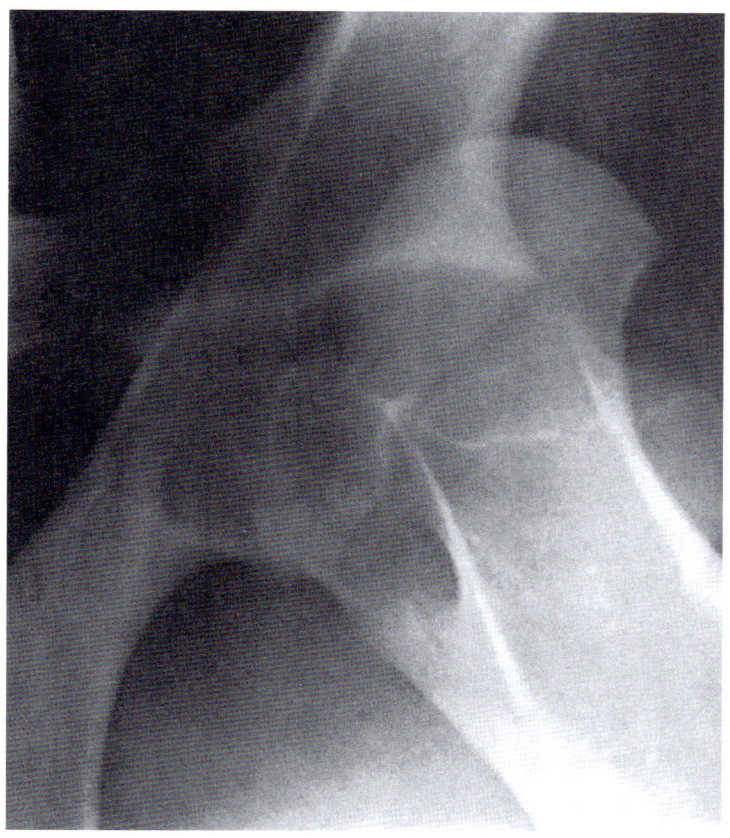

672 Left hip joint, ventrodorsal view: close-up.

Warmblood, 2 years.

Complete recent luxation of the left hip joint with craniodorsal displacement of the femur and overriding of the dorsal rim of the acetabulum.

The small, well defined radiopacity superimposed on the caudal aspect of the trochanter major and the corresponding indentation of the caudolateral acetabular border indicate that dislocation occurred together with associated chip fracture of the dorsal rim of the acetabulum.

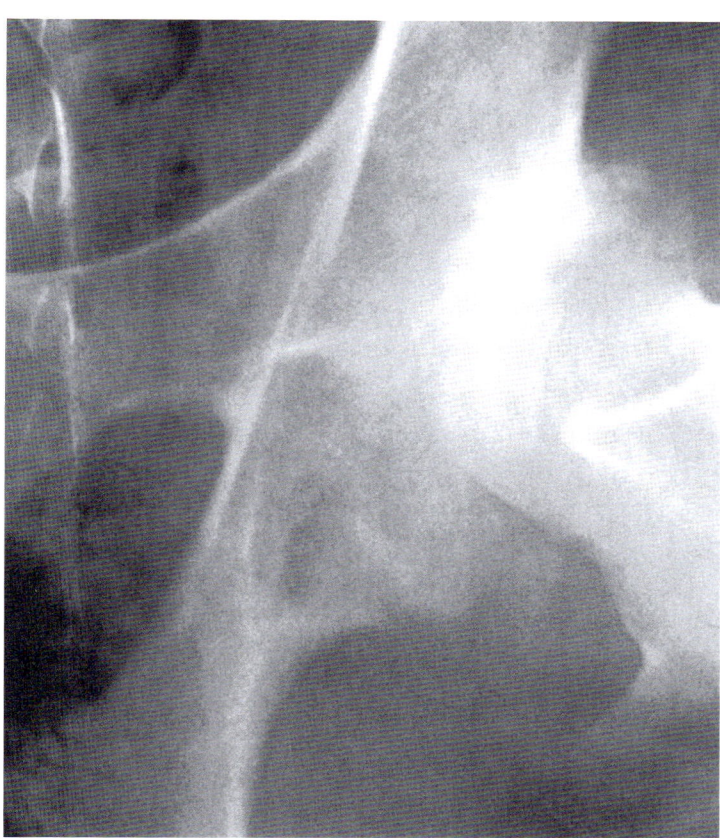

673 Left hip joint, ventrodorsal view: close-up.

Warmblood, 2 ½ years.

Complete luxation of the left hip joint, with craniodorsal displacement of the femur and overriding of the dorsal rim of the acetabulum.

The sclerosis and irregularity of the femoral head, irregularity of the acetabular border, and ill defined periarticular soft tissue calcification indicate that the luxation is not recent and resulted in coxofemoral osteoarthrosis.

The traumatic injury occurred 6 months prior to the examination.

Osteoarthrosis

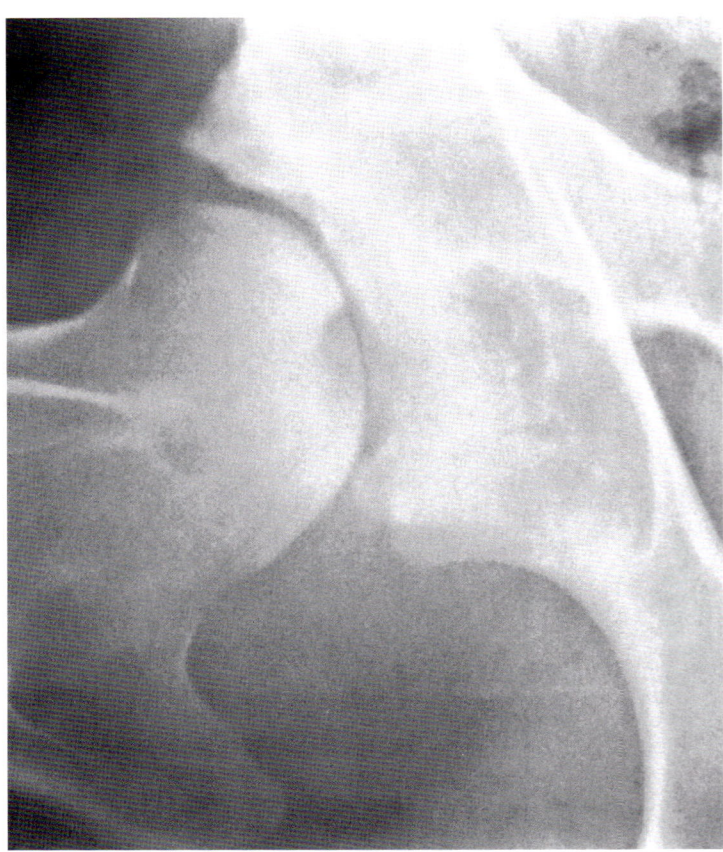

674 Right hip joint, ventrodorsal view: close-up.

Friesian horse, 1 ½ years.

Marked flattening, sclerosis and irregularity of the right acetabulum, flattening and sclerosis of the femoral head, and periarticular soft tissue swelling, indicating coxofemoral osteoarthrosis. The absence of traumatic lesions, i. e. fracture or luxation of the coxofemoral joint, or necrosis of the femoral head, and the unilateral occurrence of the disease suggest that osteoarthrosis probably resulted from joint instability associated with a rupture of the round ligament between the femoral head and the acetabulum.

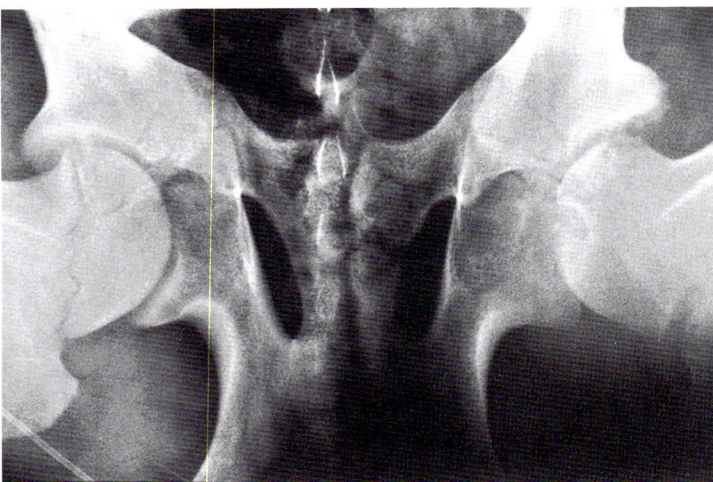

675 Pelvis, ventrodorsal view: close-up.

Foal, 5 months.

Obvious irregularity of the right acetabulum and less prominent irregularity of the contour of the corresponding femoral head and fovea capitis, representing coxofemoral osteoarthrosis due to rupture of the round ligament sustained 3 weeks previously.

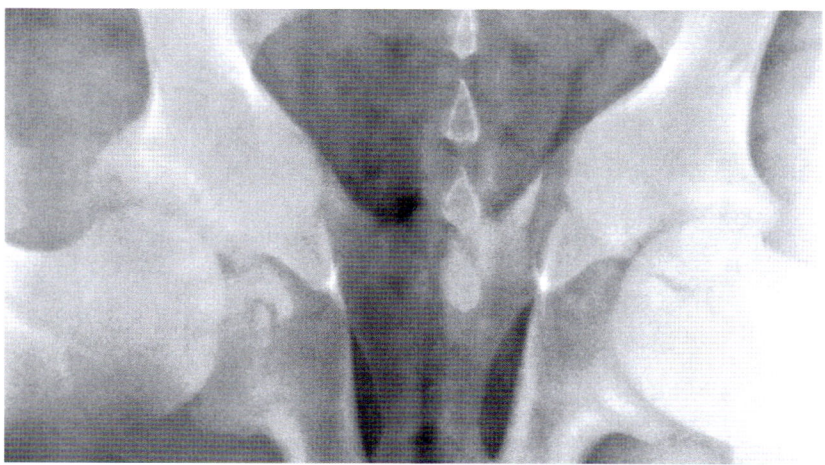

676 Pelvis, ventrodorsal view.

Foal, 4 months.

The right coxofemoral joint space is widened. The irregular contour of the dorsal acetabular rim and irregular radiolucent texture of the acetabulum indicate subchondral bone destruction. The radiographic changes are characteristic of an intermediate stage of infectious arthritis.

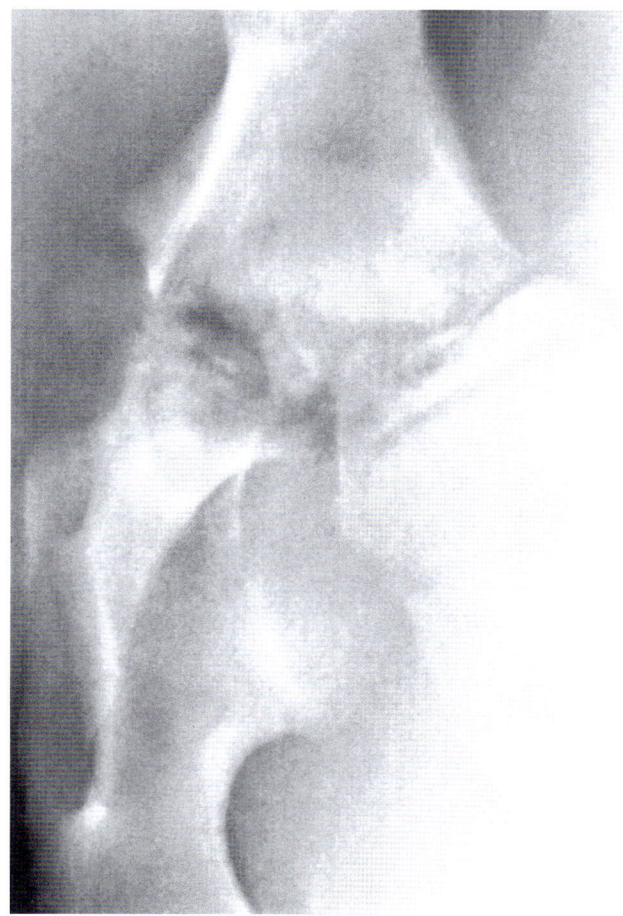

677 Left hip joint, ventrodorsal view: close-up.

Foal, 3 weeks.

The disrupted appearance of the left hip joint and mottled radiolucency of the corresponding portion of the ilium indicate extensive bone destruction, due to infectious arthritis. Joint infection resulted from extension of periarticular abscess formation.

Osteomyelitis

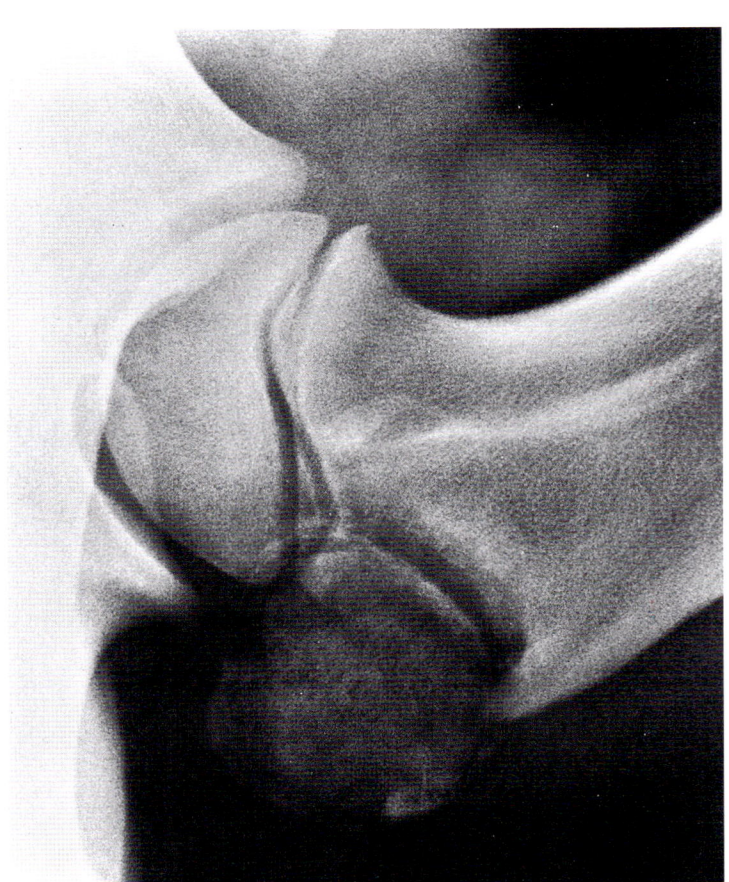

678 Left hip joint, ventrodorsal view: close-up.

Foal, 4 weeks.

Irregular radiolucency of the trochantor major, a seldom occuring manifestation of haematogenous osteomyelitis type P in a young foal.

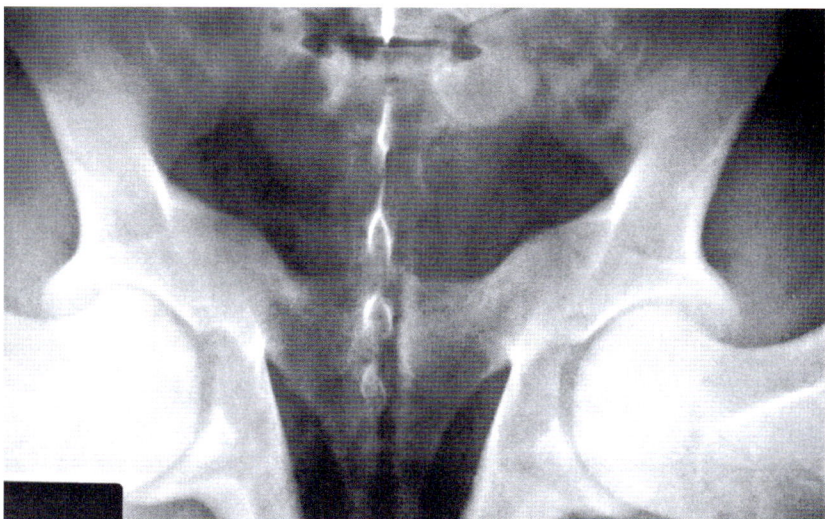

679 Pelvis, ventrodorsal view.

Foal, 7 months.

Two indistinct cystic radiolucent areas **(1)** within the subchondral bone of the cranial aspect of the right femoral head, adjacent to the fovea capitis **(2)**, indicating osteochondrosis.

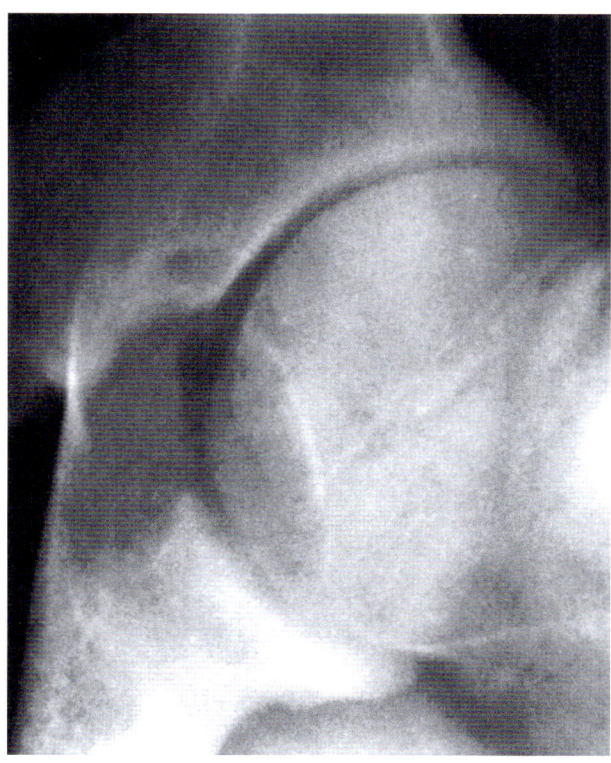

680 Left hip joint, ventrodorsal view: close-up.

Foal, 8 months.

The small cystic area of radiolucency **(1)** within the subchondral bone of the femoral head, adjacent to the cranial aspect of the fovea capitis **(2)**, is a manifestation of osteochondrosis.

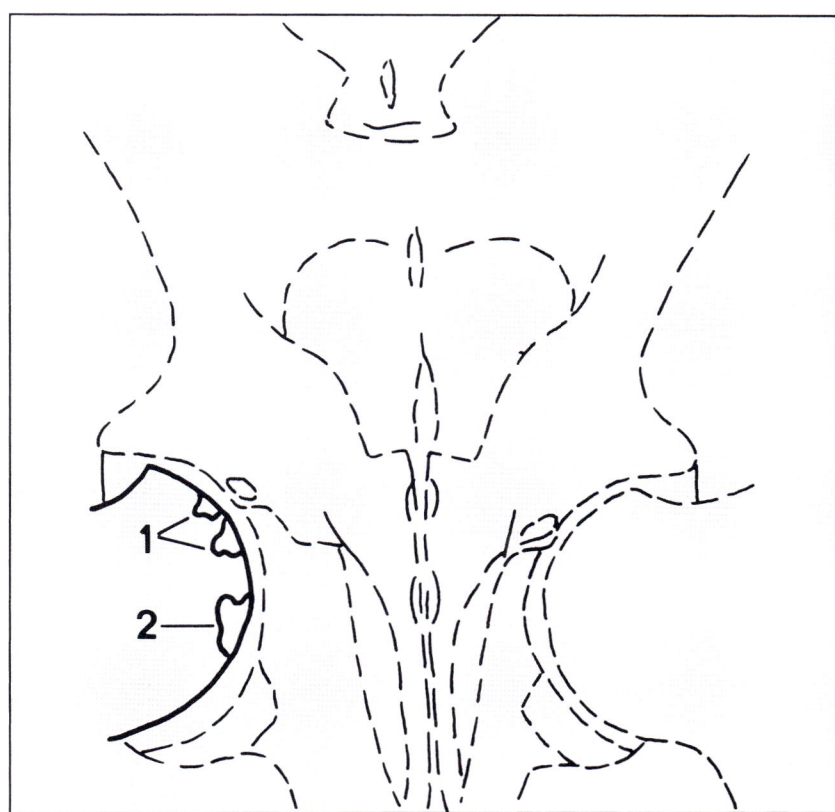

679 a Schematic drawing

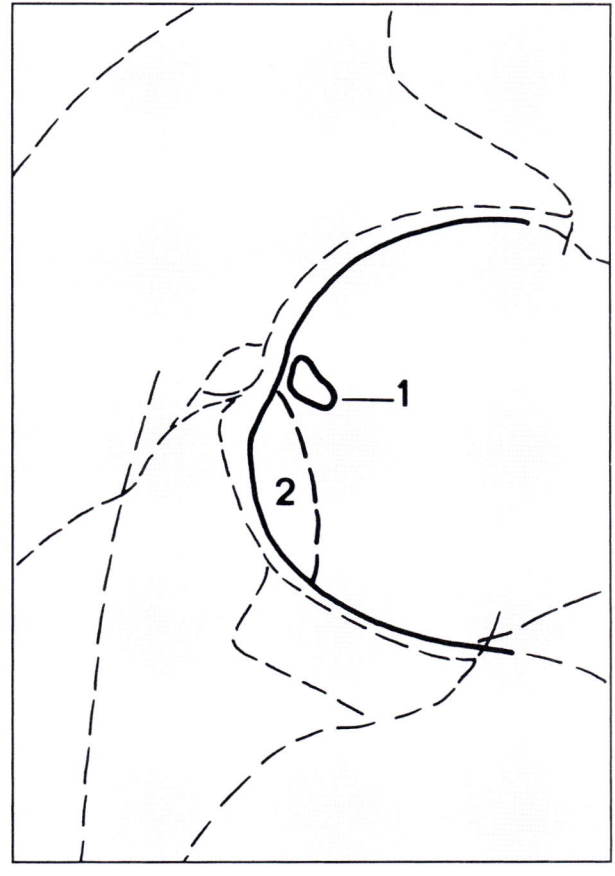

680 a Schematic drawing

Femoral head necrosis

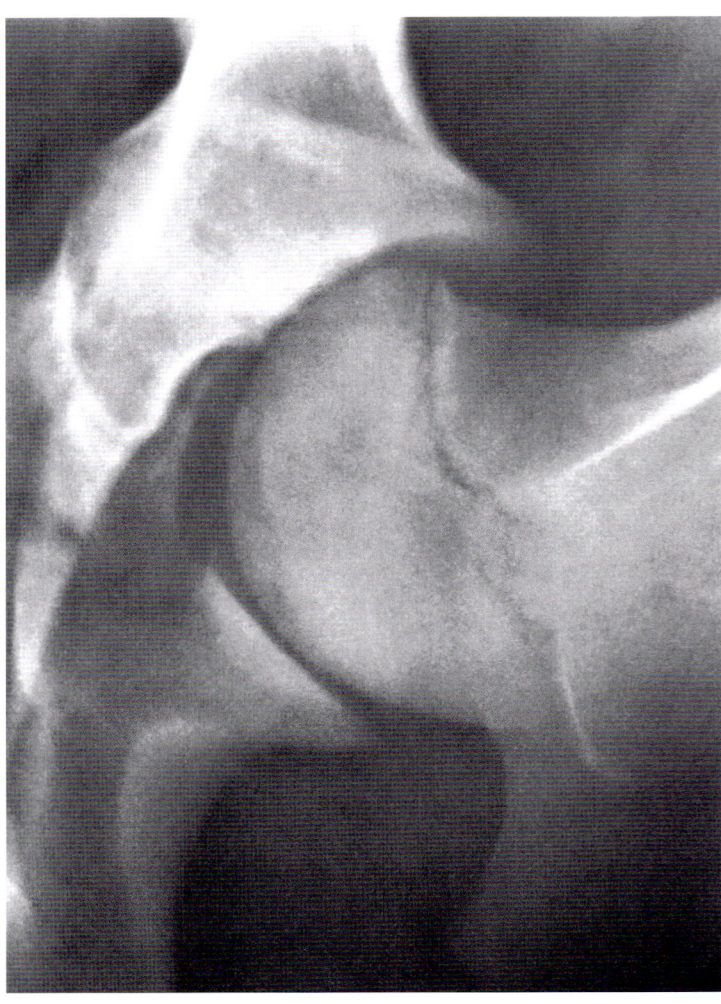

681 Left hip joint, ventrodorsal view: close-up.

Foal, 9 months.

The crescent-shaped radiolucent zone in the central aspect of the femoral head, adjacent to the articular surface, indicates separation of subchondral bone and represents an early sign of ischaemic bone necrosis (synonym: Calvé-Legg-Perthes disease).

Hip dysplasia

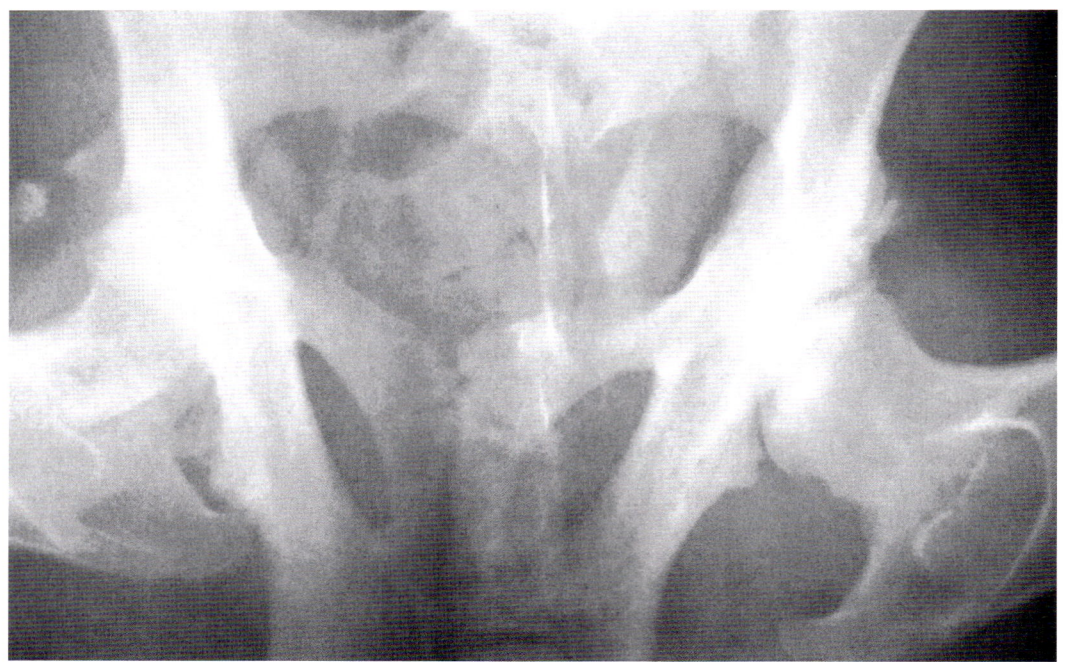

682 Pelvis, ventrodorsal view.

Pony, 2 years.

Marked flattening and deformity of both acetabula, resulting from dysplasia. The right femoral head is luxated and periaticular soft tissue calcification is visible cranial and caudal to the femoral head. Although not luxated, the left femoral head is flattened, and new bone formation on the lateral aspect of the ilium adjacent to the acetabulum indicates chronic joint instability.